Handbook of Experimental Pharmacology

Continuation of Handbuch der experimentellen Pharmakologie

Vol. 70/II

Pharmacology of Intestinal Permeation II

Contributors

J. G. Banwell · P. Bass · T. Z. Csáky · A. M. Dawson · J. M. Dietschy
K. Ewe · G. W. Gullikson · T. R. Hendrix · S. Hughes
N. N. Jezuitova · F. Lauterbach · M. Lucas · J. S. McKay
K. J. Moriarty · G. Nell · W. Rummel · L. F. Smirnova · M. Staritz
A. B. R. Thomson · L. A. Turnberg · A. M. Ugolev · V. Varró
R. Wanitschke · D. Winne

Editor

T. Z. Csáky

Springer-Verlag
Berlin Heidelberg New York Tokyo 1984

TIHAMÉR Z. CSÁKY, M.D.
Professor of Pharmacology
Department of Pharmacology
University of Missouri-Columbia
School of Medicine
Columbia, MO 65212
USA

With 149 Figures

Library of Congress Cataloging in Publication Data. Main entry under title: Pharmacology of intestinal permeation. (Handbook of experimental pharmacology; vol. 70/I–II) Includes bibliographical references and index. 1. Intestinal absorption. 2. Gastrointestinal agents – Physiological effect. I. Armstrong, W. McDermott (William McDermott) II. Csáky, T. Z. III. Series: Handbook of experimental pharmacology; v. 70/I–II. [DNLM: 1. Intestinal Absorption. 2. Intestines – metabolism. 3. Cell Membrane Permeability – drug effects. 4. Drugs – metabolism. W1 HA51L v. 70 pt. 1–2/WI 402 P536] QP905.H3 vol. 70/I–II 615′.1 s 84-5558 [QP156] [612′.33]

ISBN-13: 978-3-642-69510-0 e-ISBN-13: 978-3-642-69508-7
DOI: 10.1007/978-3-642-69508-7

Softcover reprint of the hardcover 1st edition 1984

2122/3130-543210

List of Contributors

J. G. BANWELL, Department of Medicine, Division of Gastroenterology, Case Western School of Medicine, Cleveland, OH 44106, USA

P. BASS, School of Pharmacy, University of Wisconsin, 425 N. Charter Street, Madison, WI 53706, USA

T. Z. CSÁKY, Professor of Pharmacology, Department of Pharmacology, University of Missouri-Columbia, School of Medicine, Columbia, MO 65212, USA

A. M. DAWSON, Department of Gastroenterology, St. Bartholomew's Hospital, West Smithfield, London, EC1A 7BE, Great Britain

J. M. DIETSCHY, Department of Internal Medicine, University of Texas, Health Science Center, Southwestern Medical School, Dallas, TX 75235, USA

K. EWE, I. Medizinische Klinik und Poliklinik, Johannes Gutenberg Universität, Postfach 3960, Langenbeckstraße 1, 6500 Mainz, FRG

G. W. GULLIKSON, Research Investigator, Department of Biological Research, Searle Research and Development, Division of G. D. Searle & Co., Box 5110, Chicago, IL 60680, USA

T. R. HENDRIX, Department of Medicine, Chief Gastroenterology Division, The John Hopkins University School of Medicine, 600 North Wolfe Street, Baltimore, MD 21205, USA

S. HUGHES, Department of Medicine, Hope Hospital, (University of Manchester School of Medicine), Eccles Old Road, Salford M6 8HD, Great Britain

N. N. JEZUITOVA, J.-O. Pavlov Institute of Physiology, The Academy of Sciences of the USSR, Nab. Makarova, 6, Leningrad, 199164, USSR

F. LAUTERBACH, Institut für Pharmakologie und Toxikologie, Ruhr-Universität Bochum, Postfach 102148, 4630 Bochum 1, FRG

M. LUCAS, Institute of Physiology, The University of Glasgow, Glasgow, W.2 Great Britain

J. S. MCKAY, Department of Medicine, Hope Hospital, (University of Manchester School of Medicine), Eccles Old Road, Salford M6 8HD, Great Britain

K. J. MORIARTY, Department of Gastroenterology, St. Bartholomew's Hospital, West Smithfield, London, EC1A 7BE. Present address: Department of Medicine, Hope Hospital (University of Manchester School of Medicine), Eccles Old Road, Salford M6 8HD, Great Britain

G. Nell, Institut für Pharmakologie und Toxikologie der Universität des Saarlandes, 6650 Homburg (Saar), FRG

W. Rummel, Institut für Pharmakologie und Toxikologie der Universität des Saarlandes, 6650 Homburg (Saar), FRG

L. F. Smirnova, I. P. Pavlov Institute of Physiology, The Academy of Sciences of the USSR, Nab. Makarova, 6, Leningrad, 199164, USSR

M. Staritz, I. Medizinische Klinik und Poliklinik, Langenbeckstraße 1, 6500 Mainz, FRG

A. B. R. Thomson, University of Alberta, Edmonston, Alberta, CDN

L. A. Turnberg, Department of Medicine, Hope Hospital, (University of Manchester School of Medicine), Eccles Old Road, Salford M6 8HD, Great Britain

A. M. Ugolev, I. P. Pavlov Institute of Physiology, The Academy of Sciences of the USSR, Nab. Makarova, 6, Leningrad, 199164, USSR

V. Varró, First Department of Medicine, University Medical School, P.B. 469, 6701 Szeged, Hungary

R. Wanitschke, I. Medizinische Klinik und Poliklinik, Johannes-Gutenberg-Universität, Postfach 3960, Langenbeckstraße 1, 6500 Mainz, FRG

D. Winne, Abt. für Molekularpharmakologie, Pharmakologisches Institut der Universität Tübingen, Wilhelmstraße 56, 7400 Tübingen 1, FRG

Preface

The intestine, particularly the small bowel, represents a large surface (in the adult human approximately 200 m^2) through which the body is exposed to its environment. A vigorous substrate exchange takes place across this large surface: nutrients and xenobiotics are absorbed from the lumen into the bloodstream or the lymph, and simultaneously, the same types of substrate pass back into the lumen. The luminal surface of the intestine is lined with a "leaky" epithelium, thus the passage of the substrates, in either direction, proceeds via both transcellular and intercellular routes. Simple and carrier-mediated diffusion, active transport, pinocytosis, phagocytosis and persorption are all involved in this passage across the intestinal wall.

The term "intestinal permeation" refers to the process of passage of various substances across the gut wall, either from the lumen into the blood or lymph, or in the opposite direction. "Permeability" is the condition of the gut which governs the rate of this complex two-way passage.

The pharmacologist's interest in the problem of intestinal permeation is twofold: on the one hand, this process determines the bioavailability of drugs and contributes significantly to the pharmacokinetics and toxicokinetics of xenobiotics; on the other hand, the pharmacodynamic effects of many drugs are manifested in a signigicant alteration of the physiological process of intestinal permeation.

The material in these volumes was collected in order to present some of the fundamental aspects of the permeability and the permeation of the intestine. An attempt has been made to include morphological, physicochemical, physiologic, biophysical, biochemical, pharmacologic and toxicologic aspects. Clearly, intestinal permeation cannot be properly studied from the perspective of one or a few disciplines; the subject cuts across a wide spectrum of disciplines. Consequently, it is hoped that the information provided in these volumes will be useful to scientists working in a variety of specialties.

I would like to express my thanks to those colleagues who accepted my invitation and contributed to this publication. It is somewhat unfortunate that the collection of the material required a considerable amount of time, but in a publication of this size, with a large number of contributors, some delay is inevitable. One prospective contributor was prevented from completing his task by a fatal heart attack, while others had to be excused because they failed to find enough time for the work. Fortunately, outstanding replacements were secured, but not without some holdup. Our knowledge of fundamental principles seldom changes in a revolutionary fashion, thus, despite the spread in time, it is hoped that these volumes will provide the reader with the information necessary to form a correct contemporary image of the complex process of intestinal permeation and the conditions of permeability.

Finally, I would like to thank my wife for lending me a helping hand, admist her own professional duties, in various aspects of the editorial work.

T. Z. CSÁKY

Contents

CHAPTER 18

Intestinal Absorption of Xenobiotics. T. Z. CSÁKY. With 5 Figures

CHAPTER 19

Role of Digestive Enzymes in the Permeability of the Enterocyte
A. M. UGOLEV, N. N. IEZUITOVA, and L. F. SMIRNOVA. With 26 Figures

CHAPTER 20

The Surface pH of the Intestinal Mucosa and its Significance in the Permeability of Organic Anions. M. LUCAS. With 14 Figures

CHAPTER 21

The Role of the Unstirred Water Layer in Intestinal Permeation
A. B. R. THOMSON and J. M. DIETSCHY. With 55 Figures

CHAPTER 22

Intestinal Permeation of Organic Bases and Quaternary Ammonium Compounds. F. LAUTERBACH. With 12 Figures

CHAPTER 23

Role of Blood Flow in Intestinal Permeation. D. WINNE. With 8 Figures

CHAPTER 24

Hormonal Effects on Intestinal Permeability. V. VARRÓ

Contents of Companion Volume 70, Part I

CHAPTER 18

Intestinal Absorption of Xenobiotics

T. Z. CSÁKY

A. Introduction

A xenobiotic is a substance which is foreign to the living organism, but exposure to it affects the functions of the body. The effect can be therapeutically beneficial, i.e., pharmacologic, or harmful, i.e., toxic. The difference between pharmacologic and toxic action is more quantitative than qualitative. Essentially all therapeutically effective agents (drugs) can exert toxic effects in high enough doses. Consequently, in this chapter the expression "pharmacologic" will be used for basic properties of all xenobiotics, be they pharmacologic or toxic. Similarly, the expression "drug" will refer to xenobiotics in general. Several monographs have been published on the subject of drug absorption (BINNS 1964; HOUSTON and WOOD 1980; LEVINE 1971; PRESCOTT and NIMMO 1979).

B. Drug Absorption and Pharmacologic Response

According to modern pharmacologic concepts, the vast majority of drug actions are the consequence of an interaction between the drug and a specific bodily receptor. The microcosmos in the immediate vicinity of the receptor is called the biophase. Usually the quantitative action of given drug depends on its concentration in the biophase. This, in turn, is determined by pharmacokinetics, viz., the absorption, distribution, and elimination of the drug in the body. Thus, the absorption process ultimately influences markedly the quantitative action of all xenobiotics.

Most drugs act reversibly, i.e., at equilibrium the rates of formation and dissociation of the drug-receptor complex are equal. Moreover, these rates are so high that they parallel the changes of the concentration of the drug in the biophase and, in turn, in the tissue water. The latter is in rapid equilibrium with the concentration of the unbound drug in the plasma. Consequently, the quantitative action of many drugs is directly related to their concentration in the plasma (BRODIE and MITCHELL 1973).

In humans, the gastrointestinal absorption of a given drug or drug product is usually expressed by the term "bioavailability" which is a measure of the rate and extent to which a drug is transferred from the gastrointestinal tract to the systemic circulation. Bioavailability ist quantitated by the determination of the concentration of the drug in the blood plasma at given intervals following administration. Figure 1 indicates the information which can be obtained from the data. The following parameters are usually taken into consideration:

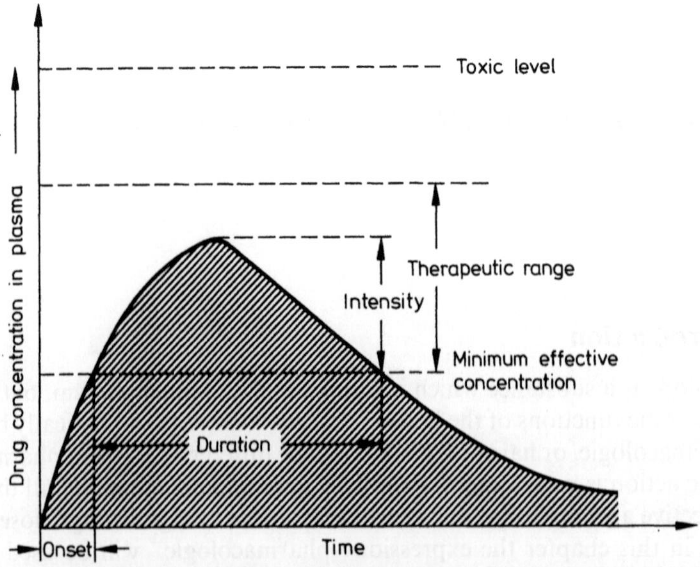

Fig. 1. Relationship between the effectiveness of the drug and its concentration in the blood plasma following oral administration. The AUC is shaded

1. The peak height to plasma or serum concentration.
2. The rate of absorption, i.e., the time between the administration and the achievement of the peak height concentration.
3. Total amount absorbed. This is measured from the area under the plasma or serum concentration–time curve and is expressed as AUC (area under curve).
4. Additional information can be obtained concerning the time needed for the onset, the duration, and the intensity of action.

Figure 2 illustrates how the variation of these parameters affects the quantitative action of the drug. Figure 2a depicts three hypothetical cases for the same drug in which the rate of absorption varied while the total amount absorbed (AUC) was unchanged. Figure 2b depicts three cases in which the rate was the same, but the fraction of the amount absorbed varied. Form the analysis of these cases it is clear that the drug absorption is of particular concern in cases of drugs, such as analgesics, spasmolytics, or antiasthmatics, which are administered in a single dose for the purpose of reaching rapidly a definite plasma concentration level. Within this category, particularly if the drug has a narrow margin of safety, monitoring the plasma level is advisable. On the other hand, in case of drugs which are given in multiple doses to achieve and maintain a relatively constant plasma level, the rate of absorption is less a determining factor, but the total amount absorbed (AUC) may be significant.

C. The Side of Drug Absorption

As will be seen, passive diffusion appears to be the most common process in the intestinal absorption of xenobiotics. In this process the rate is determined by the

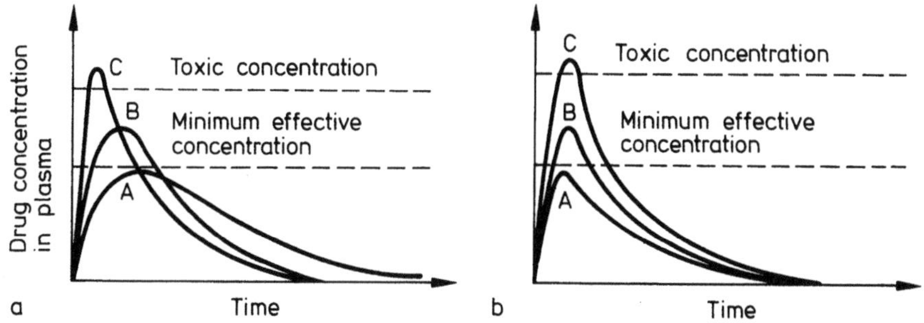

Fig. 2 a, b. Influence of the variation in the rate of absorption (**a**) and in the fraction of the amount absorbed (**b**) upon the pharmacologic effectiveness. **a** Three hypothetical cases for the same drug in which the rate of absorption varied while the total amount absorbed (AUC) was unchanged. *A*, Drug level did not reach therapeutic effectiveness; *B*, therapeutic level was achieved; *C*, toxic level was obtained. **b** Three cases in which the rate was the same, but the fraction of the amount absorbed varied. *A*, Therapeutic level not reached; *B*, therapeutic level reached; **C**, toxic level obtained. *Broken lines*, the minimum blood level at which therapeutic or toxic effects, respectively, are achieved

area of the absorptive surface and the concentration difference between the lumen and the bloodstream. In the gastrointestinal tract the small intestine represents the largest absorptive surface, about 200 m^2 in an adult human (WILSON 1962), and is endowed with an abundant blood supply. Because of its much larger surface and better blood supply, the small intestine plays a significantly greater role than the stomach in the absorption of xenobiotics. This is true even with drugs which are fat soluble,such as ethanol(MAGNUSSEN 1968), or with weak acids, e.g., aspirin (SIURULA et al. 1969), which in the acid stomach are nonionized, thus becoming lipid soluble. Drugs and other xenobiotics can be absorbed also from the large intestine which represents a smaller area with less abundant blood supply. In living subjects after oral administration the drug absorption from the small intestine is sufficiently vigorous so that little reaches the large intestine.

Lipid-soluble drugs are readily absorbed from the rectum. The principal difference between intestinal and rectal absorption is that the veins from the intestine empty into the portal circulation, while the blood from the rectum is carried to a large extent through the hemorrhoidal veins into the vena cava, thus bypassing the liver. However, in humans this is not so clear-cut: a venous plexus collects the blood from the mucosa of the rectum. From this the upper hemorrhoidal veins carry the blood into the portal system, while the lower hemorrhoidal veins empty it via the iliac veins into the vena cava. Thus, in humans part of the rectally absorbed drug may end up in the portal system and part will be transported directly into the inferior vena cava. The situation is further complicated by individual variations which render the prediction of the circulatory fate of the rectally administered drug rather uncertain (DE BOER and BREIMER 1979).

D. The Intestinal Barrier and its Permeability

One can consider the intestine as a complex biologic membrane: it is composed essentially of the mucosal epithelial cells, the tight junction and intercellular

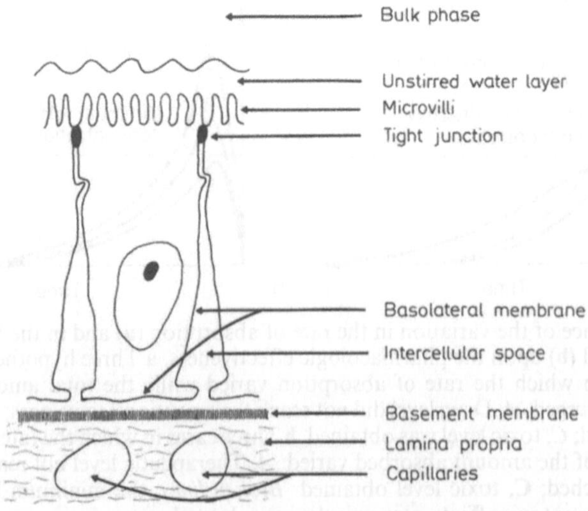

Fig. 3. Schematic representation of the intestinal permeability barriers

spaces, the glycocalyx covering the luminal face of the brush border, and the unstirred water layer immediately adjacent to the luminal face of the glycocalyx (Fig. 3). The overall permeability of the gut is then a composite of the permeability properties of its constituents. The primary function of the intestine is absorption. Consequently the anatomic structure and permeability properties of the gut are differentiated toward directional transport from the lumen into the subepithelial space. Let us consider the influence of these individual barriers upon the intestinal absorption of xenobiotics.

I. The Unstirred Water Layer

The layer of water adjacent to the mucosal surface of the absorbing epithelium is essentially unstirred (see also Chap. 22). It can be visualized as a series of water lamellae each progressively more stirred from the surface of the cell toward the bulk phase. From the point of view of functional significance, a finite thickness can be assigned to the unstirred water layer (UWL) through which solutes pass by simple diffusion. Because of the complex anatomic structure of the luminal surface of the intestinal mucosa, the thickness of the UWL can be more than 400 nm. Owing to its thickness, the UWL may represent a significant permeability barrier. Because the passage through the UWL occurs by simple diffusion, the flux rate J for a given solute across this layer will be proportional to the difference of concentration at the luminal bulk phase c_1 and at the aqueous–lipid interface on the brush border membrane c_2, and the free diffusion coefficient D; it is inversely proportional to the UWL thickness d.

$$J = \frac{(c_1 - c_2)D}{d}.$$

Thus, the resistance of the UWL depends on three factors: (a) effective thickness; (b) effective surface layer; (c) diffusion coefficient of the substrate (DIETSCHY and WESTERGAARD 1975). The resistance of the UWL is usually greater in the in vivo perfused rat (WINNE 1976) and human jejunum (READ et al. 1977) than in the in vitro preparation. If the rate of permeation of the solute through the brush border is fast (as in the case of a highly passively permeable solute, rapid intracellular metabolism, or active transport) then the rate-limiting step in the absorption is diffusion across the UWL. It is likely that the resistance of the UWL limits the absorption of long-chain fatty acids and steroids, such as bile acids, cholesterol, or steroid hormones. Orally administered drugs are generally fat soluble. Consequently it can be assumed that the flux across the UWL will influence their intestinal absorption.

As we have seen the flux of a given solute across the UWL is inversely proportional to the thickness of this layer. Consequently reduction of the UWL should have a positive influence on the flux. Experimentally, the thickness of the UWL can be effectively reduced by vigorous stirring of the luminal phase. In vivo it can be assumed that intestinal motility, particularly the contraction of the villi, may modify the UWL. However, it is difficult to assess the quantitative contribution of this factor. In some animal species, such as the dog, or in humans, the anatomic structure of the villi is such that their contraction contributes to the stirring of the surface. This may be responsible for the slight ($\sim 20\%$) increase in the rate of glucose absorption from a loop of small intestine of the dog following the increase in the rate of villous contraction produced by an intraduodenal injection of hydrochloric acid (KOKAS and LUDÀNY 1938). It is not known whether such manipulation influences the absorption of xenobiotics.

II. The Transcellular Route

Passage through the cells involves permeation across the brush border, the intracellular space, and the basolateral membrane. The principal permeability barrier is represented by the brush border. Information about possible intracellular barriers is lacking. According to present knowledge the role of the basolateral membrane in drug absorption is passive: substrates permeate across this membrane according to their relative lipid solubility.

The brush border is a membrane of complex structure composed of the microvilli (see Chap. 1). Its permeability properties are influenced, among others, by the many enzymes herein located (see Chap. 20 on membrane digestion). The luminal surface of the brush border is covered with a filamentous coating composed of sulfated acid mucopolysaccharides (ITO 1964, 1965). The possible role of this surface coating, referred to as "fuzzy coat", in the acid microvironment of the surface of the brush border (see Sect. D. II. 1. b) is not yet firmly established.

Despite its complex anatomic structure the brush border can be considered, as far as its permeability property is concerned, as a lipid barrier. Consequently lipid-soluble substances permeate it readily by diffusion, while polar substances pass only by an interaction with a specific transport mechanism, viz., carrier mediation or pinocytosis.

1. Diffusion

a) Lipid Partition Theory

The majority of orally administered drugs or other ingested xenobiotics are lipid soluble, and thus are absorbed from the intestine via diffusion. The kinetics of this process is determined by the factors expressed in Fick's law. According to this law the rate of diffusion $\mathrm{d}n/\mathrm{d}t$, i.e., the number of particles (molecules) $\mathrm{d}n$ crossing an area A in time $\mathrm{d}t$ over a distance ($\mathrm{d}x$) is proportional to the concentration difference $\mathrm{d}c/\mathrm{d}x$.

$$\frac{\mathrm{d}n}{\mathrm{d}t}=DA\frac{\mathrm{d}c}{\mathrm{d}x},$$

where D is the diffusion constant. When a lipid membrane is interposed in the path of diffusion, the rate of permeation across the membrane will be determined by the area, the thickness of the membrane, the concentration difference between the two interfaces of the membrane, and by the relative lipid solubility of the permeant.

Assuming that the intestinal cells represent basically a lipid barier, it would follow that the lipid solubility of the xenobiotic molecule will play a significant role in the transcellular intestinal transport. Experimentally the classical work of BRODIE and co-workers (for summary of this work see BRODIE 1964 and SCHANKER 1962, 1971) verified the basic correctness of this assumption. By definition the kinetics of intestinal absorption of a lipid-soluble substrate is diffusional, represented by a straight line relationship between the rate and the initial intraluminal concentration. Figure 4 shows this simple relationship between the intestinal absorption and initial luminal concentration of ethanol, a typical lipid-soluble drug.

Many drugs and other xenobiotics are weak organic acids and bases; they are highly polar in the ionized form, but more lipid soluble in the nonionized form. Consequently, the nonionized species of these compounds is expected to permeate the intestinal epithelial barrier, but not the ionized species. The extent of ionization of a given weak acid or base depends on the dissociation constant $\mathrm{p}K_\mathrm{a}$ and the pH of the medium as expressed in the Henderson–Hasselbalch equation (HENDERSON 1909; HASSELBALCH 1917)

$$\mathrm{pH}=\mathrm{p}K_\mathrm{a}+\log X$$

$$X \text{ for weak acids}=\frac{\text{ionized}}{\text{nonionized}}$$

$$X \text{ for weak bases}=\frac{\text{nonionized}}{\text{ionized}}$$

In animal experiments, the correctness of this assumption has been reasonably well verified as shown in the example in Table 1. Accordingly, the permeation across the intestinal brush border of weak acids and bases depends upon the degree of ionization, the membrane presenting little resistance to the permeation of

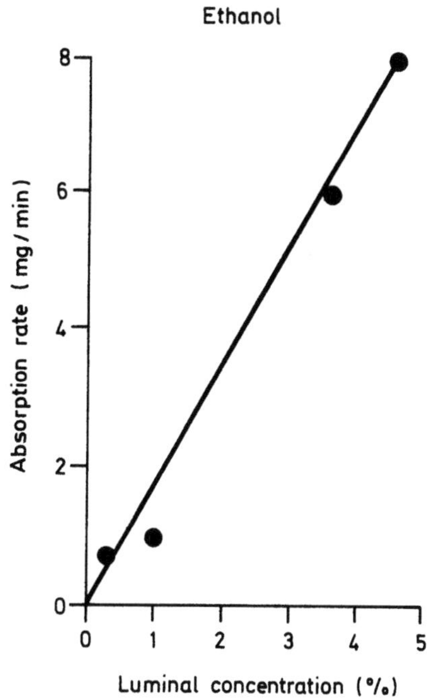

Fig. 4. Relationship between the rate of intestinal absorption and initial luminal concentration of ethanol

Table 1. Correlation between pK_a and intestinal absorption[a] in the rat (modified from Schanker et al. 1958)

Acid	pK_a	Absorption (%)	Base	pK_a	Absorption (%)
5-Sulfosalicylic	Strong	< 2	Acetanilide	0.3	42
Phenol red	Strong	< 2	Theophylline	0.7	29
			p-Nitroaniline	1.0	68
o-Nitrobenzoic	2.2	5	Antipyrine	1.4	32
5-Nitrosalicylic	2.3	9	*m*-Nitroaniline	2.5	77
Tromexan	2.9	35	Aniline	4.6	54
Salicylic	3.0	60	Aminopyrine	5.0	33
m-Nitrobenzoic	3.4	53	*p*-Toluidine	5.3	59
Acetylsalicylic	3.5	20	Quinine	8.4	15
Benzoic	4.2	51	Ephedrine	9.6	7
Phenylbutazone	4.4	65	Tolazoline	10.3	6
Acetic	4.7	42	Mecamylamine	11.2	3
Thiopental	7.6	55			
Barbital	7.8	30			
p-Hydroxy-propiophenone	7.8	61	Tetraethyl-ammonium	Strong	< 2
Phenol	9.9	51	Tensilon	Strong	< 2

[a] Percentage change of concentration of drug in saline perfused for 7 min at 1.5 ml/min through the entire small intestine

the nonionized species while rejecting the ionized species. Experimental findings (HOGBEN et al. 1959; SCHANKER et al. 1958; SCHANKER 1971) verified the general correctness of this tenet, for which MILNE et al. (1958) coined the term "nonionic diffusion".

b) Surface pH

However, under close scrutiny the classical nonionic diffusion or pH partition theory does not hold accurately for the small intestine because the quantitative rate of absorption of weak acids and bases frequently does not agree with the calculated values. A typical example is the intestinal absorption of salicylates. The pK_a of salicylic acid is 3.0, the average pH of the human jejunal luminal content is 6.5. At this pH 99.968% of the salicylic acid molecules are ionized, and thus should scarcely be absorbed at all. Yet, it is known that the acid administered in enterocoated tablet form, which bypasses the stomach unaltered and disintegrates in the small intestine, is very well absorbed. This is even true in animal experiments: 59% of the salicylic acid was found to be absorbed from the small intestine of the rat in 1 h. To explain this discrepancy, HOGBEN et al. (1959) proposed the existence of a microenvironment on the mucosal surface of the intestinal epithelium with a pH of approximately 5.3. Subsequently, this proposal was experimentally verified with the aid of a small flat microelectrode applied to the surface of the intestinal mucosa, pH values of 4.5–5 were measured (LUCAS et al. 1976; LUCAS 1976; see also Chap. 21). At a surface pH of 5, 1% of the salicylic acid would be present in a nonionized, lipophilic form which would allow absorption by diffusion through the cells.

If the pH at the lipid–water interface on the brush border is actually acid, the intestinal absorption of weak bases should be seriously hindered. For example, quinine, or its optical isomer, quinidine, have pK_a 8.4. About 2.5% of the drug is nonionized in the bulk phase of the intestine at pH 6.6, which, according to the classical pH partition theory would allow absorption of the drug. However, at the lipid–water interface on the brush border at pH 5.0, only 0.032% of the drug is nonionized which does not favor diffusional transport across the lipid membrane. Yet, it is known that both quinine and quinidine are well absorbed from the intestine. There are several reasonable explanations for this apparent paradox. There is a high probability that bases can be absorbed in ionized form through the paracellular route (see Sect. D. III. 1). Another possible mechanism for the intestinal absorption of ionized bases emerges from the observation of TURNHEIM and LAUTERBACH (1980) who found that organic cations are actively secreted from the blood into the lumen of the intestine. They also suggest that the carrier involved in the secretory process may facilitate the lumen–blood transepithelial transport of organic bases in their cationic form.

Thus, the classical pH partition theory for the intestinal absorption of organic acids and bases is still applicable, whith certain modifications. The relatively acidic pH microenvironment at the surface of the brush border will allow a distribution of ionic and nonionic species of organic acids favorable for permeation across the lipid membrane. Thus, acids can be absorbed by simple diffusion across the epithelial layer. On the other hand, organic bases are absorbed in the ionized form, which is prevalent at the low surface pH, either through the paracellular sheets, or through the cells via carrier mediation. Furthermore, it should be noted that some organic anions can also be absorbed by a specific, carrier-mediated transport mechanism or via the intercellular channels (see Sect. D. III. 1).

2. Specific Transport Mechanisms

a) Carrier Mediation

Epithelia which are differentiated primarily for transporting are those of the intestine, kidney tubules, and choroid plexus. The kidney tubular cells are endowed with specific transport mechanisms for organic acids and bases and they can transport sugars in both directions, actively absorbing and secreting them. The choroid plexus also has specific mechanisms for the transport of bases, such as morphine, organic acids, and a system for the transport of sugars. Until recently, no specific transport mechanism was known for organic acids and bases in the enterocytes. However, it has been demonstrated that organic bases are actively secreted from the blood into the lumen of the intestine (TURNHEIM and LAUTERBACH 1980). Apparently, the same carrier which mediates this active secretion may be involved in the intestinal absorption of organic bases. This arrangement could explain the paradoxical fact that basic drugs are well absorbed from the small intestine, despite the acid pH existing at the lumen–brush border interface. At acid pH the bases would be mostly in the ionized form creating, according to the classical pH partition theory, an unfavorable condition fot their absorption.

As far as the intestinal transport of organic acids is concerned, active intestinal secretion was demonstrated by SUND and LAUTERBACH (1978). In this regard the enterocyte seems to display similarity to the kidney tubular epithelial cell. The kidney tubule transports penicillin actively. In the intestine, so far, no specific transport mechanism has been detected for penicillin; however, there is good evidence for the specific intestinal transport of some semisynthetic penicillin derivatives. Cyclacillin (1-amino-cyclohexylpenicillin) was found to be actively transported from the mucosal compartment into the serosal one in the everted small intestine of the rat (DIXON and MIZEN 1977). This conclusion was drawn from the following findings: (a) cyclacillin is concentrated in the serosal compartment at 37 °C, but not at 19 °C; (b) the transport is saturable; (c) there is a flux asymmetry favoring mucosal–serosal flux. In addition there is evidence that the intestinal absorption of another aminopenicillin, amoxicillin, is also carrier mediated, but it is not an active process. The two aminopenicillins share most likely a common carrier as they mutually inhibit each other's absorption (KIMURA et al. 1978).

Many features of the kinetics of the intestinal absorption of cardioactive glucosides are not compatible with the simple diffusion or pH partition theory. Thus, the parallelism between the relative lipid solubility and the rate of absorption does not always hold for these compounds. Mutual inhibition of the absorption among these compounds was also demonstrated (SEIDENSTÜCKER and LAUTERBACH 1976; SEIDENSTÜCKER 1978; LAUTERBACH 1981). A decline of the rate of this intestinal absorption by metabolic inhibitors was also shown (DAMM and WOERMANN 1974). It is now recognized that cardiac glucosides are actively secreted from the blood into the lumen of the intestine (LAUTERBACH 1975, 1977), and there is further evidence that they are not absorbed exclusively by simple diffusion but, at least in part, by carrier mediation.

b) Pinocytosis

Little is known about the possible role of pinocytosis in the intestinal absorption of drugs and toxic substances. It has been postulated that pinocytosis is involved in the intestinal absorption of vitamin B_{12} (ABELS et al. 1959; WILSON 1963). It is likely that large molecules, such as proteins, are absorbed by pinocytosis. The well-known toxicity of orally ingested botulinus toxin (molecular weight 900,000) is a typical example which can be quoted for intestinal absorption of high molecular weight proteins.

III. The Intercellular Route

1. Tight Junction and Paracellular Channels

On the brush border side, the neighboring epithelial cells come into close contact. With the electron microscope it appears as if the brush border membranes were fused. The area of close contact was designated by the morphologists as the occluding zonules (zonulae occludentes) or the tight junctions (FARQUHAR and PALLADE 1963). Yet functionally the tight junctions do not appear tight but permeable to water, electrolytes, and other charged or uncharged molecules up to a certain size.

The epithelial lining of the small intestine belongs to the group of "leaky epithelia". Besides the intestine, the epithelia of the proximal tubule, gallbladder, and choroid plexus are also leaky (DIAMOND 1974). These epithelia are characterized by low resistance, e.g., 100 Ω cm^2 in the rabbit ileum (FRIZELL and SCHULTZ 1972) and small open-circuit potential (0–4 mV). In contrast, the "tight" epithelia represented by the distal and collecting tubules of the kidney, the urinary bladder, and frog skin, display high transepithelial resistance (300–80,000 Ω cm^2) and high transepithelial potential (20–90 mV).

The junctional channels in the leaky epithelia, such as the small intestine, are permeable to cations, anions, some uncharged molecules, and water. From studies concerning the effect of pH upon the cation and anion conductance, it was conluded that the channels are lined with negative and positive charges which influence their cation or anion permeability (MORENO and DIAMOND 1974). At neutral pH the small intestinal channel is preferentially cation sensitive (DIAMOND 1978).

A junctional pore radius has been calculated for the gallbladder of the rabbit (5 Å) and of the bullfrog (8 Å). These values can be taken as an approximation of the molecular size of substances which can permeate the intercellular channels of a leaky epithelium. The apparent radii of the intestine are not necessarily constant. The channel can be further opened by the use of calcium chelators and by increased pH to the extent that large particles, such as polyethylene glycol, can pass from the blood to the lumen (CSÁKY and AUTENRIETH 1975).

Information concerning the intestinal absorption of xenobiotics via the junction–intercellular route is scanty and not sufficient to provide a quantitative assessment of the significance of this route. The permeability measurements of MORENO and DIAMOND (1974) performed in the gallbladder on a number of organic bases indicated that the intercellular route could be significant in the permeability of a leaky epithelium, such as the small intestine. Thus, it could be assumed that both the ionized and nonionized species of a weak organic base can be absorbed in the intestine, the nonionized mainly through the brush border and intracellular route, the ionized species primarily through the tight junction and intercellular route. Although at neutral pH the intercellular channel displays some permeability preference for bases, weak organic acids can also be transported through this route. There has been a proposal for a three-compartment model for the permeation of weak electrolytes in the gut (JACKSON et al. 1974; JACKSON and KUTCHER 1977).

It was also observed that cardioactive glycosides permeate across the stripped mucosal layer of the guinea pig ileum from the lumen to the serosal side at the same rate as inulin. Since inulin does not enter the cell, this observation was interpreted as evidence that the permeation across paracellular shunts represents an important pathway for the absorption of cardioactive glycosides (KILIAN and LAUTERBACH 1979).

2. Persorption

Powdered quartz, lycopodium spores, plant pollens, diatomaceous earth particles, and starch granules in particle size up to 150 nm have been recovered in the blood plasma following an oral gavage. It is assumed and also experimentally shown that these large particles enter the subepithelial space at the tip of the villi between two cells which are ready to be sloughed off. The particles then enter the lymph and ultimately end up in the blood. This process is called persorption (VOLKHEIMER 1972).

It can be assumed that particles of potentially toxic substances (e.g., asbestos fibers) may also be absorbed via persorption. At this time, the potential pharmacotoxicologic significance of persorption has not been fully assessed. Thus it cannot be judged whether this phenomenon should be considered a curiosity or something with pharmacotoxicologic significance. It is generally assumed that persorption has little, if any, nutritional significance.

IV. Absorption via the Lymph

It is not unrealistic to visualize the lamina propria as the place where the lymph originates. Essentially all substances which pass through the epithelial layer either by the transcellular or intercellular path ultimately reach the lamina propria which is richly endowed with a net of blood capillaries. These capillaries are fenestrated (CLEMENTI and PALLADE 1969) and allow the passage of particles up to a certain size, regardless of whether they are polar or lipid soluble. Thus, theoretically, the particle size and not the lipid solubility of the absorbed substrate would determine whether it would be primarily absorbed into the blood or into the lymph. Experimental evidence seems to justify such an assumption (DEAK 1977). Botulinus type A toxin, molecular weight 900,000 (PUTNAM et al. 1946), is absorbed into the lymph. Consequently the animals can be protected from the toxic effect after oral administration by cannulating the mesenteric lymph vessels and preventing their emptying into the blood circulation (MAY and WHALER 1958). In the newborn calf, large amounts of globulins are absorbed from the colostrum. These proteins appear in the thoracic duct and not in the portal vein (COMLINE et al. 1951).

A number of drugs appear preferentially in the lymph; the mechanism by which they appear in the lymph is still not clear. *p*-Aminosalicylic acid and tetracycline can be detected in the mesenteric lymph after duodenal administration. The concentration of *p*-aminosalicylic acid is higher in the mesenteric lymph than in the plasma. However, this is not significant as far as the total net absorption is concerned because of the great difference between the flow of lymph and blood (DEMARCO and LEVINE 1969). It has been known for some time (ASELLIUS 1627) that if an animal is fed fat this appears in the lymph and renders it milky. However, the absorbed fat does not end up preferentially in the lymph because of its lipid nature, but because it is enclosed in relatively large particles called chylomicrons.

E. Factors Which Influence the Intestinal Absorption of Xenobiotics

I. Factors Inherent to the Drug Molecule

1. Solubility

The basic rule of the alchemists, *"corpora non agunt, nisi fluida"* (i.e., substances are not active unless they are fluids), applies with slight modification to the absorption of drugs. Xenobiotics have to be in true solution or at least in very fine emulsion to gain access to the absorptive surface of the gut. Solubility is one of the physicochemical features which determines intestinal absorption. Since many drugs are absorbed by diffusing through the epithelial layer, the relative lipid solubility is another determining factor.

2. pK_a

The lipid solubility is often determined by the degree of ionization in which the pK_a of the molecule plays a determining role.

3. Molecular Weight and Structure

The passage of drugs through the paracellular pathway and across the capillaries is influenced by the size of the molecule, while the three-dimensional molecular structure and the number of charges on the molecule seem to be significant in the passage across the intercellular junctions (MORENO and DIAMOND 1974).

II. Factors Inherent of Pharmaceutical Formulation

Few drugs are routinely administered in dissolved form, most formulations are solid: tablets, capsules, pills, etc. In the pharmaceutical formulation of these solids usually one or more vehicles are involved, binding materials are necessary to hold the formulation together, etc. The rate of disintegration and dissolution of these solid formulations depends on a number of physicochemical parameters. Over the past decades the study of the effect of pharmaceutical formulation upon the bioavailability of drugs has gained great significance. In fact, a new science called "biopharmaceutics" has evolved to embrace these studies. The discussion of the results of biopharmaceutical research is beyound the scope of this review. Several summaries can be found in the literature (WAGNER 1971; MATTOK et al. 1977).

III. Factors Inherent to Intestinal Permeability

Under physiologic conditions, large amounts of water are discharged into the upper alimentary tract in the form of salivary, gastric, pancreatic, and intestinal secretion. In a healthy adult this may amount to 7–8 l/day. In addition, another 1–2 l are consumed in the diet. Since relatively small amounts of water are lost in the stool (100–200 ml), the intestine absorbs nearly 10 l/day. Can this large water absorption influence the absorption of drug in the form of solvent drag? A positive answer to this question was suggested from the finding that in the rat intestine, perfused in situ with solutions of varying tonicity, the absorption of sulfanilamide, sulfisoxazole, and metoclopramide was increased with increasing transmural fluid movement from lumen to blood and decreased when the movement of water was directed from the blood to the lumen (KITAZAWA et al. 1975).

1. Solvent Drag

The question of the effect of solvent drag upon the intestinal absorption of xenobiotics was systematically studied by OCHSENFAHRT and WINNE (1974a, b) by examining the effect of increased as well as retarded lumen–blood water flux upon the appearance in the mesenteric blood of both acidic (benzoic, salicylic) and basic drugs (amidopyrine, antipyrine). The intestinal water flow was varied by placing hypo-, iso-, or hypertonic solutions in the lumen. The absorption of both acidic and basic drugs, as measured by their rate of appearance in the intestinal venous blood, was increased when the net water absorption increase (Fig. 5). The authors argue that the solvent drag is the result of the interaction of water with the solutes within the lipid membrane.

IV. Factors Inherent to the Patient

1. Gastric Emptying

This problem has been reviewed extensively by PRESCOTT (1974a, b) and NIMMO (1976, 1979). As discussed in Sect. C., because of its much larger surface the small bowel is more important in the absorption of drugs and other xenobiotics than

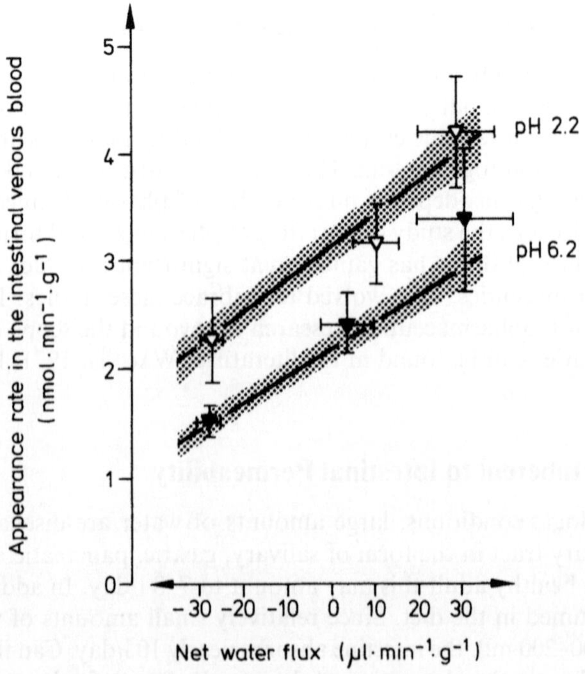

Fig. 5. Interdependence of the absorption of salicylic acid and net water flux in the intestine of the rat (Ochsenfahrt and Winne 1974b)

the stomach. Consequently, the rate of gastric emptying may significantly modify the rate of absorption. In human subjects, in whom the rate of gastric emptying and the absorption of acetaminophen (paracetamol) was simultaneously monitored, a very close parallelism was found between the rates (Prescott et al. 1977).

The more frequently used clinical methods for studying gastric emptying have been reviewed by Sheiner (1975). A simple method was developed based on the assumption that the rate of ethanol absorption is determined by the rate of gastric emptying (Finch et al. 1974). Ethanol is administered by mouth and its rate of appearance in the body is followed by monitoring the amount of ethanol in the expired air. A series of estimations over 2.5 h yielded ethanol curves with little variation within the same subject. Metoclopramide increased and propantheline decreased the rate of appearance of ethanol in the expired air. Physiologic, pathologic, and pharmacologic factors may influence the gastric emptying.

a) Physiologic Factors

Among the physiologic factors, gastric distension or liquids in the stomach enhance the emptying. On the other hand, solids in the stomach (particularly fats), increased acidity, or high osmolarity all retard the gastric emptying. A number of autacoids, e.g., gastrin, secretin, cholecystokinin, glucagon, decrease the rate of gastric emptying, but it is uncertain what role they play in normal physiologic conditions.

Several pathologic factors were found to delay gastric emptying: laparatomy (DUDLEY 1975), trauma, head injury, gastric ulcer, diabetes (RIMMER 1966), and myocardial infarction. In several of these cases the patient was treated with drugs which may have be themselves modified gastric emptying (see NIMMO 1976, 1979). For example, it was found that women in labor experience delayed gastric emptying (DAVISON et al. 1970), and this may influence the absorption of some antibiotics, thereby preventing the reaching of therapeutic plasma concentration (BUCKINGHAM et al. 1975). However, upon closer scrutiny, it was found that absorption of paracetamol was normal in labor when no other drug treatment was involved, indicating normal gastric emptying; the gastric emptying was delayed only after the woman in labor was given a narcotic analgesic (NIMMO et al. 1975).

b) Pathologic Factors

On the other hand, certain pathologic conditions, such as calcular cholecystitis (VAN DAM 1972) and duodenal ulcer (GRIFFITH et al. 1968) increase the rate of gastric emptying.

c) Pharmacologic Factors

Drugs may either delay or promote gastric emptying (PRESCOTT 1974A; NIMMO 1976). Drugs which delay gastric emptying are: anticholinergics, ganglionic blocking agents, narcotic analgesics, phenothiazines, antiparkinsonian drugs, isoniazid and iproniazid, nitrites, chloroquine, alcohol, phenytoin. Drugs which enhance gastric emptying are: metoclopramide, reserpine, anticholinesterases. Antacids have a variety of actions connected to their influence on gastric emptying (see Sect. E IV. 1. d).

d) Effect on Drug Absorption

Factors which slow gastric emptying usually decrease the rate of xenobiotic absorption. On the other hand, factors which speed up gastric emptying increase the rate of absorption from the alimentary tract. In certain instances, delay in gastric emptying may actually enhance intestinal absorption. This is the case when a drug preparation is dissolved slowly, aided by the acid pH of the stomach juice. Longer residence in the stomach will cause the drug to become dissolved. For example, a propantheline enhances the absorption of digoxin, but only if administered in tablet form, not in solution, while metoclopramide has the opposite effect (MANNINEN et al. 1973). Similar observations were made with hydrochlorothiazide (BEERMAN and GROSCHINTSKY-GRIND 1978) and nitrofurantoin (JAFFE 1975).

Some drugs are administered in the form of inactive precursor (prodrug); the conversion to the active form may take place in the acid stomach. If the gastric emptying is very rapid, the conversion may be insufficient. Such a case was found with clorazepate which is inactive and is converted in the stomach to the active desmethyldiazepam. The prodrug is poorly absorbed and is inactive. At rapid gastric emptying it was found that the preparation was pharmacologically less effective (SHADIR et al. 1978; ABRUZZO et al. 1977).

2. Intestinal Motility

It is difficult to find drugs which act exclusively on the intestinal motility without affecting gastric emptying or splanchnic blood flow, which by themselves may affect the absorption of drugs. As mentioned previously, longer residence in the intestine would allow more time for the drug to be absorbed. Thus, slowing the intestinal motility through pharmacologic means would enhance the rate of drug absorption. On the other hand, drugs which may increase the intestinal and, in particular, the villous motility will decrease the thickness of the UWL which in turn favors a more rapid drug absorption. Because of the difficulty in finding highly selective drugs which influence certain aspects of intestinal motility alone, these theoretical considerations await experimental verification.

3. Splanchnic Blood Flow

The majority of drugs are absorbed by the transepithelial route, either by simple or carrier-mediated diffusion. In either case, as long as in the mediated transport the carrier is unsaturated, the flux of the drug across the mucosal cell is primarily determined by the concentration difference between the two sides of the epithelial "membrane", viz., the brush border–water interface and the lamina propria. The content of the lamina propria is cleared in two directions: the blood and the lymph. The rate of blood flow is several magnitudes larger than that of the lymph flow, thus, the significant factor which determines the concentration of a solute in the lamina propria is the rate of the subepithelial blood flow and the concentration of the free (not protein-bound) solute in the arterial blood. In the case of drugs and other xenobiotics, plasma binding increases the concentration difference of the free compound between the brush border interface and the blood, thus secondarily the lamina propria.

a) Measurement

By the method of Rb distribution (SAPIERSTEIN 1958), it was estimated that in the rat about 7% of the cardiac output flows through the entire gastrointestinal tract. This figure includes the entire blood supply; i.e., the blood that flows through the capillary bed of the submucosal connective tissue and muscle layers as well. Clearly, not all of this blood is in immediate exchange with the lamina propria. From the point of view of intestinal drug absorption the capillary blood circulation immediately adjacent to the lamina propria is the most significant. This "effective" subepithelial circulation has been determined by CSÁKY and VARGA (1975) in the following way: barbital is a weak acid (pK_a 7.78) which is not appreciably metabolized in the animal body, is not transported across biologic membranes by specific carrier mediation, and is not bound to any extent to plasma proteins. In previous experiments it was observed that the intestinal lumen in the rat can be exposed to an alkaline pH up to 9.5 without appreciably altering the permeability properties of the gut (CSÁKY and AUTENRIETH 1975). ^{14}C-labeled barbital was injected into the blood circulation of an anesthetized rat and the gut lumen was perfused with an isotonic buffer of pH 9.5. Assuming that the blood pH is approximately 7.4, at this pH about 30% of the barbital is present in the nonionized form and can readily permeate across the epithelial layer into the lumen. The luminal perfusion was buffered at pH 9.5 and its rate was kept vigorous (~25 ml/min) to minimize the unstirred layer effect. At pH 9.5, 98% of the barbital is ionized and therefore trapped in the lumen. Thus, the clearance of the barbital was calculated in the following way.

$$\text{Barbital clearance} = \frac{V_{\text{perf}}\,C_{\text{perf}}}{C_{\text{plasma}}\,tw},$$

where V_{perf} is the volume of the perfusate, and C is the concentration of the drug, t is the time, and w the gut wet weight. It was found by this method that 50% ±5% of the total blood flow was diverted to the subepithelial circulation. This percentage was found to be rather constant, even if the cardiac output and the regional blood flow through the gastrointestinal tract were altered as in aged animals or in animals in which the body temperature was artificially lowered.

b) Effect on Drug Absorption

Blood flow influences the intestinal absorption of drugs primarily by draining the blood from the site of absorption and thereby maintaining a large lumen-blood concentration gradient of the absorbed drug. Furthermore, the intestine represents a tissue with very active metabolism, consequently, adequate blood supply is essential for its functional integrity. As expected from the assumption that the most important effect of the blood flow is the maintenance of the lumen-blood concentration difference, the absorption of substances that permeate the intestinal wall readily is more blood flow dependent. This was actually verified experimentally. The absorption of triated water and lipid-soluble compounds, such as aniline, antipyrine, ethanol, sulfaethidole, salicylamide, or sulfisoxazole, is blood flow dependent while the absorption of relatively polar substrates is not (WINNE 1973, 1978; WINNE and REMISCHOWSKY 1970, 1971 a; OCHSENFAHRT and WINNE 1969, 1974 a, b; CROUTHAMEL et al. 1975; BARR and RIEGELMAN 1970).

4. Diseases Causing Drug Malabsorption

a) Celiac Disease

The absorption of antibiotics in celiac disease has been examined by PARSONS and colleagues (PARSONS and PADDOCK 1975; PARSONS et al. 1975, 1976 a, b). Four patterns were observed: increased, reduced, delayed, and normal absorption. Several factors may be involved in the mechanism of altered drug absorption in celiac disease (PARSONS 1977): increased rate of gastric emptying (MOBERG and CARLBERGER 1974), increased intraluminal pH which decreases the solubility of certain drugs, e.g., practolol (PARSONS and KAYE 1974), increased intestinal mucosal permeability, altered intestinal drug hydrolysis and metabolism, malabsorption of lipid-soluble drugs (steatorrhea), and reduced enterohepatic circulation of bile acids.

b) Other Malabsorptive States

Steatorrhea impairs the absorption of digoxin (HEIZER et al. 1971) while it does not affect the absorption of several antibiotics (DAVIES 1975). The absorption of cephalexin is reduced in cystic fibrosis (PARSONS and PADDOCK 1975). In lactose intolerance the absorption of drugs may be delayed (JUSSILA et al. 1970). Acute shigellosis may cause malabsorption of ampicillin and nalidixic acid in infants and children (NELSON et al. 1972). Diarrhea may cause a failure of oral contraception by inhibiting the absorption of the contraceptive drug (JOHN and JONES 1975). Crohn's disease produces a thickening of the gut wall and the reduction of the intestinal absorptive surface. It is, therefore, expected that these anatomic changes may impede the intestinal absorption of drugs. Actually it was found that the time to reach peak plasma concentration was about doubled in Crohn's disease for lincomycin, trimethoprim, and sulfamethoxazole (PARSONS et al. 1976a, b).

5. Interaction with Food

Solid and liquid foods alter the rate of gastric emptying and thereby may influence the intestinal absorption of xenobiotics. Dietary fiber may act similarly to ion exchange resins which form complexes with steroids, thereby inhibiting the absorption of bile acids, thus lowering the plasma cholesterol level. At the same time, however, the fibers form complexes with steroidal drugs, such as digoxin, and inhibit their absorption as well (BROWN et al. 1977).

The presence of food may influence the absorption of several drugs. The absorption of penicillin K, benzylpenicillin (G), oxacillin, 2-biphenylpenicillin, and lincomycin was retarded if taken with food (HEATLEY 1956; KLEIN et al. 1963; SABATH et al. 1963; MCCALL et al. 1967). Similarly, the absorption of certain sulfonamide preparations (sulfadimethoxine, sulfamethoxypyridazine, sulfisoxazole) was delayed if taken with solid food (MCDONALD et al. 1967).

The bioavailability of theophylline is reduced by food (PIAFSKI and OGILVIE 1975). The anticholinergic propantheline is used as an antispasmodic in treatment of peptic ulcer. The efficacy of the drug is judged by its decreasing action on the salivary secretion; viz., appearance of dry mouth. It was found that the decrease of the salivary flow was greater when propantheline was administered on an empty stomach than after a meal (GIBALDI and GRUNDHOFER 1975).

Tetracyclines avidly chelate with polyvalent metals such as Ca, Mg, Fe, Al, Zn (ALBERT and REES 1955, 1956). Consequently, foods with high content of these metals inhibit the absorption of tetracycline antibiotics. Milk and milk products (buttermilk, cottage cheese) are rich in calcium. These products markedly decrease the bioavailability of tetracyclines (SCHEINER and OLTEMEIER 1962; NEUVONEN et al. 1971). Doxycycline has a slightly lesser tendency to form chelates, therefore milk reduces its bioavailability somewhat less (ROSENBLATT et al. 1966; SCHACH VON WITTENAU 1968).

On the other hand, under certain conditions food may enhance the absorption of drugs. This applies in particular to drugs which have to remain in the stomach to be dissolved; in this case the retardation of the emptying of the stomach by the food is the reason for the promotion of absorption. This may be the explanation of the unusual finding (BATES et al. 1974) that food enhances the bioavailability of nitrofurantoin, but only if it is administered in a macrocrystalline, not in a microcrystalline formulation. The former requires more time to go into solution in the acid stomach. The absorption of griseofulvin, a systemic antifungal agent, is enhanced by food with high fat content (CROUNSE 1961; KABASAKALIAN et al. 1970).

6. Interaction with Drugs

One drug may modify the absorption of another. The clinical pharmacodynamic consequence of such interaction may not always be as dramatic as a fatal bleeding, which is the consequence of interference with the metabolism and distribution of an anticoagulant. It may not even be recognized unless particularly looked for (PRESCOTT et al. 1977). Nonetheless, interference with the absorption may occasionally cause therapeutic failure or toxic reactions.

a) Physicochemical Interactions

α) Changing the Intestinal pH. According to the classical ion partition theory, intraluminal alkalization enhances the lipid solubility and thus theoretically increases the rate of absorption of bases, while acidification has the same effect upon the absorption of weak acids. As we have already seen, the ion partition theory is complicated by the possible existence of mediated transport and by absorption via the intercellular channels. Thus the pH alone may have little influence upon the absorption. However, in some instances, the solubility of a given drug is substantially modified by the pH of the environment to the extent that it may represent the limiting factor in the absorption. The pH effect upon solubility may be opposite to what is expected according to the classical ion partition theory. For example, the rate of absorption of quinine is reduced by alkalies, while the acid form of pentobarbital or sulfadiazine is more rapidly absorbed if the acidity of the stomach is lowered by an antacid because of the greater solubility of these drugs at higher pH levels (HURWITZ 1974).

β) Formation of Complexes with Low Solubility. Perhaps the most significant complexes in this regard are produced by the chelation of tetracyclines with a number of polyvalent cations and by complex formation of drugs with cholestyramine. It has been shown by ALBERT and REES (1955, 1956) that a number of polyvalent cations, namely aluminum, bismuth, calcium, iron, magnesium, and zinc, form complexes with tetracycline which are much less soluble, therefore much less readily absorbed from the gut. Clinically, it has been demonstrated that the absorption of tetracyclines was reduced by the simultaneous administration of aluminum- or magnesium-containing antacids (WAISBREN and HUECKEL 1950; SEED and WILSON 1950; MICHEL et al. 1950), by iron preparations (NEUVONEN and PENTTILA 1974), by foods containing high calcium, levels such as milk, buttermilk, and cottage cheese (NEUVONEN et al. 1971), and by zinc (PENTTILA et al. 1975; ANDERSSON et al. 1976).

Cholestyramine is a basic, nonabsorbable exchange resin. In therapy it is used because it binds bile acids in the gut and thus prevents their absorption. This, in turn, causes an increase of the rate of conversion of cholesterol to bile acid, resulting in a decrease in the serum cholesterol level. In addition, cholestyramine binds cholesterol in the gut lumen and inhibits its absorption. The resin binds a variety of drugs in the intestine, thus inhibiting their absorption: digitalis glucosides (HALL et al. 1977; BAZZANO and BAZZANO 1972b), thyroxine (NORTHCUTT et al. 1969), oral anticoagulants (BENJAMIN et al. 1970; GALLO et al. 1965; KOCH-WESER and SELLERS 1971), loperamide (TI et al. 1978) and, in particular, acidic drugs such as aspirin, phenylbutazone (GALLO et al. 1965), sodium fusidate (JOHNS and BATES 1972), and flufenamic or mefenamic acids (ROSENBERG and BATES 1974). Cholestipol (tetraethylenepentamine polymer) has an effect similar to cholestyramine.

γ) Adsorption. Activated charcoal can reduce absorption of a drug. In one study, a watery suspension of activated charcoal (50 g) was administered after the oral administration of six drugs in therapeutic doses: digoxin, phenytoin, carbamazepine, phenobarbital, aspirin, and phenylbutazone. The absorption was determined by following the blood concentration at given times. The blood concentration AUC was reduced more than 95% when the charcoal was given 1 h after the administration of the drug (NEUVONEN et al. 1978; NEUVONEN and ELONEN 1980). The degree of the inhibition of absorption by charcoal does not follow a fixed drug : charcoal ratio; e.g., when 1 g aspirin was ingested together with 10 g charcoal, about 80% of the drug was absorbed. But when 5 g aspirin was given together with 50 g charcoal, only 20% was absorbed (LEVY and TSUCHIYA 1972). Other adsorbens, such as kaolin, pectin, etc., may act similarly to charcoal. Certain antacid gel formations can also adsorb a number of drugs (see Sect. D.IV.6.a.δ).

δ) Effects of Antacids. Antacids interfere with the intestinal absorption of drugs in several ways:

1. They change the luminal pH and thus alter the degree of ionization. In view of the importance of the surface pH, upon which the antacids have little influence, the role of this change upon the absorption is probably minimal.
2. They may change the solubility of the drug. The solubility of many compounds depends on the pH of the environment. For example, sulfadiazine in acidic form, if administered orally together with magnesium hydroxide, is absorbed significantly better, whereas magnesium hydroxide has little effect upon the absorption of the sodium salt of sulfadiazine (HURWITZ 1971). The reason for this is that the free acidic form of sulfadiazine is sparingly soluble while the ionized form is very soluble.
3. They may alter the gastric emptying. Antacids, particularly aluminum salts generally slow gastric emptying. Trivalent metals (aluminum, lanthanum, etc.) markedly diminish the contraction produced by acetylcholine in the isolated stomach muscle of rats or humans (HAVA and HURWITZ 1973).
4. They form complexes with altered solubility. The chelation of tetracyclines with metals (Ca, Mg, Al, Fe, Bi, Zn) is now well documented (see Sect. E.IV.6.a.β). These chelates are more sparingly soluble than the mother compound; consequently their absorption is impeded. On the other hand, chelation may produce complexes which are better absorbed than the parent drug, e.g., the dicumarol-Mg chelate (AMBRE and FISCHER 1973; AKERS et al. 1973).
5. Drugs may be adsorbed on the surface of the antacid gels and thereby their absorption is impeded. Such interaction was demonstrated for chlorpromazine (FANN et al. 1973; PINELL et al. 1978), dexamethasone (NAGGAR et al. 1978), digoxin (KHALIL 1974; BROWN et al. 1976; MCELNAY et al. 1978), and indomethacin (NAGGAR et al. 1976; GALEAZZI 1977).

6. They may inhibit the conversion of a prodrug to an active metabolite. For example, clorazepate is a poorly absorbed prodrug which in the acid stomach is rapidly converted to the active desmethyldiazepam. The conversion is more rapid at acid pH and is delayed if the pH of the stomach is raised by an antacid; thus the hydrolysis may not be completed before the prodrug reaches the small intestine from which it is absorbed very poorly (SHADIR et al. 1978; ABRUZZO et al. 1977).
7. A rather unusual antacid interaction has been described when the cation exchange resin, sodium polystyrene sulfonate, was concurrently administered with magnesium hydroxide or magnesium aluminum hydroxide. It was found that the ion exchange resin reacted in the gut with magnesium forming a magnesium polystyrene sulfonate and sodium chloride. As a consequence, the bicarbonate ions, which are normally secreted into the gut, are not neutralized but absorbed into the circulation, producing alkalosis (SCHROEDER 1969; FERNANDEZ and KOVNAT 1972).

b) Physiologic Interactions

Drugs may affect the absorption of other drugs by changing gastric emptying, gastrointestinal motility, or splanchnic blood flow. Such effects are discussed under the basic functions which are involved in the absorption (see Sect. E.IV). No evidence is available about the possible alteration by drugs of the surface pH or the intracellular channels.

Transport Mechanisms of the Enterocytes. A number of metabolic inhibitors may decrease the rate of absorption of many drugs (DAMM and WOERMANN 1974). Some drugs, e.g., neomycin, *p*-aminosalicylic acid, and colchicine, exert toxicity upon the intestinal mucosa, thus decreasing the absorption of drugs, particularly of those which utilize specific transport mechanisms such as digoxin, folate, and vitamin B_{12} (NEUVONEN 1979). Competitive inhibition is also possible between two ore more drugs utilizing the same transport carrier for absorption, e.g., cyclacillin and amoxycillin mutually inhibit each other's absorption (KIMURA et al. 1978).

7. Aging

This subject has been reviewed by BENDER (1968), TRIGGS and NATION (1975), CROOKS et al. (1976), RICHEY and BENDER (1977), VESTAL (1978), and CROOKS and STEVENSON (1979).

a) Definition of Aged

It is customary to classify as aged every subject older than 60 years. This classification is far from being scientifically satisfactory. Old age does not come about suddenly. It is a process which commences with birth and continues throughout life. The rate by which the various stages of morphological and physiologic changes related to aging occur varies considerably from individual to individual. Because of this a few basic rules should be observed when examining the effect of age on any given physiologic or pharmacologic parameter, including drug absorption:

1. Biologic age cannot be equated, in general, with the calendar age. Some individuals age considerably more rapidly than others.
2. Because of this, very large variations can be expected in many biologic parameters within a group of individuals belonging to a given calendar age group.
3. These large variations gradually diminish as age progresses. Consequently a group composed of a "senescent" (>80 year-old) individuals yield more reliable information than a group of "aged" (>60 year-old) subjects.

However, as far as the intestine is concerned, this tissue is continuously renewed: the average life span of a human intestinal epithelial cell is about 5–7 days (SHORTER et al. 1964; MACDONALD et al. 1964). Consequently, the gut epithelium is basically a young tissue. Although it is speculated that the rate of cell renewal in the intestinal mucosa is gradually declining with age, accurate quantitative data in this regard are not available. In the gut of senescent (>80 year-old) individuals atrophic changes are frequently detected.

The clinical finding that adverse drug reactions are relatively more frequent in the elderly (HURWITZ 1969) directed the interest toward pharmacokinetics in the elderly. Intestinal absorption is part of pharmacokinetics. Systemic human studies in which the drug was introduced directly into the small intestine with bypass of the stomach have not yet been carried out to any large extent. Consequently the occasional finding that the rate of appearance in the blood or the peak drug level after a single oral dose is lower in the elderly, as was found with diazepam (GARATTINI et al. 1973), does not necessarily reflect impaired intestinal absorption, but perhaps delayed gastric emptying or slower dissolution in the stomach.

b) Changes in Blood Flow

The majority of drugs are lipid soluble and thus are most likely absorbed across the lipid barriers of the intestine by simple diffusion. The rate of this process is largely determined by the concentration difference between the intestinal lumen and the bloodstream; the latter depends upon the rate of blood flow in the splanchnic area. The splanchnic blood perfusion is derived from the cardiac output and the regional blood flow.

Many details about the relationship between blood flow and intestinal absorption have been obtained primarily from studies on animals. There is no reason, however, why these results could not be extended, with certain precautions, to humans. It was observed in animal studies that the absorption of most fat-soluble substances is blood flow dependent. On the other hand, it was found that, in the rat, both the cardiac output and the subepithelial blood flow decrease with age: the cardiac output decreased from a value of 450 ml min^{-1} kg^{-1} in a 100 g young Sprague-Dawley male animal to 126 ml min^{-1} kg^{-1} in a 566 g old rat (VARGA and CSÁKY 1976). In humans, the cardiac output decreases by 30%–40% between the ages of 25 and 65 years (BRAUNDFONBREUER et al. 1955). It is speculated that the age-related decrease of cardiac output results in a reduced splanchnic blood flow (BENDER 1965).

Based on the these observations it would be expected that the rate of intestinal absorption of many drugs is significantly decreased in aging individuals. However, in studies conducted in various groups of aged persons, no significant change was found in the intestinal absorption of aspirin and quinine (SALEM and STEVENSON 1977), propicillin K (SIMON et al. 1972), indomethacin (TRAEGER et al. 1973), sulfamethizole and acetaminophen (TRIGGS et al. 1975), theophylline (CUSACK et al. 1979a), and digoxin (CUSACK et al. 1979b).

c) Experimental Findings and Interpretations

Two features of drug absorption in the elderly emerge from these studies: (1) in most instances the scatter of the values obtained with older subjects belonging to a given calendar age group is quite high and this renders the quantitation of the observed values rather difficult; (2) the plasma concentration AUC is in most instances significantly larger in the older than in the younger groups. This, however, is not necessarily a reflection upon the absorption, but most likely upon a slower rate of elimination either by metabolism, or renal excretion, or both. Because of the larger scatter, a sizeable number of measurements have to be performed to obtain meaningful data. For this reason the results of many of the studies quoted should be considered preliminary. The possibility exists that with studies performed in numbers sufficient for meaningful statistical evaluation, differences in the elderly in the rate of absorption of some drugs may be established (STEVENSON et al. 1979).

References

Abels H, Vegter JJM, Woldring M, Jous JH, Nieweg HO (1959) The physiologic mechanism of vitamin B_{12} absorption. Acta Med Scand 165:105–113
Abruzzo CW, Macasieb T, Weinfeld R, Rider JA, Kaplan SA (1977) Changes in the oral absorption characteristics in man of dipotassium clorazepate at normal and elevated gastric pH. J Pharmacokinet Biopharm 5:377–390
Akers MA, Lach JL, Fischer LJ (1973) Alteration in the absorption of dicoumarol by various excipient materials. J Pharm Sci 62:391–395
Albert A, Rees CW (1955) Incompatibility of aluminium hydroxide and certain antibiotics. Br Med J 2:1027
Albert A, Rees CW (1956) Avidity of the tetracyclines for the cations of metals. Nature 177:433:434
Ambre JJ, Fischer IJ (1973) Effect of coadministration of aluminium and magnesium hydroxydes on absorption of anticoagulants in man. Clin Pharmacol Ther 14:231–237
Andersson K-E, Bratt L, Dencker H, Kamme C, Lanner E (1976) Inhibition of tetracycline absorption by zinc. Eur J Clin Pharmacol 10:59–62
Asellius G (1627) De lactibus sive lacteis venis quarto vasorum mesaraicorum genere novo invento dissertatio. I. B. Bidelius, Milan
Bates TR, Sequeira JA, Thembo AV (1974) Effect of food on nitrofurantion absorption. Clin Pharmacol Ther 16:63–68
Barr WH, Riegelman S (1970) Intestinal drug absorption and metabolism. I: comparison of methods and models to study physiological factors of in vitro and in vivo intestinal absorption. J Pharm Sci 59:154–163
Bazzano G, Bazzano GS (1972a) Effect of digitalis-binding resins on cardiac glycoside plasma levels. Clin Res 20:24
Bazzano G, Bazzano GS (1972b) Digitalis intoxication. Treatment with a new steroid-binding resin. JAMA 220:828–830
Beerman B, Groschinsky-Grind M (1978) Enhancement of the gastrointestinal absorption of hydrochlorothiazide by propanthaline. Eur J Clin Pharmacol 13:385–387
Bender AD (1965) The effect of increasing age on the distribution of peripheral blood flow in man. J Am Geriat Soc 13:192–198

Bender AD (1968) Effect of age on intestinal absorption: implications for drug absorption in the elderly. J Am Geriat Soc 16:1331–1339
Benjamin D, Robinson DS, McCormack JJ (1970) Cholestyramine binding of warfarin in man and in vitro. Clin Res 18:336
Binns TB (ed) (1964) Absorption and Distribution of Drugs. Williams and Wilkins, Baltimore
Brandfonbreuer M, Landowne M, Shock NW (1955) Changes in cardiac output with age. Circulation 12:557–566
Brodie BB (1964) Physico-chemical factors in drug absorption. In: Binns TB (ed) Absorption and distribution of drugs. Williams and Wilkins, Baltimore, pp 16–48
Brodie BB, Mitchell JR (1973) The value of correlating biological effects of drugs with plasma concentration. In: Davis DS, Pritchard BNC (eds) Biological effects of drugs in relation of their plasma concentration. University Park Press, Baltimore, pp 1–12
Brown DD, Juhl Rp, Lewis K, Schrott M, Bartel B (1976) Decreased bioavailability of digoxin due to antacids and kaolin-pectin. N Engl J Med 295:1034–1037
Brown DD, Juhl RP, Warner SL (1977) Decreased bioavailability of digoxin produced by dietary fiber and cholestyramine. Am J Cardiol 39:297
Buckingham M, Welply G, Miller JF, Elstein M (1975) Gastro-intestinal absorption and transplacental transfer of amoxycillin during labour and the influence of metoclopramide. Curr Med Res Opin 3:392–396
Clementi F, Pallade GE (1969) Intestinal Capillaries I. Permeability to peroxidase and ferritin. J Cell Biol 41:33
Comline TS, Roberts HE, Titchen DA (1951) Route of absorption of colostrum globulin in the newborn animal. Nature 167:561–562
Crooks J, Stevenson IH (eds) (1979) Drugs and the elderly: perspectives in geriatric clinical pharmacology. Macmillan, London
Crooks J, O'Malley K, Stevenson IH (1976) Pharmacokinetics in the elderly. Clin Pharmacokinet 1:280–296
Crounse RG (1961) Human pharmacology of griseofulvin: the effect of fat intake on gastrointestinal absorption. J Invest Dermatol 37:529–533
Crouthamel WG, Diamond L, Dittert LW, Doluisio JT (1975) Drug absorption VII. Influence of mesenteric blood flow on intestinal drug absorption in dogs. J Pharm Sci 64:664–671
Csáky TZ, Autenrieth B (1975) Transcellular and intercellular intestinal transport. In: Csáky TZ (ed) Intestinal absorption and malabsorption. Raven, New York, pp 177–185
Csáky TZ, Varga F (1975) Subepithelial capillary blood flow estimated from blood-to-lumen flux of barbital in ileum of rats. Am J Physiol 229:549–552
Cusack B, Kelly J, Lavan J, Noel J, O'Malley K (1979a) The effect of age and smoking on theophylline kinetics. Br J Clin Pharmacol 8:384P–385P
Cusack B, Kelly J, O'Malley K, Noel J, Lavan J, Horgan J (1979b) Digoxin in the elderly; pharmacokinetic consequences of old age. Clin Pharmacol Ther 25:772–776
Damm KH, Woermann C (1974) The effect of probenecid on the in vitro absorption of cardiac glycosides. Eur J Pharmacol 28:157–163
Davies JA (1975) Absorption of cephalexin in diseased and aged subjects. J Antimicrob Chemother [Suppl] 1:69–70
Davison JS, Davison MC, Hay DM (1970) Gastric emptying time in late pregnancy and labour. Br J Obstet Gynecol 77:37–41
Deak ST (1977) Factors regulating the intestinal lymphatic absorption of nutrients and drugs. Ph D thesis, University of Kentucky
Deboer AG, Breimer DD (1979) Rectal absorption: portal or systemic? In: Prescott LF, Nimmo WS (eds) Drug Absorption. Adis, New York, pp 61–72
Demarco TJ, Levine RR (1969) Role of the lymphatics in the intestinal absorption and distribution of drugs. J Pharmacol Exp Ther 169:142–151
Diamond JM (1974) Tight and leaky junctions of the epithelia. Fed Proc 33:2220–2224
Diamond JM (1978) Channels in epithelial cell membranes and junctions. Fed Proc 37:2639–2644

Dietschy JM, Westergaard H (1975) The effect of unstirred water layers on various transport processes in the intestine. In: Csáky TZ (ed) Intestinal Absorption and Malabsorption. Raven, New York, pp 197–207
Dixon C, Mizen LW (1977) Absorption of amino penicillins from everted rat intestine. J Physiol 269–549–559
Dudley HAF (1975) Laparatomy. Br J Hosp Med 14:577–589
Fann WE, Davis JM, Janowsky DS, Sekerke HJ, Schmidt DM (1973) Chlorpromazine: effects of antacids on its gastrointestinal absorption. J Clin Pharmacol 13:388–390
Farquhar MG, Pallade GE (1963) Functional completexes in various epithelia. J Cell Biol 17:375–412
Fernandez PC, Kovnat PJ (1972) Metabolic acidosis reversed by the combination of magnesium and a cation-exchange resin. N Engl J Med 286:23–25
Finch JE, Kendall MJ, Mitchard M (1974) An assessment of gastric emptying by breathalyser. Br J Clin Pharmacol 1:233–236
Frizell RA, Schultz SA (1972) Ionic conductances of extracellular shunt pathway in rabbit ileum. J Gen Physiol 59:318–346
Galeazzi RL (1977) The effect of an antacid on the bioavailability of indomethacin. Eur J Clin Pharmacol 12:65–68
Gallo DG, Bailey KR, Sheffner AL (1965) The interaction between cholestyramine and drugs. Proc Soc Exp Biol Med 120:60–65
Garattini S, Marcucci F, Morselli PL, Mussini E (1973) The significance of measuring blood levels of benzodiazepines. In: Davies DS, Prichard BNC (eds) Biological effects of drugs in relation to their plasma concentrations. University Park Press, Baltimore, pp 211–225
Gibaldi M, Grundhofer B (1975) Biopharmaceutic influences on the anticholinergic effects of propantheline. Clin Pharmacol Ther 18:457–461
Griffith GH, Owen GM, Campbell H, Shields R (1968) Gastric emptying in health and in gastroduodenal disease. Gastroenterology 54:1–7
Hall WH, Shappell SD, Doherty JE (1977) Effect of cholestyramine on digoxin absorption and excretion in man. Am J Cardiol 39:213–216
Hasselbalch KA (1917) Die Berechnung der Wasserstoffzahl des Blutes aus der freien und gebundenen Kohlensäure desselben, und die Sauerstoffbindung des Blutes als Funktion der Wasserstoffzahl. Biochem 78:112–144
Hava M, Hurwitz A (1973) The relaxing effect of aluminium and lanthanum on rat and human gastric smooth muscle in vitro. Eur J Pharmacol 22:156–161
Heatley NG (1956) Comparative serum concentration and excretion experiments with benzyl penicillin (G) and phenoxymethyl penicillin (V) on a single subject. Antibiot Med 2:33–41
Henderson LJ (1909) Das Gleichgewicht zwischen Basen und Säuren im tierischen Organismus. Ergeb Physiol 8:254–325
Heizer WD, Smith TW, Goldfinger SE (1971) Absorption of digoxin in patients with malabsorption syndromes. N Engl J Med 285:257–259
Hogben CAM, Tocco DJ, Brodie BB, Schanker LS (1959) On the mechanism of intestinal absorption of drugs. J Pharmacol Exp Ther 125:275–282
Houston JB, Wood SG (1980) Gastrointestinal absorption of drugs and other xenobiotics. In: Bridges JW, Chasseaud LF (eds) Progress in drug metabolism, vol 4. Wiley, Chichester, pp 57–129
Hurwitz N (1969) Predisposing factors in adverse reactions to drugs. Br Med J 1:536–539
Hurwitz A (1971) The effects of antacids on gastrointestinal drug absorption. II. Effect on sulfadiazine and quinine. J Pharmacol Exp Ther 179:485–489
Hurwitz A (1974) Gastrointestinal drug absorption: effects of antacids. In: Morselli PL, Garattini S, Cohen SN (eds) Drug interactions. Raven, New York, pp 21–31
Ito S (1964) The surface coating of enteric microvilli. Anat Rec 148:294
Ito S (1975) The enteric surface coat of cat intestinal microvilli. J Cell Biol 27:475–491

Jackson MJ, Kutcher LM (1977) The three-compartment system for transport of weak electrolytes in the small intestine. In: Kramer M, Lauterbach F (eds) Intestinal permeation. Excerpta Medica, Amsterdam, pp 65–73
Jackson MJ, Shiau YF, Bane S, Fox M (1974) Intestinal transport of weak electrolytes. Evidence in favor of a three-compartment system. J Gen Physiol 63:187–213
Jaffe JM (1975) Effect of propantheline on mitrofurantoin absorption. J Pharm Sci 64:1729–1730
John AH, Jones A (1975) Gastroenteritis causing failure of oral contraception. Br Med J 3:207–208
Johns WH, Bates TR (1972) Drug-cholestyramine interactions II: influence of cholestyramine on GI absorption of sodium fusidate. J Pharm Sci 61:735–739
Jussila J, Mattila MJ, Takki S (1970) Drug absorption during lactose-induced intestinal symptoms in patients with selective lactose malabsorption. Ann Med Exp Biol Fenn 48:33–37
Kabasakalian P, Katz M, Rosenkrantz B, Townley E (1970) Parameters affecting absorption of griseofulvin in a human subject using urinary metabolite excretion data. J Pharm Sci 59:595–600
Khalil SAH (1974) The uptake of digoxin and digitoxin by some antacids. J Pharm Pharmacol 26:961–967
Kilian U, Lauterbach F (1979) Intestinal secretion of drugs by isolated mucosae of the small and largeintestine of guinea pig and man. Gastroenterol Clin Biol 3:178–179
Kimura T, Endo H, Yoshikawa M, Muranishi S, Sezaki H (1978) Carrier-mediated transport systems for aminopenicillins in rat small intestine. J Pharm Dyn 1:262–267
Kitazawa S, Ito H, Sezaki H (1975) Transmucosal fluid movement and its effect on drug absorption. Chem Pharm Bull 23:1856–1865
Klein JO, Sabath LD, Finland M (1963) Laboratory studies of oxacillin. II. Absorption and urinary excretion in young men. Am J Med Sci 245:399–412
Koch-Weser J, Sellers EM (1971) Drug interactions with coumarin anticoagulants. N Engl J Med 285:487–498, 547–558
Kokas E, Ludány G (1938) Relation between the "villikinine" and the absorption of glucose from the intestine. Q J Exp Physiol 28:15–22
Lauterbach F (1975) Resorption und Sekretion von Arzneistoffen durch die Mukosaepithelien des Gastrointestinal Traktes. Arzneim Forsch 25:479–488
Lauterbach F (1977) Intestinal secretion of organic ions and drugs. In: Kramer M, Lauterbach F (eds) Intestinal permeation. Excerpta Medica, Amsterdam, pp 173–194
Lauterbach F (1981) Intestinal absorption of secretion of cardiac glucosides. In: Greff K (ed) Handbook of experimental pharmacology, vol 56/II. Springer, Berlin Heidelberg New York, pp 105–139
Levine RR (1971) Intestinal absorption. In: Rabinowitz JL, Myerson RM (eds) Absorption Phenomena, vol 4. Topics in medicinal chemistry. Wiley, New York, pp 27–95
Levy G, Tsuchiya T (1972) Effect of activated charcoal on aspirin absorption in man. Clin Pharmacol Ther 13:317–322
Lucas ML (1976) The association between acidification and electrogenic events in the rat proximal jejunum. J Physiol 257:645–662
Lucas ML, Blair JA, Cooper BT, Cooke WT (1976) Relationship of the acid micro-climate in rat and human intestine to malabsorption. Biochem Soc Trans 4:154–156
MacDonald WC, Trier JS, Everett NB (1964) Cell proliferation and migration in the stomach, duodenum, and rectum of man: radioautographic studies. Gastroenterology 46:405–417
Magnussen MP (1968) The effect of ethanol on the gastrointestinal absorption of drugs in the rat. Acta Pharmacol Toxicol 26:130–144
Manninen V, Spajalahti A, Melia J, Karesoya M (1973) Altered absorption of digoxin in patients given propantheline and metoclopramide. Lancet 1:398:401
Mattok GL, Lovering EG, McGilveray IJ (1977) Bioavailability and drug dissolution. In: Bridges JW, Chasseaud LF (eds) Progress in drug metabolism, vol 2. Wiley, London, pp 259–308

May AJ, Whaler BC (1958) The absorption of clostridium botulinum type A toxin from the alimentary canal. Br J Exp Pathol 39:307–316
McCall CE, Steigbigel NH, Finland M (1967) Lincomycin: activity in vitro and absorption and excretion in normal young men. Am J Med Sci 254:144–155
McDonald H, Place VA, Falk H, Darden MA (1967) Effect of food on absorption of sulfonamides in man. Chemotherapie 12:282–285
McCelnay JC, Harron DWB, D'Arcy PF, Eagle MRG (1978) Interaction of digoxin with antacid constitutents. Br Med J 1:1554
Michel JC, Sayer RJ, Kirby WMM (1950) Effect of food and antacids on blood levels of aureomycin and terramycin. J Lab Clin Med 36:632–634
Milne MD, Scribner BH, Crawford MA (1958) Non-ionic diffusion and the excretion of weak acids and bases. Am J Med 24:709–729
Moberg S, Carlberger G (1974) Gastric emptying in healthy subjects and in patients with various malabsorption states. Scand J Gastroenterol 9:17–21
Moreno JH, Diamond JM (1974) Discrimination of monovalent inorganic cations by "tight" junctions of gallbladder epithelium. J Membr Biol 15:277–318
Naggar VF, Khalil SA, Daabis NA (1976) The in vitro adsorption some anti-rheumatics on antacids. Pharmazie 31:461–465
Naggar VF, Khalil SA, Gouda MW (1978) Effect of concomitant administration of magnesium triscilicate on GI absorption of dexamethasone in humans. J Pharm Sci 67:1029–1030
Nelson JD, Shelton S, Kusmiesz HT, Haltalin KC (1972) Absorption of ampicillin and nalidixic acid by infants and children with acute shigellosis. Clin Pharmacol Ther 13:897–886
Neuvonen PJ (1979) Drug absorption interactions. In: Prescott LF, Nimmo WS (eds) Drug absorption. Adis, New York
Neuvonen PJ, Elonen E (1980) Effect of activated charcoal on absorption and elimination of phenobarbitone, carbamazepine and phenylbutazone in man. Eur J Clin Pharmacol 17:51–57
Neuvonen PJ, Penttilä O (1974) Effect of oral ferrous sulphate on the half-life of doxycycline in man. Eur J Clin Pharmacol 7:361–363
Neuvonen P, Mattila M, Gothoni G, Hackman R (1971) Interference of iron and milk with absorption of tetracycline. Scand J Clin Lab Invest [Suppl 27] 116:76
Neuvonen PJ, Elfving SM, Elonen E (1978) Reduction of absorption of digoxin, phenytoin and aspirin by activated charcoal in man. Eur J Clin Pharmacol 13:213–218
Nimmo WS (1976) Drugs, diseases and altered gastric emptying. Clin Pharmacokinet 1:189–203
Nimmo WS (1979) Gastric emptying and drug absorption. In: Prescott LF, Nimmo WS (eds) Drug absorption. Adis, New York, pp 11–20
Nimmo WS, Wilson J, Prescott LF (1975) Narcotic analgesics and delayed gastric emptying during labour. Lancet 1:890–893
Northcutt RC, Stiel JN, Hollifield JW, Stant EG (1969) The influence of cholestyramine on thyroxine absorption. J Am Med Assoc 208:1857–1861
Ochsenfahrt H, Winne D (1969) Der Einfluß der Durchblutung auf die Resorption von Arzneimitteln aus dem Jejunum der Ratte. Naunyn Schmiedebergs Arch Pharmacol 264:55–75
Ochsenfahrt H, Winne D (1974a) The contribution of solvent drag to the intestinal absorption of the basic drugs amidopyrine and antipyrine from the jejunum of the rat. Naunyn Schmiedebergs Arch Pharmacol 281:175–196
Ochsenfahrt H, Winne D (1974b) The contribution of solvent drag to the intestinal absorption of the acidic drugs benzoic acid and salicylic acid from the jejenum of the rat. Naunyn Schmiedebergs Arch Pharmacol 281:197–217
Parsons RL (1977) Drug absorption in gastrointestinal disease with particular reference to malabsorption syndromes. Clin Pharmacokinet 2:45–60
Parsons RL, Kaye CM (1974) Plasma propranolol and practolol in adult coeliac disease. Br J Clin Pharmacol 1:348P

Parsons RL, Paddock GM (1975) Absorption of two antibacterial drugs, cephalexin and co-trimoxazole in malabsorption syndromes. J Antimcrob Chemother [Suppl] 1:59–67
Parsons RL, Hossack GA, Paddock GM (1975) The absorption of antibiotics in adult patients with coeliac disease. J Antimicrob Chemother 1:39–50
Parsons RL, Jusko WJ, Lewis GP (1976a) Pharmacokinetics of antibiotic absorption in coeliac disease. J Antimicrob Chemother 2:214–215
Parsons RL, Kaye CM, Raymond K, Trounce JR, Turner P (1976b) Absorption of propranolol and practorol in coeliac disease. Gut 17:139–143
Parsons RL, Paddock GM, Hossack GA, Hailey DM (1976c) Antibiotic absorption in Crohn's disease. In: Williams ID, Geddes AM (eds) Chemotherapy, vol 4: Pharmacology of antibiotics. Plenum, New York, pp 219–229
Pentillä, Hurme H, Neuvonen PJ (1975) Effect of zinc sulphate on the absorption of tetracycline and doxycycline in man. Eur J Clin Pharmacol 9:131–134
Piafsky KM, Ogilvie RI (1975) Dosage of theophylline in bronchial asthma. N Engl J Med 292:1218–1222
Pinell OC, Fenimore DC, Davis CM, Moreira O, Fann WE (1978) Drug-drug interaction of chlorpromazine and antacid. Clin Pharmacol Ther 23:125
Prescott LF (1974a) Gastric emptying and drug absorption. Br J Clin Pharmacol 1:189–190
Prescott LF (1974b) Drug absorption interactions – gastric emptying. In: Morselli PL, Garattini S, Cohen SN (eds) Drug interactions. Raven, New York, pp 11–20
Prescott LF, Nimmo WS (eds) (1979) Drug absorption. Adis, New York
Prescott LF, Nimmo WS, Heading RC (1977) Drug absorption interactions. In: Grahame-Smith DG (ed) Drug interactions. University Park Press, Baltimore, pp 45–51
Putnam FW, Lamanna C, Sharp DG (1946) Molecular weight and homogeneity of crystalline botulinus A toxin. J Biol Chem 165:735–736
Read NW, Barber DC, Levin RJ, Holdsworth CD (1977) Unstirred layer and kinetics of electrogenic glucose absorption in the human jejunum in situ. Gut 18:865–876
Richey DP, Bender AD (1977) Pharmacokinetic consequences of aging. Ann Rev Pharmacol Toxicol 17:49–65
Rimmer DG (1966) Gastric retention without mechanical obstruction. Arch Intern Med 117:287–299
Rosenberg HA, Bates TR (1974) Inhibitory effect of cholestyramine on the absorption of flufenamic and mefanamic acids in rats. Proc Soc Exp Biol Med 145:93–98
Rosenblatt JE, Barrett JE, Brodie JL, Kirby WMM (1966) Comparison of in vitro activity and clinical pharmacology of doxycycline with other tetracyclines. Antimicrob Agents Chemother 134:141
Sabath LD, Klein JO, Finland M (1963) Ancillin (2-biphenylpenicillin) antibacterial activity and clinical pharmacology. Am J Med Sci 246:129–146
Salem SAM, Stevenson IH (1977) Absorption kinetics of aspirin and quinine in elderly subjects. Br J Clin Pharmacol 4:397
Sapirstein LA (1958) Regional blood flow by fractional distribution of indicators. Am J Physiol 193:161–168
Schach von Wittenau M (1968) Some pharmacokinetic aspects of doxycycline metabolism in man. Chemotherapy [Suppl] 13:41–50
Schanker LS (1962) Passage of drugs across body membranes. Pharmacol Rev 14:501–530
Schanker LS (1971) Absorption of drugs from the gastrointestinal tract. In: Brodie BB, Gilette JR (eds) Concepts in biochemical pharmacology. Springer, Berlin Heidelberg New York, pp 9–24 (Handbook of experimental pharmacology, vol 28/1)
Schanker LS, Tocco DJ, Brodie BB, Hogben CAM (1958) Absorption of drugs from the rat small intestine. J Pharmacol Exp Ther 123:81–88
Scheiner J, Oltemeier WA (1962) Experimental study of factors inhibiting absorption and effective therapeutic levels of declomycin. Surg Gynecol Obstet 114:9–14
Schroeder EG (1969) Alkalosis resulting from combined administration of a "nonsystemic" antacid and a cation-exchange resin. Gastroenterology 56:868–874

Seed JC, Wilson CE (1950) The effect of aluminium hydroxide on serum aureomycin concentrations after simultaneous oral administration. Bull Johns Hopkins Hosp 86:415–418
Seidenstücker R (1978) Beziehungen zwischen enteraler Sekretion und Resorption herzwirksamer Glycoside. Ph D Thesis Bochum
Seidenstücker R, Lauterbach F (1976) Mediation of intestinal absorption of cardiotonic steroids by a secretory transfer mechanism. Naunyn Schmiedebergs Arch Pharmacol 293:R45
Shadir RI, Georgotas A, Greenblatt DJ, Harmatz JS, Allen MD (1978) Impaired absorption of desmethyldiazepam from clorazepate by magnesium aluminum hydroxide. Clin Pharmacol Ther 24:308–315
Sheiner HJ (1975) Gastric emptying tests in man. Gut 16:235–247
Shorter RG, Moertel CG, Titus JL, Reitemeier RJ (1964) Cell kinetics in the jejunum and rectum of man. Am J Dig Dis 9:760–763
Simon C, Malerczyk V, Müller U, Müller G (1972) Zur Pharmakokinetik von Propicillin bei geriatrischen Patienten im Vergleich zu jüngeren Erwachsenen. Dtsch Med Wochenschr 97:1999–2003
Siurula M, Mustala O, Jussila J (1969) Absorption of acetylsalicylic acid by a normal and an atrophic gastric mucosa. Scand J Gastroenterol 4:269–273
Stevenson IH, Salem SAM, Shepherd AMM (1979) Studies on drug absorption and metabolism in the elderly. In: Crooks J, Stevenson IH (eds) Drugs and the elderly. Macmillan, London, pp 51–63
Sund RB, Lauterbach F (1978) intestinal secretion of sulphanilic acid by the isolated mucosa of guinea pig jejunum. Acta Pharmacol 43:331–338
Ti TY, Giles HG, Sellers EM (1978) Probable interaction of loperamide and cholestyramine. Can Med Assoc J 119:607–608
Traeger A, Kunze M, Stein G, Ankermann H (1973) Zur Pharmakokinetik von Indomethazin bei alten Menschen. ZFA (Dresden) 27:151–155
Triggs EJ, Nation RL (1975) Pharmacokinetics in the aged: a review. J Pharmacokinet Biopharm 3:387–418
Triggs EJ, Nation RL, Long A, Ashley JJ (1975) Pharmacokinetics in the elderly. Eur J Clin Pharmacol 8:55–62
Turnheim K, Lauterbach F (1980) Interaction between intestinal absorption and secretion of monoquaternary ammonium compounds in guinea pigs – a concept for the absorption kinetics of organic cations. J Pharmacol Exp Ther 212:418–424
van Dam APM (1972) Gastric emptying utilizing the gamma camera. Thesis University of Nijmegen
Varga F, Csáky TZ (1976) Changes in the blood supply of the gastrointestinal tract in rats with age. Pfluegers Arch 364:129–133
Vestal RE (1978) Drug use in the elderly: a review of problems and special considerations. Drugs 16:358–382
Volkheimer G (1972) Persorption. Thieme Stuttgart
Wagner JG (1971) Biopharmaceutics and relevant pharmacokinetics. Drug Intelligence Publications, Hamilton
Waisbren BA, Hueckel JS (1950) Reduced absorption of aureomycin caused by aluminum hydroxide gel (Amphojel). Proc Soc Exp Biol Med 73:73–75
Wilson ITH (1962) Intestinal absorption. Saunders, Philadelphia
Wilson TH (1963) Intestinal absorption of vitamin B_{12}. Physiologist 6:11–26
Winne D (1973) The influence of blood flow on the absorption of L and D-phenylalanine from the jejunum of the rat. Naunyn Schmiedebergs Arch Pharmacol 277:113–138
Winne D (1976) Unstirred layer thickness in perfused rat jejunum in vivo. Experientia 32:1278–1279
Winne D (1978) Blood flow in intestinal absorption models. J Pharmacokinet Biopharm 6:55–78
Winne D, Remischovsky J (1970) Intestinal blood flow and absorption of non-dissociable substances. J Pharm Pharmacol 22:640–641

Winne D, Remischovsky J (1971 a) Der Einfluß der Durchblutung auf die Resorption von Harnstoff, Methanol und Äthanol aus dem Jejunum der Ratte. Naunyn Schmiedebergs Arch Pharmacol 268:392–416
Winne D, Remischovsky J (1971 b) Der Einfluß der Durchblutung auf die Resorption von Polyalkoholen aus dem Jejunum der Ratte. Naunyn Schmiedebergs Arch Pharmacol 270:22–40

CHAPTER 19

Role of Digestive Enzymes in the Permeability of the Enterocyte

A. M. Ugolev, N. N. Iezuitova, and L. F. Smirnova

A. Introduction

During the last few decades ideas on the functions of the enterocytes have undergone significant changes. This concerns primarily the concept of intestinal absorption. However, of hardly less importance for the understanding of the mechanisms of absorption were findings of late 1950s which confirmed the existence of a special type of digestion, membrane digestion, occurring directly on the resorptive surface. Subsequently, in the late 1960s and early 1970s these data led to a view of the enterocyte as a system responsible not only for transport, but also for digestive functions. As will be shown in this chapter, discovery of membrane digestion influenced the two main dogmas of gastroenterology: (1) the two-stage scheme of the alimentary system (luminal digestion–absorption) was replaced by the three-stage scheme (luminal digestion–membrane digestion–absorption); (2) the generally accepted view of digestion being performed in the intestinal lumen and absorption by the intestinal mucosa as two autonomous processes was abandoned. Instead, a concept of the digestive transport conveyor with spatial, time and functional integration of the final stages of digestion and initial stages of absorption on the lipoprotein membrane surface of the enterocytes has been proposed. The purpose of this chapter is to define the role of the hydrolases of the apical membrane of the enterocytes in the function of the transport system. It will be demonstrated that absorption may be controlled by the membrane enzymes in several ways. These enzymes provide: (1) the intermediate and final stages of a transformation of nonabsorptive food substances into transportable forms, i.e. splitting of poly- and oligosaccharides and poly- and oligopeptides to monosaccharides and amino acids, respectively; (2) destruction of transportable forms and conversion into less transportable forms, i.e. hydrolysis of conjugated bile acids; (3) direct cooperative interactions with the carriers as a result of allosteric effects; and (4) energetics of the transport systems.

The analysis of the mechanism of interaction between the enzymatic and transport systems of the apical membrane of the enterocytes permitted one to account for many peculiarities of the transport of monomers released by hydrolysis of poly- and oligomers. The transport of monomers released during digestion is usually termed transport of released monomers, enzyme-related transport, enzyme-dependent transport or hydrolysis-dependent transport. In contrast, the transport of free monomers is referred to as enzyme-independent transport.

In this chapter, an attempt will be made not only to characterize interactions between the membrane hydrolysis and transport, but also to differentiate as far as possible between the accepted facts and hypotheses requiring additional testing. The results from numerous studies carried out in many countries served as a basis for the modern concept of the digestive transport membrane. Interesting and often paradoxical features of the enzyme-dependent transport of monomers will be distinguished from the hypotheses and the models proposed for their interpretation.

The discussion of self-regulation of the processes of membrane digestion and transport at the molecular and cellular levels is beyond the scope of this chapter. Therefore, in the concluding section of the chapter, the main principles of self-regulation will be mentioned. The problem is developing so rapidly both in the field of fundamental science and as applied to medicine that it is impossible to embrace all its aspects in such a brief review.

B. Relationship Between the Hydrolytic and Transport Systems of the Enterocytes

The major organic food components, including proteins, carbohydrates and fats enter the gastrointestinal tract in unabsorbed form. Some of them, in particular proteins, possess pronounced antigenic properties which must be eliminated before entering the internal medium of the organism. The essence of the digestive process is a transformation of nontransportable substances into transportable ones (devoid of species specificity), largely monomers (glucose, amino acids, fatty acids etc.). Absorption of dimers and trimers (di- and tripeptides), monoglycerides etc. has also been demonstrated. Besides, there are strong arguments in favour of absorption of small amounts of native intact molecules (for reviews see MORRIS 1974; WALKER and ISSELBACHER 1974; IMMUNOLOGY OF THE GUT 1977; GÖTZE and ROTHMANN 1978; HEMMINGS and WILLIAMS 1978; TAGESSON et al. 1978; Ferguson 1979; Walker 1979) and even supramolecular aggregations – persorption (for reviews see VOLKHEIMER 1972, 1974, 1977, 1978). Digestion represents a system of hydrolytic processes accomplished by a wide complex of enzymes attacking various bonds in different food substances. Three basic types of digestion are now recognized and their relation to transport processes differs.

I. The Basic Types of Digestion and Their Relation to Absorption

The modern interpretation of the basic types of digestion is represented in a generalized form in Fig. 1. There exist three types of digestion depending on a spatial relation to the absorptive cell: extracellular, intracellular (two kinds) and membrane digestion.

Extracellular (luminal) digestion is produced by hydrolytic enzymes acting outside the cell (in higher animals this occurs in special digestive lumens). The distribution of enzymes in the aqueous phase occurs by thermal transport. By virtue of this, the spatial organization of the enzymatic sequences is either impossible or restricted. Extracellular digestion allows for any orientation of the active centres of enzymes relative to the molecules attacked by them. This provides favourable conditions for the action of the enzymes dissolved in the aqueous phase on

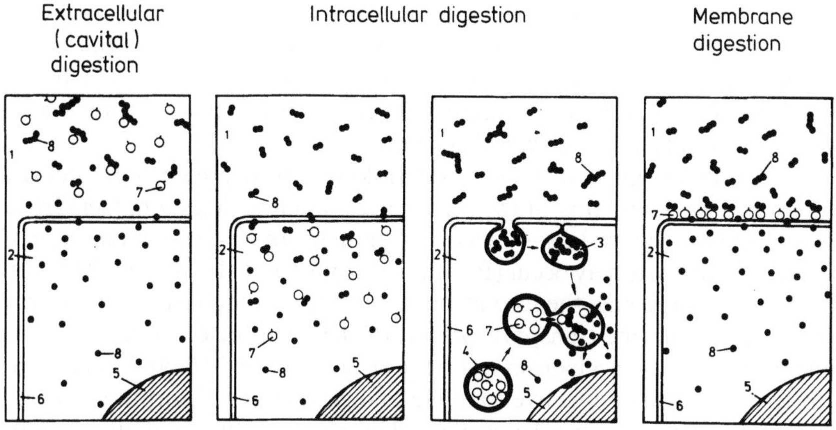

Fig. 1. Location of hydrolysis of nutrients during different types of digestion. *1*, extracellular fluid; *2*, intracellular fluid; *3*, intracellular vacuole; *4*, lysosomes; *5*, nucleus; *6*, cell membrane; *7*, enzymes; *8*, substrates and their hydrolysis products. UGOLEV et al. (1979 a)

large molecules and supramolecular aggregations. The enzymes ensuring luminal digestion in humans and higher animals are mostly endohydrolases. The production of the final (transportable) substances by luminal digestion is insignificant. Moreover, these have no direct contact with the absorptive surface.

Intracellular digestion occurs after penetration of hydrolytic substrates inside the cell. Thus, it requires a preliminary absorption which may be achieved by endocytosis (phagocytosis and pinocytosis). In this case, a formed vesicle contains substrates, and the digestive enzymes are derived from the lysosome interacting with it by producing a common structure, the phagosome, where hydrolysis and subsequent absorption of food substances occur. This process appears to be too slow to provide the high rates of assimilation characteristic of higher animals. Another type of intracellular hydrolysis is associated with the transport of intact molecules through the membrane as a result of diffusion across the water pores or a transfer by means of the carriers, the existence of which has been demonstrated in higher animals and, in particular, in prokaryotes (for reviews see GILVARG 1972; PAYNE 1972, 1977; MATTHEWS and PAYNE 1975; MATTHEWS 1977).

Membrane digestion is accomplished by the enzyme systems of the cell membrane (in humans and other mammals by the enzymes of the apical membrane of the enterocytes). Membrane digestion is spatially an intermediate type between extracellular and intracellular digestion. Immobilization of enzymes by the membrane structures enables the complex enzyme and enzyme transport systems to be formed that distinguish fundamentally this type of digestion from the extracellular one. Membrane digestion is effected by the structures of the same membrane which is involved in transport processes. This provides highly favourable conditions for the coupling of the final stages of digestion and the initial stages of absorption. As will be shown in Sect. E.III, it is reached not only owing to a spatial proximity but also to functional interactions between the elements releasing transportable products and those responsible for their transmembrane transfer.

Each of these three types of digestion has its advantages and limitations. Thus, extracellular digestion ensures an effective breakdown of large molecules, with respect to which immobilized membrane enzymes are ineffective. On the other hand, luminal digestion fails to interact efficiently with the membrane transport systems, in contrast to membrane digestion.

The real assimilation of food macromolecules is at present interpreted as a complex process consisting of the three stages: luminal digestion, membrane digestion and absorption. In some cases, at the stage of absorption one type of intracellular hydrolysis may occur (Peptide Transport and Hydrolysis 1977). As follows from the foregoing, the second and third stages of food assimilation are performed by the enzyme transport systems of the enterocytes. In this case, membrane digestion is a mechanism not only of the intermediate and final stages of hydrolysis, but also of effective coupling of digestion and absorption which until very recently were considered as separated in space and time and functionally autonomous. A consideration of transport processes is not the purpose of this chapter. These are described in detail in a number of reviews (SMYTH 1974; MARKIN and CHIZMADZHEV 1974; CSÁKY and AUTENRIETH 1975; ROBINSON 1976; KINNE and MURER 1976; SEMENZA and CARAFOLI 1977; NIKOLSKY 1977; GUIDOTTI et al. 1978; HOFFMAN 1978; OGSTON and MICHEL 1978; WILSON 1978; DEVES and KRUPKA 1979; LAUGER 1979; SCHULTZ 1979).

II. Membrane Digestion and Digestive-Absorptive Functions of the Enterocyte Membrane

The present three-stage scheme of assimilation of food substances as well as the concept of membrane digestion appeared in late 1950s and early 1960s. The molecular mechanism underlying the interactions between the enzyme and transport systems of the enterocytes was investigated later and even now this problem, equally important for both the physiology and pathology of the alimentary system, cannot be regarded as completely resolved.

To understand the reasons for introducing the concept of membrane digestion, one should take into account the following important circumstances. (1) Early in twentieth century when modern gastroenterology was developed owing to the efforts of outstanding investigators such as Claude Bernard, Carl Ludwig, P.H. Heidenhain, I.P. Pavlov, W.M. Bayliss and E.H. Starling, the two-stage scheme of the assimilation of nutrients (luminal digestion absorption) was adopted. This scheme remained predominant until the mid 1960s (for reviews see BERNARD 1877; MALI 1886; PAVLOV 1911–1912; LONDON 1916; BABKIN 1927, 1960; STRAUB 1960; CONSOLAZIO and IACONO 1963; KALSER 1964). (2) At the end of the nineteenth and in the early twentieth century attention was drawn to the fact that many enzymes responsible for the final stages of hydrolysis (disaccharidases, dipeptidases etc.) are present only sparingly in the secretions of the digestive glands, although they are present in great amounts in the intestinal cells (BIERRY 1912; KOSKOWSKY 1926; PIERCE et al. 1935). This led to the idea that the final stages of digestion were accomplished under the influence of enzymes entering the small intestinal lumen after desquamation and degradation of the enterocytes (LEUBE 1868, WRIGHT et al. 1940; FLOREY et al. 1941; Shlygin 1952, 1964). In this case, a suggestion has been made that formation of monomers may not occur and many nutrients are absorbed in the form of oligomers, in particular, as oligopeptides (for reviews see LONDON 1916; FISHER 1954). However, most attention has been attracted by the possibility of the final hydrolysis of small molecules (e.g. oligopeptides and oligosaccharides) during their absorption as a result of intracellular digestion (CAJORI 1933). This point of view received wide recognition in the 1950s and early 1960s as a feasible mechanism for the uptake of oligomers (BORGSTRÖM et al. 1957; NEWEY and SMYTH 1957, 1959, 1960a, 1960b, 1961, 1962; BORGSTRÖM and DAHLQVIST 1958; DAHLQVIST and BORGSTRÖM 1961; DAHLQVIST and BRUN 1962; for reviews see SMYTH 1961; WILSON 1962; ISSELBACHER and SENIOR 1964; WISEMAN 1964). According to this view, intact oligomers are capable of crossing the membrane into the absorptive cells where they are transformed to monomers. This concept of intracellular digestion accounts for both the absence from the intestinal contents of many enzymes accomplishing the final stages of hydrolysis and their high concentration in the enterocytes. Moreover, it provides a satisfactory explanation for the phenomenon that many substances, after disappearing from the small intestinal lumen as oligomers, appear in the blood or serosal fluid in the form of monomers (monosaccharides, amino acids etc.).

The evidence for the existence of fundamental distinctions between the real rates of oligosaccharide absorption and respective enzyme activity of the luminal contents of the small intestine played an important role in the formulation of modern concepts of digestion. In particular, it has been estimated that it would take about 100 h to complete the hydrolysis of ingested lactose. However, only 3–4 h are required for disappearance of the latter from the human small intestine (BORGSTRÖM et al. 1957; DAHLQVIST and BORGSTRÖM 1961). This could indicate the presence of a hydrolytic mechanism distinct from intraluminal digestion.

At the same time histochemical investigations have revealed that at least some digestive enzymes are concentrated in the brush border region of the enterocytes (GOMORI 1941; DEANE and DEMPSEY 1945; DEMPSEY and DEANE 1946; EMMEL 1946; MARTIN and JACOBY 1949; BRADFIELD 1950; BARRNETT 1959; NACHLAS et al. 1960; ZETTERQVIST and HENDRIX 1960; ASHWORTH et al. 1963; CLARK 1961a, b; PADYCULA 1962; JOS et al. 1967; MOOG and GREY 1967). On the basis of these findings, the concept of apical intracellular digestion was formulated and later developed with a great degree of consistency (MILLER and CRANE 1961a, b, 1963; CRANE 1966).

The possibility of the existence of the third type of digestion, membrane digestion, was first demonstrated by UGOLEV. The first strong proof of this new type of digestion was obtained in 1958 (UGOLEV 1960a, b). It has been found that pancreatic amylase adsorbed on the luminal surface of the enterocytes is involved in hydrolysis of starch. During a reversible immobilization of this enzyme, its properties undergo changes (e.g. thermal stability and resistance to acid increase, specific activity; i.e. the ability to split large polysaccharide molecules decreases, and the activity with respect to smaller molecules increases). It has concurrently been demonstrated that enteric enzymes completing the hydrolysis of peptides and disaccharides also take part in membrane digestion. Thus, membrane digestion is effected by enzymes of two origins: (1) enteric enzymes synthesized by a particular epithelial cell and incorporated into their membrane; and (2) adsorbed enzymes synthesized by other cells (mainly by pancreatic cells), secreted into the small intestinal lumen and then adsorbed by the cell surface structures.

Membrane digestion has sometimes been interpreted with reference to our work as digestion due to adsorbed enzymes. This point of view is not valid. Thus, in 1960 in *Nature* and in 1965 in *Physiological Reviews* membrane digestion was characterized as follows:

In previous papers, it was shown that cavital (chyme) digestion is probably not the sole or main mechanism underlying the hydrolysis of food. It was suggested that the surface of the intestine presents a living porous reactor (the pores being formed by microvilli), on the surface of which intensive hydrolysis occurs on account of enzymes (self-contained and adsorbed) on the external side of the cellular membrane (UGOLEV 1960 b p. 588).

Membrane digestion is due to enzymes adsorbed from chyme and enzymes structurally associated with the membrane of the intestinal cells (UGOLEV 1965 p. 587).

Membrane digestion as a main mechanism responsible for the intermediate and final stages of hydrolysis and coupling of digestive and transport processes was subjected to severe criticism in the first half of 1960s. Subsequently, however, membrane digestion received complete confirmation first for carbohydrates and later in the 1970s for proteins. Some evidence for the important role of membrane digestion as a mechanism for the assimilation of triglycerides has also been reported (for reviews see UGOLEV 1968, 1972 a, 1974). However, until recently consideration has only been given to their luminal and intracellular digestion in the small intestine (for reviews see BORGSTRÖM 1974, 1977; BRINDLEY 1974; HOLDSWORTH and SLADEN 1979).

For characterization of membrane hydrolysis and transport of food substances in the enterocytes as well as their relationships, various methodological approaches were used, each possessing both advantages and limitations. The use of the brush border preparations first introduced by MILLER and CRANE (1961 a, b) and especially preparations of the apical and basolateral membrane proved very fruitful (for reviews see Chap. 6; SEMENZA 1968; 1977 a, b, 1979 a, b, c; ISSELBACHER 1974; LOUVARD et al. 1973, 1975 a; KENNY 1977; NORÉN et al. 1977; WACKER and SEMENZA 1977; CRANE 1977; MOOG 1979). However, investigations of brush border enzyme activity supplemented by determination of the kinetic characteristics of the brush border enzymes did not at first confirm membrane digestion but refuted it. Indeed, MILLER and CRANE (1961 a) in their first report subtitled "An intracellular locus of disaccharide and sugar phosphate ester hydrolysis" showed that the enzymes splitting disaccharides (sucrose and maltose) and glucose-1-phosphate are localized in the apical part of the enterocyte. These data are in agreement with the histochemical results indicating the intestinal brush border location of alkaline phosphatase and aminopeptidase. However, these findings have failed to show whether these enzymes are available in the core of microvilli or in the brush border membrane. Further analysis using the concentration criterion and glucose oxidase led MILLER and CRANE (1961 b) to the conclusion that intracellular rather than membrane location is characteristic of hydrolytic enzymes.

Later, CRANE (1975) regretted the inadequancy of the title of his article which suggested membrane rather than intracellular location of hydrolases. However, at the time the concept of membrane digestion was formed, CRANE and his colleagues wrote:

Hydrolysis occurs at a site from which diffusion into the tissue occurs more rapidly than diffusion into the medium. The only conclusion that it seems possible to draw is that the hydrolases are intracellular enzymes (MILLER and CRANE 1961 a, p. 291).

. . . The fact that here the tissue levels do exceed those in the medium, at least initially, is strong evidence against the theory that glucose is formed by hydrolysis outside the tissue ... if digestive hydrolysis with the formation of glucose takes place in the medium or the cell surface, glucose should be oxidized as it is formed, and the amount taken up by the tissue should be decreased. This is not happen.

In all the experiments essentially similar results were obtained using disaccharides, sucrose and maltose, and the sugar phosphate ester, glucose-l-phosphate. Tissue uptake of the monosaccharides resulting from digestive hydrolysis does not depend on the liberation of these sugars in the incubation medium or the free surface of the tissue. Hydrolysis takes place at a site from which sugar diffusion into the tissue occurs more readily than its diffusion into the medium. The only conclusion that seems possible is that these rehydrolases are intracellular enzymes (MILLER, CRANE 1963, pp. 222–223).

The concept of intracellular digestion inevitably leads to the conclusion that transport systems, particularly those for monosaccarides, are localized not in the apical membrane of the enterocyte, but intracellularly. ISSELBACHER and SENIOR (1964) examined this and commented on the characteristic features of intracellular apical digestion:

A series of ingenious experiments were carried out by Crane and his associates to suggest that indeed the disaccharide splitting enzymes are intracellular... Additional support for the concept that the disaccarides enter the mucosal cells before hydrolysis came from a study in vitro in which glucose oxidase was present in the medium. Thus, the maltose must have been split primarily within the cells rather than in the medium... The final evidence for the intracellular concept of disaccharide hydrolysis, came from further experiments in which Miller and Crane were effectively able to isolate the "brush border" fraction of the cell (pp. 289–290).

Experimental testing of the concepts of intracellular and membrane digestion has demonstrated that in the process of evolution a predominant system was developed in which hydrolysis on the membrane surface preceded transport through it. Peculiarities and specificity of this mechanism will be discussed in Sect. E.III.

III. Classification of Digestive Processes

Recently, a number of investigators (JOSEFSSON, KIM, MATTHEWS, PARSONS, UGOLEV) have reexamined the classification of digestive processes, in particular the terms "membrane" and "cytosol" digestion (Peptide Transport and Hydrolysis 1977). PARSONS recommended the following classification developed from the example of peptide hydrolysis: (1) extracellular digestion: enzymes are acting in solution; (2) cellular digestion: enzymes form a part of or are attached to the cell. In the first case, enzymes are synthesized in the cell and form part of its structure, e.g. as the components of a membrane; in the second case, enzymes may be adsorbed to the cell surface and synthesized by the cells of other organs, e.g. pancreatic enzymes adsorbed to the cells of the intestinal epithelium. Cellular digestion may be divided into membrane digestion and intracellular digestion.

In the case of membrane digestion, if the active sites are located on the outside of the plasma membrane, the process can be called surface digestion. If the active sites are located in the depth of the membrane, the process may be intramembrane digestion. If the active sites are on the internal membrane surface, we are concerned with inner surface digestion. The enzymes responsible for intracellular digestion are not an integral part of the plasma membrane (brush border membrane) and their active sites are not associated with the membrane.

As early as the 1960s a classification based on two basic types of digestion was proposed (UGOLEV 1965, 1968).

1. Extracellular digestion is accomplished by the enzymes secreted by the cells and acting beyond their limits. It may be: (a) luminal when food substances undergo splitting in special digestive lumens; (b) extraluminal (bacteria, protozoa) when the hydrolytic enzymes are secreted into the fluid surrounding the organism, or it may occur directly in the food substrates themselves.

2. Cellular digestion is characterized by hydrolysis of food substances by the enzymes associated with the cell structures. It may be subdivided into: (a) intracellular and (b) membrane. Intracellular digestion takes place in special intracellular spaces and may be characterized as vacuolar or intracellular extraplasmic digestion; in the cytosol; in special subcellular structures (granular digestion); on the inner face of the cell membrane (submembrane digestion).

Insofar as membrane digestion occurs on the external surface of the cell membrane, it bears a certain resemblance to extracellular digestion. However, in many respects it is similar to intracellular digestion since it is performed by the enzymes associated with the cell structures.

The discovery of the glycocalyx and development of the concept of a "thick" membrane in the functioning of systems of different complexity allowed the following types of membrane digestion, within the basic scheme, to be distinguished:

1. Premembrane (matrix or glycocalyx) digestion carried out mainly by the pancreatic enzymes adsorbed to different layers of the glycocalyx
2. Superficial membrane digestion largely due to the membrane enzymes synthesized by the ribosomal apparatus of the cell and acting in the composition of the apical membrane and partly by the enzymes adsorbed to the lipoprotein membrane
3. Submembrane digestion performed by the enzymes associated with the inner membrane surface
4. Intramembrane digestion due to the enzymes associated with the catalytic sites within the membrane

IV. The Enzyme Apparatus of Membrane Digestion

The enzymes performing membrane digestion in the small intestine in mammals may be of two origins: (1) adsorbed to the intestinal mucosa predominantly of pancreatic origin; (2) enteric enzymes of the microvillous membrane synthesized in the enterocytes (Table 1). The enzymes responsible for the intermediate stages of hydrolysis of the main groups of nutrients are adsorbed to the surface of the small intestine. Enteric enzymes of the apical membrane of the enterocytes generally accomplish the final stages of hydrolysis of carbohydrates, proteins and possibly fats as well as coupling of the final stages of digestion and the initial stages of absorption (UGOLEV 1960a, b; for reviews see UGOLEV 1963, 1965, 1968, 1972a, b, 1974; CODE 1968a, b; UGOLEV and DE LAEY 1973; SMYTH 1974; Peptide Transport and Hydrolysis 1977; UGLEV et al. 1979a).

The adsorbed enzymes seem to be predominantly associated with the glycocalyx structures while enteric enzymes constitute an integral part of the plasma membrane of the enterocytes. Nevertheless, the enzymes entering the intestinal lumen may be adsorbed to the lipoprotein membrane surface whereas enteric enzymes may be inserted at least partially into the glycocalyx.

1. Adsorbed Enzymes

A variety of pancreatic enzymes are adsorbed to the surface intestinal mucosal structures in humans and animals (Tables 1 and 2). The adsorbed pancreatic enzymes, as a rule, contain one polypeptide chain and have relatively low molecular mass varying from 12,700 (ribonuclease) to 45,000 daltons (α-amylase).

Reversible adsorption of enzymes to the cell structures of the small intestine was first demonstrated in rat pancreatic amylase (UGOLEV 1960a, b) and confirmed by experiments on different animals and humans (for reviews se UGOLEV 1963, 1965, 1968, 1972a, 1974; RAKHIMOV 1965; DE LAEY 1966; a, b, c, d, 1967a, b, c; ALPERS and SOLIN 1970; KOJEZKÝ and MATLOCHA 1973; ZLATKINA et al. 1973, 1976; MASEVICH et al. 1975; MATLOCHA and KOJEZKÝ 1976; UGOLEV et al. 1977a). Adsorption of lipase, ribonuclease, elastase, trypsin and chymotrypsin has also been demonstrated (GOLDBERG et al. 1968, 1971; WOODLEY and KENNY 1969; VALENKEVICH 1973; VALENKEVICH et al. 1978; UGOLEV et al. 1978, 1979d; for reviews see UGOLEV 1968, 1972a, 1974; UGOLEV et al. 1977a). It is important

Table 1. The main enzymes responsible for membrane digestion in the small intestine in mammals (from various sources)

Origin	Enzyme	EC
Adsorbed pancreatic enzymes	α-Amylase	3.2.1.1
	Lipase	3.1.1.3
	Trypsin	3.4.21.4
	Chymotrypsin	3.4.21.1
	Carboxypeptidase A	3.4.12.2
	Carboxypeptidase B	3.4.12.3
	Elastase	3.4.21.11
	Ribonuclease	3.1.4.22
Enteric enzymes	Maltase	3.2.1.20
	Sucrase	3.2.1.48
	Isomaltase	3.2.1.10
	γ-Amylase	3.2.1.3
	Lactase	3.2.1.23
	Alkaline phosphatase	3.1.3.1
	Monoglyceride lipase	3.1.1.23
	Peptidase	3.4.11–15
	Aminopeptidase	3.4.11.2
	Dipeptidylaminopeptidase	3.4.14.1
	Carboxypeptidase	3.4.12.4
	Enteropeptidase	3.4.21.9
	γ-Glutamyltranspeptidase	2.3.2.2
	Cholesterolesterase	3.1.1.13

Table 2. Adsorption of pancreatic amylase by the enterocyte surface in different animal species (from various sources; UGOLEV 1972a)

Mammals	Human, monkey, dog, horse, cow, sheep, pig, rabbit, hamster, rat, mouse, guinea-pig
Birds	Pigeon, duck, hen, chick
Amphibians	Frog
Fish	Trout, carp
Cyclostomata	Lamprey
Invertebrates	Insects (pine hawkmoth caterpillar), helminths (cestoid worms) of cattle (adsorb enzymes from host's chyme through body surface structures)

that the adsorbed enzymes not only participate in the intermediate stages of the hydrolysis of polymers, but also facilitate a passage of oligomers through the glycocalyx to the lipoprotein membrane. A preliminary desorption of α-amylase decreases the utilization of starch 8–10-fold, without affecting the uptake of maltose and glucose (for review see UGOLEV et al. 1977a).

The important role of adsorbed enzymes in the digestive processes has been shown for pancreatic amylase when comparing the rates of starch hydrolysis in the intestine at different steps of enzyme desorption. The efficiency of the hydrolysis of this substrate was greatly decreased during the desorption of amylase from the small intestinal mucosal surface. During readsorption of this enzyme to the intestinal mucosal surface a recovery of the initial effects may be observed (for reviews see UGOLEV 1963, 1968, 1972a, 1974; JESUITOVA et al. 1964; UGOLEV et al. 1977a; ZARIPOV et al. 1978).

The activity of pancreatic amylase in the small intestinal lumen is rather high. In the period of intensive digestion the activity of amylase in the small intestinal lumen and on the surface in dogs was approximately 50% and 50% (IEZUITOVA et al. 1967) and in rats 40% and 60%, respectively. In humans starch hydrolysis by luminal amylase proceeds for some minutes (DAHLQVIST and BORGSTRÖM 1961; FOGEL and GRAY 1973). However, the roles of enzymes acting in the small intestinal lumen and adsorbed to the surface differ. The first ensures the initial and the second the intermediate stages of the hydrolysis of polymers, including polysaccharides. The role of adsorbed enzymes increases with the depolymerization of polymers. Thus, if intact starch molecules are split in the lumen of the small intestine, then polyglucosidic sequences of 30 or more glucosidic residues will be hydrolysed both in the lumen and on the surface of the small intestine. Dextrins of 8–20 glucosidic residues are subjected to splitting predominantly in the brush border zone (UGOLEV and MARAUSKA 1964). Under normal conditions, hydrolysis of starch in the small intestine occurs without the accumulation of dextrins. The comparison of amylolysis spectra in vivo and in vitro has shown that in the first case no accumulation of dextrins occurs. Dextrins are formed in the brush border zone when passing across the glycocalyx.

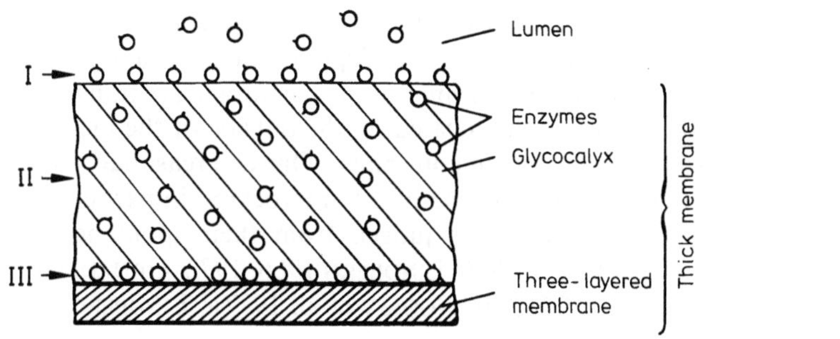

Fig. 2. The distribution of adsorbed enzymes on (I) and inside (II, III) the glycocalyx (simplified scheme). UGOLEV et al. (1977 a)

The stability of binding of pancreatic enzymes to the structures of the intestinal mucosa is different in various animal species. Thus, desorption of α-amylase occurs more readily in rats than in guinea-pigs. Hamsters and white mice occupy an intermediate position (for reviews see UGOLEV 1968, 1972a, 1974). It has been shown that the adsorption of amylase is a regulated process. In fed animals there is more bound amylase and the rate of desorption is lower than in fasting animals (RAKHIMOV 1965; DE LAEY 1967 a).

Precise localization of adsorbed enzymes in the structures of the small intestine still remains to be elucidated. A number of suggestions have been brought forth (for reviews see UGOLEV 1972a; UGOLEV et al. 1977 a). Enzymes penetrating into the glycocalyx may be: (1) adsorbed to the membrane of the enterocytes; (2) distributed throughout the entire glycocalyx space; or (3) adsorbed mainly to the luminal surface of the glycocalyx (Fig. 2).

We have recently succeeded in a preparative separation of the apical glycocalyx from the plasma membrane of the enterocytes in rats without destroying the membrane (UGOLEV et al. 1978, 1979d). The pancreatic enzymes such as α-amylase and trypsin, as was shown, localized predominantly in the apical part of the glycocalyx: make up 62.0% ± 3.3% and 86.5% ± 3.0%, respectively. At the same time a significant amount of these enzymes (some 40% for α-amylase and 15% for trypsin) may be inserted deeper into the intermicrovillous glycocalyx, possibly partly on the lipoprotein membrane. These data confirm the previous view on the role of adsorbed enzymes performing the function of intermediate hydrolysis of nutrients. Enteric enzymes (invertase, γ-amylase, di- and tripeptidases) are generally associated with the lipoprotein membrane fraction. However, alkaline phosphatase, known as membrane integral enzyme, is also present in the apical glycocalyx (up to 20%) (UGOLEV et al. 1978, 1979d).

2. Enteric Enzymes

The enteric enzymes which are involved in membrane digestion are synthesized by the enterocytes themselves and exert the digestive effect in the composition of the apical membrane (see Table 1). This group is represented by many enzymes acting on different substrates. Enteric enzymes represent exohydrolases (e.g. disaccharidases, γ-amylase, aminopeptidase) and form transportable products, mainly monomers. It is suggested that intestinal dipeptidases also take part in the intracellular hydrolysis of dipeptides (Peptide Transport and Hydrolysis 1977).

The majority of enteric enzymes of the membrane are transmembrane integral proteins with the active site located on the outside of the membrane and orientated towards the external aqueous phase. One can reasonably suggest that some enzymes of the apical membrane of the enterocytes, in particular, certain dipeptidases may be peripheral, as judged from their spontaneous solubilization (JOSEFSSON and SJÖSTROM 1966; LINDBERG 1966, 1972; GRUZDKOV et al. 1970; for reviews see UGOLEV 1972a, b; UGOLEV et al. 1977a; LINDBERG et al. 1975).

Table 3. Molecular mass of some mammalian enteric enzymes

Enzyme	Animal	Molecular mass (daltons)		Reference
		Integral form	Individual subunits	
Alkaline phosphatase (detergent form)	Pig	120,000–130,000	63,000– 65,000	COLBEAU and MAROUX (1978)
Alkaline phosphatase (papain form)		120,000–130,000	60,000– 61,000	
Aminopeptidase	Pig	280,000	130,000 97,000 49,000	MAROUX et al. (1973)
Aminopeptidase	Rat	280,000		KIM and BROPHY (1976); KIM et al. (1976); KIM (1977)
γ-Amylase	Human	210,000		KELLY and ALPERS (1973)
Maltase–sucrase	Human	185,000		HEATON (1970)
Sucrase–isomaltase	Human	200,000–220,000		CUMMINS et al. (1968); YAMASHIRO and GRAY (1970)
Sucrase–isomaltase	Human	200,000–350,000		CONCLIN et al. (1975)
Isomaltase (large)	Human	330,000		YAMASHIRO and GRAY (1970)
Sucrase–isomaltase	Human	220,000		YAMASHIRO and GRAY (1970)
Sucrase			110,000	
Isomaltase			110,000	
Sucrase–isomaltase	Rabbit	211,000		SEMENZA and KOLINSKA (1968)
Sucrase–isomaltase	Rabbit	235,000		TAKESUE et al. (1967); NISHI et al. (1968); TAKESUE and KASHIWAGI (1969)
Sucrase–isomaltase	Rabbit	220,000–221,000		COGOLI et al. (1972, 1973)
Sucrase			110,000–120,000	MOSIMANN et al. (1973)
Isomaltase			110,000–120,000	SEMENZA (1977a)
Sucrase–isomaltase	Rabbit		140,000	SIGRIST et al. (1975)
Sucrase (complex)	Rabbit	312,000		KRETCHMER et al. (1979)
Maltase–glucoamylase	Rat	250,000–500,000	134,000–480,000	FLANAGAN and FORSTNER (1978)
β-Galactosidase (neutral)	Rat	360,000–510,000		KRAML et al. (1969)
Lactase	Human	280,000		GRAY and SANTIAGO (1969)
Lactase	Human	350,000–420,000		ASP (1971)

The enzymatically active proteins of the enterocyte membrane usually have high molecular mass and in most cases an oligomeric structure (Table 3); in a few cases they represent enzymatic heterologous complexes; e.g. sucrase–isomaltase. Most enteric enzymes are tightly bound to the plasma membrane. Their separation from the membrane may be achieved either by protease or neutral detergents treatment. The latter seem to release the integral molecule bound to the lipid matrix (for review see HELENIUS and SIMONS 1975) whereas proteases hydrolyse peptide bonds and liberate only the catalytic part. In the next sections a more detailed characterization of the main properties of these enzymes will be given.

3. The Subcellular Distribution of Enteric Enzymes

The method of differential centrifugation with subsequent analysis of the distribution of particular enzymes between the brush border and cytosol fractions is widely used for the assessment of the relative role of the enterocyte enzymes in membrane and intracellular digestion. With this method it has been demonstrated that about 90% of all disaccharidase activities are concentrated in the brush border. Thus, it has been shown that the enterocyte brush border fraction in hamsters contains up to 90% of maltase and sucrase activities (MILLER and CRANE 1961 b, 1963); some 96% of sucrase activity (GALLO and TREDWELL 1963) and 66% of all maltase activities (RUTTLOFF et al. 1964) were found in the enterocyte brush border in rats. In guinea-pigs, the brush border of the intestinal cells contains about 74% (HÜBSHER et al. 1965) and in rabbits 75%–80% (GITZELMAN et al. 1964) of sucrase activity.

About 80%–90% of maltase activity of the enterocyte brush border is associated with the membrane fraction (EICHHOLZ and CRANE 1965; OVERTON et al. 1965). According to some evidence sucrase activity in the cytoplasm of the pig intestinal cells contains only 1% of the total enzyme activity in the whole mucosal homogenate. The sucrase activity in the microvillous membrane fraction in the rat is 15 times higher than in the whole homogenate, while the maltase and sucrase activities in the same fraction in hamster are 33-fold higher (RHODES et al. 1977). Thus, the brush border disaccharidase activity varies in different animal species. The level of enterocyte brush border invertase activity has been shown to depend on the functional state of the organism. In particular, in fed rats, the enzyme activity is higher than in fasting animals (MITYUSHOVA 1970).

The use of histochemical and immunological techniques has also revealed that in the small intestine in humans and different animals the maltase, sucrase and lactase activities are associated with the brush border (for reviews see LOJDA 1974; KRAML and LOJDA 1977; SLABY et al. 1977). As for the small intestinal alkaline phosphatase, it has been reported that it is predominantly a component of the apical membrane of the enterocytes (FOSSET et al. 1974; LOUVARD et al. 1975 a; COLBEAU and MAROUX 1978) and may be found in the glycocalyx (ITO 1965, 1969; UGOLEV et al. 1978, 1979 d). After homogenization and centrifugation of the guinea-pig intestinal mucosa it was found that the brush border contains only 40% of alkaline phosphatase activity (HÜBSHER et al. 1965).

Recent studies of the location of peptidases in the enterocytes will contribute to further elucidation of their role in digestion and absorption of proteins. The brush border contains a number of enzymes possessing peptidase activity. At least one of these enzymes is more active relative to tri- and higher peptides than to dipeptides (PETERS 1970; WOJNAROWSKA and GRAY 1975). Besides, peptidase activity in the brush border appears to be different from that in the cytosol (HEIZER and ISSELBACHER 1970, HEIZER et al. 1972; UGOLEV 1972a; KIM et al. 1974; LINDBERG et al. 1975; UGOLEV et al. 1977c), although there are communications about great similarity between the brush border peptidases and intracellular hydrolases (O'CUINN et al. 1974). The brush border oligopeptidase activity is rather high, indicating its digestive functions. However, most of the dipeptidase activity is concentrated intracellularly (O'CUINN and FOTTRELL 1975; PIGGOTT and FOTTRELL 1975).

Using the method of differential centrifugation it has been shown that the brush border contains 6%–10% (for reviews see PETERS 1970, 1975), and in some cases about 15% of dipeptidase activity of the enterocytes (FUJITA et al. 1972). A hypothesis had earlier been proposed that some elements of the brush border membrane structure, including many dipeptidases may be loosely bound to membranes and, as mentioned, readily solubilized during subcellular fractionation (for reviews see LINDBERG 1966, 1972; UGOLEV, 1972a, b; UGOLEV et al. 1977c; JODL and LINDBERG 1979). After density gradient centrifugation it has been revealed that in rats the brush border comprises one-half and in guinea-pigs one-third of dipeptidase activity of the enterocytes (WELLS et al. 1979).

High tripeptidase activity: 20%–80% from some data (PETERS 1970, 1975; KIM et al. 1972; KIM 1977) and practically all from other data (WELLS et al. 1979) is located in the brush border region. All the tetra-, penta- and hexapeptidase activities are also associated with the brush border fraction (for review see PETERS 1975). Arylamidase, isolated from the brush border as shown, is capable of reproducing almost the whole spectrum of dipeptidase activity of the enterocytes (NOACK et al. 1975). The brush border location of aminopeptidase and glycylprolyl-β-naphthylamidase has histochemically been demonstrated in the enterocytes in humans, rats, guinea-pigs and pigs (LOJDA 1976; LOJDA et al. 1978).

It is known that the final products of extracellular digestion of protein (dipeptides) may be subjected to hydrolysis in two regions of the enterocytes: (1) on the brush border membrane surface with subsequent transport of formed hydrolysis products (amino acids) by the digestive transport conveyor; (2) intracellularly after penetration of peptides through the brush border membrane (Peptide Transport and Hydrolysis 1977).

At present, there is evidence suggesting the physiological significance of the active transport of small peptides through the membrane of the enterocytes and their subsequent intracellular hydrolysis (for reviews see MATTHEWS 1972, 1975a, b; BURSTON et al. 1977). However, the problem of differentiation of the two types of digestion in the animal small intestine is very difficult and is still far from being resolved as to peptides because of ambiguous conclusions which can be made using the experimental criteria (for review see UGOLEV et al. 1977c).

For assessing the roles of membrane and intracellular peptidases of the small intestine in splitting peptides we have recently used the so-called anoxic criterion first proposed by NEWEY and SMYTH (1962). the essence of this criterion is as follows: (1) in the case of intracellular hydrolysis of dipeptides one may expect that under anaerobic conditions in experiments in vitro there will be less dipeptide hydrolysis products in the incubation medium than under aerobic conditions because anoxia inhibits the active transport of peptides to the site of their hydrolysis inside the cells; (2) in the case of membrane hydrolysis of dipeptides and under both aerobic and anaerobic conditions no difference in the concentration of hydrolysis products should be observed in the incubation medium since the site of hydrolysis (the brush border membrane surface) is in both cases equally accessible to dipeptides. It is noteworthy that anoxia has no direct effect on dipeptidase activity (NEWEY and SMYTH 1962; CHENG et al. 1971). Using this criterion, it has been demonstrated that Gly-Gly and L-Met-L-Met are transported through the membrane of the enterocytes and are hydrolysed intracellularly (NEWEY and SMYTH 1962; CHENG et al. 1971; for review see MATTHEWS 1972).

However, it has been shown in our laboratory that anoxia does not influence the hydrolysis of many dipeptides of the intact intestinal mucosa. This suggests that the enzymes splitting such dipeptides as Gly-L-Val, Gly-L-Leu, Gly-L-Phe, L-Ala-L-Ala, Gly-L-Ala, L-Leu-Gly, Gly-Gly, Gly-L-Pro are predominantly located on the external surface of the apical membrane of the enterocytes rather than intracellularly (SMIRNOVA et al. 1976; MOOZ et al. 1978; for review see UGOLEV et al. 1977c). In contrast to other dipeptides, the rate of transport of L-Pro-Gly remained unaffected by anoxia. L-Pro-Gly appears to enter the enterocytes by passive transport down the concentration gradient and is hydrolysed intracellularly (MOOZ et al. 1978). This is consistent with the data on the absence from the enterocyte brush border of enzymes which split proline-containing dipeptides (DAS and RADHAKRISHNAN 1972; HUECKEL and ROGERS 1972; for reviews see RUBINO and GUANDALINI 1977; JOSEFSSON et al. 1977). Moreover, many authors have reported that proline-containing dipeptides may be transported intact into the small intestinal cells (BOULLIN et al. 1973; SAIDEL and EDELSTEIN 1974; HEADING et al. 1977). Although the absence of membrane hydrolysis of L-Pro-Gly in the small intestine is now more rarely questioned, there is indirect evidence suggesting that in some cases Gly-L-Pro may be hydrolysed on the brush border membrane surface (RUBINO et al. 1971; LANE et al. 1975; WIESMAN 1977); this is in agreement with our results obtained using the anoxic criterion (MOOZ et al. 1978).

It is not possible at present to evaluate quantitatively the significance of the membrane and intracellular mechanisms of peptide hydrolysis. Moreover, their roles may be expected to vary in animals of different levels of organization and depending on the type of feeding. However, the attempt to demonstrate an exclusive role of intracellular peptidases at the final stages of the splitting of dietary peptides in the small intestine (Peptide Transport and Hydrolysis 1977) led to a recognition of the important digestive function of peptidases located on the external surface of the apical membrane of the enterocytes.

The view is now widely accepted that the physiological role of various enzymes of the enterocytes in the hydrolysis of nutrients is proportional to its content in one or another subcellular fraction. This implies that the hydrolysis of disaccharides is exclusively due to membrane digestion while that of peptides occurs mostly intracellularly. However, as will be shown in Sect. B.IV.4, spatial relationships and vectorial direction of the process can considerably change the role of the enzyme systems. Thus, a small amount of the enzymes localized on entry into the enterocyte (on the apical membrane) may play an important or even dominant part in the peptide hydrolysis. These data obtained from the analysis of real processes have been characterized as a "sequential" model of peptide hydrolysis.

4. The Sequential Model of the Final Stages of Hydrolysis

A sequential (multicompartment) mathematical model for peptide uptake in the small intestine has recently been proposed and a possible role of several peptidase barriers has been demonstrated (UGOLEV et al. 1977c; MOOZ et al. 1978). To build a model the following assumptions have been made: the hydrolysis of substrate influenced by enzymes is considered as a chemical reaction of the first order; the diffusive properties of the brush border zone and cytosol are the same; the enzymes are absent from the small intestinal lumen, but distributed regularly in the brush border and cytosol at the same concentration, taking into account the relationship between the volume of the brush border and that of the cell itself. The latter assumption means that the total amount of enzymes in the cytosol is one order of magnitude higher than in the brush border.

The relative distribution of the initial substrate concentration along the cell (U) in the direction from the lumen to the basal membrane may be described by the following equation

$$U(x,t) = U\left(t - \int_0^x \frac{dx}{D(x)}\right) \exp\left(-\int_0^x \frac{E(x)}{D(x)} dx\right),$$

where $D(x)$ is the diffusion coefficient, $E(x)$ is the enzyme concentration, x is the spatial coordinate and t is the time.

Figure 3 shows the two modes of substrate distribution with respect to high enzyme activity or low diffusion rate (curve I) and with respect to relatively low enzyme activity or high diffusion rate (curve II). As can be seen, in the first case the hydrolysis of substrates occurs predominantly in the brush border zone. The reverse relationship is peculiar to low enzyme activity or high diffusion rate. However, in this case the relative role of the membrane hydrolysis is greater than the relative content of the enzyme in the brush border region. It can be demonstrated that these regularities will be expressed more distinctly if we keep in mind the presence of diffusive resistance of the microvillous membrane separating the glycocalyx space from the cytosol.

Thus, the study of the model made it possible to conclude that even in the case when the enzymes are concentrated in the cytosol, membrane hydrolysis by the enzymes localized in the brush border zone may play an important role and depends on a relationship between the rate at which substrates pass through the cell and that of enzymatic splitting of this substrate. At the same time the intracellular peptidases of the small intestine, except for a participation in the catabolism of proteins, may possibly perform the function of a third barrier (after glycocalyx and lipoprotein membrane enzymes) in the way of dietary peptides.

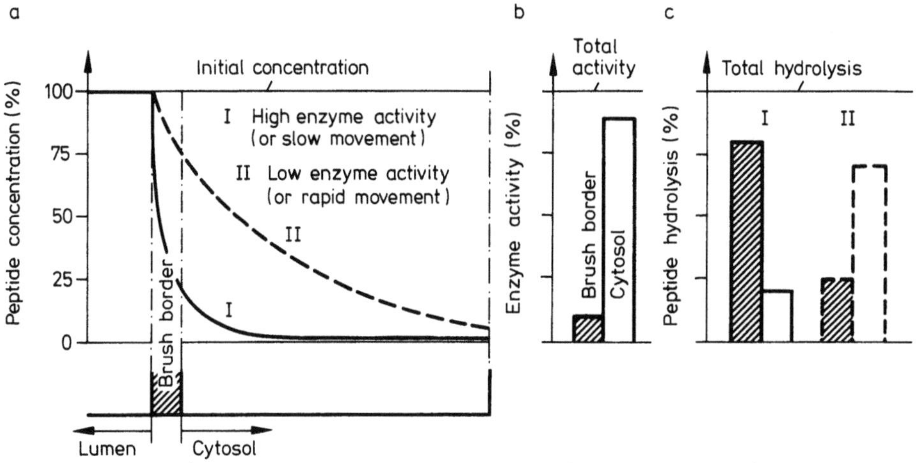

Fig. 3 a–c. A subsequent model of peptide transport. **a** decrease in peptide concentration during passage across the cell; **b** brush border and cytosol enzymatic activities; **c** level of dipeptide hydrolysis in the brush border and cytosol. MOOZ et al. (1978)

V. Membrane Digestion in Normal Function of the Gastrointestinal Tract

Membrane digestion is a universal mechanism which can be found in mammals, birds, fish and many groups of invertebrates. In humans and higher animals it occurs on the surface of the enterocytes forming the brush border by the microvilli. The latter are covered by the lipoprotein membrane on the external surface of which there is a layer of acid mucopolysaccharide filaments forming the glycocalyx.

The external surface of the lipoprotein membrane and, possibly, the glycocalyx contain some nonenzymatic factors such as immunoglobulins (PLAUT 1972; WALKER and ISSELBACHER 1974; IMMUNOLOGY OF THE GUT 1977; BROWN 1978, for review see WALKER 1979), CA^{2+} binding proteins (WASSERMAN et al. 1966; TAYLOR et al. 1970; WASSERMAN and TAYLOR 1971; Bredderman and WASSERMAN 1974; for reviews see BAUMAN 1977; WASSERMAN 1974; FEHER and WASSERMAN 1979), Zn^{2+} binding proteins (KOWARSKI et al. 1974), folate (LESLIE and ROWE 1972), intrinsic factor-vitamin B_{12} complex (TOSKES and DEREN 1973; KATZ and COOPER 1974; MATHAN et al. 1974), hormone binding specific receptors (probably glycoproteins) (for reviews see ROBINSON et al. 1971; PITOT and YATVIN 1973), inhibitors (WILSON et al. 1978).

The structure of the membrane fragment with the glycocalyx as well as different enzymes and the transport apparatus (carriers) are represented in Fig. 4. The zone of membrane digestion is permeable to relatively small molecules, whereas large molecules, supramolecular aggregations and, what is more important, bacteria cannot penetrate into this region. Thus, the initial stages of digestion are accomplished exclusively in the digestive lumen. Once some critical limit of breakdown is reached, small molecules enter the sterile brush border zone where they undergo gradual splitting to the final products and then are transported into the

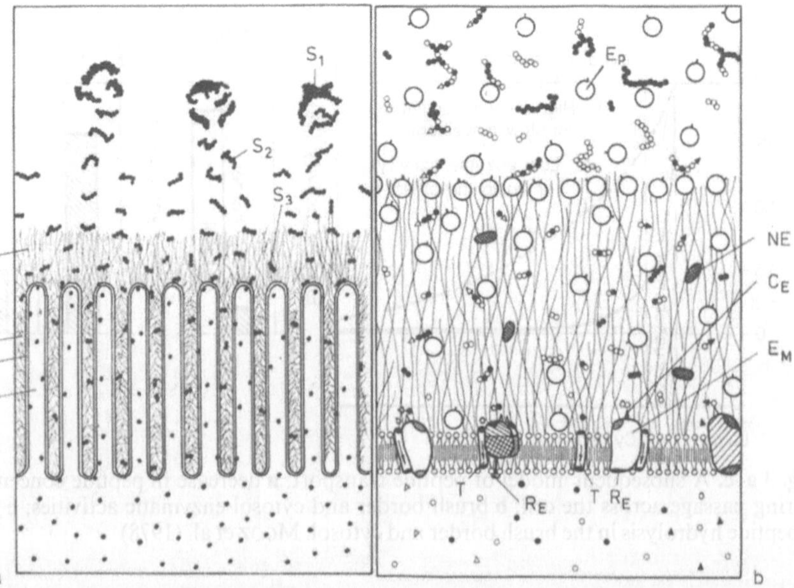

Fig. 4a, b. A scheme of interactions between luminal and membrane digestion. **a** scheme of subsequent depolymerization of food substances in the lumen and on the small intestinal surface; **b** fragment of lipoprotein membrane with adsorbed and enteric enzymes. *M*, membrane; *MV*, microvilli; Gl_a, apical glycocalyx; Gl_i, lateral glycocalyx; S_1, S_2, S_3, substrates; E_P, pancreatic enzymes; E_M, membrane enzymes; *T*, transport systems of the membrane; R_E, regulatory sites of the enzymes; C_E, catalytic sites of the enzymes; NE nonenzymatic factors. UGOLEV et al. (1979a)

circulation. Owing to membrane digestion, first, the intermediate and final stages of the hydrolysis of nutrients and second, the effective coupling of the digestive and transport processes are realized.

Functionally, membrane digestion occupies an intermediate position in the three-stages scheme of functioning of the digestive apparatus (luminal digestion–membrane digestion–absorption). This suggests that membrane digestion plays a part as a mechanism which may be an acceptor relative to intralumen hydrolysis and a donor relative to absorption. Thus, intraluminal digestion cannot be of significant importance without membrane digestion for absorption in this case is impossible because of the lack of adequate substrates (substances formed during enzymatic transformation). Along with this the role of luminal digestion cannot be underestimated since common dietary food substances are incapable of penetrating into the brush border zone and the glycocalyx space without a preliminary treatment in the digestive lumen. Therefore with the enzyme apparatus ensuring membrane digestion being fully retained the latter may be defective if there are severe disorders in luminal hydrolysis.

For the correct evaluation of the role of membrane digestion some factors which were not considered in traditional gastroenterology may be important.

1. Enzymes responsible for membrane digestion are structurally bound. In view of this, a spatial organization is possible both for the proper enzyme systems

ensuring digestion and the enzyme transport systems (providing a functional integration for the final stages of digestion and initial stages of absorption).

2. The zone of membrane digestion possesses special physicochemical properties, in particular, pH (Chap. 20; UGOLEV 1972a; LUCAS et al. 1975, 1978; KONDER et al. 1977; PARSONS 1977; LUCAS and BLAIR 1978), concentration of organic and inorganic ions, unstirred fluid layer (Chap. 21; WILSON and DIETSCHY 1974; DIETSCHY and WESTERGAARD 1975; WINNE 1976, 1977; THOMSON and DIETSCHY 1977; WINNE et al. 1979; for reviews see UGOLEV 1972a; LEVIN 1979).

3. Structurally bound enzymes possess peculiar properties. In particular, after separation of enzymes from the membrane (for analysis) their catalytic and regulatory properties change significantly (for reviews see UGOLEV 1972a; UGOLEV and KOLTUSHKINA 1975; KRAML and LOJDA 1977).

4. Membrane digestion occurs in a zone inaccessible to bacteria that prevents the uptake by them of easily assimilated food substances of low molecular mass (oligomers and monomers).

5. Owing to the enzyme apparatus the glycocalyx layer is a highly specific filter. This layer is permeable to those substances for which there are adequate enzymes on the surface and inside the glycocalyx and impermeable to other substances with the same molecular size.

6. The data on the contractility function of the brush border regulated by Ca^{2+} (MOOSEKER 1974) are also important for the understanding of transmembrane permeability and efficiency of membrane digestion. It has been shown that the microvillous microfilaments performing these functions contain actin and myosin and are associated with the apical membrane of the enterocytes (MOOSEKER and TILNEY 1975; BRETCHER and WEBER 1978; MOOSEKER et al. 1978).

C. Enzyme Apparatus of the Apical Membrane of the Enterocytes

For the understanding of the role of the digestive enzymes in the transport of substances through the apical membrane of the enterocytes it is necessary first of all to characterize the structure and functions of the plasma membrane (in the composition of which these enzymes perform their functions) and also the location, molecular structure and properties of these enzymes.

I. Fine Location of Membrane Hydrolases

Membrane structure has been described at length in a number of articles and reviews (HENDLER 1971; ROTHFIELD 1971; BANGHAM 1972; FINEAN 1972; GREEN 1972; FLEISCHER and PACKER 1974; CHAPMAN 1974; LENAZ 1974; SINGER 1974, 1977; BERGELSON 1975; FARIAS et al. 1975; GULIK-KRZYWICKI 1975; HARRISON and LUNT 1975; ROBINSON 1975; TROSHIN 1975; CHAPMAN and WALLACH 1976; QUINN 1976; RACKER 1976; SEMENZA and CAROFOLI 1977; GENNIS and JONAS 1977; MCINTOSH et al. 1977; NILSSON and DALLNER 1977; PETERS and RICHARDS 1977; FINEAN et al. 1978; SANDERMANN 1978; ZWAAL 1978; ELEZKY and TSYBULEVSKY 1979).

According to the modern concept, the plasma membrane has a lipoprotein structure. It consists of the phospholipid bilayer in the composition of which other lipids, proteins and polysaccharides are incorporated. Proteins comprise about 50% of the apical membrane of the enterocytes (for review see CRANE 1977). The phospholipid membrane matrix is formed by phospholipids and glycosphingolipids together with cholesterol. The molar ratio of cholesterol, phospholipids and glycosphingolipids is 2:1:1 (FORSTNER and WHERRETT 1973). In contrast to other plasma membranes, the membranes of the enterocytes are characterized by a relatively high content of cholesterol (BILLINGTON and NAYUDU 1976, 1978).

Lipid-soluble substances, including lipid hydrolysis products can cross the phospholipid bilayer of the membrane owing to diffusion. However, the membrane represents an essential barrier for diffusion of water-soluble compounds, including hexoses, because they do not readily penetrate through the phospholipid matrix and are too large to pass through the water channels of the membrane. The equivalent radius of the pores of the membrane is about 4–6 Å (LINDEMANN and SOLOMON 1962; SMYTH and WRIGHT 1966; SOLOMON 1968; for review see SCHULTZ 1979). There exist water channels between the cells which are permeable to ions and small readily soluble organic compounds as well as molecules of the size of a hexose (for review see SCHULTZ 1979).

The barrier properties of the membrane are generally determined by fatty acid residues composing the internal part of the phospholipid bilayer. The specific functions of recognition, binding, hydrolysis and transfer of substances through the membrane are largely performed by its protein and glycoprotein components.

The data based on X-ray structural analysis, use of paramagnetic resonance, spin and fluorescent probes has demonstrated that the charged heads of phospholipids orientated towards the internal and external faces of the membrane, are fixed rather firmly although the lipid matrix of the membrane as a whole is in a liquid crystalline state. Fluidity of the membrane is of great importance (for reviews see HOCHACHKA and SOMERO 1973; BRESLER and BRESLER 1974; BERGELSON 1975; ROBINSON 1975; CHERRY 1976; RACKER 1976; SCHREIER 1978). This provides a possibility for mobility of the lipid molecules and for incorporation into phospholipid bilayer protein molecules, including transmembrane proteins and supramolecular complexes to which hydrolases and carriers are referred; these processes are different. It has been shown that some proteins and polypeptides are capable of migrating both in lateral (FRYE and EDIDIN 1970; DEVAUX and MCCONNEL 1972; LEE et al. 1973; SACKMAN et al. 1973; LEE 1975; for reviews see GULIK-KRZYWICKI 1975; ROBINSON 1975; CHERRY 1976; RACKER 1976; OSTROVSKI 1977) and vertical directions (KORNBERG and MCCONNEL 1971; BOROCHOV and SHINITZKY 1976; BENZ et al. 1977; OVCHINNIKOV and IVANOV 1977). Attachment of enzymes and other proteins to the membrane is achieved in different ways: Ca^{2+} bridges, ionic and hydrogen bonds and hydrophobic interactions. The latter play a particularly important role.

Membrane proteins, including enzymes, have a vectorial distribution in the membrane (for reviews see SINGER 1974, 1977; STECK 1974; BRETSCHER and RAFF 1975; CARRAWAY 1975; MARCHESI et al. 1976; ROTHMAN and LENARD 1977; SANDERMANN 1978; ZWAAL 1978). Carbohydrates are located mostly on the external face of the membrane and are either the components of glycolipids or of glycoproteins. Carbohydrates associated with proteins or lipids of the surface coat differ along the small intestine (LOUVARD et al. 1973). They act as binding sites for many lectins (ETZLER and BRANSTRATOR 1974; GARRIDO 1975) as well as for cholera toxins (WALKER et al. 1974).

It is important that most intestinal enzymes are glycoproteins, including carbohydrases (COGOLI et al. 1972, 1973; KELLY and ALPERS 1973; MOSIMANN et al. 1973; CRITCHLEY et al. 1975; SIGRIST et al. 1975; BRAUN et al. 1977; FLANAGAN and FORSTNER 1978; TSUBOI et al. 1979), aminopeptidase (KIM and BROPHY 1976; LOUVARD et al. 1976), alkaline phosphatase (COLBEAU and MAROUX 1978). Sucrase–isomaltase complex (COGOLI et al. 1972) contains about 15%, alkaline phosphatase (FOSSET et al. 1974) some 12% of carbohydrates. In contrast, γ-amylase (KELLY and ALPERS 1973) and enterokinase (MAROUX et al. 1971) amount to more than 30%, and aminopeptidase (MAROUX et al. 1973) 23% of carbohydrates.

Several types of location of proteins in the apical membrane are suggested. The spatial distribution of proteins is now considered in terms of the present views on the structure and functions of the plasma membrane. Recent views on location of proteins in the membrane (including enzymes and carriers) have been described in a number of reviews (ISSELBACHER 1974; SINGER 1974, 1977; KENNEDY 1978; SANDERMANN 1978; ZWAAL 1978; DESNUELLE 1979). There seem to exist several types of membrane integral proteins.

1. Peripheral proteins located on the external or internal membrane surface and only partly embedded within the phospholipid matrix.

2. Transmembrane integral proteins, spanning the membrane, with the hydrophilic segments projected on either side of the membrane and with the hydrophobic segment between them submerged into the lipid matrix of the membrane. The substitute group of enzyme molecules (one or more oligosaccharide chains) has an external position in the membrane and protrudes into the intestinal lumen, possibly participating in formation of the glycocalyx structure, reception of biologically active substances and binding of substrates.

3. Quaternary transmembrane proteins with the water channels between subunits (Fig. 5). It is this type to which specific transport proteins of the membrane are attributed.

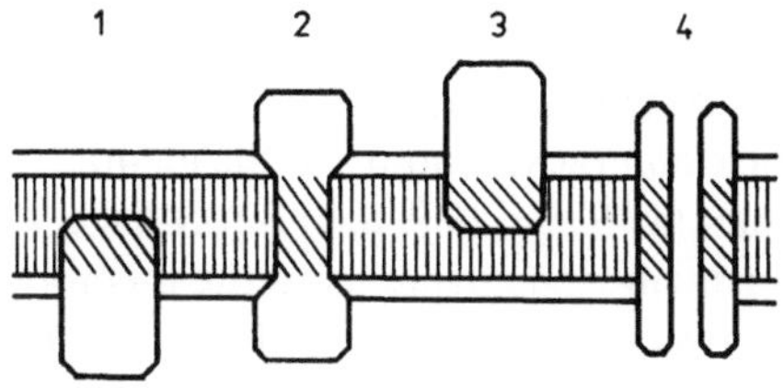

Fig. 5. A scheme of different types of location of integral proteins in the membrane: peripheral proteins (*1,3*); transmembrane protein (*2*); transmembrane transport protein with a water channel (*4*). SINGER (1977)

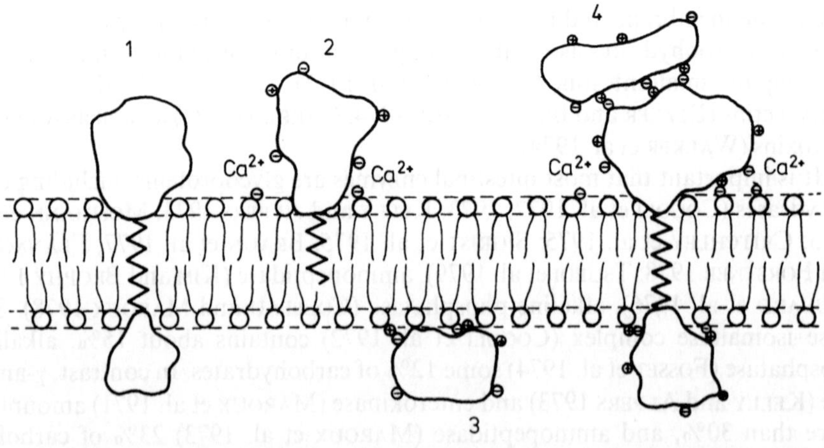

Fig. 6. A scheme of different interactions of proteins with the phospholipid membrane: transmembrane proteins (*1,4*); peripheral integral protein (*2*); peripheral protein (*3*). ZWAAL (1978)

A suggestion has been made (for review see CRANE 1977) that in contrast to enzymes and transport proteins which are transmembrane integral proteins and folate binding proteins, Ca^{2+} and Zn^{2+} binding proteins and intrinsic factor–vitamin B_{12} complex are peripheral.

ZWAAL (1978) described the interactions of proteins, including enzymes, with the membrane (Fig. 6). There exist several types of binding of proteins to the membrane. Some proteins are characterized by polar bonds and Ca^{2+} bridges, while others, including transmembrane proteins, are distinguished by the presence of hydrophobic bonds to the phospholipid matrix of the membrane. It is important that in a few cases proteins interact with the membrane by more than one type of binding. Nonhydrophobic interactions are essential for the peripheral type of binding while hydrophobic interactions with the hydrophobic matrix of the membrane are significant for the transmembrane type of binding. For hydrophobic interactions the α-helical structure is important.

Most enteric enzymes are transmembrane oligomeric proteins (glycoproteins) with the active site orientated towards the small intestinal lumen. In a number of cases, it has been shown that each subunit of enzyme oligomer has its anchor part. However, there may be one common anchor for the whole complex. For example, in the sucrase–isomaltase complex, binding to the membrane is due to the isomaltase subunit alone (SEMENZA 1977c, 1979a, b; BRUNNER et al. 1978, 1979).

The binding of transmembrane proteins to the membrane is stable because it is due to interactions between the phospholipid matrix and the hydrophobic part of the enzyme and becomes more stable owing to the external hydrophilic part. Moreover, at least in some instances different types of polar interactions may occur between the enzymatically active hydrophilic part of the enzyme and charged heads of phospholipids.

By combining the electron microscopic, biochemical and immunological approaches, it has been shown that sucrase, maltase, lactase and leucylnaphthylamidase form knob-like structures on the external membrane surface (MAESTRACCI et al. 1975; MAESTRACCI 1976). It is important that a part of the enzyme can project onto the membrane. This has been demonstrated, in particular, by the example of sucrase, maltase and some other enzymes (LOUVARD et al. 1975b; NISHI and TAKESUE 1978a, b; TAKESUE and NISHI 1978; VASSEUR et al. 1978). There is evidence suggesting that at least the protein part of the sucrase–isomaltase complex projects onto the three-layered membrane surface of the enterocytes by about 150 Å (NISHI and TAKESUE 1978a, b), and that of β-naphthylamidase by 100 Å (TAKESUE and NISHI 1978). The data presented have made possible a better understanding of interactions between the enzymatic and transport system. They indicate that all the hydrolases studied form monomers on the external rather than internal surface of the apical membrane of the enterocytes.

The evidence on fine location of the enzymes is interesting to correlate with a recent characterization of location of the transport protein for glucose. On the basis of experiments with closed intact and open penetrating membrane vesicles obtained from the rabbit intestinal brush border and treated by inhibitors of phlorhizin H^3 binding to the membrane, a suggestion has been made that the sugar carrier is a transmembrane asymmetric protein (KLIP et al. 1979). The molecular mass of the carrier estimated from direct evidence amounts to about 100,000 daltons. A comparison of the number of carrier molecules per milligram vesicular protein with the number of glucose molecules has revealed that the transport cycle of a carrier may be approximately 20–40 s^{-1} (for review see SEMENZA 1979c).

The results demonstrating that the catalytic site and entry into the transport system are localized on the external surface of the apical membrane of the enterocytes have confirmed previous suggestion that on this surface an integration of the enzymatic and transport processes takes place. However, building a correct model of the enzyme transport complex requires the knowledge of the molecular structure both of hydrolysis and transport mechanisms. A brief summary of the molecular structure of the membrane enzymes of the enterocytes will be given in Sect. C.II.

II. The Amphipathic Structure of Membrane Enzymes

Most enteric enzymes are transmembrane amphipathic proteins consisting of hydrophobic and hydrophilic parts. This is true for maltase 2 and 3, aminopeptidase and alkaline phosphatase. The evidence comes mostly from studies on enzymatically active proteins solubilized from the membrane preparations by treatment with proteolytic enzymes or neutral detergents. (The mechanism of action of detergents has been described in the review by HELENIUS and SIMONS 1975). The detergents, in particular Triton X-100, liberate the integral enzyme molecules which aggregate in their absence. Proteases release the hydrophilic part which is soluble in aqueous medium in the absence of detergent. Papain and, in a few cases, trypsin

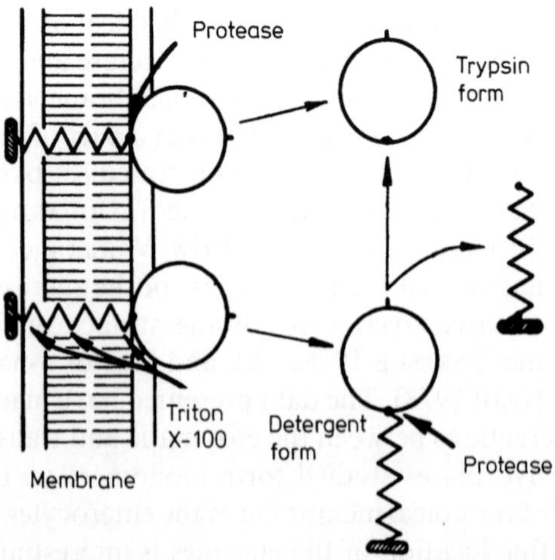

Fig. 7. A model of integration of intestinal hydrolases in the apical membrane of the enterocytes. MAROUX et al. (1975)

can transform the detergent form of the enzyme into a protease-like form by splitting the molecule into two parts (Fig. 7). The hydrophilic part includes carbohydrate residues and a catalytically active site. It makes up the bulk of the enzyme, 90%–95%. The hydrophobic part possesses other properties which will be considered in Sect. C.II and C.III. An increased understanding of the molecular structure and functions of membrane hydrolases stems from a consideration of the characteristics of individual enzymes.

1. Maltases

The intestinal enzymes of the maltase group (EC 3.2.1.20) are glycoproteins providing hydrolysis of maltose, sucrose and isomaltose. These enzymes also participate in hydrolysis of polysaccharides, splitting the final products of amylolysis – maltose and isomaltose.

The enzymes of this group exist as complexes: sucrase–isomaltase, maltase–glycoamylase and others (YAMASHIRO and GRAY 1970; COGOLI et al. 1972, 1973; KOLINSKA and KRAML 1972; MOSIMANN et al. 1973; COGOLI and SEMENZA 1975; SIGRIST et al. 1975; QUARONI and SEMENZA 1976; BRAUN et al. 1977; BRUNNER et al. 1977/78, 1979; GREEN and HADORN 1977; SEMENZA 1977a, b, 1979a, b; SLABY et al. 1977; FLANAGAN and FORSTNER 1978). Such complexes are located on the external membrane surface of the enterocytes and project above its level by approximately 150 Å (NISHI and TAKESUE 1978a, b). The complexes dissociate into separate subunits with molecular mass varying from 110,000 to 120,000 daltons (YAMASHIRO and GRAY 1970; COGOLI et al. 1972, 1973; MOSIMANN et al. 1973; COGOLI and SEMENZA 1975; SEMENZA 1977a) or about 140,000 daltons (SIGRIST et al. 1975; FLANAGAN and FORSTNER 1978).

The structures of maltases 2 and 3 are very much alike (MAROUX et al. 1973, 1975; MAROUX and LOUVARD 1976). An analysis of the detergent and trypsin forms of the enzymes has shown that the former contains a short fragment of hydrophobic nature. The hydrophobic parts proved to be NH_2 terminal. Three NH_2 terminal amino acid residues: Ala, Leu and Lys were found in the detergent form which seem to correspond to three subunits of the enzyme. After trypsin treatment, two hydrophobic fragments with NH_2 terminal residues Phe and Lys were identified.

The sucrase–isomaltase complex is associated with the membrane by a hydrophobic fragment of the isomaltase subunit (SEMENZA 1977c, 1979a, b; BRUNNER et al. 1978). A sequence of 37 amino acid residues in the NH_2 terminal region of the isomaltase subunit has recently been deciphered (FRANK et al. 1978). The hydrophobic part was shown to consist predominantly of hydrophobic amino acids. The fragment of this part between amino acid residues 12 and 31 probably makes contact with the hydrophobic matrix of the phospholipid bilayer of the brush border membrane. This fragment has a poorly expressed β-sheet conformation.

The hydrophilic part of the sucrase–isomaltase complex is orientated towards the aqueous phase and makes up more than 90% of the total mass (BRUNNER et al. 1978, 1979). The molecular mass of a small hydrophobic part incorporated into the phospholipid bilayer amounts to 8,000–10,000 daltons (MAROUX et al. 1975; MAROUX and LOUVARD 1976), while that of the whole complex represents about 200,000 daltons (see Table 3).

The hydrophilic part performs a catalytic function and is nearly completely protruded into the small intestinal lumen (LOUVARD et al. 1975a). It may be separated from the surface of the membrane phospholipid bilayer by more than 10 Å and is bound to it by means of "stalk" (BRUNNER et al. 1977, 1979). The hydrophilic nature of the catalytic part of the enzyme may be accounted for by the presence of many carbohydrate chains forming the structure in the direction of the intestinal lumen where the substrates come from (LOUVARD et al. 1975b; MAROUX and LOUVARD 1976).

2. Aminopeptidase

Aminopeptidase of the small intestine (EC 3.4.11.2) accounts for much of the brush border peptidase activity. It is also responsible for arylamidase activity and total aminopeptidase activity relative to oligopeptides as well as one-half of tripeptidase activity and has a slight but undoubted relation to a part of dipeptidase activity (MAROUX et al. 1973; NOACK et al. 1975; KIM 1977; SMITHSON and GRAY 1977; ANTONOWICZ 1979).

The enzyme of the pig intestinal mucosa is a glycoprotein and contains 77% amino acid residues, 23% sugars (15% neutral and 8% amino saccharides), 0.3% sialic acid and two atoms of zinc per molecule. The molecular mass of aminopeptidase is about 280,000 daltons. The enzyme appears to involve three subunits with molecular mass 130,000, 97,000 and 49,000 daltons, respectively (MAROUX et al. 1973).

Two similar aminopeptidases with molecular mass about 280,000 daltons (KIM et al., 1976; KIM and BROPHY 1976; for reviews see KIM 1977) were purified from the intestinal brush border of the rat. Both enzymes are glycoproteins of analogous chemical composition, antigenic properties, substrate specificity and kinetic characteristics. In contrast to other enzymes, the rat intestinal aminopeptidase contains glucose. It has been demonstrated that each brush border form of the enzyme is composed of two subunits of equal molecular mass. The molecular mass of aminopeptidase in the rabbit intestinal mucosa is somewhat less and amounts to 225,000 daltons (TAKESUE 1975).

Aminopeptidase is an amphipathic enzyme and has a hydrophilic and a hydrophobic part (MAROUX et al. 1975; LOUVARD et al. 1975a, b; MAROUX and LOUVARD 1976; LOUVARD et al. 1976; PATTUS et al. 1976; VANNIER et al. 1976; for review see DESNUELLE 1979). The hydrophobic fragment is many times smaller than the hydrophilic one and involves hydrophobic amino acid residues such as Leu, Ile, Ala and Val. Its molecular mass amounts to about 8,500–10,000 daltons.

In the hydrophilic part of the enzyme (its trypsin form) the three terminal amino acid residues (Ala, Ser, Val) were revealed. In the detergent form of aminopeptidase, instead of NH_2 terminal Val, Ala was found which splits off from a detergent molecule together with its respective hydrophobic peptide after trypsin treatment. The hydrophobic part of the enzyme is free from disulphide bridges (MAROUX et al. 1975; MAROUX and LOUVARD 1976).

It is suggested that most of the aminopeptidase molecule protrudes out of the external surface of the membrane phospholipid bilayer (LOUVARD et al. 1975a, b; for review see DESNUELLE 1979). Immunologically, it has been demonstrated that aminopeptidase is a transmembrane protein with the hydrophobic segment partly embedded within the lipid matrix of the membrane and partly projecting onto its inner face (LOUVARD et al. 1976). An assumption can be made that if the polypeptide chain of the molecule has an α-helix structure in the hydrophobic internal part of the membrane (40–50 Å according to SEGREST and FELDMAN 1974) and consists of 80 amino acid residues, then the internal side of the membrane will contain up to 40–50 amino acid residues. However, physicochemical considerations and some indirect data led to the idea that the terminal fragment of the hydrophobic part of the enzyme projected on the internal membrane surface would on the whole possess hydrophilic properties. This suggests its localization not in the hydrophobic matrix, but on the side facing the cytoplasm, and increase the stability of enzyme fixation.

3. Alkaline Phosphatase

Alkaline phosphatase (EC 3.1.3.1) is a glycoprotein and participates in the splitting of orthophosphorous acid esters on the membrane external surface of the enterocytes. A suggestion has been made (SKILLEN and RAHBANI-NOBAR 1979) that despite the nonidentity of membrane-bound alkaline phosphatase und Ca^{2+}, Mg^{2+}-ATPase, alkaline phosphatase may act as ATPase, being an integral part of the membrane.

Alkaline phosphatase may be released from the membrane by detergents or papain treatment in two different forms (LOUVARD et al. 1975a). Alkaline phosphatase purified from different tissues in animals of various species is unlike many hydrolases, a symmetrical dimer (SUSSMAN and GOTTLIEB 1969; CHAPPELET-TORDO et al. 1974; FOSSET et al. 1974; OHKUBO et al. 1974; CATHALA et al. 1975; BOOTH and KENNY 1976; COLBEAU and MAROUX 1978).

The molecular mass of the detergent and papain forms of alkaline phosphatase from pig intestinal mucosa is 120,000–130,000 daltons (COLBEAU and

MAROUX 1978). Each form of the enzyme is composed of two subunits with molecular mass of 63,000–65,000 and 60,000–61,000 daltons, respectively. Thus, the discrepancy between these two forms amounts to 3,000–4,000 daltons. Such distinctions may be accounted for by the presence of the hydrophobic part in the detergent form of the enzyme which is lacking in the papain form. As each native subunit of alkaline phosphatase has a hydrophobic part, binding of the enzyme to the membrane is accomplished by two anchors that lend a certain rigidity to the enzyme and greater stability to the integrated system. By this specific fixation COLBEAU and MAROUX (1978) also explain difficulties arising while separating alkaline phosphatase from the membrane.

The identity of NH_2 terminal dipeptides (Phe-Ile) in subunits of the papain and detergent forms permitted the suggestion (COLBEAU and MAROUX 1978) that these are localized not on the NH_2 terminal end, as in the aminopeptidase molecule from pig and rabbit intestinal mucosa as well as in maltases 2 and 3 of pig intestinal mucosa, but on the COOH terminus. Therefore, the modes of integration of membrane proteins, attributed to the same class of hydrolases, are not identical for all membranes.

4. Molecular Structure of Membrane Hydrolases

From the foregoing, despite similarity in the molecular structure of various hydrolases, there exist definite distinctions. In particular, in aminopeptidase and maltases 2 and 3, the hydrophobic part is located on the NH_2 terminal end of the molecule. Such a location suggests that the hydrophobic part may be a "signal peptide" and take part in the process of transmembrane transfer at the stage of synthesis of a polypeptide chain. However, the hydrophobic part of alkaline phosphatase is located at the COOH terminal end. Therefore the location of the hydrophobic part in the molecule may vary in different enzymes which may be accounted for by their independent evolutionary origins.

Variations have also been noted in the structure of hydrophobic fragments. Thus, the composition of amino acid residues in maltase 2 as well as aminopeptidase hydrophobic fragments differ, although the total number of these residues is equal. The NH_2 terminal residues of the detergent and trypsin forms of these enzymes are different.

Attention has been drawn to the structural and topological similarity of the brush border aminopeptidases of the enterocytes and those of the renal tubular cells of the pig (VANNIER et al. 1976). Each enzyme consists of a hydrophilic catalytically active part which emerges almost entirely from the membrane and a much smaller hydrophobic part in the NH_2 terminal region of one of the enzyme subunits providing a fixation of the enzyme to the phospholipid matrix of the membrane. Along with this, there exist differences in the composition of amino acid residues of the hydrophobic parts and in some other properties of both enzymes. In particular, the hydrophobic polypeptides of the renal and intestinal aminopeptidases have the same amino acid composition except for two Val residues and two Tyr residues, which are absent from the first enzyme. Further, NH_2 terminal amino acid residues in the detergent form of renal aminopeptidase are Gly, Ser, Gly; in its trypsin form they are Gly, Ser, Val; and in intestinal aminopeptidase they are Ala, Ser, Ala and Ala, Ser, Val, respectively. There are inessential differences in the molecular mass of both enzymes, in neutral and amino saccharides as well as sialic acid content.

Finally, there exist differences in the modes of fixation of various hydrolases to the membrane. As mentioned, alkaline phosphatase consists of two symmetrical subunits, each attached to the membrane by its own hydrophobic fragment. However, in the sucrase–isomaltase complex, only the isomaltase subunit has a hydrophobic part, which is associated with the membrane (Semenza 1977c, 1979 a, b; Brunner et al. 1978, 1979). Thus, the sucrase subunit has no hydrophobic part of its own and uses the isomaltase subunit as an anchor. It appears that only one of aminopeptidase subunits has an anchor (Maroux and Louvard 1976).

III. Functions of the Hydrophobic Part of Intestinal Enzymes

The main functional characteristics of the enzymes (hydrolytic, antigenic, functions of recognition and binding of substrates etc.) are generally associated with the hydrophilic part of the enzyme. In the opinion of many investigators, the hydrophobic part of the enzyme plays a part in the interactions with the phospholipid matrix of the membrane and fixation of the hydrophilic catalytically active part of the enzyme (anchor function) (Maroux et al. 1975; Maroux and Louvard 1976; Pattus et al. 1976; Wacker and Semenza 1977; Brunner et al. 1978, 1979; Colbeau and Maroux 1978; Frank et al. 1978). In this case, the hydrophobic part of the protein is embedded within the hydrophobic matrix of the phospholipid bilayer. Such a mode of fixation makes it possible to understand a lateral migration of proteins in the membrane. Participation of the hydrophobic part in attachment of the enzyme to the phospholipid matrix of the membrane has been reported in a number of papers. Thus, it was found that the detergent form of pig intestinal aminopeptidase possessing a hydrophobic fragment is readily inserted into liposomes and forms a lipid–protein film at the water–air interface, whereas the trypsin form of the enzyme lacks this ability (Pattus et al. 1976). It has also been demonstrated that the rabbit small intestinal aminopeptidase and the sucrase–isomaltase complex as well as porcine renal aminopeptidase in their integral (detergent) forms interact with lecithin as a result of which stable lipoprotein complexes are formed (Wacker and Semenza 1977; Brunner et al. 1977).

Some investigators suggest a participation of the hydrophobic part of the enzyme in the transport of monomers formed during hydrolysis of oligomer (Maroux et al. 1973, 1975; Maroux and Louvard 1976; Louvard et al. 1976). However, the transport function of the enzyme's hydrophobic part has yet to be demonstrated, although there are no results dispelling this suggestion.

The function of the hydrophobic part of the enzyme seems to be much wider. Thus, we have demonstrated in our laboratory some vital functions of the hydrophobic part of hydrolytic enzymes and a particularly important one in the maintenance of optimal conformation of the enzymatically active hydrophilic part. This function was realized when comparing the kinetic properties of the Triton and trypsin forms of carbohydrases and alkaline phosphatase of the rat enterocytes and after complexing of the trypsin form of the enzymes with lecithin liposomes (Gozitte et al. 1976; Egorova et al. 1977; Ugolev et al. 1979b, c). Con-

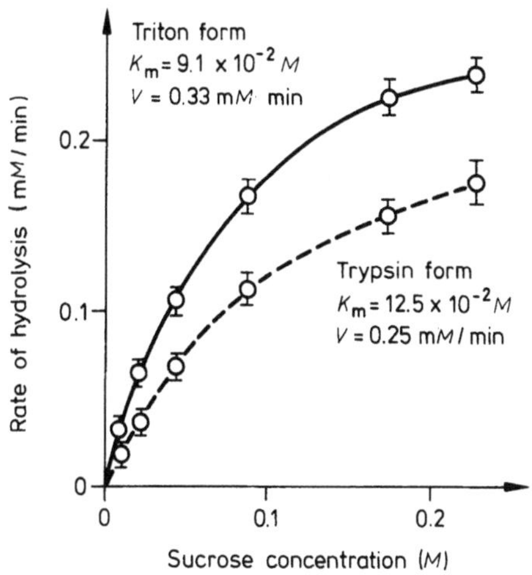

Fig. 8. Activity of the Triton and trypsin forms of sucrase at different substrate concentrations. UGOLEV et al. (1979 b)

version of the Triton form of the enzyme into the trypsin form or removal of the hydrophobic part have been shown to change the kinetic properties (Fig. 8). Thus, V for the Triton form of sucrase is higher than for the trypsin form and K_m is lower. For γ-amylase, K_m of the Triton form is also lower than for the trypsin form. It is important that the activity of the γ-amylase Triton form at low concentrations of substrate is higher and at high concentrations is lower than for the trypsin form. It follows from this that the hydrophobic part of the enzyme is essential for the maintenance of optimal conformation of its catalytic hydrophilic part.

The hydrophobic part of the enzyme also appears to stabilize its structure when exposed to the action of different factors. Thus, studying pH function of the rat small intestinal carbohydrases, it was found that the zone of high activity was wider for the Triton form of the enzymes than for the trypsin form. These findings are consistent with the observations of stabilization of enzymatic activity in the presence of ligands and during sorption on artificial or native membranes (for review see UGOLEV and KOLTUSHKINA 1975). It is assumed that the hydrophobic part binding the catalytic subunit to the membrane may change the properties of the hydrophilic part of the enzyme molecule in the same direction as the membrane does.

Finally, the hydrophobic part of the enterocyte membrane enzymes has been revealed to be important for their allosteric properties. The allosteric properties of the intestinal enzymes have been demonstrated in our laboratory in experiments with a selective disturbance of the regulatory sites of the intestinal enzymes without affecting the catalytic ones. Thus, in many cases, a separation of the hydrophobic part of the enzyme from the hydrophilic part resulted in a loss of sensitivity to some allosteric modifiers (GOZITTE et al. 1976; EGOROVA et al 1977; UGOLEV et al. 1979 b, c). After solubilization of γ-amylase and alkaline phosphatase by Triton X-100 the regulatory properties of these enzymes are maintained whereas solubilization by trypsin or papain leads to a loss of sensitiv-

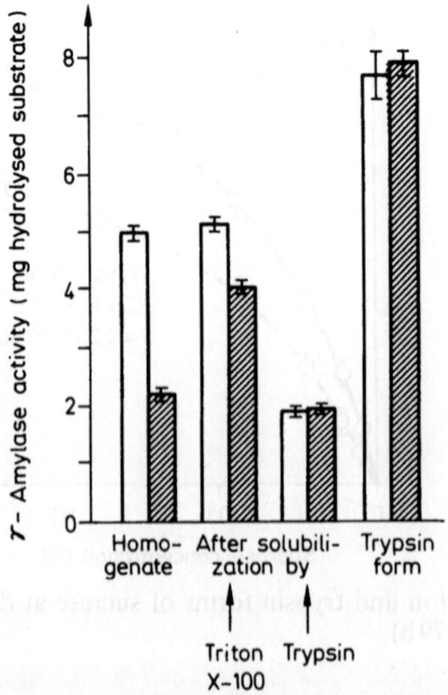

Fig. 9. The effect of tributyrine on γ-amylase activity of various preparations of the rat small intestine. UGOLEV et al. (1979 b) *Open bars* activity in the absence of a modifier; *hatched bars* activity in the presence of a modifier

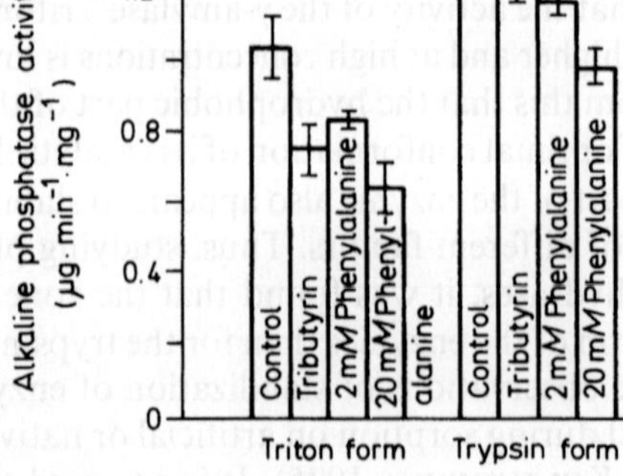

Fig. 10. The effect of modifiers on the activity of the Triton and trypsin forms of alkaline phosphatase. UGOLEV et al. (1979 b)

ity of the enzymes to the action of modifiers: complete in the case of γ-amylase and significant in the case of alkaline phosphatase (Figs. 9, 10). These data indicate that the catalytic and regulatory subunits of the small intestinal hydrolases are associated with the membrane of the enterocytes by two subsequent bonds: one sensitive to the action of proteases and another to the action of detergents. In this case, the regulatory part of the enzyme is assumed to be located between these two bonds (for review see UGOLEV 1972a), since the hydrophobic part of the enzyme is located between the zone of action of Triton X-100 and that of trypsin. Therefore, the conclusion can be drawn that the regulatory properties of the intestinal enzymes are largely accounted for by their hydrophobic parts (Fig. 11).

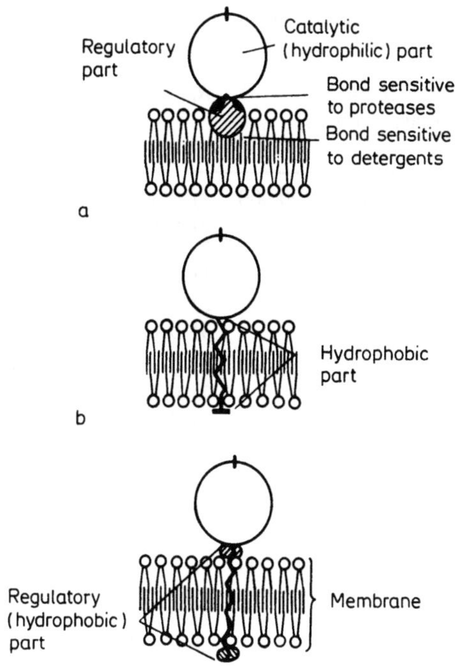

Fig. 11 a–c. Different models of microvillous enzymes. **a** original model of the enzyme with catalytic and regulatory parts; **b** model of MAROUX et al. (1975) in which no regulatory properties in the hydrophobic part of the enzymes are assumed; **c** scheme of the amphipathic enzyme in which regulatory properties are taken into account. UGOLEV et al. (1977 b)

IV. Characterization of Hydrolases [1]

Attention has already been given to some differences in the properties of highly purified microvillous enzymes (their detergent and protease forms). One may think that these differences reflect species adaptations of similar enzymes or different functional properties of various enzymes acting in the same membrane. However, it is not excluded that certain differences might be accounted for by nonidentity of purification procedures or other technical characteristics of experiments.

In order to demonstrate a relationship between the molecular structure of the enzymes and their properties depending on the functional and evolutionary differences and to give a deeper insight into the species pecularities of the functions of the hydrophobic part of the membrane integral enzymes, a cycle of experiments has been carried out in our laboratory under identical methodological conditions. A comparative study has been made of the properties of the Triton and trypsin

1 The authors of this section are Dr. H. Hütter (Institute of Clinical Biochemistry, Martin Luther University, Halle, German Democratic Republic), Dr. V. V. Egorova, Dr. A. A. Nikitina and Prof. A. M. Ugolev (Pavlov Institute of Physiology, Leningrad, U. S. S. R.)

Table 4. Characterization of the Triton and trypsin forms of alkaline phosphatase and alaninaminopeptidase of the dog and rabbit small intestine

Enzyme	Animal	Form of enzyme	Molecular mass (daltons)	R_f	K_m (mM)	V (U/l)	E_{act} (cal/mol)	pH optimum
Alkaline phosphatase	Dog	Triton	2,000,000–3,000,000	1) 0.00 2) 0.18 3) 0.29	0.143	62	7,500	9.0
		Trypsin	165,000	1) 0.00 2) 0.10 3) 0.17	0.710	100	5,600	8.5–9.0
	Rabbit	Triton	2,000,000–3,000,000	1) 0.00 2) 0.12 (weak) 3) 0.24 (weak) 0.43	0.072	37	9,350	9.0
		Trypsin		0.26	0.042	42	8,400	9.0
Alaninaminopeptidase	Dog	Triton	1,000,000–2,000,000	0.00	0.050	471	16,220	9.2
		Trypsin	295,000	0.444	0.021	719	14,860	8.85
	Rabbit	Triton	1,000,000–2,000,000	1) 0.00 2) 0.333 (weak)	0.017	169	19,220	8.7
		Trypsin	280,000	0.333			15,790	8.7

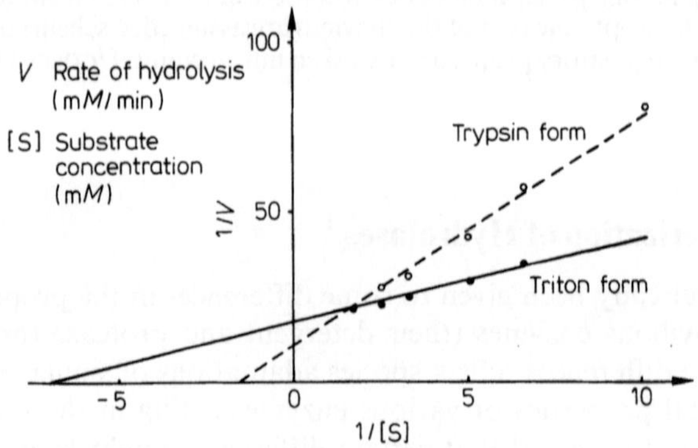

Fig. 12. Lineweaver–Burk plot for the Triton and trypsin forms of alkaline phosphatase in the dog small intestine

forms of the enterocyte brush border alkaline phosphatase and aminopeptidase in rabbits and dogs, two kinds of animals distinguished by their diet. The main results are summarized in Table 4 and in Figs. 12, 13, and 14. As can be seen, there are certain distinctions between the Triton and trypsin forms of both enterocyte enzymes in these animal species. (Identification of the detergent and protease forms of the enzymes by gel electrophoresis has confirmed the availability of each of these two forms.)

It is now recognized that the molecular mass of the hydrophobic part of alkaline phosphatase and aminopeptidase does not exceed 10,000 daltons. Theoretically, a similarity in the molecular masses of the Triton and trypsin forms might be expected. Nevertheless, significant differences have been revealed. In particular, the molecular mass of the trypsin form of alkaline phosphatase of the dog intestinal mucosa amounts to 165,000 and that of aminopeptidase somewhat less 300,000 daltons. (These data are not at variance with the results obtained by us and other investigators for some other animal species.) However, the molecular mass of the Triton form of enzymes proved to be unexpectedly large: $2–3 \times 10^6$ daltons for the rabbit and dog enterocyte alkaline phosphatase and $1–2 \times 10^6$ daltons for the intestinal aminopeptidase of the same animals. Such an abnormally high molecular mass may be interpreted as a result of association of molecules into aggregates, possibly owing to the interactions of hydrophobic parts, that is compatible with the absence of such an aggregation after separation of these parts from the whole enzyme molecule. A possibility of aggregation after dissociation of oligomeric enzymes was confirmed. Thus, after a purification of the maltase–glucoamylase complex of the rat small intestine, anomalously high molecular mass of fragments (134,000–480,000 daltons) has also been revealed following a dissociation of the complex with molecular mass 250,000–500,000 daltons (FLANAGAN and FORSTNER 1978). It was suggested that a monomer might be in an aggregated state. In this case, it is not a single polypeptide chain but a stable macromolecular aggregate.

In a few cases we were able to demonstrate that the presence of the hydrophobic part of the enzyme changes the properties of the hydrophilic part in the same direction as binding of the trypsin form of the enzyme-deprived hydrophobic part with the phospholipid bilayer (for reviews see UGOLEV and KOLTUSHKINA 1975; EGOROVA et al. 1977; UGOLEV et al. 1979c). In fact, in both instances a decrease in K_m was observed. Changes in V are also similar.

As for carbohydrases, alkaline phosphatase and aminopeptidase of the small intestine of the rat, it had earlier been demonstrated that separation of the hydrophobic part of the enzyme leads to an increase in K_m and in a number of cases to a decrease in V (GOZITTE et al. 1976; EGOROVA et al. 1977; UGOLEV et al. 1979c). However, the present study has shown that the influence of the hydrophobic part may be more variable depending on the animal species and the type of enzyme. In particular, a low value of K_m of alkaline phosphatase from rabbit small intestine compared with that of dogs attracts notice. Differences in V are of the same character but less marked.

In all the experiments, V for the trypsin form of dog enterocyte alkaline phosphatase is higher than for the Triton form, while values of V for both forms of rabbit small intestinal alkaline phosphatase are approximately equal. The K_m value for the trypsin form of this enzyme in dog small intestine is higher than for the Triton form. On the contrary, in rabbits, the K_m value of alkaline phosphatase of the enterocytes for the Triton form is higher than for trypsin. Thus, the presence of the hydrophobic part results in a decrease in K_m values for alkaline phosphatase of dog small intestine and an increase of this value in rabbits.

The effect of temperature on the enzymatic activity was investigated within the range 0 °–70 °C. Energy of activation was estimated by an Arrhenius plot. On the whole, the trypsin form of the small intestinal alkaline phosphatase and aminopeptidase of both animal species is characterized by a lower energy of activation than the Triton form. Along with this, in many cases the energy of activation of the Triton and trypsin forms of alkaline phosphatase of the rabbit small intestinal mucosa does not differ significantly. However, the differences between the Triton and trypsin forms of intestinal aminopeptidase in these animals seem essential. In this case, the trypsin form of the enzyme is characterized by lower energy of activation.

A determination of energy of activation gave unexpected results. Thus, it has been simultaneously shown that membrane-bound alkaline phosphatases of rabbit and dog small intestine possess a higher energy of activation. A more detailed analysis of the thermodynamic characteristics of the enzymes, particularly enthalpy and entropy, is possibly required. It should be noted, that membrane-bound and Triton forms of the enzymes are characterized by changes in a slope of the Arrhenius plot, suggesting conformational changes while the trypsin form has a constant energy of activation over the whole temperature range.

The influence of pH on the membrane-bound, Triton and trypsin forms of the small intestinal alkaline phosphatase of dogs and rabbits is illustrated in Figs. 13 and 14 where some distinctions are seen. Membrane-bound enzyme possesses a narrow zone of optimal values pH, although along with a decrease in the activity in the left side of the curve, an increase in resistance may be observed in the alkaline zone. The unexpected feature is a narrowing of the zone of optimal pH values as well as a shift in membrane-bound enzyme optimum activity toward a zone of nonphysiological values of pH.

The data obtained confirm the fact that the hydrophilic part of the enzymes carries enzymatic activity. In all the cases, certain differences were found in the catalytic properties of the Triton and trypsin forms. In particular, the kinetic characteristics of the enzymes vary after separation of the hydrophobic part. Furthermore, some characteristics of the Triton and trypsin forms have proved to be very close or identical, for example, the pH function for both forms of the enzymes of rabbit and dog small intestine.

Besides, the available evidence indicates that the hydrophobic part of the enzyme in all cases (in various animal species and different types of enzymes) not only performs an anchor function, but has a significant effect on the catalytic activity of the hydrophilic part. In other words, the hydrophobic part of the enzyme is a regulator of the catalytic properties. The same function is fulfilled by the matrix of the membrane with respect to membrane-bound enzymes. The properties and nature of the effects of the hydrophobic part of the enzymes are genetically determined. In contrast, the influence of the membrane on the enzymatic activity may vary with the change in the composition of the phospholipid bilayer.

The principle of doubling of functions, including the functions of regulation and control was developed by BARCROFT (1937). In the case of the control of enzymatic activity of membrane-bound enzymes, this principle holds true at the membrane level. Besides, there exist fundamental differences in the characterization of both controlling effects. The influence of the hydrophobic part, since it is determined by a definite structural gene is similar owing to the stereospecificity of matrix synthesis. The effect of the membrane depends on its composition which

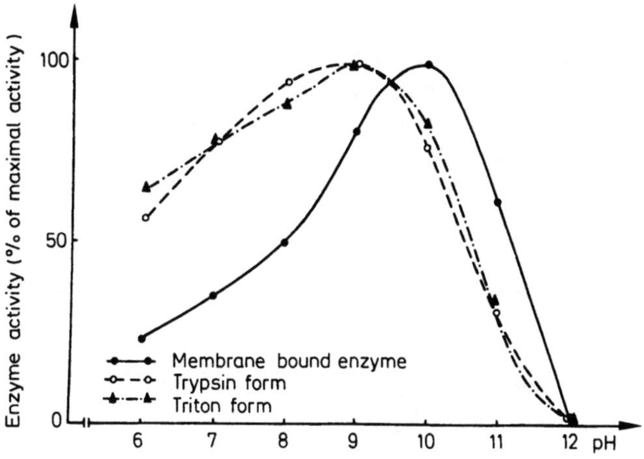

Fig. 13. The pH function of alkaline phosphatase of the dog small intestine

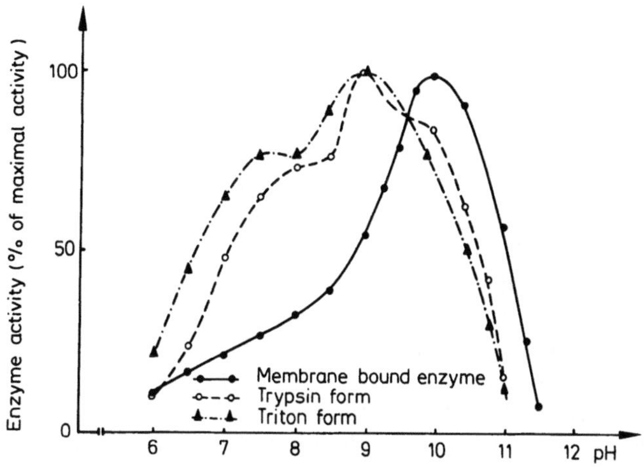

Fig. 14. The pH function of alkaline phosphatase of the rabbit small intestine

in turn may vary under different conditions, including a degree of saturation of phospholipid fatty acid residues. Thus, genotype information is realized in the hydrophobic part of the enzyme, whereas in the membrane matrix both genotype and phenotype information may be realized. The functions of the hydrophobic part, and the effects on the catalytic properties of the enzyme may change during evolution and species adaptation.

The information available suggests that the hydrophilic and hydrophobic parts of the membrane integral enzymes perform different functions. The external hydrophilic parts appear to fulfil predominantly catalytic functions and, possibly, those of receptors. The hydrophobic parts participate in: (1) maintenance of the optimal conformation of the hydrophilic part of the enzyme acting like a phospholipid matrix; (2) stabilization of enzyme structure; (3) realization of the regulatory function, either affecting the conformation of the hydrophilic fragments of the enzyme, in particular their regulatory sites, or being carriers for the regulatory sites; and (4) realization of anchor functions.

At present there is no adequate evidence, however, one may think that the hydrophobic parts of the membrane enzymes possibly have some other functions: (1) participation in the transport processes; (2) species and individual adaptations, a certain joint effect being reached by a combination of the effects of the phospholipid bilayer of the membrane and the hydrophobic part of the enzyme; and (3) a hypothetical transfer of signals through the membrane.

D. Characterization of the Transport of Free Monomers and Hydrolysis-Released Monomers

According to the classical two-stage scheme of function of the alimentary system in higher animals a release of monomers subjected to absorption occurs in the digestive lumen. Then, by convection and diffusion monomers reach the enterocyte surface where they come into contact with the transport systems of the apical membrane. A decrease in the rate and efficiency of the process in the metabolic chains by reason of diffusion in the digestive apparatus has recently been reinvestigated (UGOLEV et al. 1976b; SHNOL et al. 1979).

The discovery of membrane digestion has made possible the suggestion that spatial proximity of the enzyme and transport systems as parts of a single membrane surface of the enterocytes should lead to more intensive interactions between the final stages of hydrolysis and initial stages of transport (Fig. 15). Nevertheless, a certain loss in efficiency and rate can remain owing to diffusion.

For the last few decades, experimental investigations of the transport processes in the small intestine of higher animals and humans have revealed some characteristics of absorption of hydrolysis-released monomers compared with free monomers, which may seem paradoxical from the point of view of the classical concepts of digestive transport interactions.

This section will deal with a consideration of these characteristics in order to give a modern interpretation of the enzyme transport conveyors and, as far as

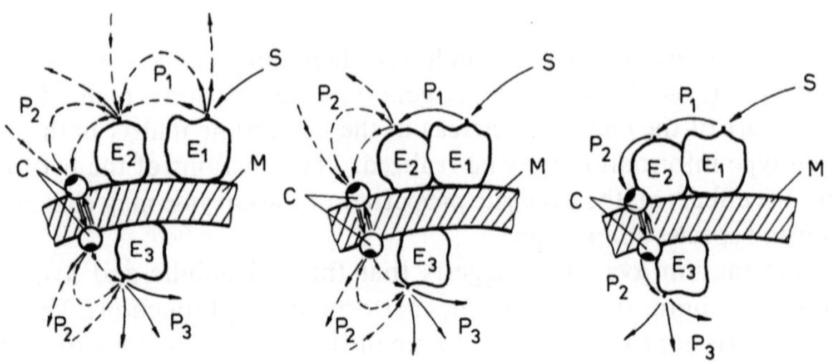

Fig. 15. Different types of transfer of reaction products along the enzyme transport chain. E_{1-3} enzymes; *S*, substrates; P_{1-3}, products; *C*, carriers; *M*, membrane; *broken line*, diffusion stages; *full line*, direct transfer of substances. UGOLEV et al. (1976b)

possible, to elucidate the molecular structure and principles of function of the enzyme transport complexes. Briefly, the essence of the phenomena discussed is that during absorption monomers released by hydrolysis gain advantages over free monomers. As will be shown, this is valid for both water-soluble (carbohydrate and protein hydrolysis products) and apparently for fat-soluble substances (in particular, triglyceride hydrolysis products).

The advantages of enzyme dependent transport are seen when comparing the rates of absorption of different oligomers and equivalent mixtures of constituent monomers. These advantages can be discovered by studying the kinetic properties of transport, e.g. K_m and V, competition for a common transport system and some other characteristics. Besides, differences in the transport mechanisms of monomers formed during hydrolysis and free monomers may be observed in studying the sensitivity of these processes to various modifiers, for example, to the action of phlorhizin, the presence of Na^+ as well as the composition of basic diets.

I. Comparison of the Rates of Absorption of Oligomers and Monomers

The experimental data indicating a facilitation and acceleration of absorption of hydrolysis-released monomers compared with free monomers are summarized in Tables 5 and 6. As can be seen, only in some studies were hexoses found to be absorbed more rapidly than equivalent amounts of corresponding di- and oligosaccharides (Table 5). In most cases di- and oligosaccharides are absorbed at the same or even higher rates than monosaccharides.

When these data were first obtained, they seemed unlikely and the possibility of artifacts could not be excluded. However, a comparison of the transport of hexoses from maltose, sucrose, trehalose, starch and other solutions with that of equivalent mixtures of monosaccharides was made using various techniques to minimize methodological errors. Such criteria were used as the rates of disappearance of substances from the small intestinal lumen, rates of accumulation of monomers in the intestinal tissues, and the rates of entry of absorbed substances into blood and serosal fluid bathing isolated preparations of the small intestine in vitro. Along with humans, many animal species including rat, hamster, rabbit, frog and toad have been investigated.

By now a great many comparisons of peptide and amino acid intestinal transport have been made (Table 6). As can be seen, in most cases transport of amino acids formed during hydrolysis of di- and oligopeptides is more rapid than that of equivalent amounts of the corresponding amino acids. A relationship between the rates of oligomer and monomer transport depends to a large extent on the concentration of substances in the fluid bathing the small intestinal mucosa. In a number of studies oligomers were absorbed more rapidly than monomers at higher initial concentrations of the respective substances.

Of particular interest is a comparison of the rates of transport of amino acids in the human small intestine from partial protein hydrolysates consisting predom-

Table 5. Rates of absorption of di-, oligo-, polysaccharides and equivalent corresponding monosaccharides in the animal small intestine

Substrate	Concentration	Absorptive period (min)	Transportable substance	Rate of absorption	Animal	Technique	Reference
Dextrose monohydrate	50.0 g	22.3	Hexose	139 mg/100 ml	Human	In vivo, study of the level of hexoses in blood after peroral loads by carbohydrates	DODDS et al. (1959)
Sucrose	45.4 g	21.2	Hexose	136 mg/100 ml			
Glucose	56.8 g	20.4	Hexose	134 mg/100 ml			
Starch incomplete hydrolysate	0.5%	60	Glucose	0.96 mg	Rat	In vitro, perfusion technique from FISHER and PARSONS (1949)	CHAIN et al. (1960)
Glucose	0.5%	60	Glucose	1.18 mg			
Sucrose	0.5%	60	Glucose	0.3 mg			
			Fructose	0.17 mg			
Glucose + fructose	0.5%	60	Glucose	0.57 mg			
			Fructose	0.06 mg			
Sucrose	800 mg	60	Glucose	200 mg	Rat	In vivo, study of the difference between substance perorally injected into the intestine and eliminated from it	DAHLQVIST and THOMSON (1963a)
			Fructose	112 mg			
Glucose + fructose	800 mg	60	Glucose	228 mg			
			Fructose	119 mg			
Maltose	800 mg	60	Glucose	271 ± 35 mg	Rat	In vivo, study of the difference between substance perorally injected into the intestine and eliminated from it	DAHLQVIST and THOMSON (1963b)
Trehalose	800 mg	60	Glucose	235 ± 27 mg			
Glucose	800 mg	60	Glucose	297 ± 19 mg			
Maltose	800 mg	180	Glucose	~800 mg			
Trehalose	800 mg	180	Glucose	~550 mg			
Glucose	800 mg	180	Glucose	~800 mg			
Starch	5%	15	Hexose	45 mg	Rat	In vivo, study of the level of hexoses in blood after an injection of	JEZUITOVA et al. (1965); UGOLEV
Maltose	5%	15	Hexose	76.1 ± 4.8 mg			
Glucose	5%	15	Hexose	75.4 ± 9.2 mg			

Sucrose	5%	15	Hexose	89.9 ± 5.8 mg		carbohydrates in the small intestine	(1968)
Glucose + fructose	5%	15	Hexose	51.0 ± 10.6 mg			
Lactose	5%	15	Hexose	25.7 ± 8.0 mg			
Maltose	200 mg-%	60	Glucose	53 ± 4 μg/ml	Frog	In vitro, perfusion technique from FISHER and PARSONS (1949)	PARSONS and PRICHARD (1965)
Glucose	200 mg-%	60	Glucose	66 ± 4 μg/ml			
Sucrose	2 g/kg body weight	120	Glucose	69 ± 3.9 mg-%	Human	In vivo, study of the level of hexoses in blood after peroral loads by carbohydrates	MACDONALD and TURNER (1968)
			Fructose	9.8 ± 1.25 mg-%			
Glucose + fructose	2 g/kg body weight	120	Glucose	8.1 ± 5.3 mg-%			
			Fructose	6.3 ± 0.54 mg-%			
Sucrose	2 g/kg body weight	120	Glucose	88 ± 3.8 mg-%	Human (women)		
			Fructose	8.4 ± 0.62 mg-%			
Glucose + fructose	2 g/kg body weight	120	Glucose	85 ± 5.8 mg-%			
			Fructose	4.8 ± 0.62 mg-%			
Maltose	90 g/70 kg body weight	90	Glucose	8.0 ± 11.1 mg-%	Human	In vivo, study of the level of glucose in blood after peroral loads by carbohydrates	MATTHEWS et al. (1968 a)
Glucose	90 g/70 kg body weight	90	Glucose	8.7 ± 9.1 mg-%			
Maltose	90 g/70 kg body weight	120	Glucose	7.9 ± 8.6 mg-%			
Glucose	90 g/70 kg body weight	120	Glucose	2.2 ± 7.7 mg-%			
Maltose	5.56 m*M*	15	Glucose	292 ± 24 μ*M*	Frog	In vitro, perfusion technique from FISHER and PARSONS (1949)	PARSONS and PRICHARD (1968)
Glucose	11.11 m*M*	15	Glucose	368 ± 22 μ*M*			
Maltose	5.56 m*M*	15	Glucose	98 ± 1 μ*M*			
Glucose	11.11 m*M*	15	Glucose	114 ± 2 μ*M*			
Maltose	0.2%	10	Glucose	106 ± 10 mg-%	Rat	In vitro, accumulating mucosal preparation from UGOLEV et al. (1970)	NOIM et al. (1970)
Glucose	0.2%	10	Glucose	46 ± 18 mg-%			
Maltose	0.2%	20	Glucose	187 ± 21.2 mg-%			
Glucose	0.2%	20	Glucose	228 ± 18 mg-%			
Maltose	0.2%	30	Glucose	196 ± 16 mg-%			
Glucose	0.2%	30	Glucose	236 ± 21 mg-%			

Table 5 (continued)

Substrate	Concentration	Absorptive period (min)	Transportable substance	Rate of absorption	Animal	Technique	Reference
Maltose	2.78 m*M*	At steady state	Glucose	111.2 ± 2.3 μmol h^{-1} g^{-1}	Frog	In vitro, perfusion of the intestine combined with vascular perfusion	PARSONS and PRICHARD (1971)
Glucose	5.56 m*M*		Glucose	175.1 ± 4.4 μmol h^{-1} g^{-1}			
Maltose	2.78 m*M*		Glucose	156.5 ± 1.3 μmol h^{-1} g^{-1}			
Glucose	5.56 m*M*		Glucose	175.0 ± 2.1 μmol h^{-1} g^{-1}			
Starch	200 mg-%	30	Glucose	102.7 ± 23.1 mg-%	Rat	In vitro, method of everted sac from WILSON and WISEMAN (1954); modification UGOLEV (1972a)	UGOLEV (1972a)
Maltose	200 mg-%	30	Glucose	287.7 ± 52.8 mg-%			
Glucose	200 mg-%	30	Glucose	177.6 ± 29.3 mg-%			
Starch	0.2%	60	Glucose	205 ± 37 mg-%	Rat	In vitro, accumulating mucosal preparation from UGOLEV et al. (1970)	UGOLEV (1972a)
Maltose	0.2%	60	Glucose	435 ± 31 mg-%			
Glucose	0.2%	60	Glucose	455 ± 38 mg-%			
Maltose	1 g/kg body weight	15	Glucose	48 ± 10 mg-%	Human	In vivo, study of the level of hexoses in blood after peroral loads by carbohydrates	RYBAKOVA et al. (1973)
Glucose	1 g/kg body weight	15	Glucose	47 ± 9 mg-%			
Maltose	1 g/kg body weight	30	Glucose	78 ± 18 mg-%			
Glucose	1 g/kg body weight	30	Glucose	80 ± 10 mg-%			
Maltose	1 g/kg body weight	60	Glucose	49 ± 24 mg-%			
Glucose	1 g/kg body weight	60	Glucose	53 ± 12 mg-%			
Glucose	50 g	60	Glucose	6,184 ± 592 mg-%	Human	In vivo, study of the level of hexoses in blood after peroral loads by carbohydrates	WAHLQVIST et al. (1978)
Pentasaccharide	50 g	60	Glucose	6,925 ± 330 mg-%			

Starch	50 g	60	Glucose	6,369 ± 319 mg-%			
Glucose	50 g	120	Glucose	4,388 ± 973 mg-%			
Penta-saccharide	50 g	120	Glucose	5,243 ± 561 mg-%			
Starch	50 g	120	Glucose	5,434 ± 750 mg-%			
Glucose	50 g	180	Glucose	4,223 ± 289 mg-%			
Penta-saccharide	50 g	180	Glucose	4,474 ± 222 mg-%			
Starch	50 g	180	Glucose	4,800 ± 99 mg-%			
Glucose	50 g	240	Glucose	4,392 ± 292 mg-%			
Penta-saccharide	50 g	240	Glucose	4,496 ± 84 mg-%			
Starch	50 g	240	Glucose	4,815 ± 52 mg-%			
Glucose	50 g	300	Glucose	4,583 ± 241 mg-%	Human	In vivo, study of the level of hexoses in blood after peroral loads by carbohydrates	Wahlqvist et al. (1978)
Penta-saccharide	50 g	300	Glucose	4,871 ± 102 mg-%			
Starch	50 g	300	Glucose	4,890 ± 50 mg-%			
Glucose	50 g	60	Glucose	7,590 mg-%			
Maltose	50 g	60	Glucose	7,306 mg-%			
Glucose	50 g	120	Glucose	6,218 mg-%			
Maltose	50 g	120	Glucose	4,163 mg-%			
Glucose	50 g	180	Glucose	5,100 mg-%			
Maltose	50 g	180	Glucose	4,700 mg-%			
Glucose	50 g	240	Glucose	5,213 mg-%			
Maltose	50 g	240	Glucose	4,710 mg-%			
Glucose	50 g	300	Glucose	5,273 mg-%			
Maltose	50 g	300	Glucose	4,980 mg-%			

Table 6. Rates of absorption of di-, oligopeptides and equivalent corresponding amino acids in the animal small intestine

Substrate (L-form)	Concentration (mM)	Absorptive period (min)	Transportable substance	Rate of absorption	Animal	Technique	Reference
Gly–Gly	3.75	30	Gly	64 ± 4.0 μM	Rat	In vitro, method of everted sac from WILSON and WISEMAN (1954)	NEWEY and SMYTH (1962)
Gly	7.55	30	Gly	54 ± 6.2 μM			
Gly–Gly	7.5	30	Gly	88 ± 2.0 μM			
Gly	15.1	30	Gly	94 ± 4.3 μM			
Gly–Gly	15.1	30	Gly	108 ± 5.0 μM			
Gly	30.2	30	Gly	130 ± 5.3 μM			
Gly–Gly	30.2	30	Gly	144 ± 12.0 μM			
Gly	60.4	30	Gly	162 ± 9.6 μM			
Gly–Gly–Gly	88	5	Gly	6.63 ± 0.48 μmol/cm	Rat	In vivo, tied loops of the small intestine	MATTHEWS et al. (1968b)
Gly–Gly	133	5	Gly	6.88 ± 0.44 μmol/cm			
Gly	267	5	Gly	4.24 ± 0.33 μmol/cm			
Met	25	10	Met	0.87 ± 0.33 μmol/cm	Rat	In vivo, tied loops of the small intestine	CRAFT et al. (1969)
Met–Met–Met	8.3	10	Met	0.99 ± 0.01 μmol/cm			
Met	50	10	Met	1.60 ± 0.07 μmol/cm			
Met–Met	25	10	Met	1.47 ± 0.13 μmol/cm			
Met	100	10	Met	2.42 ± 0.075 μmol/cm	Rat	In vivo, tied loops of the small intestine	CRAFT et al. (1969)
Met–Met	50	10	Met	3.42 ± 0.33 μmol/cm			
Met	150	10	Met	2.73 ± 0.22 μmol/cm			
Met–Met	75	10	Met	4.86 ± 0.36 μmol/cm			
Met	200	10	Met	3.43 ± 0.25 μmol/cm			
Met–Met	100	10	Met	5.69 ± 0.25 μmol/cm			
Gly	100	10	Gly	3.59 ± 0.06 μmol/cm			
Met + Gly	100	10	Met	2.86 ± 0.16 μmol/cm			
	+ 100		Gly	2.54 ± 0.12 μmol/cm			
Gly–Met	100	10	Met	3.43 ± 0.07 μmol/cm			
			Gly	2.81 ± 0.12 μmol/cm			
Met–Gly	100	10	Met	3.47 ± 0.14 μmol/cm			
			Gly	2.64 ± 0.14 μmol/cm			
Gly–Met	50	10	Met	2.52 ± 0.08 μmol/cm	Rat	In vivo, tied loops of the small intestine	MATTHEWS et al. (1969)
			Gly	2.45 ± 0.08 μmol/cm			

Met+Gly	50	10	Met	2.43±0.11 µmol/cm			
	+50		Gly	1.63±0.06 µmol/cm			
Gly−Met	100	10	Met	3.94±0.10 µmol/cm			
			Gly	3.53±0.12 µmol/cm			
Met−Gly	100	10	Met	3.97±0.14 µmol/cm			
			Gly	3.36±0.14 µmol/cm			
Met+Gly	100	10	Met	3.42±0.19 µmol/cm			
	+100		Gly	2.54±0.12 µmol/cm			
Gly−Met	150	10	Met	4.26±0.18 µmol/cm	Rat	In vivo, tied loops of the small intestine	Matthews et al. (1969)
			Gly	3.87±0.29 µmol/cm			
Met+Gly	150	10	Met	3.28±0.19 µmol/cm			
	+150		Gly	2.40±0.16 µmol/cm			
Met−Gly−Met	100	10	Met	5.48±0.30 µmol/cm			
			Gly	2.74±0.15 µmol/cm			
Met+Gly	200	10	Met	3.57±0.17 µmol/cm			
	+100		Gly	1.72±0.19 µmol/cm			
Met−Met	0.625	5	Met	3.6±0.16 µmol/g dry weight	Rat	In vitro, everted rings of the small intestine from Agar et al. (1954)	Cheng and Matthews (1970)
Met	1.25	5	Met	3.3±0.44 µmol/g dry weight			
Met−Met	1.25	5	Met	4.2±0.25 µmol/g dry weight			
Met	2.5	5	Met	5.0±0.83 µmol/g dry weight			
Met−Met	2.5	5	Met	6.8±0.44 µmol/g dry weight			
Met	5.0	5	Met	6.3±0.46 µmol/g dry weight			
Met−Met	5.0	5	Met	9.2±0.65 µmol/g dry weight			
Met	10.0	5	Met	7.8±1.30 µmol/g dry weight			
Met−Met	10.0	5	Met	11.4±0.60 µmol/g dry weight			
Met	20.0	5	Met	11.3±2.60 µmol/g dry weight			
Gly−Leu	50	55	Gly	114±17 µM	Human	In vivo, perfusion technique of the small intestine	Adibi (1971)
			Leu	298±20 µM			
Gly+Leu	50	55	Gly	67± 5 µM			
	+50		Leu	220±17 µM			
Gly−Leu	50	85	Gly	140±11 µM			
			Leu	327±32 µM			
Gly+Leu	50	85	Gly	101± 9 µM			
	+50		Leu	263±21 µM			
Gly−Gly	50	55	Gly	606±25 µM			
Gly	100	55	Gly	140±19 µM			
Gly−Gly	50	85	Gly	707±52 µM			
Gly	100	85	Gly	250±33 µM			

Table 6 (continued)

Substrate (L-form)	Concentration (mM)	Absorptive period (min)	Transportable substance	Rate of absorption	Animal	Technique	Reference
Met – Met	20	5	Met	21.5 ± 3.5 µmol/g per 5 min	Rat	In vitro, everted rings of the small intestine from AGAR et al. (1954)	CHENG et al. (1971)
Met	40	5	Met	15.6 ± 1.2 µmol/g per 5 min			
Met – Met	40	5	Met	26.2 ± 4.0 µmol/g per 5 min			
Met	80	5	Met	13.6 ± 3.2 µmol/g per 5 min			
Met – Gly	0.5	5	Met	1.0 ± 0.2 µmol/g per 5 min			
			Gly	0.5 ± 0.1 µmol/g per 5 min			
Met + Gly	0.5	5	Met	1.1 ± 0.1 µmol/g per 5 min			
	+ 0.5		Gly	0.7 ± 0.2 µmol/g per 5 min			
Met – Gly	1.0	5	Met	2.8 ± 0.2 µmol/g per 5 min			
			Gly	3.2 ± 0.6 µmol/g per 5 min			
Met + Gly	1.0	5	Met	2.8 ± 0.2 µmol/g per 5 min	Rat	In vitro, everted rings of the small intestine from AGAR et al. (1954)	CHENG et al. (1971)
	+ 1.0		Gly	1.9 ± 0.6 µmol/g per 5 min			
Met – Gly	2.0	5	Met	4.6 ± 0.7 µmol/g per 5 min			
			Gly	6.1 ± 1.1 µmol/g per 5 min			
Met + Gly	2.0	5	Met	4.4 ± 1.1 µmol/g per 5 min			
	+ 2.0		Gly	–			
Met – Gly	5.0	5	Met	7.0 ± 0.7 µmol/g per 5 min			
			Gly	6.7 ± 1.0 µmol/g per 5 min			
Met + Gly	5.0	5	Met	4.8 ± 0.4 µmol/g per 5 min			
	+ 5.0		Gly	1.9 ± 0.1 µmol/g per 5 min			
Met – Gly	10.0	5	Met	10.5 ± 0.04 µmol/g per 5 min			
			Gly	8.9 ± 0.8 µmol/g per 5 min			
Met + Gly	10.0	5	Met	6.0 ± 0.6 µmol/g per 5 min			
	+ 10.0		Gly	2.7 ± 1.0 µmol/g per 5 min			
Met – Met	100	10	Met	70.0 ± 4.8 µmol/g wet weight	Rat	In vivo, tied loops of the small intestine	LIS et al. (1971)
Met	200	10	Met	34.1 ± 1.8 µmol/g wet weight			
Met – Met	100	10	Met	61.1 ± 4.0 µmol/g wet weight	Polecat		
Met	200	10	Met	41.3 ± 4.4 µmol/g wet weight			
Met – Met	100	10	Met	44.0 ± 3.7 µmol/g wet weight	Rabbit		
Met	200	10	Met	34.9 ± 1.4 µmol/g wet weight			
Met – Met	100	10	Met	38.0 ± 2.2 µmol/g wet weight	Guinea-		
Met	200	10	Met	[illegible]	pig		

Met – Met	100	10	Met	107.0 ± 15.0 µmol/g wet weight	Mouse		
Met	200	10	Met	100.0 ± 3.0 µmol/g wet weight			
Glu – Glu	2.5	10	Glu	2.1 ± 0.43 µmol/g	Rat	In vitro, everted rings of the small intestine from AGAR et al. (1954)	BURSTON and MATTHEWS (1972)
Glu	5	10	Glu	1.9 ± 0.17 µmol/g			
Met – Glu	5	10	Glu	3.3 ± 0.66 µmol/g			
			Met	5.8 ± 0.58 µmol/g			
Met + Glu	5	10	Glu	0.35 ± 0.23 µmol/g			
	+ 5		Met	6.25 ± 0.65 µmol/g			
Lys – Glu	5	10	Glu	8.5 ± 1.6 µmol/g			
			Lys	15.0 ± 2.7 µmol/g			
Glu + Lys	5	10	Glu	5.2 ± 0.5 µmol/g			
	+ 5		Lys	5.6 ± 1.7 µmol/g			
Gly – Gly	50	35	Gly	57.2 mg/min per 30 cm	Human	In vivo, method of perfusion of the small intestine	COOK (1972)
Gly	100	35	Gly	43.5 mg/min per 30 cm			
Gly – Leu	10	60	Gly	8.72 ± 1.23 m*M*	Rat	In vitro, method of everted sac from WILSON and WISEMAN (1954) modification UGOLEV (1972 a)	SMIRNOVA and UGOLEV (1972)
Gly + Leu	10	60	Gly	4.44 ± 0.30 m*M*			
	+ 10						
Gly – Gly	10	60	Gly	14.9 ± 2.6 m*M*			
Gly	20	60	Gly	15.9 ± 1.8 m*M*			
Gly – Leu	3	5	Gly	5.84 ± 0.39 m*M*	Chicken	In vitro, accumulating mucosal preparation from UGOLEV et al. (1970)	KUSHAK et al. (1973)
Gly + Leu	3	5	Gly	4.60 ± 0.51 m*M*			
	+ 3						
Gly – Leu	3	30	Gly	9.19 ± 0.37 m*M*			
Gly + Leu	3	30	Gly	6.72 ± 0.50 m*M*			
	+ 3						
Gly – Leu	3	45	Gly	8.48 ± 0.49 m*M*			
Gly + Leu	3	45	Gly	7.44 ± 0.86 m*M*			
	+ 3						
Gly – Leu	3	60	Gly	7.65 ± 0.72 m*M*			
Gly + Leu	3	60	Gly	6.12 ± 0.76 m*M*			
	+ 3						
Gly – Val	11.48	5	Gly	14.47 ± 1.10 m*M*			
Gly + Val	11.48	5	Gly	5.78 ± 0.65 m*M*			
	+ 11.48						

Table 6 (continued)

Substrate (L-form)	Concentration (mM)	Absorptive period (min)	Transportable substance	Rate of absorption	Animal	Technique	Reference
Gly − Val	11.48	10	Gly	16.56 ± 1.35 mM			
Gly + Val	11.48 + 11.48	10	Gly	7.14 ± 0.44 mM			
Gly − Val	11.48	30	Gly	16.21 ± 1.83 mM			
Gly + Val	11.48 + 11.48	30	Gly	8.17 ± 0.96 mM			
Gly − Val	11.48	60	Gly	10.85 ± 1.44 mM			
Gly + Val	11.48 + 11.48	60	Gly	9.99 ± 0.21 mM			
Gly − Trp	0.24	15	Trp	19.03 ± 3.10 mM	Chicken	In vitro, accumulating mucosal preparation from UGOLEV et al. (1970)	KUSHAK et al. (1973)
Gly + Trp	0.24 + 0.24	15	Trp	29.70 ± 1.80 mM			
Gly − Trp	0.24	60	Trp	278.90 ± 14.70 mM			
Gly + Trp	0.24 + 0.24	60	Trp	571.40 ± 278.90 mM			
Gly − Leu	5	60	Leu	182 ± 17 μmol/g dry weight per 1 h	Frog	In vivo, perfusion of intestine in combination with vascular perfusion from ROBINSON (1970)	CHEESEMAN and PARSONS (1974)
			Gly	174 ± 16 μmol/g dry weight per 1 h			
Gly + Leu	10	60	Leu	123 ± 17 μmol/g dry weight per 1 h			
	+ 10		Gly	58 ± 8 μmol/g dry weight per 1 h			
Gly − Pro	10	At steady state	Gly	3.97 ± 0.43 μmol/g wet weight per 5 min	Rat	In vivo, perfusion technique of the small intestine	LANE et al. (1975)
			Pro	4.11 ± 0.45 μmol/g wet weight per 5 min			

Gly + Pro	10		Gly	3.05 ± 0.36 μmol/g wet weight per 5 min			
	+ 10		Pro	3.13 ± 0.35 μmol/g wet weight per 5 min			
Pro – Gly	10		Gly	2.06 ± 0.45 μmol/g wet weight per 5 min			
			Pro	2.09 ± 0.44 μmol/g wet weight per 5 min			
Pro + Gly	10		Gly	3.37 ± 0.18 μmol/g wet weight per 5 min			
	+ 10		Pro	3.63 ± 0.18 μmol/g wet weight per 5 min			
Gly – Leu	10	At steady state	Gly	172.8 ± 20.8 μmol/g dry weight per 1 h	Frog	In vivo, perfusion technique of the intestine in combination with vascular perfusion from Boyd et al. (1975)	Cheeseman and Parsons (1976)
			Leu	162.0 ± 12.2 μmol/g dry weight per 1 h			
Leu – Gly	10		Gly	115.1 ± 11.6 μmol/g dry weight per 1 h			
			Leu	133.8 ± 18.7 μmol/g dry weight per 1 h			
Gly + Leu	10		Gly	33.2 ± 3.7 μmol/g dry weight per 1 h			
	+ 10		Leu	106.0 ± 10.4 μmol/g dry weight per 1 h			
Gly – Leu	10	60	Gly	15.0 ± 1.4 m*M*	Rat	In vitro, accumulating mucosal preparation from Ugolev et al. (1970)	Smirnova (1978)
Gly + Leu	10 + 10	60	Gly	11.4 ± 0.7 m*M*			
Gly – Gly	10	60	Gly	20.7 ± 1.3 m*M*			
Gly	20	60	Gly	26.8 ± 1.1 m*M*			
Gly – Pro	10	60	Gly	16.4 ± 0.89 m*M*	Rat	In vitro, accumulating mucosal preparation from Ugolev et al. (1970)	Mooz et al. (1978)
Gly + Pro	10 + 10	60	Gly	17.6 ± 1.89 m*M*			
Pro – Gly	10	60	Gly	5.3 m*M*			
Pro + Gly	10 + 10	60	Gly	10.5 m*M*			

inantly of small peptides and from equivalent mixtures of amino acids, simulating these proteins. In this case, absorption of hydrolysis-released monomers was no less efficient than that of free monomers. Thus, MARRS et al. (1975) investigated an increase in α-amino nitrogen in the blood plasma of normal subjects 45 min after an ingestion of equivalent amounts of trypsin hydrolysate of casein and the mixture of amino acids simulating casein and found that an increase in α-amino nitrogen in blood plasma amounted to 31 μmol/l, and 23 μmol/l, respectively. Similar results have been obtained using a perfusion technique (SILK et al. 1975; for review see SILK 1977). Moreover, it has been demonstrated that some amino acids are absorbed at equal rates from both partial casein hydrolysates and equivalent mixtures of amino acids, while other amino acids (Phe, Lys, Glu, Ala, Ser, His, Gly, Asp) are absorbed more rapidly from casein hydrolysate.

A relationship of the rates of absorption of fat-soluble substances formed during hydrolysis and free substances is far less well investigated. However, judging from the publications available, triglycerides are absorbed faster than free fatty acids (BORGSTRÖM et al. 1951; LONG and BROOKS 1965; BARRY et al. 1966; for reviews see UGOLEV 1965, 1968, 1972a, 1974). These data would be difficult to account for by the widely accepted concept that the brush border enzymes of the enterocytes are not involved in the splitting of triglycerides to monoglycerides and fatty acids (for review see HOLDSWORTH and SLADEN 1979). However, membrane hydrolysis of triglycerides influenced by adsorbed pancreatic lipase and monoglyceride lipase of the brush border surface has been demonstrated in our laboratory in rats (CHERNYAKHOVSKAYA and UGOLEV 1969; for reviews see UGOLEV 1972a, 1974). Subsequently these results were confirmed by studies on humans (VALENKEVICH 1973; VALENKEVICH et al. 1978).

II. Factors Affecting the Relationship Between Oligomer and Monomer Transport

The relationship between the rates of absorption of oligomers and monomers varies greatly (Tables 5 and 6, Figs. 16 and 17). Thus, Figs. 16 und 17 illustrate different relationships between the rates of transport of free glucose and glucose formed during hydrolysis of maltose in the rat small intestine. These differences depend to a certain extent on the methodological approach. It is now realized that a relationship between enzyme-dependent and enzyme-independent transport is in some measure a physiological property of the enterocyte. In particular, the effectiveness of enzyme-dependent transport differs along the small intestine (MATTHEWS et al. 1971; UGOLEV 1972a; CRAMPTON et al. 1973). Figure 16 shows that after all the periods of incubation of everted segments of the rat small intestine, the transport of glucose from maltose was more rapid than from glucose alone in the upper and middle ileum. In more distal segments of the small intestine no changes were observed in transport of the two substances. Studies on peptide and amino acid transport in vivo in rats have revealed that the greatest differences in the transport of amino acids formed during hydrolysis of dipeptides and free amino acids are observed in the jejunum. These decrease distally and completely

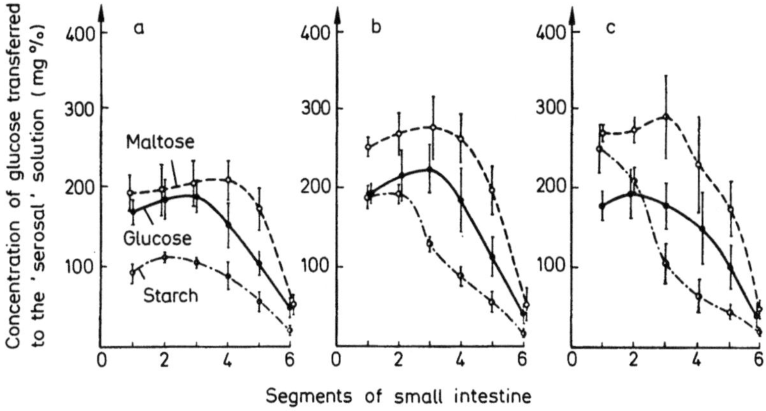

Fig. 16a-c. Transport of glucose, maltose and starch by different segments of the white rat small intestine after three subsequent incubations: 0–30 min (**a**); 30–60 min (**b**); 60–90 min (**c**). UGOLEV (1972a)

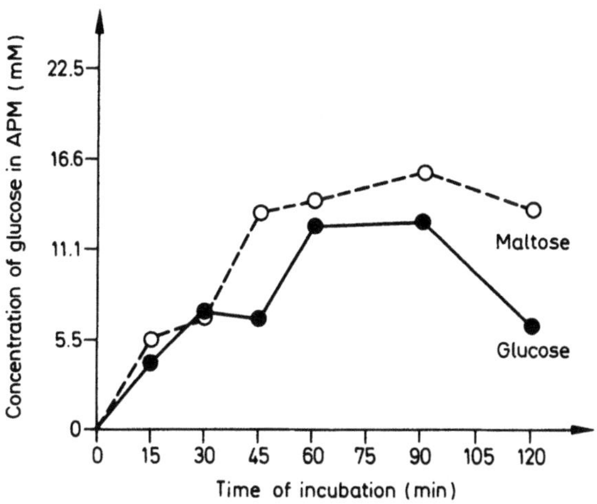

Fig. 17. Accumulation of glucose in accumulating preparation of mucosa (APM) during incubation in equivalent solutions of glucose and maltose. UGOLEV et al. (1976b)

disappear in the most distal segment of the ileum (MATTHEWS et al. 1971; CRAMPTON et al. 1973). Besides, duration of function of the small intestine in the experiment had a varied effect on the transport of oligomers and monomers. After prolonged incubations of the rat small intestinal segments in equivalent solutions of maltose and glucose one could observe a stimulation of maltose transport, while glucose transport had a tendency to decrease (Fig. 17).

There is a great deal of evidence that monomer transport defects may occur in some diseases of the small intestine (e.g. Hartnup disease), whereas oligomer transport remains unaffected (for reviews see MATTHEWS 1972, 1975a, b; MATTHEWS and ADIBI 1976). Thus, in most cases (but not always), absorption of hydrolysis-released monomers has an advantage over free monomers. A relationship between oligomer and monomer transport may change, depending on the functional state and topography of the small intestine and possibly on animal species. However, the techniques applied may be of some importance.

III. Kinetic Characteristics of Oligomer and Monomer Transport

There is no need to reemphasize that the intact enterocyte (and even more so, the intact intestinal mucosa) represents too complex a dynamic system to determine the true kinetic characteristics of the enzyme and transport systems of the apical membrane. Therefore, K_m and V (for transport systems K_t and J_{max}, respectively) are apparent and include a variety of distorting factors such as the presence or absence of convective flows, an increase or decrease in the thickness of unstirred layers in the proximity of the membrane surface or the effect of local pH (for reviews see Chaps. 20 and 21; UGOLEV 1972a; PARSONS 1976; LEVIN 1979; SCHULTZ 1979). However, differences found when comparing K_t and J_{max} for oligomer and monomer transport under the same experimental conditions, for theoretical reasons, depend to a great degree on the properties of the enzyme and transport systems of the enterocytes.

In most cases, when membrane hydrolysis and transport at the surface of the apical membrane of the brush border microvilli are functionally autonomous the main characteristics for oligomer and monomer transport should be the same

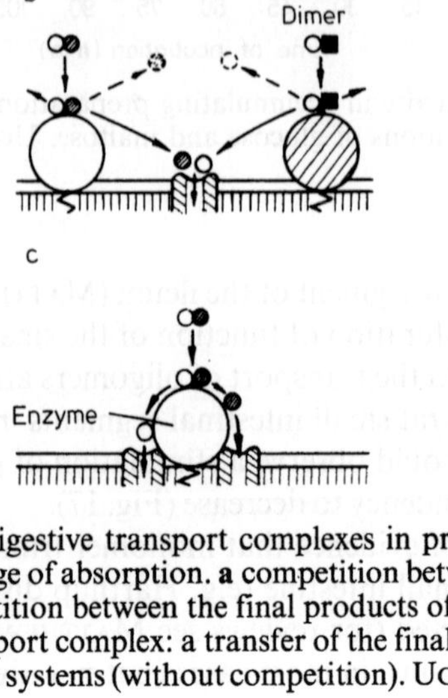

Fig. 18 a–c. Role of the digestive transport complexes in prevention of competition between monomers at the stage of absorption. **a** competition between monomers for the same transport system; **b** competition between the final products of hydrolysis for the transport system; **c** the enzyme transport complex: a transfer of the final products of hydrolysis from the enzyme to the transport systems (without competition). UGOLEV et al. (1976b)

Table 7. Kinetic characteristics of the transport of monosaccharides, free and released during disaccharide hydrolysis

Substrate	K_t	J_{max}	Animal	Technique	Reference
Maltose	0.45×10^{-3} *M*	71 µ*M*	Frog	In vitro, perfusion technique from FISHER and PARSONS (1949)	PARSONS and PRICHARD (1965)
Glucose	0.32×10^{-3} *M*	83 µ*M*			
Maltose	2.90 g/100 ml	0.59 g/min per 30 cm	Human	In vivo, method of intubation from SCHEDL and CLIFTON (1961)	MCMICHAEL et al. (1966); Data on glucose from HOLDSWORTH and DAWSON (1964)
Glucose	2.90 g/100 ml	0.59 g/min per 30 cm			
Lactose	2.15 g/100 ml	0.36 g/min per 30 cm			
Maltose	0.38 m*M*	86.7 µmol h^{-1} g^{-1}	Frog	In vitro, perfusion technique from FISHER and PARSONS (1949)	PARSONS and PRICHARD (1968)
Glucose	0.45 m*M*	137.0 µmol h^{-1} g^{-1}			
Maltose	0.45 m*M*	70.0 µmol h^{-1} g^{-1}	Toad		
Glucose	0.54 m*M*	76.0 µmol h^{-1} g^{-1}			
Trehalose	0.88 m*M*	204.0 µmol h^{-1} g^{-1}	Frog		
Glucose	0.83 m*M*	233.0 µmol h^{-1} g^{-1}			

(Fig. 18). However, as a result of direct estimations of K_t values and J_{max} for transport of some substances in experiments both in vitro and in vivo using different technical approaches it has been demonstrated that these constants for oligomer and monomer transport may differ significantly (Tables 7 and 8). Moreover, it can be seen that K_t is often lower (MATTHEWS et al. 1968b, 1969; PARSONS and PRICHARD 1968; CHENG et al. 1971; HIMUKAI et al. 1978), and J_{max} higher (MATTHEWS et al. 1968 b, 1969; CHENG et al. 1971; ADIBI and SOLEIMANPOUR 1974; ADIBI 1975) for oligomer transport compared with monomer transport.

The differences in kinetics of oligomer and monomer transport have been demonstrated not only in mammals, but also in the lowest vertebrates, in particular in amphibia (PARSONS and PRICHARD 1965, 1968). It is interesting that the relationship between K_t and J_{max} for transport of the two groups of substances may vary in such relatively close species of animals as frog and toad, suggesting an ecological dependence of the kinetic features for oligomer and monomer transport.

IV. Competitive Interactions Between Free and Hydrolysis-Released Monomers

When studying the transport of substances in the small intestine CORI (1925, 1926) paid attention to the fact that substances of similar structure (in particular, glucose and galactose) compete at the stage of absorption. It was later demonstrated for monosaccharides and amino acids that the most widespread observation is a competition for a common carrier (for reviews see CORI 1925; FISCHER and PARSONS 1953; WISEMAN 1964, 1968, 1974; SEMENZA 1968; UGOLEV 1972a; GRAY 1975; GUIDOTTI et al. 1978). Competition is especially powerful at high concentrations

Table 8. Kinetic characteristics of the transport of amino acids, free and released during oligopeptide hydrolysis

Substrate	Transportable substance	K_t	J_{max}	Animal	Technique	Reference
Gly	Gly	91 m*M*	5.5 µmol/cm per 5 min	Rat	In vivo, tied loops of the small intestine	MATTHEWS et al. (1968b)
Gly – Gly	Gly	328 m*M*	10.0 µmol/cm per 5 min			
Gly – Gly – Gly	Gly	260 m*M*	8.3 µmol/cm per 5 min			
Gly	Gly	233 m*M*	9.9 µmol/cm per 10 min	Rat	In vivo, tied loops of the small intestine	MATTHEWS et al. (1969)
Met	Met	66 m*M*	4.8 µmol/cm per 10 min			
Met – Met	Met	137 m*M*	7.1 µmol/cm per 10 min			
Gly – Met	Gly	62 m*M*	5.5 µmol/cm per 10 min			
Gly – Met	Met	88 m*M*	7.0 µmol/cm per 10 min			
Met – Met	Met	2.9 µmol/ml	14.2 µmol/g per 5 min	Rat	In vitro, everted rings of the small intestine from AGAR et al. (1954)	CHENG et al. (1971)
Met	Met	2.5 µmol/ml	9.7 µmol/g per 5 min			
Gly – Pro	Gly	1.43 m*M*	0.91 µmol cm^{-2} h^{-1}	Rabbit	In vitro, method of accumulation in tissue	RUBINO et al. (1971)
Gly	Gly	1.26 m*M*	0.86 µmol cm^{-2} h^{-1}			
Gly – Gly	Gly	43.3 m*M*	837 µmol/min per 15 cm	Human	In vivo, method of perfusion of the small intestine	ADIBI and SOLEIMANPOUR (1974)
Gly	Gly	42.7 m*M*	590 µmol/min per 15 cm			
Gly – Gly	Gly	3.4 m*M*	57.4 nmol cm^{-2} min^{-1}	Guinea-pig	In vitro, everted rings of the small intestine	HIMUKAI et al. (1978)
Gly	Gly	27.0 m*M*	290.0 nmol cm^{-2} min^{-1}			

of substances under conditions of saturation of the transport systems. Besides, competition can take place owing to limitations in the energy required for active transport (NEWEY and SMYTH 1964; SMYTH 1970; SCHULTZ 1979). Finally, allosteric competition for different sites of a common carrier has ben demonstrated, for example, during simultaneous transport of glucose and amino acids (for reviews see ALVARADO 1978; ALVARADO and ROBINSON 1979). Studies of all three types of mutual inhibition are important for analysis of the structural and functional features of intestinal transport.

For the understanding of differences in the transport mechanisms of hydrolysis-released and free monomers the analysis of competition for a common carrier is of particular importance. However, it happens that competition in the small intestine between monomers sharing the same carrier (e.g. between glucose and galactose, two neutral amino acids) is sharply decreased or completely avoided, if they are released by oligomer splitting during absorption. Formally, the point is that monomers competing in a free state do not compete for the same carrier if they make contact with the apical membrane of the enterocyte in the form of a dimer. For example, L-leucine is a strong inhibitor of glycine transport in the small intestine. In experiments in vitro using the everted sac technique, the rates of glycine uptake by the rat small intestine were compared in the case when there were equivalent amounts of glycine, mixtures of glycine and L-leucine and glycyl-L-leucine in the mucosal fluid (SMIRNOVA and UGOLEV 1972). As can be seen from Fig. 19, L-leucine in a mixture of free amino acids powerfully inhibits (by approximately 60%) absorption of glycine. However, the inhibition is considerably decreased if amino acids are transported from dipeptide solution. Similar phenomena have also been observed by other authors (MATTHEWS et al. 1969; CHENG et al. 1971; CHEESEMAN and PARSONS 1974, 1976; for reviews see MATTHEWS 1972, 1975a, b).

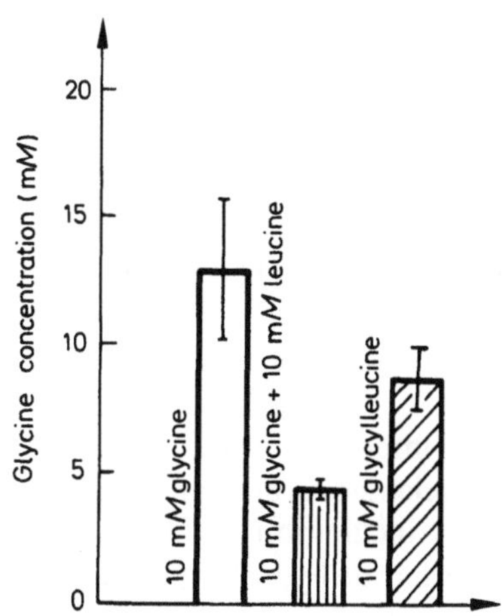

Fig. 19. The concentration of glycine in serosal fluid after 60 min incubation of the rat small intestinal segments in solution: 10 m*M* glycine; 10 m*M* glycine + 10 m*M* leucine; and 10 m*M* glycylleucine. UGOLEV et al. (1976b)

Moreover, competition will appreciably decrease if identical structurally similar molecules in the form of oligomers and monomers come simultaneously into contact with the surface of the intestinal mucosa. In particular, free monosaccharides have no effect on the transport of disaccharide-bound monomers (CRANE et al. 1970; MALATHI et al. 1973; RAMASWAMY et al. 1974) and amino acids on the transport of dipeptide-bound monomers (RUBINO et al. 1971; DAS and RADHAKRISHNAN 1974; CHEESEMAN and PARSONS 1974, 1976).

The presence of competitive inhibition is an important argument favouring the conclusion that the same transport system is used by monomers. It is logical to infer that the absence of competition between oligomers and monomers during the transport of oligomers consisting of monomers which generally compete in a free form implies independent transport pathways for free monomers and monomers formed by hydrolysis.

It may be assumed that the digestive transport conveyors (see Sec. E) provide separate flows of monomers through the apical membrane of the enterocytes and bring about a decrease in inhibition by the substrate external to a given conveyor. Of great importance is the circumstance that competition between substrates released within a single transport conveyor is practically absent or minimized.

V. Role of Na^+ in the Transport of Hydrolysis-Released and Free Monomers

After a demonstration in the pioneer studies (RIKLIS and QUASTEL 1958; CLARKSON and ROTHSTEIN 1960; CSÁKY and THALE 1960; CURRAN 1960; CSÁKY et al. 1961) that monosaccharide and amino acid intestinal transport is Na^+ dependent, this dependence was subjected to thorough experimental analysis (for reviews see WILSON 1962; WISEMAN 1964; CRANE 1968a, b, 1974, 1977; SEMENZA 1968; CSÁKY 1969; MÜLLER et al. 1972; ALVARADO and MAHMOOD 1974; ALVARADO 1976, 1978; MURER et al. 1978; REMKE et al. 1978; ALVARADO and ROBINSON 1979; LEVIN 1979; SCHULTZ 1979; CSÁKY and FISHER 1981).

At present there exist several hypotheses for the explanation of a coupling of the transport of Na^+ and organic substances in the small intestine. However, irrespective of interpretation, the basis for them provides a fundamental finding that elimination of Na^+ from the incubation medium in vitro results in almost complete inhibition of active transport. The elimination of Na^+ from the luminal solution in vivo does not significantly affect Na^+-dependent transport because it is mainly due to microcirculation of endogenous Na^+ (MOTHES and MÜLLER 1979).

Unexpected and highly important for the interpretation of the transport mechanisms for hydrolysis-released monomers and free monomers was evidence that removal of Na^+ from the incubation medium has little effect on the transport of glucose liberated by disaccharide hydrolysis in the hamster small intestine (RAMASWAMY et al. 1974; CASPARY 1972, 1976, 1978). Thus, enzyme-dependent transport does not require the presence of Na^+ and released glucose does not intermix with luminal glucose before entering the cell. More recently it has been demonstrated that the effect of Na^+ on the intestinal transport of dipeptides is insignificant compared with amino acids (CHEESEMAN and PARSONS 1974; 1976; HIMUKAI et al. 1978). This evidence testifies to the independence of transfer pathways of free and hydrolysis-released monomers across the apical membrane of enterocytes.

We have made an attempt to systematize the information available on the peculiarities of intestinal transport of hydrolysis-released monomers in comparison with free monomers. Numerous observations of high rates of absorption of hydrolysis-released monomers are in good agreement with the concept of membrane digestion. In accord with this concept, the systems responsible for liberation of transported products and those responsible for their transfer into the cell are brought close together at the membrane surface. However, a previous hypothesis on the enzyme and transport systems as closely interacting but not integrated has failed to account for phenomena of facilitation and acceleration of the enzyme-dependent transport.

The higher rates of amino acid transport from dipeptides have been interpreted in terms of the hypothesis of intact oligomer transport through the membrane of enterocytes by special transport systems, distinct from the transport systems for amino acids. This point of view is consistent with the fact that intestinal dipeptidases are predominantly located intracellularly and suggests that hydrolysis of dipeptides occurs after their transfer through the membrane. Many other properties of peptide transport (i.e. absence of competition between constituent amino acids as well as between amino acids and dipeptides etc.) are explicable in terms of this hypothesis. However, all the peculiarities of oligomer transport were also demonstrated for disaccharides for which the amount of intracellular hydrolases was insufficient. Moreover, as already mentioned, the active sites of intestinal carbohydrases are located on the outer surface of the apical membrane of the enterocytes. This suggests that monomers are being transferred across the membrane. Thus, difficulties in explaining many fundamental characteristics of oligomer transport may be encountered in studying dipeptides.

In order to explain how it happens that the monomers released by hydrolysis on the external membrane surface do not compete with each other and with free monomers during transport, one should assume that there exist independent transport systems for free monomers and the monomers released during membrane hydrolysis. The transport systems of the latter interact with the enzymes completing hydrolysis, allowing a differentiation to be made between the formed monomers and analogous free monomers available in the microenvironment. For this it is necessary to admit the existence on the apical membrane surface of enterocytes with special structures providing a direct transfer of hydrolysis products from the final enzyme to the transport sites. This structure, called the enzyme transport complex (for reviews see UGOLEV 1963, 1968, 1972a, 1974; UGOLEV et al. 1977c) will be discussed in Sect. E. It should be pointed out that enzyme-dependent transport or hydrolase-related transport has been considered from a somewhat different viewpoint in a number of studies (for reviews see CRANE 1968 a, b, 1975; 1977; MALATHI et al. 1973; RAMASWAMY et al. 1974, 1976; SEMENZA 1968; MEISTER 1973; MEISTER et al 1976, 1977).

E. The Enzyme Transport Complexes of the Apical Membrane of the Enterocytes

In the previous section, the characteristics of enzyme-dependent transport as compared with the transport of free monomers have been presented. We will now attempt to consider possible molecular and supramolecular structures of the enzyme transport complexes which could account for these characteristics. A consideration will first be made of data concerned with the transport of glucose released during membrane hydrolysis of di- and oligosaccharides for a number of reasons: (1) in contrast to many other cases of oligomer transport, it is established that glucose is released on the external surface of the apical membrane of the enterocytes; (2) glucose released by hydrolysis of poly- and oligosaccharides has the same conformation after entering into the aqueous phase as free glucose; (3) subcellular location and some properties of the transport system for glucose are known; and (4) many properties and some molecular characteristics of the enzymes releasing glucose during membrane hydrolysis of di- and oligosaccharides on the membrane surface of the enterocytes have been determined.

Figure 18 shows that if the final enzyme and transport system are located on the surface of the same membrane and transfer of hydrolysis products the transport system occurs by diffusion through the aqueous phase, then the transport of hydrolysis-released monomers will not be quantitatively different from that of free monomers. If the enzyme transport system (see Fig. 18c) is realized, when the final enzyme and transport system are spatially and functionally integrated, then it will be possible for a direct transfer of reaction products to the transport system to occur without their liberation into the aqueous phase. On the basis of this simplified scheme many pecularities of behaviour of hydrolysis-released monomers during transport can be accounted for. In particular, one can understand the high efficiency of such transport because of the absence of diffusion effects and loss of substances by dissipation in the aqueous phase. Since a spatial orientation of hydrolysis-released molecules is feasible competition between them can be prevented. As will be shown later in this section the hypothesis of the enzyme transport complex appears to hold for each supposed mechanism of transport: a mobile carrier, a carrier functioning by a change of conformation and, finally, a channel.

However, in order to explain many other properties of the enzyme-dependent transport in terms of the concept on the enzyme transport complex, an assumption should be made that its enzymatic and transport parts, allosterically interacting with each other, form a cooperative system. In this case an explanation could be given of the advantages gained by hydrolysis-released monomers during their transport and of the absence or decrease in competition between monomers and oligomers for a carrier.

A suggestion that the final enzyme and the carrier form an allosteric system is an expression of the universal mode of self-regulation at the molecular level. Along with the original concept of allosteric enzymes (MONOD et al. 1963, 1965; KOSHLAND et al. 1966; KOSHLAND and NEET 1968; KIRTLEY and KOSHLAND 1968; for reviews see ATKINSON 1970; KOSHLAND 1969, 1970; KURGANOV 1978), many properties of the transport system of the apical membrane of the enterocytes may be accounted for by the concept of allosteric regulation (ALVARADO and ROBINSON 1979). We have proposed the hypothesis of an allosteric system which combines enzymatic and transport elements of the membrane (for reviews see UGOLEV 1968; UGOLEV et al. 1977c, 1979a). There is a great deal of indirect evidence that the enzyme transport complex may exist and exhibit allosteric properties. In particular, during the last few years this suggestion has received convincing though indirect confirmation in both clinical and experimental observations. Many studies have demonstrated that most hydrolases of the enterocyte apical membrane are oligomers and have an amphipathic structure (see Sec. D). As already mentioned, French scientists have suggested that the hydrophobic part of these enzymes may perform transport functions.

It has been demonstrated in our laboratory that many microvillous enzymes are allosteric. Their regulatory sites have also been identified (for reviews see UGOLEV 1972a, UGOLEV et al. 1975a, b, 1977b, c, 1979b, c; EGOROVA et al. 1977). However, all these indirect arguments in favour of the possibility of allosteric effects within the enzyme transport complex were not substantiated until very recently.

I. Cooperative Interactions Between Enzymatic and Transport Parts

When the enzyme and transport system form a quaternary structure or cooperative system, there must be kinetic signs of such cooperativity. It is known that sigmoid kinetics is characteristic of allosteric enzymes and cooperative systems (for reviews see ATKINSON 1970; KOSHLAND 1970; CORNISH-BOWDEN 1976; KURGANOV 1978; TAKAGI and SASAKI 1979). On the contrary, functioning of noncooperative systems, and independent enzymes and carriers, may be described by a hyperbolic curve consistent with Michaelis kinetics (for reviews see ALVARADO 1976; NIKOLSKY 1977; ATKINS and GARDNER 1977; PRITCHARD and PORTEOUS 1977).

The typical hyperbolic curves have been obtained in our laboratory (UGOLEV et al. 1976c) in studying accumulation of free glucose in the rat small intestinal mucosa (Fig. 20). The behaviour of highly purified maltase, γ-amylase, and sucrase from the rat intestinal mucosa also follows Michaelis kinetics (UGOLEV et al. 1976 a; UGOLEV 1977, 1978). It could be suggested that attachment of enzyme to the phospholipid bilayer would result in transformation of the hyperbolic kinetics of the enzymatic action into a sigmoid form. However, as seen from Fig. 21, incorporation of enzymes into the lecithin liposomes increases their activity without affecting the form of the kinetics (UGOLEV and KOLTUSHKINA 1975). Analogous results were obtained for various microvillous enzymes of a different degree of purity (SEMENZA et al. 1965; for reviews see SEMENZA 1968; UGOLEV and KOLTUSHKINA 1975; ALVARADO 1976; ATKINS and GARDNER 1977). It should be emphasized that the absence of sigmoid kinetics does not exclude the presence of different types of cooperativities, although it makes it less likely.

A suggestion has recently been made and supported experimentally that a pronounced cooperativity of the enzyme transport complex requires undisturbed interactions between catalytic and transport parts of the complex. In fact, it has

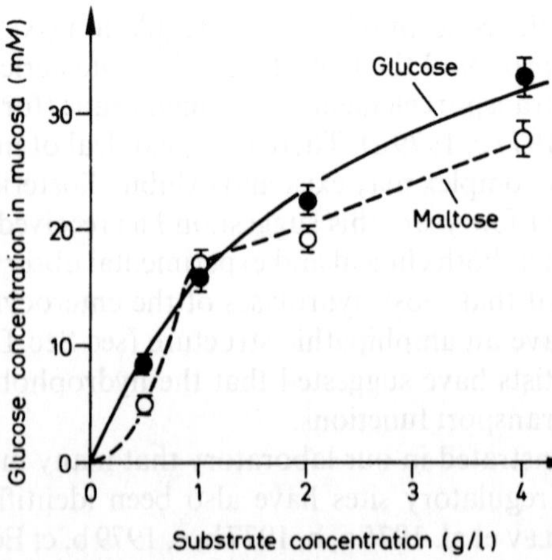

Fig. 20. Accumulation of glucose in the intestinal mucosa from glucose and maltose solutions at different concentrations. UGOLEV (1977)

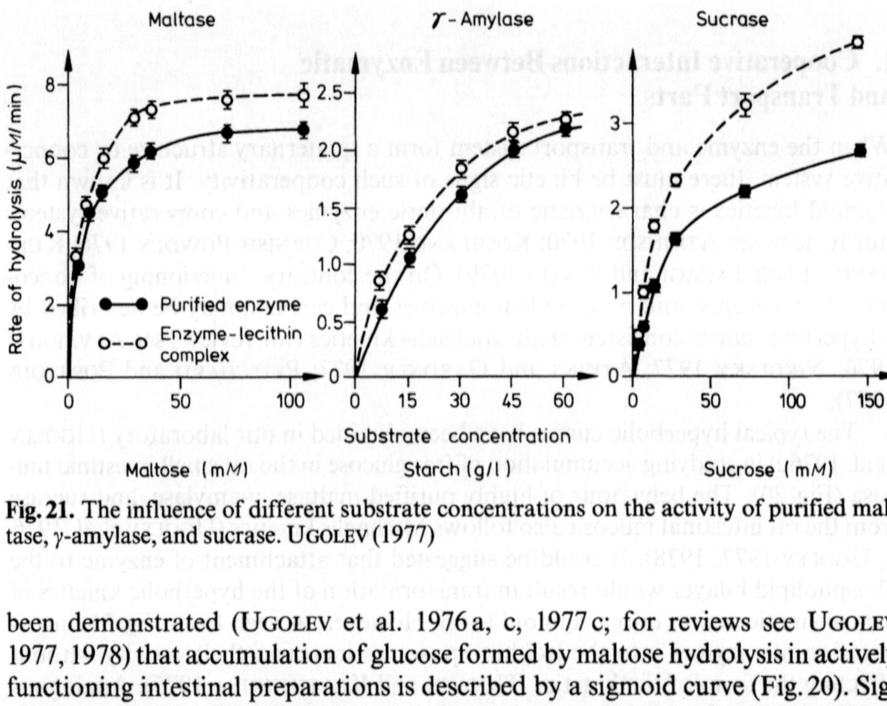

Fig. 21. The influence of different substrate concentrations on the activity of purified maltase, γ-amylase, and sucrase. UGOLEV (1977)

been demonstrated (UGOLEV et al. 1976a, c, 1977c; for reviews see UGOLEV 1977, 1978) that accumulation of glucose formed by maltose hydrolysis in actively functioning intestinal preparations is described by a sigmoid curve (Fig. 20). Sigmoid kinetics has also been found for accumulation of glucose formed by hydrolysis of other sugars (sucrose and starch). It is important that not only the kinetics of accumulation, but also that of hydrolysis of sugars is described by a sigmoid curve, if an interaction between the enzymatic and transport systems takes place (Fig. 22).

Switching off the active transport of glucose by substitution of oxygen for nitrogen, the sigmoid curves of carbohydrate hydrolysis are transformed into hyperbolic ones. Of greater importance is the transformation of sigmoid curves into

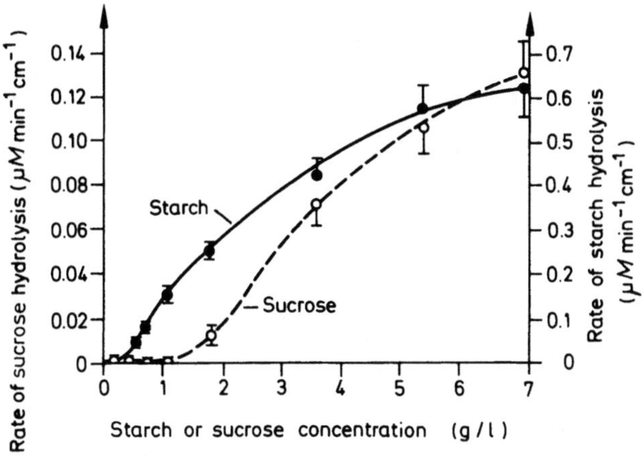

Fig. 22. The influence of different substrate concentrations on the activity of γ-amylase and sucrase from rat small intestine during active transport. UGOLEV et al. (1976 b)

hyperbolic ones under a specific blockage of the glucose transport system by phlorhizin (for reviews see UGOLEV 1977, 1978; UGOLEV et al. 1977 c). It was earlier demonstrated, by the group led by SEMENZA and independently by our group, that phlorhizin does not directly affect the activity of carbohydrases, in particular, sucrase and γ-amylase (for reviews see SEMENZA 1968; UGOLEV and GOZITTE 1972; UGOLEV 1972 a). These results may serve as direct proof of enzyme transport interactions of the allosteric type in the apical membrane of the enterocytes. These interactions may be expressed in the existence of positive cooperativities. Their possible functional importance will be discussed in Sect. E.II. The possibility of transforming sigmoid kinetics of hydrolysis into hyperbolic form by switching off the active transport indicates that any interpretation other than that proposed will be rather difficult.

II. Allosteric Interactions Between Enzyme and Transport Parts

A simpler scheme, taking into account both experimental data in favour of allosteric interactions between the enzyme and transport parts of the complex and the characteristics of the enzyme-dependent transport, is shown in Fig. 23. At rest, the active site of the enzyme and the carrier binding site are not congruent to their substrates. Thus, we extend the principle of induced fit proposed by Koshland for enzymes (KOSHLAND et al. 1966; KIRTLEY and KOSHLAND 1968; KOSHLAND and NEET 1968; for reviews see KOSHLAND 1969; 1970) to the functioning of carriers.

Figure 23 b illustrates that as a result of interactions between substrate and enzyme, in the molecule of the latter there occur conformational changes required for substrate binding. In particular this has been demonstrated for some hydrolases by combining X-ray structural analysis and subsequent computer analysis of closure of the cleft where the active site is located, at the moment of substrate binding (ANDERSON et al. 1979). It is assumed that at this step in the enzymatic reaction, or at the next one when the enzyme transport complex is being

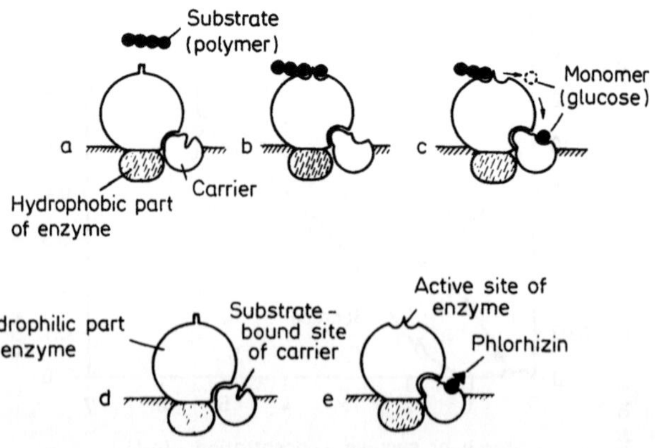

Fig. 23 a–e. A simplified scheme of allosteric interactions between the enzyme and transport parts of the complex. **a–c** allosteric effects of the enzyme on the transport system; **d, e** allosteric effects of the state of the transport system on the enzyme activity. **a** decreased affinity of the carrier contact site for hydrolysis product; **b, c** increased affinity of the carrier contact site for hydrolysis product; **d** less active state of the catalytic site of the enzyme; **e** more active state of the catalytic site of the enzyme. UGOLEV (1977)

formed, conformational changes in the enzyme molecule induce an allosteric fit of the carrier binding site (or opening of a channel, if we accept the channel hypothesis) to the reaction product (for reviews see UGOLEV 1977, 1978; UGOLEV et al. 1977c). The released product is transferred to the transport system which at that moment has a high affinity for it (Fig. 23b). Release of monosaccharide on the internal face of the enterocyte membrane (in cytoplasm) leads to a return of the system to the initial state. It appears that "transported product–carrier" complex is capable of maintaining, by a feedback mechanism, a conformation of the enzyme molecule which differs from that at rest. The studies already described with phlorhizin lend support for this suggestion.

Figures 23d and 23e show how the changes in kinetics of the enzyme (γ-amylase of the enterocytes) occur as a result of attachment of phlorhizin to an actively functioning transport system. As can be seen, attachment of phlorhizin (a powerful substrate-like inhibitor of transport) to the carrier contact site (Fig. 23d) induces conformational changes in the active site of the enzyme. Therefore, affinity of the carrier for hydrolysis product manifests itself at a certain stage of the enzymatic cycle. Since there exist definite relationships between conformations of enzyme and carrier, although the enzyme itself is insensitive to phlorhizin, sensitivity to it may arise due to an integration with the actively functioning transport system. Thus, the state of the transport system may also exert an allosteric effect on the catalytic activity of the enzyme. The hypothesis proposed offers various opportunities for interactions between enzyme and transport parts of the enzyme transport complex of the apical membrane of the enterocytes.

The molecular interpretation of such a system will be presented in Sect. E.III. It should be pointed out that the model proposed is based on two important concepts of modern molecular biology and membranology: (1) the concept of induced fit; and (2) the concept of allosteric interactions. We have made some essential additions. It is necessary to admit that in a given heterologous complex, an interaction takes place between the elements of different functional importance: enzyme and carrier. It is also necessary to assume the existence of two types of induced fit: direct or isosteric induction and allosteric induction. There seem to exist systems which may be induced by both means or by one of them. The suggestion that the structural fit of the transport part of the complex to its substrate may only be induced by the enzyme rather than as a result of direct contact with substrate permits one to explain how molecules released during hydrolysis within the enzyme transport complex can be distinguished from identical molecules present in free form in the surrounding medium.

A number of important implications follow from the foregoing. A slight competition which may sometimes be observed between hydrolysis-released and free monomers seems to occur in the independent transport system, but not within the limits of the enzyme transport complex (Fig. 24). Furthermore it becomes clear why under some forms of pathology of the small intestine, e.g. Hartnup disease, the transport of hydrolysis-released amino acids may be maintained while the transport of free amino acids is disturbed. We assume that in this case, amino acid transport is accomplished only by those carriers which are involved in peptidase transport complexes. Since these carriers are induced only during splitting of the

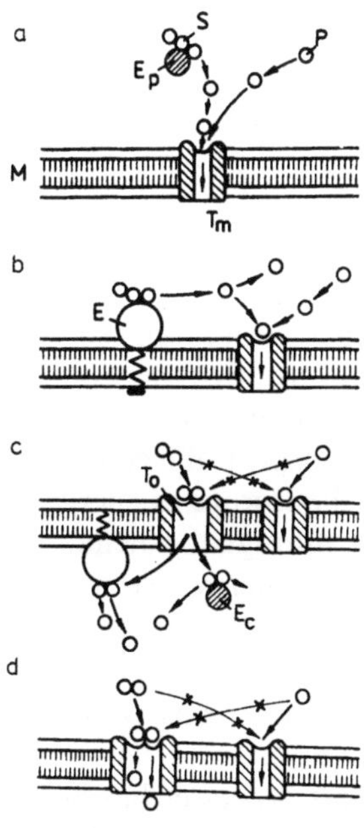

Fig. 24 a–d. Different spatial and functional interactions between the enzyme and transport systems of the membrane. **a** luminal digestion (enzyme-independent transport); **b** independent systems of hydrolysis and transport; **c** intracellular hydrolysis of dimers; **d** enzyme-dependent transport (enzyme transport complex); *M*, membrane; E_p, pancreatic enzyme; *S*, substrate; *P*, reaction product; *E*, membrane enzyme; E_c, cytosol enzyme; T_m, transport system for monomers; T_o transport system for oligomers

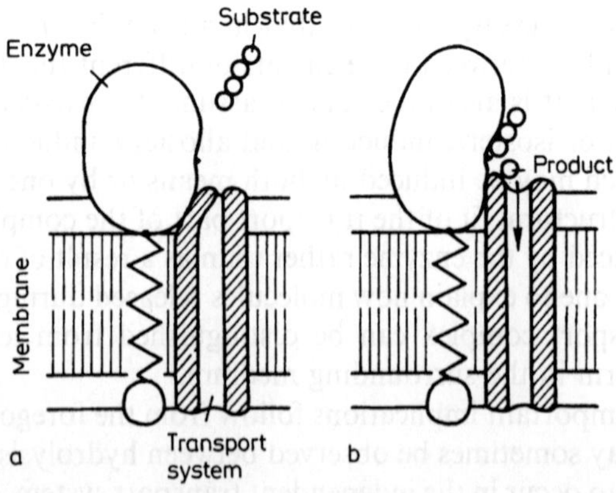

Fig. 25 a, b. A scheme of induction of a channel in the phospholipid bilayer of the membrane during activation of the enzyme by a substrate. **a** enzyme transport complex at rest; **b** enzyme transport complex in the active state

corresponding oligopeptides they are efficient only for amino acids released within a functioning enzyme transport complex.

The analysis of possible principles of the function of enzyme transport complexes led to the conclusion that membrane-bound hydrolases are regulators of cell permeability for under their actions the actively transported molecules are formed directly on the absorptive surface of the enterocytes. At the same time, for the transport systems, these hydrolases serve as allosteric regulators, ensuring induction of their affinity for a transported substrate (Fig. 25). Finally, one more point cannot be neglected. The enzyme transport cooperativities may play a role not only in induced permeability, but also in energizing the transport system within the enzyme transport complex.

Three basic hypotheses have been proposed to account for the mechanism of transformation and conservation of free energy in biological systems: (1) chemical coupling; (2) chemiosmotic coupling; and (3) conformational coupling. In the first case, the energy of the transport of electrons is stored in high energy bonds of ATP. In the second case, the storage of energy occurs as a result of a transfer of ions, in particular protons, through the membrane. In the third case, which has been less thoroughly studied, the energy is stored as conformational changes from low to high energy states. The latter hypothesis postulates a subsequent transformation of the energy of conformational change into ATP energy as a result of phosphorylation of ADP or into the energy of membrane charge by transfer of cations, or as structural changes.

The energizing of transport processes has been described in a number of reviews (Chap. 8; Biological Membranes 1975; Intestinal Ion Transport 1976; RACKER 1976; Biochemistry of Membrane Transport 1977; CRANE 1977; ATKINSON 1977; CAULSON et al. 1978; WILSON 1978; CASTILLO et al. 1979).

The hypothesis set for by us from the foregoing consists in the possibility of transduction of the energy released from hydrolysis of peptide and glucosidic bonds in substrate molecules and initially accumulated as conformational changes of the enzyme on the carrier. This energy is supposedly sufficient for transfer of substances into the cell. It is also possible that in this case a coupled transfer of ions through the membrane will take place.

III. Possible Molecular Models

We have presented the characteristics of enzyme-dependent transport and the abstract model of the system which is able to provide such a transport. The question arises: what kind of molecular structure is capable of realizing the processes we have represented as a functional model? One complexity of the solution of this problem is caused by the possibility of several interpretations of the enzyme transport complex.

1. The complex may comprise one molecule of rather complex structure. In this cases one part of the molecule will fulfil enzymatic and another transport functions.
2. The enzyme transport complex may be an oligomer. As a transport system the channel between subunits may be used, closing or opening as a result of conformational changes in the active site of the enzyme in the course of enzymatic cycle. It is possible that in this case, on changing the conformation of an enzyme, each reaction product will enter its own channel. This model reminds one a little of SINGER'S (1977) model of the membrane with a channel for the transport of ions.
3. The complex can be formed as a supramolecular structure in which an interaction occurs between active enzymatic and transport proteins. It is this case that is represented in our scheme, although it is not obligatory.

The next two models are based on the supposition that during activation of the enzyme by a substrate a temporary channel is induced. Two versions can be assumend: (1) a channel is formed between the subunits of the oligomer molecule; (2) a channel is induced in the phospholipid bilayer as a result of transposition of constituent molecules. Each of the molecular schemes considered has definite advantages. Therefore it is not exluded that for various substances, and possibly for a single substance in specific animal cells, different molecular structures of the enzyme transport complex may be realized.

IV. The Permeome

Transport processes in the small intestine are the result of the structural and functional integration of membrane hydrolytic enzymes and transport systems, including a source of energy. In recent years, in a number of branches of biology and medicine consideration of systems in terms of their integration with other systems has acquired an increasing popularity. Thus, geneticists along with the notion "gene" use a term "genome". In ecology and general biology along with the notion "organism" and "population" a term "biome" is used for geological, climatic and biological components forming an integrated structure.

For a designation of the smallest aggregate of molecules responsible for a certain physiological process, in this case for a transfer of substances through the

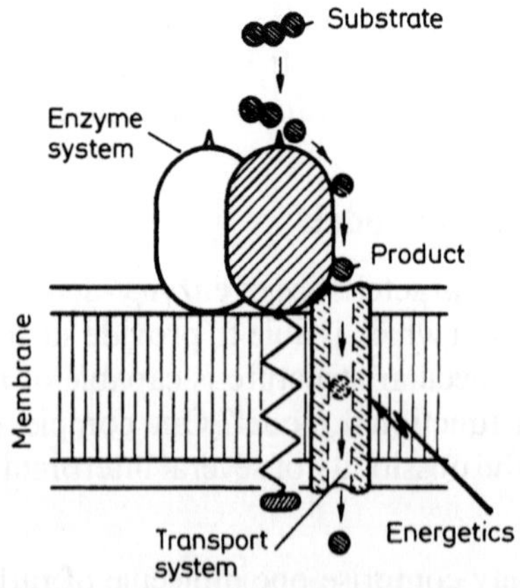

Fig. 26. A scheme of the permeome of the apical membrane of the enterocyte. UGOLEV (1977)

membrane, the term "ergome" (UGOLEV 1977) has been introduced. Many fundamental properties are characteristic of the whole ergome rather than its separate elements. Therefore the task of studying structure and function at the level of the ergome under normal and pathological conditions seems very important.

Such ideas have a definite prehistory. Many membrane enzymes are so unlike the relatively simple enzymes of the ribonuclease type that one may wish to introduce a special term for them. For example, SEMENZA (1968) proposed the term "hyphezyme". However, the fact is that membrane hydrolysis is coupled with transport and is accomplished by neither enzymes nor hyphezymes, but by a higher level structure, comprising an enzyme as one of its elements. For the understanding of the process occurring at this level a new notion "ergome" has been introduced; then the ergomes participating in the transport should be called "permeomes" with an indication of the substrate transferred. In other words, there exist glucose, sucrose, maltose, lactose and other permeomes. Permeomes provide not only transfer of substances, but in a number of instances (e.g. in the case of sucrose, maltose and lactose permeomes) the integration of transport with the process of splitting.

A typical permeome of the enterocyte membrane consists of enzymatic and transport systems (Fig. 26). A complex enzyme has an oligomeric structure and, as a rule, more than one active site. The active sites of the enzymes may be homologous (maltase) or heterologous (sucrase). In the latter case the enzyme possesses an active site splitting sucrose and a site splitting maltose. Each subunit of the enzyme consists of hydrophilic and hydrophobic parts, performing not only catalytic, but also regulatory functions.

Many properties of the permeome are determined by its usual membrane component. Finally, the permeome involves an energy source. It is important that the permeome hypothesis may account for a number of physiological processes, for example, transfer of substances through the membrane, including their transformation. Thus, when a release of monomers from oligomers in the small intestine precedes transport through the apical membrane of the enterocytes, explanation of the peculiarities of the process requires one to postulate the existence of enzyme transport complexes in which the formation and transport of substances are integrated. In order to describe the main features of enzyme-dependent transport and its advantages over the transport of free monomers one must take into account that the enzyme transport complex should possess the following features: (1) a transfer of hydrolysis products from the enzyme onto the transport part of the complex should occur without their liberation into the aqueous phase; (2) the transport part of the complex must have a high affinity for analogous molecules present in the microenvironment; (3) the enzyme and transport parts of the complex must form a cooperative system with direct and reversed allosteric effects.

At present the data available are insufficient to give an adequate molecular interpretation of the function of the enzyme transport complex. However, knowledge of the principles of its operation at this stage allows for a better understanding and prediction of many characteristics of enzyme-dependent transport under normal and pathological conditions.

As a confirmation of the important role of enzymes in transmembrane transfer of substances one may take the model experiments in which, during incorporation of a purified sucrase–isomaltase complex into black phospholipid membranes impermeable to sucrose and fructose, an increase in permeability is observed for sucrose hydrolysis products, but not for free glucose and fructose (STORELLI et al. 1972).

In conclusion it should be noted that participation of membrane-bound γ-glutamyltranspeptidase has been demonstrated in transmembrane transfer of oligopeptides, and possibly amino acids, through the intestinal mucosa. This possibility has been shown in a number of studies, including those by MEISTER and his co-workers (for reviews see MEISTER 1973; MEISTER et al. 1976, 1977; PRUSINER et al. 1976.

F. Conclusion

Let us attempt to summarize the current views on the role and peculiarities of integration of the enterocyte membrane systems responsible for the final stages of hydrolysis of different food substances and subsequent transport of released products; in other words, the systems of membrane hydrolysis and transport. There seem to exist several mechanisms of the enzyme transport interactions which vary from substrate to substrate, from tissue to tissue and among different animal species, ensuring in the last case species and ecological specialization. The main types of interaction between the enzymatic and transport processes have already been described and can be summarized as: (1) transport of oligomers through the membrane with subsequent hydrolysis to monomers inside the cell; and (2) hydrolysis of oligomers which precedes transmembrane transfer of formed monomers. In the second case hydrolysis and transport may be realized by means of functionally independent structures and a transfer of hydrolysis products to the cell occurs by diffusion. However, in a number of cases the existence of special integrated supramolecular structures – the enzyme transport complexes – has been demonstrated on the surface of the apical membrane of the enterocytes. Then no loss of substances nor reduction in the rate of transmembrane transfer of hydrolysis products occurs by diffusion and the enzyme and transport parts of the complex interact as a cooperative system. This mode of assimilation of nutrients appears to be most highly adopted and efficient.

In fact, a comparison of the mechanisms of the enzyme transport interactions in bacteria and higher animals leads to a realization that enzyme transport complexes of the membrane have, in the course of evolution, largely or completely superseded all other mechanisms of interaction between hydrolytic and transport processes. This is not surprising if we take into account that in higher animals the proportion of enterocytes to the total number of cells in the organisms amounts to approximately 10^{-5}. In other words, to meet the requirements of the organism an enterocyte has to provide some 100,000 cells with energy and structural material.

It should be emphasized that the processes of membrane hydrolysis and transport ensure not only an effective transition from the stage of transformation to that of translocation, but also a reliable protection of the internal medium from penetration of heterologous substances. The fact that the fundamental hydrolysis products, at least in higher forms of living organisms, are monomers, in particular monosaccharides and amino acids, may be interpreted from different points of view. These forms of nutrients have adequate transport systems both in the enterocyte membranes and somatic cell membranes. However, there is another, possibly more important circumstance. Monomers are the main elements which participate in different types of metabolism, including the processes of energy generation and protein synthesis. In view of the efficiency of the evolutionary process one cannot ignore the fact that one of its manifestations is an identity of utilized monomeric forms as the fundamental elements of intermediate metabolism.

I. Adaptability and Regulation of the Enzyme Transport Complexes

In this chapter the characteristics of enzyme-dependent transport have been demonstrated. The scope of this work did not permit us to consider one of the most important properties of such a mechanism: its dynamics and adaptability. These properties have been discussed at length in many reviews (UGOLEV 1972a; DOWLING and RIECKEN 1974; UGOLEV 1975, 1976; Development of Mammalian Absorptive Processes 1979).

There exist several mechanisms producing changes in the rate of absorption of the final products of the hydrolysis of nutrients by enterocytes as a result of changes in the activity of membrane hydrolases. The latter may in turn be accounted for by variations in synthesis and degradation of intestinal enzymes. Besides, as many key enzymes of the apical membrane of the enterocytes are allosteric, their levels of activity may be controlled by allosteric regulation. Owing to this regulation, after natural polysubstrate feeding at every site of the gastrointestinal tract, treatment of one or more (but not all) ingested substrates occurs. As a consequence, at the molecular level a definite temporal and spatial sequence (along the small intestine) of hydrolysis and absorption of the components of complex food mixture takes place. It is important that many products of membrane hydrolysis are allosteric (or isosteric) inhibitors of the enzymes releasing them. This mechanism ensures a feedback maintenance of constant hydrolysis rates, the activity of the hydrolytic system of the membrane not exceeding the maximal activity of the transport system. Finally, disturbances in the regulatory properties of intestinal enzymes have been demonstrated under some forms of experimental and clinical pathology.

In contrast to rapid adaptations at the level of enzyme activity, adaptations at the level of their synthesis and degradation occur less rapidly. However, even in this case the effects are observed in a few hours or perhaps days (for review see UGOLEV 1972a, ULSHEN and GRAND 1979). Essential changes in hydrolysis and transport of different types of food polymers occur owing to adaptive synthesis of the enzymes controlled by both the food composition and hormonal mechanisms (i.e. direct substrate and mediator effects). Such changes have been demonstrated in more detail during the transition of different animals from milk to definitive nutrition (for reviews see UGOLEV 1972a; DOWLING and RIECKEN 1974; Development of Mammalian Absorptive Processes 1979) as well as when the proportions of proteins, fats and carbohydrates in the food of adult animals are changed (for reviews see UGOLEV 1972a; DOWLING and RIECKEN 1974; ULSHEN and GRAND 1979). At present, however, there are strong arguments suggesting that changes in the relationships of different types of enzymes are associated not only with the induction or repression of their synthesis, but also with intensification or deterioration of their degradation (DAS and GRAY 1970; ALPERS and GOODWIN 1971; ALPERS 1972, 1977; ULSHEN and GRAND 1979; MCNURLAN and GARLICK 1980). The mechanism of control at the stage of degradation of enzymes is not yet fully clarified. However, it has been recently shown that some hormones, in particular, cholecystokinin, are able to bring about a solubilization of enzymatic and transport elements of the apical membrane of the enterocytes (NIKITINA et al. 1979).

II. The Enzyme Transport Complexes of the Membrane in Pathology

In various forms of pathology, disturbances in absorption may be induced by changes in the synthesis of membrane hydrolases. Numerous deficiencies of membrane carbohydrases, especially inherent and acquired lactase deficiencies are now well known. Deficiencies of other carbohydrases are more rarely observed. The genetic, biochemical and gastroenterological characteristics of the defects in hydrolysis and transport are presented in a number of reviews (UGOLEV 1972a; MILNE 1974). Disturbances in the final stages of protein hydrolysis have also been revealed.

Enzymatic deficiencies should be considered as a specific malabsorption as a consequence of membrane maldigestion. A special case is Hartnup disease in which the capacity of the enterocytes for absorption of free amino acids, including phenylalanine is lost. At the same time the capacity for absorption of analogous amino acids in the form of di- and oligopeptides is fully or largely retained (for reviews see MATTHEWS 1972, 1975a, b). This problematical form of pathology was initially interpreted as proof of a transmembrane transfer of unsplit dipeptides. However, it has received a new explanation in terms of the peculiarities of function of the enzyme transport complexes of the enterocyte membrane. This hypothesis has been developed by PARSONS and UGOLEV (for reviews see UGOLEV 1972a; Peptide Transport and Hydrolysis 1977).

III. Concluding Remarks

However complex the metabolic chains of living systems may be, two fundamental types of element can be distinguished: (1) transformational, when the molecular structure of the substrate is changed; and (2) transport, when a molecule is transferred from one site to another. However effective the mechanisms providing for the processes of transformation and transport may be, perfection of metabolic chains is on the whole impossible without an effective transition from one process to another. From this point of views one begins to understand the important and unique features of interactions between enzyme and transport systems of membranes which have been analysed in this chapter for the example of the apical membrane of the enterocytes. These features may be of general biological significance.

References

Adibi SA (1971) Intestinal transport of dipeptides in man: relative importance of hydrolysis and intact absorption. J Clin Invest 50:2266–2275

Adibi SA (1975) Dipeptide absorption and hydrolysis in human small intestine. In: Matthews DM, Payne JW (eds) Peptide transport in protein nutrition. North-Holland, Amsterdam, pp 147–166

Adibi SA, Soleimanpour MR (1974) Functional characterization of dipeptide transport system in human jejunum. J Clin Invest 53:1368–1374

Agar WT, Hird FJR, Sidhu GS (1954) The uptake of amino acids by the intestine. Biochim Biophys Acta 14:80–84

Alpers DH (1972) Protein synthesis in intestinal mucosa: the effect of route of administration of precursor amino acid. J Clin Invest 31:167–173

Alpers DH (1977) Protein turnover in intestinal villus and crypt brush border membranes. Biochem Biophys Res Commun 75:130–135

Alpers DH, Goodwin C (1971) Effect of size and anatomic location on the degradation rate of intestinal brush border proteins. Gastroenterology 60:760 (Abstr)

Alpers DH, Solin M (1970) The characterization of rat intestinal amylase. Gastroenterology 58:833–842

Alvarado F (1976) Sodium transport: a re-evaluation of the sodium-gradient hypothesis. In: Robinson JWL (ed) Intestinal ion transport. Medical and Technical Publishing, Lancaster, pp 117–152

Alvarado F (1978) Resolution by graphical methods of the equations for allosteric competitive inhibition and activation in Michaelian enzyme and transport systems. Application to the competitive inhibition of glucose transport in brain by phlorizin and phloretin. J Physiol (Paris) 74:633–639

Alvarado F, Mahmood A (1974) Contransport of organic solutes and sodium ions in the small intestine: a general model. Amino acid transport. Biochemistry 13:2882–2890

Alvarado F, Robinson JWL (1979) A kinetic study of the interactions between amino acids and monosaccharides at the intestinal brush-border membrane. J Physiol (London) 295:457–475

Anderson CM, Zucker FH, Steiz TA (1979) Spacefilling models of kinase clefts and conformation changes. Science 204:375–381

Antonowicz I (1979) The role of enteropeptidase in the digestion of protein and its development in human fetal small intestine. In: Development of mammalian absorptive processes. Ciba Found Symp 70: 169–183

Ashworth CT, Luibel FJ, Stewart SC (1963) The fine structural localization of adenosine triphosphatase in the small intestine, kidney and liver of the rat. J Cell Biol 17:1–18

Asp N-G (1971) Small-intestinal β-galactosidases. Characterization of different enzymes and application to human lactase deficiency. Studentenliteratur, Lund

Atkins GL, Gardner ML (1977) The computation of saturable and linear components of intestinal and other transport kinetics. Biochim Biophys Acta 468:127–145

Atkinson DE (1970) Enzymes as control elements. In: Boyer PD (ed) The enzymes, vol 1. Structure and control. Academic, New York, pp 461–489

Atkinson DE (1977) Cellular energy metabolism and its regulation. Academic, New York

Babkin BP (1927) External secretion of digestive glands (in Russian). Gosizdat, Moscow

Babkin BP (1960) Secretory mechanism of digestive glands (in Russian). Medgiz, Leningrad

Bangham AD (1972) Lipid bilayers and biomembranes. Annu Rev Biochem 41:753–776

Barcroft DK (1937) Basic character of the architecture of physiological functions (in Russian). Biomedgiz, Moscow

Barrnett RJ (1959) The demonstration with the electron microscope of the end-products of histochemical reactions in relation to the fine structure of cells. Exp Cell Res [Suppl] 7:65–89

Barry RJC, Jackson MJ, Smyth DH (1966) Handling of glycerides of acetic acid by rat small intestine in vitro. J Physiol (London) 185:667–683

Bauman VK (1977) Absorption of divalent cations (in Russian). In: Physiology of absorption. Nauka, Leningrad, pp 152–222

Benz R, Fröhlich O, Läuger P (1977) Influence of membrane structure on the kinetics of carrier-mediated ion transport through lipid bilayers. Biochim. Biophys Acta 464:465–481

Bergelson LD (1975) Biological membranes (in Russian). Nauka, Moskow

Bernard CL (1877) Leçons sur la diabete et la glycogenese animale. Baillière, Paris

Bierry H (1912) Saccharose spaltende Fermente. Biochem 44:415–425

Billington T, Nayudu PRV (1976) Studies on the brush border membrane of mouse duodenum. II. Membrane protein metabolism. J Membr Biol 27:83–100

Billington T, Nayudu PRV (1978) Studies on the brush border membrane of mouse duodenum: lipids. Aust J Exp Biol Med Sci 56:25–29

Booth AG, Kenny AJ (1976) Proteins of the kidney microvillus membrane. Identification of subunits after sodium dodecyl sulphate/polyacrylamide gel electrophoresis. Biochem J 159:395–407

Borgström B (1974) Fat digestion and absorption In: Smyth DH (ed) Intestinal absorption. (Biomembranes, Vol 4 A). Plenum, London, pp 555–620

Borgström B (1977) Digestion and absorption of lipids. In: Crane RK (ed) Gastrointestinal physiology II. (International review of physiology, Vol 12). University Park Press, Baltimore, pp 305–323

Borgström B, Dahlqvist A (1958) Cellular localisation, solubilization and separation of intestinal glycosidases. Acta Chem Scand 12:1997–2006

Borgström S, Borgström B, Rottenberg M (1951) Intestinal absorption and distribution of fatty acids and glycerides in the rat. Acta Physiol Scand 25:120–139

Borgström B, Dahlqvist A, Lundh G, Sjövall J (1957) Studies of intestinal digestion and absorption in the human. J Clin Invest 36:1521–1536

Borochov H, Shinitzky M (1976) Vertical displacement of membrane proteins mediated by changes in microviscosity. Proc Natl Acad Sci USA 73:4526–4530

Boullin DJ, Crampton RF, Heading CE, Pelling D (1973) Intestinal absorption of dipeptides containing glycine, phenylalanine, proline, β-alanine or histidine in the rat. Clin Sci Mol Med 45:849–858

Boyd CAR, Cheeseman CI, Parsons DS (1975) Amino acid movements across the wall of anuran small intestine perfused through the vascular bed. J Physiol (London) 250: 409–429

Bradfield JRG (1950) The localization of enzymes in cells. Biol Rev 25:113–157

Braun H, Cogoli A, Semenza G (1977) Carboxyl group at the two active centers of sucrase-isomaltase from rabbit small intestine. Eur J Biochem 73:437–442

Bredderman PJ, Wasserman RH (1974) Chemical composition, affinity for calcium, and some related properties of the vitamin D dependent calcium-binding protein. Biochemistry 13:1687–1694

Bresler SE, Bresler VM (1974) On liquid-cristalline structure of biological membranes (in Russian). Dokl Akad Nauk SSSR 214:936–939

Bretscher A, Weber K (1978) Localization of actin and microfilament-associated proteins in the microvilli and terminal web of the intestinal brush border by immunofluorescence microscopy. J Cell Biol 79:839–845

Bretscher MS, Raff MC (1975) Mammalian plasma membranes. Nature 258:43–49

Brindley DN (1974) The intracellular phase of fat absorption. In: Smyth DH (ed) Intestinal absorption. Plenum, London, pp 621–672

Brown WR (1978) Relationships between immunoglobulins and the intestinal epithelium. Gastroenterology 75:129–138

Brunner J, Hauser H, Semenza G, Wacker H (1977) Incorporation of pure hydrolases isolated from brush border membrane in single-bilayer lecithin vesicles. In: Semenza G, Carafoli E (eds) Biochemistry of membrane transport, FEBS – symposium 42. Springer, Berlin Heidelberg New York, pp 105–113

Brunner J, Hauser H, Semenza G (1978) Single bilayer lipid-protein vesicles formed from phosphatidylcholine and small intestinal sucrase-isomaltase. J Biol Chem 253:7538–7546

Brunner J, Hauser H, Braun H, Wilson KJ, Wacker H, O'Neil B, Semenza G (1979) The mode of association of the enzyme complex sucrase-isomaltase with the intestinal brush border membrane. J Biol Chem 254:1821–1828

Burston D, Matthews DM (1972) Intestinal transport of dipeptides containing acidic and basic L-amino acids and a neutral D-amino acid. Clin Sci 42:4 P

Burston D, Marrs TC, Sleisenger MH, Sopahen T, Matthews DM (1977) Mechanisms of peptide transport. In: Peptide transport and hydrolysis. Ciba Found Symp 50: 79–98

Cajori FA (1933) The enzyme activity of dog's intestinal juice and its relation to intestinal digestion. Am J Physiol 104:659–668

Carraway KL (1975) Covalent labeling of membranes. Biochim Biophys Acta 415:379–410

Caspary WF (1972) Evidence for a sodium-independent transport system to glucose derived from disaccharides. In: Heinz E (ed) Na-linked transport of organic solutes. Springer, Berlin Heidelberg New York, p 99

Caspary WF (1976) Jonic dependence of glucose transport from disaccharides. In: Robinson JWL (ed) Intestinal ion transport. MTP Press London, pp 153–154

Caspary WF (1978) Disaccharide hydrolysis and absorption. In: Varro V, Balint GA (eds) Current views in gastroenterology. Hung Soc Gastroenterol, Budapest, pp 103–104

Castillo Del LF, Mason EA, Viehland LA (1979) Energy-barrier models for membrane transport. Biophys Chem 9:111–120

Cathala G, Brunel C, Chappelet-Tordo D, Lazdunski M (1975) Bovine kidney alkaline phosphatase. Purification, subunit structure, and metalloenzyme properties. J Biol Chem 250:6040–6045

Caulson RA, Herbert JD, Hernandez T (1978) Energy for amino acid absorption, transport and protein synthesis in vivo. Comp Biochem Physiol [A] 60:13–20

Chain EB, Mansford KRL, Pocchiari F (1960) The absorption of sucrose, maltose and higher oligosaccharides from the isolated rat small intestine. J Physiol (London) 154:39–51

Chapman D (1974) Biological membranes. In: Smyth DH (ed) Intestinal absorption. Plenum, London, pp 123–158

Chapman D, Wallach DFH (eds) (1976) Biological membranes vol 3. Academic, London

Chappelet-Tordo D, Fosset M, Iwatsubo M, Gache C, Lazdunski M (1974) Intestinal alkaline phosphatase. Catalytic properties and half of the sites reactivity. Biochemistry 13:1788–1795

Cheeseman CI, Parsons DS (1974) Intestinal absorption of peptides. Peptide uptake by small intestine of Rana pipiens. Biochim Biophys Acta 373:523–526

Cheeseman CI, Parsons DS (1976) The role of some small peptides in the transfer of amino nitrogen across the wall of vascularly perfused intestine. J Physiol (London) 262:459–476

Cheng B, Matthews DM (1970) Rates of uptake of amino acid from L-methionine and the peptide L-methionyl-L-methionine by rat small intestine in vitro. J Physiol (London) 210:37P–38P

Cheng B, Navab F, Lis MT, Miller TN, Matthews DM (1971) Mechanisms of dipeptide uptake by rat small intestine in vitro. Clin Sci 40:247–259

Chernyakhovskaya MYu, Ugolev AM (1969) Localization of the final stages of tributyrine hydrolysis in the epithelial small intestinal cells (in Russian). Dokl Akad Nauk SSSR 187:701–703

Cherry RJ (1976) Protein and lipid mobility in biological and model membranes. In: Chapman D, Wallach DFH (eds) Biological membranes, vol 3. Academic, London, pp 47–102

Clark SL (1961 a) Alkaline phosphatase of the small intestine studied with electron microscope in suckling and adult mice. Anat Rec 139:216

Clark SL (1961 b) The localization of alkaline phosphatase in tissues of mice, using the electron microscope. Am J Anat 109:57–61

Clarkson TW, Rothstein A (1960) Transport of monovalent cations by the isolated small intestine of the rat. Am J Physiol 199:898–906

Code CF (ed) (1968 a) Intestinal absorption. American Physiology Society, Washington DC (Handbook of physiology, sect 6. Alimentary canal, vol III.)

Code CF (ed) (1968 b) Bile; digestion; ruminal physiology. American Physiology Society, Washington DC (Handbook of physiology, sect 6. Alimentary canal, vol V)

Cogoli A, Semenza G (1975) A probable oxocarbonium ion in the reaction mechanism of small intestinal sucrase and isomaltase. J Biol Chem 250:7802–7809

Cogoli A, Mosimann H, Vock C, von Balthazar A-K, Semenza G (1972) A simplified procedure for the isolation of the sucrase-isomaltase complex from rabbit intestine. Its amino-acid and sugar composition. Eur J Biochem 30:7–14

Cogoli A, Eberle A, Sigrist H, Joss C, Robinson E, Mosimann H, Semenza G (1973) Subunits of the small intestinal sucrase-isomaltase complex and separation of its enzymatically active isomaltase moiety. Eur J Biochem 33:40–48

Colbeau A, Maroux S (1978) Integration of alkaline phosphatase in the intestinal brush border membrane. Biochim Biophys Acta 511:39–51

Conclin K, Yamashiro K, Gray G (1975) Human intestinal sucrase-isomaltase: identification of free sucrase and isomaltase and cleavage of the hybrid into active distinct subunits. J Biol Chem 250:5735–5741

Consolazio CF, Iacono JM (1963) Carbohydrates. In: Albanese AA (ed) Newer methods of nutritional biochemistry. Academic, New York, pp 290–367

Cook GC (1972) Comparison of intestinal absorption rates of glycine and glycylglycine in man and the effect of glucose in the perfusing fluid. Clin Sci 43:443–453

Cori CF (1925) The fate of sugar in the animal body. I. The rate of absorption of hexoses and pentoses from the intestinal tract. J Biol Chem 66:691–715

Cori CF (1926) The absorption of glycine and d,l-alanine. Proc Soc Exp Biol Med 24:125–126

Cornish-Bowden A (1976) Principles of enzyme kinetics. Butterworths, London

Craft IL, Crampton RF, Lis MT, Matthews DM (1969) Intestinal absorption of L-methionine, glycine and some of their peptides in the rat. J Physiol (London) 200:111–112

Crampton RF, Lis MT, Matthews DM (1973) Sites of maximal absorption and hydrolysis of two dipeptides by rat small intestine. Clin Sci 44:583–594

Crane RK (1966) Sructural and functional organization of an epithelial cell brush border. In: Intracellular transport symposia. Int Soc Cell Biol, vol 5. Academic, New York, pp 71–102

Crane RK (1968 a) Absorption of sugars. In: Code CF, Heidel W (eds) Intestinal absorption. (Handbook of physiology, sec 6. Alimentary canal, vol III). American Physiology Society Washington, pp 1323–1351

Crane RK (1968 b) Digestive-absorptive surface of the small bowel mucosa. Annu Rev Med 19:57–68
Crane RK (1974) Intestinal absorption of glycose. In: Smyth DH (ed) Intestinal absorption. Plenum, London, pp 541–553
Crane RK (1975) 15 years of struggle with the brush border. In: Csaky TZ (ed) Intestinal absorption and malabsorption. Raven, New York, pp 127–141
Crane RK (1977) Digestion and absorption: watersoluble organics. In: Crane RK (ed) Gastrointestinal physiology II. Rev Physiol 12:325–365
Crane RK, Malathi P, Caspary WF, Ramaswamy K (1970) Evidence for a second glucose transport system in hamster small intestine specific for glucose released by brush border digestive enzymes. Fed Proc 29:595 (abstr)
Critchley DR, Howell KE, Eichholz A (1975) Solubilization of brush borders of hamster small intestine and fractionation of some of the components. Biochim Biophys Acta 394:361–376
Csáky TZ (1969) Biologicial transport in epithelial cells. Atti Sem Stud Biol 4:163
Csáky TZ, Fisher E (1981) Intestinal sugar transport in experimental diabetes. Diabetes 30:568–574
Csáky TZ, Autenrieth B (1975) Transcellular and intercellular intestinal transport. In: Csáky TZ (ed) Intestinal absorption and malabsorption. Raven, New York, pp 177–185
Csáky TZ, Thale M (1960) Effect of ionic environment on intestinal sugar transport. J Physiol (London) 151:59–65
Csáky TZ, Hartzog HG, Fernald GW (1961) Effect of digitalis on active intestinal sugar transport. J Physiol (London) 200:459–460
Cummins DL, Gitzelman R, Lindenmann J, Semenza G (1968) Immunochemical study of isolated human and rabbit intestinal sucrase. Biochim Biophys Acta 160:396–403
Curran PF (1960) Na, Cl and water transport by rat ileum in vitro. J Gen Physiol 43:1139–1148
Dahlqvist A, Borgström B (1961) Digestion and absorption of disaccharides in man. Biochem J 81:411–418
Dahlqvist A, Brun A (1962) A method for the histochemical demonstration of disaccharidase activities: application to invertase and trehalase in some animal tissues. J Histochem Cytochem 10:294–302
Dahlqvist A, Thomson DL (1963 a) The digestion and absorption of sucrose by the intact rat. J Physiol (London) 167:193–209
Dahlqvist A, Thomson DL (1963 b) The digestion and absorption of maltose and trehalose by the intact rat. Acta Physiol Scand 59:111–125
Das BC, Gray GM (1970) Intestinal sucrase: in vivo synthesis and degradation. Clin Res 18:378 (abstr)
Das M, Radhakrishnan AN (1972) Substrate specificity of a highly active dipeptidase purifical from monkey small intestine. Biochem J 128:463–465
Das M, Radhakrishnan AN (1974) Studies on the uptake of glycyl-L-leucine by strips of monkey small intestine. Indian J Biochem Biophys 11:12–16
Deane HW, Dempsey EW (1945) The localization of phosphatases in the Golgi region of intestinal and other epithelial cells. Anat Rec 93:401
DeLaey P (1966 a) Development of the intestinal digestion mechanism of starch as a function of age in rats. Nature 212:78–79
DeLaey P (1966 b) Die Membranverdauung der Stärke. 1. Mitt. Der Einfluß von Seiten der Perfusionsgeschwindigkeit und der amylolytischen Aktivität des Pankreassaftes auf die „in vivo" Verdauung der Stärke. Nahrung 10:641–648
DeLaey P (1966 c) Die Membranverdauung der Stärke. 2. Mitt. Der Einfluß von Mucinen auf die Membranverdauung der Stärke. Nahrung 10:649–653
DeLaey P (1966 d) Die Membranverdauung der Stärke. 3. Mitt. Der Einfluß von alimentären Komponenten des Chymus auf die Membranverdauung der Stärke. Nahrung 10:655–663
De Laey P (1967 a) Die Membranverdauung der Stärke. 4. Mitt. Der Einfluß der Größe der intestinalen Schleimhaut auf die Membranverdauung. Nahrung 11:1–7

DeLaey P (1967b) Die Membranverdauung der Stärke. 5. Mitt. Zur Zweigestaltigkeit der Membranverdauung der Stärke. Nahrung 11:9–15

DeLaey P (1967c) Die Membranverdauung der Stärke. 6. Mitt. Die Bindung der Amylase auf der Intestinal Mucosa. Nahrung 11:17–30

Dempsey EW, Deane HW (1946) The cytological localization, substrate specificity, and pH optima of phosphatases in the duodenum of the mouse. J Cell Comp Physiol 27:159–171

Desnuelle P (1979) Intestinal and renal aminopeptidases: a model of a transmembrane protein. Eur J Biochem 101:1–11

Devaux A, McConnel H (1972) Lateral diffusion in spin-labeled phosphatidylcholine multilayers. J Am Chem Soc 94:4475–4481

Development of mammalian absorptive processes (1979) Ciba Found Symp 70. Excerpta Medica, Amsterdam

Deves R, Krupka RM (1979) A general kinetic analysis of transport. Tests of the carrier model based on predicted relations among experimental parameters. Biochim Biophys Acta 556:533–547

Dietschy JM, Westergaard H (1975) The effect on unstirred water layers on various transport processes in the intestine. In: Csáky TZ (ed) Intestinal absorption and malabsorption. Raven, New York, pp 197–206

Dodds C, Fairweather FA, Miller AL, Rose CFM (1959) Blood-sugar response of normal adults to dextrose, sucrose and liquid glucose. Lancet 1:485–488

Dowling RH, Riecken EO (eds) (1974) Intestinal adaptation. Schattauer, Stuttgart

Egorova VV, Gozitte IK, Koltushkina GG, Ugolev AM (1977) Comparative characterization of some brush border enzymes isolated from the composition of membranes by detergents and proteases (in Russian). Dokl Akad Nauk SSR 233:487–490

Eichholz A, Crane RK (1965) Studies on the organization of the brush border in intestinal epithelial cells. I. Tris disruption of isolated hamster brush border and density gradient separation of fractions. J Cell Biol 26:687–691

Elezky YuK, Tsybulevsky AYu (1979) Ultrastructural and molecular bases of the transport of substances through the enterocyte brush border of the small intestine (in Russian). Adv Modern Biol 2:304–320

Emmel VM (1946) The intracellular distribution of alkaline phosphatase activity following various methods of histologic fixation. Anat Rec 95:159–173

Etzler ME, Branstrator ML (1974) Differential localization of cell surface and secretory components in rat intestinal epithelium by use of lectins. J Cell Biol 62:329–343

Farias RN, Bloj B, Morero RD, Sineriz F, Trucco R (1975) Regulation of allosteric membrane bound enzymes through changes in membrane lipid composition. Biochim Biophys Acta 415:231–251

Feher JJ, Wasserman RH (1979) Studies on the subcellular localization of the membrane-bound fraction of intestinal calcium-binding protein. Biochim Biophys Acta 585:599–610

Ferguson A (1979) In: Duthie HL, Wormsley KG (eds) Scientific basis of gastroenterology. Livingstone, Edinburgh, pp 49–70

Finean JB (1972) The development of ideas on membrane structure. Subcell Biochem 1:363

Finean JB, Coleman R, Michell RH (1978) Membranes and their cellular functions, 2nd ed. Blackwell Scientific Publications, Oxford

Fisher RB (1954) Protein metabolism. Methuen, Willey, London

Fisher RB, Parsons DS (1949) A preparation of surviving rat small intestine for the study of absorption. J Physiol (London) 110:36–46

Fisher RB, Parsons DS (1953) Galactose absorption from the surviving small intestine of the rat. J Physiol (London) 119:224–232

Flanagan FR, Forstner GG (1978) Enzyme activity in partly dissociated fragments of rat intestinal maltase/glucoamylase. Biochem J 177:487–492

Fleischer S, Packer L (eds) (1974) Biomembranes, vol 32, part B. Characterization of membranes and membrane components, Sect I; Model membranes, Sect IV. Academic, New York, pp 3–272, 485–554

Florey HW, Wright RD, Jennings MA (1941) The secretion of the intestine. Physiol Rev 21:36–69
Fogel MR, Gray GM (1973) Starch hydrolysis in man: an intraluminal process not requiring membrane digestion. J Appl Physiol 35:263–267
Forstner G, Wherrett JR (1973) Plasma membrane and mucosal glycosphingolipids in the rat intestine. Biochim Biophys Acta 306:446–459
Fosset M, Chappelet-Tordo D, Lazdunski M (1974) Intestinal alkaline phosphatase. Physical properties and quaternary structure. Biochemistry 13:1783–1788
Frank G, Brunner J, Hauser H, Wacker H, Semenza G, Zuber H (1978) The hydrophobic anchor of small-intestinal sucrase-isomaltase. N-terminal sequence of the isomaltase subunit. FEBS Letters 96:183–188
Frye CD, Edidin M (1970) The rapid intermixing of cell surface antigens after formation of mouse-human heterokaryons. J Cell Sci 7:319–335
Fujita M, Parsons DS, Wojnarowska F (1972) Oligopeptidases of brush border membranes of rat small intestinal mucosal cells. J Physiol (London) 227:377–394
Gallo LL, Treadwell CR (1963) Localization of cholesterol esterase and cholesterol in mucosal fractions of rat small intestine. Proc Soc Exp Biol Med 114:69–72
Garrido J (1975) Ultrastructural labeling of cell surface lectin receptors during the cell cycle. Exp Cell Res 94:159–175
Gennis RB, Jonas A (1977) Protein-lipid interactions. Annu Rev Biophys Bioeng 6:195–238
Gilvarg C (1972) Peptide transport in bacteria. In: Peptide transport in bacteria and mammalian gut. Ciba Found Symp 4:11–16
Gitzelmann R, Davidson EA, Osinchak J (1964) Disaccharidase of rabbit small intestine: intracellular distribution, solubilization, purification and specificity. Biochim Biophys Acta 85:69–81
Götze H, Rothman SS (1978) Amylase transport across ileal epithelium in vitro. Biochim Biophys Acta 512:214–220
Goldberg DM, Campbell R, Roy D (1968) Binding of trypsin and chymotrypsin by human intestinal mucosa. Biochim Biophys Acta 167:613–615
Goldberg DM, Campbell R, Roy D (1971) The interaction of trypsin and chymotrypsin with intestinal cells in man and several animal species. Comp Biochem Physiol 38:697–706
Gomori G (1941) The distribution of phosphatase in normal organs and tissue. J Cell Comp Physiol 17:71–83
Gozitte IK, Koltushkina GG, Egorova VV, Ugolev AM (1976) Comparative kinetic characterization of some brush border enzymes solubilized from the membranes by means of detergents and proteases (in Russian). In: Digestive enzymes. Comm of 1st bilateral symposium USSR-Czechoslovakia, Uzhgorod, pp 31–35
Gray GM (1975) Carbohydrate digestion and absorption. Role of the small intestine. N Engl J Med 292:1225–1230
Gray GM, Santiago NA (1969) Intestinal β-galactosidases. 1. Separation and characterization of three enzymes in normal human intestine. J Clin Invest 48:716–729
Green JR (1972) Membrane structure and its biological application. Ann N Y Acad Sci 195
Green JR, Hadorn B (1977) Glycosidases of the guinea pig brush border membrane. Biochim Biophys Acta 467:86–90
Gruzdkov AA, Egorova VV, Jezuitova NN, Timofeeva NM, Tulyaganova EKh, Chernyakhovskaya MYu, Ugolev AM (1970) Distribution of some enzymatic activities of the small intestine of white rats on ultracentrifugation (in Russian). In: Physiology and pathology of the small intestine. Proc of the All-Union congr gastroenterol. Riga, pp 53–56
Guidotti G, Borghetti AF, Gazzola GC (1978) The regulations of amino acid transport in animal cells. Biochim Biophys Acta 515:329–366
Gulik-Krzywicki T (1975) Structural studies of the association between biological membrane components. Biochim Biophys Acta 415:1–28

Harrison R, Lunt GG (1975) Biological membranes: their structure and function, vol VIII. Blackie, Glasgow, p 253
Heading RC, Schedl HP, Stegink LD, Miller DL (1977) Intestinal absorption of glycine and glycyl-L-proline in the rat. Clin Sci Mol Med 52:607–614
Heaton JW (1970) Intestinal maltase-sucrase: unique alpha-glucosidase. Gastroenterology 58:1044
Heizer WD, Isselbacher KJ (1970) Intestinal peptide hydrolases: differences between brush border and cytoplasmic enzymes. Clin Res 18:382
Heizer WD, Kerley RL, Isselbacher KJ (1972) Intestinal peptide hydrolases. Difference between brush border and cytoplasmic enzymes. Biochim Biophys Acta 264:450–461
Helenius A, Simons K (1975) Solubilization of membranes by detergents. Biochim Biophys Acta 415:29–79
Hemmings WA, Williams EW (1978) Transport of large breakdown products of dietary protein through the gut wall. Gut 19:715–723
Hendler RW (1971) Biological membrane ultrastructure. Physiol Rev 51:66–97
Himukai M, Suzuki Y, Hoshi T (1978) Differences in characteristics between glycine and glycylglycine transport in guinea pig small intestine. Jpn J Physiol 28:499–510
Hochachka PW, Somero GN (1973) Strategies of biochemical adaptation. Saunders, Philadelphia
Hoffman JF (ed) (1978) Membrane transport processes, vol 1. Raven, New York
Holdsworth CD, Dawson AM (1964) The absorption of monosaccharides in man. Clin Sci 27:371–377
Holdsworth CD, Sladen GE (1979) Absorption from stomach and small intestine. In: Duthie HL, Wormsley KG (eds) Scientific basis of gastroenterology. Levingstone, Edinburgh, pp 338–397
Hübscher G, West GR, Brindley DN (1965) Studies on the fractionation of mucosal homogenates from the small intestine. Biochem J 97:629–642
Hueckel HJ, Rogers QR (1972) Prolylhydroxyproline absorption in hamster. Can J Biochem 50:782–790
Iezuitova NN, Nadirova TYa, Toropova NW, Ugolev AM (1965) The characterization of the entry of hexoses into the blood after the administration of poly-, oligo-, and monosaccharides into the gastrointestinal tract (in Russian). In: Skljarov JaP (ed) Conference on physiology and pathology of digestion. Lvov, pp 102–105
Iezuitova NN, Timofeeva NM, Chernyakhovskaya MYu, Zabelinsky EK, Ugolev AM (1967) Distribution of some enzymes (amylase, invertase, dipeptidase, lipase and monoglyceride lipase) between the small intestinal contents and mucosa in dogs and rats during digestion (in Russian). Dokl Akad Nauk SSSR 173:475–478
Immunology of the gut (1977) Ciba Found Symp 46.
Isselbacher KJ (1974) The intestinal cell surface: properties of normal, undifferentiated, and malignant cells. Harvey Lect 69:197–221
Isselbacher KJ, Senior JR (1964) The intestinal absorption of carbohydrate and fat. Gastroenterology 46:287–298
Ito S (1965) The enteric surface coat on cat intestinal microvilli. J Cell Biol 27:475–491
Ito S (1969) Structure and function of the glycocalyx. Fed Proc 28:12–25
Jesuitova NN, De Laey P, Ugolev AM (1964) Digestion of starch in vivo and in vitro in a rat intestine. Biochim Biophys Acta 86:205–210
Jodl J, Lindberg T (1979) In vitro release of intestinal dipeptidases from everted rings of rat jejunum. Acta Physiol Scand 105:248–250
Jos J, Frezal J, Rey J, Lamy M (1967) Histochemical localization of intestinal disaccharidases: application to peroral biopsy specimens. Nature 213:516–518
Josefsson L, Sjöström H (1966) Intestinal dipeptidases. IV. Studies on the release and subcellular distribution of intestinal dipeptidases of the mucosa cells of the pig. Acta Physiol Scand 67:27–33
Josefsson L, Sjöström H, Noren O (1977) Intracellular hydrolysis of peptides. In: Peptide transport and hydrolysis. Ciba Found Symp 50:199–207
Kalser MH (1964) Physiology of the small intestine. In: Bockus HL (ed) Gastroenterology, vol II, Saunders, Philadelphia, pp 10–30

Katz M, Cooper BA (1974) Solubilized receptor for intrinsic factor-vitamin B_{12} complex from guinea pig intestinal mucosa. J Clin Invest 54:733–739

Kelly JJ, Alpers DH (1973) Properties of human intestinal glucoamylase. Biochim Biophys Acta 315:113–122

Kennedy SJ (1978) Structures of membrane protein. J Membr Biol 42:265–279

Kenny AJ (1977) Endopeptidase in the brush border of the kidney proximal tubule. In: Peptide transport and hydrolysis. Ciba Found Symp 50:209–215

Kim YS (1977) Intestinal mucosal hydrolysis of proteins and peptides. In: Peptide transport and hydrolysis. Ciba Found Symp 50:151–171

Kim YS, Brophy EJ (1976) Rat intestinal brush border peptidases. I. Solubilization, purification and physicochemical properties of two different forms of the enzyme. J Biol Chem 251:3199–3205

Kim YS, Birtwhistle W, Kim YW (1972) Peptide hydrolases in the brush border and soluble fractions of small intestine mucosa of rat and man. J Clin Invest 51:1419–1430

Kim YS, Kim YW, Sleisenger MH (1974) Studies on the properties of peptide hydrolases in the brush border and soluble fractions of small intestinal mucosa of rat and man. Biochim Biophys Acta 370:283–296

Kim YS, Brophy EJ, Nicholson JA (1976) Rat intestinal brush border membrane peptidases. II. Enzymatic properties, immunochemistry and interactions with lectins of two different forms of the enzyme. J Biol Chem 251:3206–3212

Kinne R, Murer H (1976) Polarity of epithelial cells in relation to transepithelial transport in kidney and intestine. In: Intestinal ion transport. Proc Int Symp, Baltimore, pp 79–95

Kirtley ME, Koshland DE (1968) Models for cooperative effects in proteins containing subunits. J Biol Chem 242:4192–4205

Klip A, Grinstein S, Semenza G (1979) Transmembrane disposition of the phlorizin binding protein of intestinal brush border. FEBS Letters 99:91–96

Kojezky Z, Matlocha Z (1973) Možnosti studia poruch membránového traveni v klinice. Cesk Gastroenterol Vyz 27:507–513

Kolinska J, Kraml J (1972) Separation and characterization of sucrase-isomaltase and of glucoamylase of rat intestine. Biochim Biophys Acta 284:235–247

Konder H, Haberich FJ, Stöckert HG (1977) pH-values in the small intestine of rats and their possible role in the absorption of bile acids. Pflügers Arch 368 [Suppl]: R 20

Kornberg RD, McConnell HM (1971) Inside-outside transitions of phospholipids in vesicle membranes. Biochemistry 10:1111–1120

Koshland DE (1969) Conformational aspects of enzyme regulation. In: Curr Top Cell Regul 1:1–27

Koshland DE (1970) The molecular basis of enzyme regulation. In: Boyer PD (ed) The enzymes, vol 1. Structure and control, 3rd edn. Academic, New York, pp 342–397

Koshland DE, Neet KE (1968) The catalytic and regulatory properties of enzymes. Annu Rev Biochem 37:359–410

Koshland DE, Nemethy G, Filmer D (1966) Comparison of experimental binding data and theoretical models in proteins containing subunits. Biochemistry 5:365–385

Koskowski W (1926) The influence of histamine on the intestinal secretion of the dog. J Pharmacol 26:413–419

Kowarski S, Blair-Stanek CS, Schachter D (1974) Active transport of zinc and identification of zinc binding protein in rat jejunal mucosa. Am J Physiol 226:401–407

Kraml J, Lojda Z (1977) Biochemistry and immunochemistry of membrane-bound enzymes. Acta Univ Carol [Med] (Praha), Monographia 77, Part 1, pp 83–94

Kraml J, Koldovsky O, Heringova A, Jirsova V, Kacl K, Ledvina M, Pelichova H (1969) Characteristics of β-galactosidase in the mucosa of the small intestine of infant rats. Physicochemical properties. Biochem J 114:621–627

Kretchmer N, Latimer JS, Raul F, Berry K, Legum C, Sharp HL (1979) Sucrase and cellular development. In: Development of mammalian absorptive processes. Ciba Found Symp 70:117–130

Kurganov BI (1978) Allosteric enzymes (in Russian). Nauka, Moskow

Kushak RI, Zigure DR, Kopman EA (1973) Accumulation of glycine from dipeptides and equivalent amino acid mixtures in rats and chickens (in Russian). Izv Akad Nauk Latv SSR 5:97–104

Lane AE, Silk BDA, Clark ML (1975) Absorption of two proline containing peptides by rat small intestine in vivo. J Physiol (London) 248:143–149

Lauger P (1979) A channel mechanism for electrogenic ion pump. Biochim Biophys Acta 552:143–161

Lee AG (1975) Interaction within biological membranes. Endeavour 34:67–71

Lee AG, Birdsall NJM, Metcalfe JC (1973) Measurement of fast laterial diffusion of lipids in vesicles and in biological membranes by ^{1}H nuclear magnetic resonance. Biochemistry 12:1650–1659

Lenaz G (1974) Lipid-protein interactions in the structure of biological membranes. Subcell Biochem 3:167–248

Leslie GI, Rowe PB (1972) Folate binding by the brush border membrane proteins of small intestinal epithelial cells. Biochemistry 11:1696–1703

Leube W (1868) Über Verdauungsprodukte des Dünndarmsaftes. Centralbl Med Wiss 19:289–292

Levin RJ (1979) Fundamental concepts of structure and function of the intestinal epithelium. In: Duthie HL, Wormsley KG (eds) Scientific basis of gastroenterology. Livingstone, Edinburgh, pp 308–337

Lindberg T (1966) Studies on intestinal dipeptidases. Acta Physiol Scand 69 [Suppl 285]:1–38

Lindberg T (1972) In: Peptide transport in bacteria and mammalian gut. Ciba Found Symp 4:91

Lindberg T, Norén O, Sjöstrom H (1975) Peptidases in the intestinal mucosa. In: Matthews DH, Payne JW (eds) Peptide transport in protein nutrition. ASP, Amsterdam, pp 204–242

Lindemann B, Solomon AK (1962) Permeability of luminal surface of intestinal mucosal cells. J Gen Physiol 45:801–810

Lis MT, Crampton RF, Matthews DM (1971) Rates of absorption of a dipeptide and the equivalent free amino acid in various mammalian species. Biochim Biophys Acta 233:453–455

Lojda Z (1974) Cytochemistry of enterocytes and other cells in the mucous membrane of the small intestine. In: Smyth DH (ed) Intestinal absorption. Plenum, London, pp 43–123

Lojda Z (1976) The significance of histochemistry for the study of enzymes of the digestive tract (in Russian). In: Fucik M, Jablonska M et al. (eds) Digestive enzymes. Comm 1st bilateral symposium USSR–Czechoslovakia. Uzhgorod, pp 46–53

Lojda Z, Frič P, Jodl J, Lojda L (1978) Progress in the peptidase hystochemistry of the gastrointestinal tract (in Russian). In: Kojecky Z (ed) Physiology and pathology of digestion. Comm 2nd bilateral symp CSSR-SSSR. Olomouci, pp 60–70

London ES (1916) Physiology and pathology of digestion (in Russian). Practicheskaya Medizina, Petrograd

Long JF, Brooks FP (1965) Relation between inhibition of gastric secretion and absorption of fatty acid. Am J Physiol 209:447–451

Louvard D, Maroux S, Baratti J, Desnuelle P, Mutaftschiev S (1973) On the preparation and some properties of closed membrane vesicles from hog duodenal and jejunal brush border. Biochim Biophys Acta 291:747–763

Louvard D, Maroux S, Vannier Ch, Desnuelle P (1975 a) Topological studies on the hydrolases bound to the intestinal brush border membrane. I. Solubilization by papain and Triton X-100. Biochim Biophys Acta 325:236–248

Louvard D, Maroux S, Desnuelle P (1975 b) Topological studies on the hydrolases bound to the intestinal brush border membrane. II. Interactions of free and bound aminopeptidase with a specific antibody. Biochim Biophys Acta 389:389–400

Louvard D, Semeriva M, Maroux S (1976) The brush-border intestinal aminopeptidase, a transmembrane protein as probed by macromolecular photolabelling. J Mol Biol 106:1023–1035

Lucas ML, Blair JA (1978) The magnitude and distribution of the acid microclimate in proximal jejunum and its relation to luminal acidification. Proc R Soc (Lond) 200:27–41

Lucas ML, Schneider W, Haberich FJ, Blair JA (1975) Direct measurement by pH-microelectrode of the pH microclimate in rat proximal jejunum. Proc R Soc (Lond) 192:39–48

Lucas ML, Cooper BT, Lei FH, Johnson IT, Holmes GKT, Blair JA, Cooke WT (1978) Acid microclimate in coeliac and Crohn's disease: a model for folate malabsorption. Gut 19:735–742

MacDonald I, Turner LJ (1968) Serum-fructose levels after sucrose or its constituent monosaccharides. Lancet 1:841–843

Maestracci D (1976) Enzymic solubilization of the human intestinal brush border membrane enzymes. Biochim Biophys Acta 433:449:481

Maestracci D, Preiser H, Hedges T, Schmitz J, Crane RK (1975) Enzyme of the human intestinal brush border membrane. Identification after gel electrophoretic separation. Biochim Biophys Acta 382:147–156

Malathi P, Ramaswamy K, Caspary WF, Crane RK (1973) Studies on the transport of glucose from disaccharides by hamster small intestine in vitro. Biochim Biophys Acta 307:613–626

Mali R (1886) Chemistry of digestive fluids and digestion (in Russian). In: Herman L (ed) Physiology manual, vol 5. St. Petersburg

Marchesi VT, Furthmayr H, Tomita M (1976) The red cell membrane. Annu Rev Biochem 45:667–698

Markin VS, Chizmadzhev YuA (1974) Induced ion transport (in Russian). Nauka, Moskow

Maroux S, Louvard D (1976) On the hydrophobic part of aminopeptidase and maltase which bind the enzyme to the intestinal brush border membrane. Biochim Biophys Acta 419:189–195

Maroux S, Baratti J, Desnuelle P (1971) Purification and specificity of porcine enterokinase. J Biol Chem 246:5031–5039

Maroux S, Louvard D, Baratti J (1973) The aminopeptidase from hog intestinal brush border. Biochim Biophys Acta 321:282–295

Maroux S, Louvard D, Desnuelle P (1975) The intestinal brush border aminopeptidase (β-naphthyl amidase) as a model of enzyme bound to the surface of a membrane. Proceedings of the tenth FEBS meeting. Federation of European Biochemical Societies. Pergamon, Oxford, pp 55–69

Marrs TC, Addison JM, Burston D, Matthews DM (1975) Changes in plasma amino acid concentrations in man after ingestion of an amino acid mixture simulating casein, and a tryptic hydrolysate of casein. Br J Nutr 34:259–265

Martin BF, Jacoby F (1949) Diffusion phenomenon complicating the histochemical reaction for alkaline phosphatase. J Anat 83:351–363

Masevich CH, Ugolev AM, Zabelinski EK, Kisily NP (1975) Lumenal and membrane hydrolysis of starch in some diseases of the small intestine. Am J Gastroenterol 63:299–306

Mathan VI, Babior BM, Donaldson RM (1974) Kinetics of the attachment of intrinsic factor-bound cobamides to ileal receptors. J Clin Invest 54:598–608

Matlocha Z, Kojezky Z (1976) Amylase adsorption of small intestinal mucosa in prenatal time (in Russian). In: Fucik M, Jablonska M (eds) Digestive enzymes. Comm 1st bilateral symp USSR-Czechoslovakia. Uzghorod, pp 101–103

Matthews DM (1972) Rates of peptide uptake by small intestine. In: Peptide transport in bacteria and mammalian gut. Ciba Found Symp 4:71–88

Matthews DM (1975a) Intestinal transport of peptides. In: Csáky TZ (ed) Intestinal absorption and malabsorption. Raven, New York, pp 95–111

Matthews DM (1975b) Absorption of peptides by mammalian intestine. In: Matthews DM, Payne JW (eds) Peptide transport in protein nutrition. ASP, Amsterdam, pp 61–146

Matthews DM (1977) Introduction. In: Peptide transport and hydrolysis. Ciba Found Symp 50:5–14

Matthews DM, Payne JW (1975) Peptides in the nutrition of microorganisms and peptides in relation to animal nutrition. In: Matthews DM, Payne JW (eds) Peptide transport in protein nutrition. ASP, Amsterdam, pp 1–60

Matthews DM, Adibi SA (1976) Peptide absorption. Gastroenterology 71:151–161

Matthews DM, Craft LL, Crampton RF (1968 a) Intestinal absorption of saccharides and peptides. Lancet 2:49

Matthews DM, Craft LL, Geddes DM, Wise SJ, Hyde CW (1968b) Absorption of glycine and glycine peptides from the small intestine of the rat. Clin Sci 35:415–424

Matthews DM, Lis MT, Cheng B, Crampton RF (1969) Observations on the intestinal absorption of some oligopeptides of methionine and glycine in the rat. Clin Sci 37:751–764

Matthews DM, Crampton RF, Lis MT (1971) Sites of maximal intestinal absorptive capacity for amino acids and peptides: evidence for an independent peptide uptake system or systems. J Clin Pathol 24:882–883

McIntosh TJ, Waldbilling RC, Robertson JD (1977) The molecular organization of asymmetric lipid bilayers and lipid-peptide complexes. Biochim Biophys Acta 466:209–230

McMichael HB, Webb J, Dawson AM (1966) The absorption of maltose and lactose in man. Clin Sci 33:135–145

McNurlan MA, Garlick PJ (1980) Contribution of rat liver and gastrointestinal tract to whole body protein synthesis in the rat. Biochem J 186:381–383

Meister A (1973) On the enzymology of amino acid transport. Science 180:33–39

Meister A, Tate SS, Ross LL (1976) Membrane bound γ-glutamyl transpeptidase. In: Martinosi A (ed) The Enzymes of biological membranes, vol 3. Plenum, New York, pp 315–347

Meister A, Tate SS, Thompson GA (1977) The function of the γ-glutamyl cycle in the transport of amino acids and peptides. In: Peptide transport and hydrolysis. Ciba Found Symp 50:123–138

Miller D, Crane RK (1961 a) The digestive function of the epithelium of the small intestine. I. An intracellular locus of disaccharide and sugar phosphate ester hydrolysis. Biochim Biophys Acta 52:281–293

Miller D, Crane RK (1961 b) The digestive function of the epithelium of the small intestine. II. Localization of disaccharide hydrolysis in the isolated brush border portion of the intestinal epithelial cells. Biochim Biophys Acta 52:293–298

Miller D, Crane RK (1963) The digestion of carbohydrates in the small intestine. Am J Clin Nutr 12:220–227

Milne HD (1974) Hereditary disorders of intestinal transport. In: Smyth DH (ed) Intestinal absorption. Plenum, London, p 961

Mityushova NM (1970) Some problems of the method of isolation of the brush border (in Russian). In: Ugolev AM (ed) Physiology and pathology of the small intestine. Proc All-Union congr gastroenterol. Riga, pp 18–20

Monod J, Changeux J-P, Jacob F (1963) Allosteric proteins and cellular control systems. J Mol Biol 6:306–329

Monod J, Wyman J, Changeux J-P (1965) On the nature of allosteric transitions; a plausible model. J Mol Biol 12:88–118

Moog F (1979) The differentiation and redifferentiation of the intestinal epithelium and its brush border membrane. In: Development of mammalian absorptive processes. Ciba Found Symp 70:31–44

Moog F, Grey RD (1967) Spatial and temporal differentiation of alkaline phosphatase on the intestinal villi of the mouse. J Cell Biol 32:C1–C5

Mooseker MS (1974) Brush border motility: microvillar contraction in isolated brush border membrane. J Cell Biol 63:231 a

Mooseker MS, Tilney LG (1975) Organization of an actin filament-membrane complex: filament polarity and membrane attachment in the microvilli of intestinal epithelial cells. J Cell Biol 67:725–743

Mooseker MS, Pollard TD, Fujiwara K (1978) Characterization and localization of myosin in the brush border of intestinal cells. J Cell Biol 79:444–453

Mooz R, Noack R, Friedrich M, Roshchina GM, Smirnova LF, Timofeeva NM, Ugolev AM (1978) Localization of hydrolysis of dipeptides in the small intestine determined on the basis of anoxic criterion (in Russian). Izv Akad Nauk SSSR [Biol] 6:872–881

Morris IG (1974) Immunological proteins. In: Smyth DH (ed) Intestinal absorption. Plenum, London, pp 483–540

Mosimann H, Semenza G, Sund H (1973) Hydrodynamic properties of the sucrase-isomaltase complex from rabbit small intestine. Eur J Biochem 36:489–494

Mothes Th, Müller F (1979) On the Na^+-dependence of 3-0-methyl-D-glucose transport in the isolated rabbit small intestine, perfused through the lumen and the vascular bed. In: Energetics and regulation of membrane transport, Symposium, Prague

Müller F, Dettmer D, Remke H, Hartenstein H, Luppa D (1972) Intestinaler Monosaccharid-Transport. Wiss Z Karl Marx Univ Leipzig Math Naturwiss 21:536–543

Murer H, Hopfer U, Kinne R (1978) Molecular evidence for the sodium gradient hypothesis. In: Varro V, Balint GA (eds) Current views in gastroenterology. Hung Soc Gastroenterol, Budapest, pp 77–91

Nachlas MM, Monis B, Rosenblatt D, Seligman AM (1960) Improvement in the histochemical localization of leucine aminopeptidase with a new substrate, L-leucyl-4-methoxy-2-naphthylamide. J Biophys Biochem Cytol 7:261–264

Newey H, Smyth DH (1957) Intestinal absorption of dipeptides. J Physiol (London) 135:43–44P

Newey H, Smyth DH (1959) The intestinal absorption of some dipeptides. J Physiol (London) 145:48–56

Newey H, Smyth DH (1960 a) Intracellular hydrolysis of dipeptides during intestinal absorption. J Physiol (London) 152:367–380

Newey H, Smyth DH (1960 b) Absorption rates of glycine and glycyl-glycine. J Physiol (London) 152:70–71P

Newey H, Smyth DH (1961) Two-stages transfer of glycine by the intestine in vitro. J Physiol (London) 157:15–16P

Newey H, Smyth DH (1962) Cellular mechanisms in intestinal transfer of amino acids. J Physiol (London) 164:527–551

Newey H, Smyth DH (1964) Effects of sugars on intestinal transfer of amino acids. Nature 202:400–401

Nikitina AA, Zaripov BZ, Varro V, Ugolev AM (1979) Intestinal hormones and inhibition of enzyme and transport function of enterocytes membrane (in Russian). Dokl Akad Nauk SSSR 249:500–503

Nikolsky NN (1977) Absorption of sugars (in Russian). In: Physiology of absorption. Nauka, Leningrad, pp 249–284

Nilsson O, Dallner G (1977) Transverse asymmetry of phospholipids in subcellular membranes of rat liver. Biochim Biophys Acta 464:453–458

Nishi Y, Takesue Y (1978 a) Localization of intestinal sucrase-isomaltase complex on the microvillous membrane by electron microscopy using nonlabelled antibodies. J Cell Biol 79:516–525

Nishi Y, Takesue Y (1978 b) Electron microscope studies on Triton-solubilized sucrase from rabbit small intestine. J Ultrastruct Res 62:1–12

Nishi Y, Takato O, Takesue Y (1968) Electron microscope studies on the structure of rabbit intestinal sucrase. J Mol Biol 37:441–444

Noack R, Friedrich M, Proll J, Uhlig J (1975) Verdauung und Resorption von Proteinen. Nahrung 19:891–901

Noim AG, Nurks EE, Ugolev AM (1970) Characterization of the digestive and transport functions of the intestinal epithelium in fed and fasting states (in Russian). In: Ugolev AM (ed) Physiology and pathology of the small intestine. Proc of the All-Union congr gastroenterol, Riga, pp 78–80

Norén O, Sjöstrom H, Svensson B, Jeppesen L, Staun M, Josefsson L (1977) Intestinal brush border peptidases. In: Peptide transport and hydrolysis. Ciba Found Symp 50:177–191

O'Cuinn G, Donlon J, Fottrell PF (1974) Similarities between one of the multiple forms of peptide hydrolase purified from brush border and cytosol fractions of guinea pig intestinal mucosa. FEBS Letters 39:225–228
O'Cuinn G, Fottrell PF (1975) Purification and characterization of an aminoacyl proline hydrolase from guinea-pig intestinal mucosa. Biochim Biophys Acta 391:388–395
Ogston AG, Michel CC (1978) General description of passive transport of neural solute and solvent through membranes. Prog Biophys Mol Biol 34:197–217
Ohkubo A, Langerman N, Kaplan MM (1974) Rat liver alkaline phosphatase. Purification and properties. J Biol Chem 249:7174–7180
Ostrovski DN (1977) Molecular organization of biological membranes (in Russian). In: Beker ME, Dubur Gja (eds) Biomembranes. Structure, functions and methods of investigation. Zinatne, Riga, pp 7–27
Ovchinnikov YuA, Ivanov VT (1977) Recent development in the structure-functional studies of peptide ionofores. In: Semenza G, Carafoli E (eds) Biochemistry of membrane transport. FEBS symposium 42. Springer, Berlin Heidelberg New York, pp 123–146
Overton J, Eichholz A, Crane RK (1965) Studies on the organization of the brush border in intestinal epithelial cells. II. Fine structure of fractions of tris-disrupted hamster brush borders. J Cell Biol 26:693–706
Padykula HA (1962) Recent functional interpretations of intestinal morphology. Fed Proc 21:873–879
Parsons DS (ed) (1975) Biological membranes. Twelve assays on their organization, properties, and functions. Clarendon, Oxford
Parsons DS (1976) Closing summary (app 2, unstirred layer). In: Robinson JWL (ed) Intestinal ion transport. MTP Press, London, pp 429–430
Parsons DS (1977) In: Peptide transport and hydrolysis. Ciba Found Symp 50:327
Parsons DS, Prichard JS (1965) Hydrolysis of disaccharides during absorption by the perfused small intestine of amphibia. Nature 208:1097–1098
Parsons DS, Prichard JS (1968) Disaccharide absorption by amphibian small intestine in vitro. J Physiol (London) 199:137–150
Parsons DS, Prichard JS (1971) Relationships between disaccharide hydrolysis and sugar transport in amphibian small intestine. J Physiol (London) 212:299–319
Pattus F, Verger R, Desnuelle P (1976) Comparative study of the interaction of the trypsin and detergent form of the intestinal aminopeptidase with liposomes. Biochem Biophys Res Commun 69:718–723
Pavlov IP (1911–1912) Lectures for students of military-medical academy (in Russian). In: Airapetjants E Sh (ed) (1952) Complete works, vol 5, 2nd edn. Izd Akad Nauk SSSR, Moscow, pp 11–275
Payne JW (1972) Mechanisms of bacterial peptide transport. In: Peptide transport in bacteria and mammalian gut. Ciba Found Symp 4:17–32
Payne JW (1977) Transport and hydrolysis of peptides by microorganisms. In: Peptide transport and hydrolysis. Ciba Found Symp 50:305–325
Peptide transport and hydrolysis (1977) Ciba Found Symp 50
Peters TJ (1970) The subcellular localisation of di- and tri-peptide hydrolase activity in guinea pig small intestine. Biochem J 120:195–203
Peters TJ (1975) The subcellular localisation of intestinal peptide hydrolases. In: Matthews DM, Payne JW (eds) Peptide transport in protein nutrition. ASP, Amsterdam, pp 243–267
Peters K, Richards FM (1977) Chemical across-linking: reagents and problems in studies of membrane structure. Annu Rev Biochem 46:523–551
Pierce HB, Nasset ES, Murlin JR (1935) Enzyme production in a transplanted loop of the upper jejunum. J Biol Chem 108:239–250
Piggott CO, Fottrell PF (1975) Purification and characterization from guinea-pig intestinal mucosa of two peptide hydrolases which preferentially hydrolyse dipeptides. Biochim Biophys Acta 391:403–409
Pitot HC, Yatvin MB (1973) Interrelationships of mammalian hormones and enzymes levels in vivo. Physiol Rev 53:228–325
Plaut A (1972) A review of secretory immune mechanisms. Am J Clin Nutr 25:1344–1350

Pritchard PJ, Porteous JW (1977) Steady-state metabolism and transport of D-glucose by rat small intestine in vitro. Biochem J 164:1–14

Prusiner S, Doak CW, Kirk G (1976) A novel mechanism for group translocation: substrate-product reutilization by γ-glutamyl transpeptidase in peptide and amino acid transport. J Cell Physiol 89:853–863

Quaroni A, Semenza G (1976) Partial amino acid sequences around the essential carboxylate in the active sites of intestinal sucrase and isomaltase. J Biol Chem 251:3250–3253

Quinn PJ (1976) The molecular biology of cell membranes, vol X. University Park Press, Baltimore, p 229

Racker E (1976) A new look at mechanisms in bioenergetics. Academic, New York

Rakhimov KR (1965) Amylolytic activity of the rat intestine depending on functional state of the digestive organs (in Russian). In: Problems of physiology of man and animals under the conditions of hot climate. Tashkent, pp 159–163

Ramaswamy K, Malathi P, Caspary WF, Crane RK (1974) Studies on the transport of glucose from disaccharides by hamster small intestine in vitro. II. Characteristics of the disaccharidase-related transport system. Biochim Biophys Acta 345:39–48

Ramaswamy K, Malathi P, Crane RK (1976) Demonstration of hydrolase-related glucose transport in brush border membrane vesicles prepared from guinea pig small intestine. Biochem Biophys Res Comm 68:162–168

Remke H, Schellenberger W, Mothes T, Müller F (1978) Zum Mechanismus der Na^+-abhängigen Monosaccharidresorption: Kompartimentierung des resorbierten Na^+ unter in vitro-Bedingungen. Acta Biol Med Ger 37:49–57

Rhodes B, Arvanitakis C, Folscroft J (1977) Intestinal hydrolysis of disaccharides and peptides: comparison of hydrolases and perfusion studies. In: Peptide transport and hydrolysis. Ciba Found Symp 50:245–263

Riklis E, Quastel H (1958) Effect of cations on sugar absorption by isolated surviving guinea pig intestine. Can J Biochem 36:347–362

Robinson GA, Butcher RW, Sutherland EW (1971) Cyclic AMP. Academic, New York

Robinson JB (1975) Principles of membrane structure. In: Parsons DS (ed) Biological membranes. Twelve assays on their organization, properties, and functions. Clarendon, Oxford, pp 33–57

Robinson JWL (1970) Comparative aspects of the response of the intestine to its ionic environment. Comp Biochem Physiol 34:641–655

Robinson JWL (ed) (1976) Intestinal ion transport. MTP Press, London

Rothfield LI (ed) (1971) Structure and functions of biological membranes. Academic, London

Rothman JE, Lenard J (1977) Membrane asymmetry. The nature of membrane asymmetry provides clues to the puzzle of how membranes are assembled. Science 195:743–753

Rubino A, Guandalini S (1977) Dipeptide transport in the intestinal mucosa of developing rabbits. In: Peptide transport and hydrolysis. Ciba Found Symp 50:61–70

Rubino A, Field M, Shwachman H (1971) Intestinal transport of amino acid residues of peptides. 1. Influx of the glycine residue of glycyl-l-proline across mucosal border. J Biol Chem 246:3542–3548

Ruttloff H, Noack R, Friese R, Schenk G (1964) Zur Lokalisation von Carbohydrasen im Bürstensaum der Rattenmucosa. Biochem Zeitschr 341:15–22

Rybakova GS, Zlatkina AR, Ugolev AM (1973) A new method for determination of reserve functional capacities of the small intestine (in Russian). Theraupeut Arch 45:44–47

Sackmann E, Träuble H, Galla H-J, Overath P (1973) Lateral diffusion, protein mobility, and phase transitions in Escherichia coli membranes. A spin label study. Biochemistry 12:5360–5369

Saidel LJ, Edelstein I (1974) Hydrolysis and absorption of proline dipeptides across the wall of sacs prepared from everted rat intestine. Biochim Biophys Acta 367:75–80

Sandermann H (1978) Regulation of membrane enzymes by lipids. Biochim Biophys Acta 515:209–237

Schedl HP, Clifton JA (1961) Kinetics of intestinal absorption in man: normal subjects and patients with sprue. J Clin Invest 40:1079–1080

Schreier S (1978) Spin labels in membranes. Problems and practice. Biochim Biophys Acta 515:395–436

Schultz SG (1979) Transport across small intestine. In: Giebisch G (ed) Membrane transport in biology, vol IVB, Transport organs. Springer, Berlin Heidelberg New York, pp 749–780

Segrest JP, Feldmann RJ (1974) Membrane proteins: amino acid sequence and membrane penetration. J Mol Biol 87:853–858

Semenza G (1968) Intestinal oligosaccharidases and disaccharidases. In: Code CF (ed) Bile; digestion; ruminal physiology (Handbook of physiology, sec 6. Alimentary canal, vol V). American Physiological Society, Washington, pp 2543–2566

Semenza G (1977a) Glucosidases of small intestinal brush border. In: Farber E, Sigano H (eds) Pathophysiology of carcinogenesis in digestive organs. University Park Press, Baltimore, pp 207–220

Semenza G (1977b) Intestinal membrane-bound carbohydrase. In: Enzymology and its clinical use. Acta Universitatis Carolinae monographia 77, part I. University Karlova, Prague, pp 21–32

Semenza G (1977c) In: Peptide transport and hydrolysis. Ciba Found Symp 50:119

Semenza G (1979a) Mode of insertion of sucrase-isomaltase complex in the intestinal brush border membrane: implications for the biosynthesis of this stalked intrinsic membrane protein. In: Development of mammalian absorptive processes. Ciba Found Symp 70:133–144

Semenza G (1979b) The mode of anchoring of sucrase-isomaltase to the small intestinal brush-border membrane and its biosynthetic implication. In: Rapoport S (ed) Proceed 12th FEBS meeting, vol 53, Pergamon, Oxford, pp 21–28

Semenza G (1979c) Structure-function relationships in the small intestinal brush border membrane: a site of the merging of biochemistry, physiology and nutrition which Bottazzi indicated two thirds of a century ago. Bull Soc Ital Biol Sperimental 55:597–635

Semenza G, Carafoli E (eds) (1977) Biochemistry of membrane transport. FEBS Symposium 42. Springer, Berlin Heidelberg New York

Semenza G, Kolinska J (1968) An "enzyme-substrate chromatography": intestinal sucrase-isomaltase on sephadex G-200. In: Peeters H (ed) Protides of the biological fluids, Proc 15th coll. Elsevier, Amsterdam, pp 581–583

Semenza G, Auricchio S, Rubino A (1965) Multiplicity of human intestinal disaccharidases. I. Chromatographic separation of maltases and two lactases. Biochim Biophys Acta 96:487–497

Shlygin GK (1952) Secretion of intestinal enzymes (in Russian). Adv Modern Biol 33:14–32

Shlygin GK (1964) The fundamental characteristics of the enzymatic processes in the intestine (in Russian). Vestn Akad Med Nauk SSSR 5:21–31

Shnol SE, Ermakova EA, Frank GM (1979) Diffusive limitations and evolutionary sense of the formation intracellular structures (in Russian). In: Ivanitsky GR (ed) Methodological and theoretical problems of biophysics. Nauka, Moscow, pp 90–99

Sigrist H, Ronner P, Semenza G (1975) A hydrophobic form of the small-intestinal sucrase-isomaltase complex. Biochim Biophys Acta 406:433–446

Silk DBA (1977) Amino acid and peptide absorption in man. In: Peptide transport and hydrolysis. Ciba Found Symp 50:15–29

Silk DBA, Clark ML, Marrs TC, Addison JM, Burston D, Matthews DM, Clegg KM (1975) Jejunal absorption of an amino acid mixture simulating casein and an enzymic hydrolysate of casein prepared for oral administration to normal adults. Br J Nutr 33:95–100

Singer SJ (1974) The molecular organization of membranes. Annu Rev Biochem 43:805–833

Singer SJ (1977) Thermodynamics, the structure of integral membrane proteins, and transport. J Supramol Struct 6:313–323

Skillen AW, Rahbani-Nobar M (1979) ATPase and alkaline phosphatase activities of chick and rat small intestinal mucosa. Biochim Biophys Acta 571:86–93

Slaby J, Lojda Z, Kraml J, Kolinska J (1977) Immunohistochemical localization of intestinal glycosidases. Acta Univ Carol [Med] (Praha), Monographia 77, Part 1:105–112

Smirnova LF (1978) On a decrease in competition in the processes of absorption between amino acids released from dipeptides (in Russian). In: Biological bases for a rational use of the animal and plant world. Zinatne, Riga, pp 55–57

Smirnova LF, Ugolev AM (1972) Relationship between transport of some glycine-containing peptides and equivalent mixtures of constituent amino acids in the rat small intestine (in Russian). Dokl Akad Nauk SSSR 206:763–765

Smirnova LF, Timofeeva NM, Ugolev AM (1976) On the subcellular localization of dipeptide hydrolysis in small intestine (in Russian). Dokl Akad Nauk SSSR 228:992–994

Smithson KW, Gray GM (1977) Intestinal assimilation of a tetrapeptide in the rat. Obligate function of brush border aminopeptidase. J Clin Invest 60:665–674

Smyth DH (1961) Intestinal absorption. Proc Soc Med 54: 769–773

Smyth DH (1970) Mechanisms in intestinal transfer. J Clin Pathol 23:1–6

Smyth DH (ed) (1974) Intestinal absorption. Plenum, London

Smyth DH, Wright EM (1966) Streaming potentials in the rat small intestine. J Physiol (London) 182:591–602

Solomon AK (1968) Characterization of biological membranes by equivalent pores. J Gen Physiol 51:335S–364S

Steck TL (1974) The organization of proteins in the human red blood cell membrane. J Cell Biol 62:1–20

Storelli C, Vögeli H, Semenza G (1972) Reconstitution of a sucrase-mediated sugar transport system in lipid membranes. FEBS Letters 24:287–292

Straub FB (1960) Biochemie. Hungarian Akademie of Siences, Budapest

Sussman HM, Gottlieb AJ (1969) Human placental alkaline phosphatase. II. Molecular and subunits properties of the enzyme. Biochim Biophys Acta 194:170–179

Tagesson Ch, Sjödahl R, Thoren B (1978) Passage of molecules through the wall of the gastrointestinal tract. I. A simple experimental model. Scand J Gastroenterol 13:519–524

Takagi R, Sasaki T (1979) Phospholipid-deacylating enzyme of rat small intestinal mucosa. J Biochem 85:29–39

Takesue Y (1975) Purification and properties of leucine β-naphthylamidase from rabbit small-intestinal mucosal cells. J Biochem 77:103–115

Takesue Y, Kashiwagi T (1969) Solubilization and behavior toward to sephadex of rabbit intestinal sucrase. J Biochem (Tokyo) 65:427–434

Takesue Y, Nishi Y (1978) Topographical studies on intestinal microvillous leucine beta-naphthylamidase on the outer membrane surface. J Membr Biol 39:285–296

Takesue Y, Kashiwagi T, Yoshida TO (1967) Purification and properties of invertase from rabbit small intestine. 7th Int congr biochemistry V:920 (abstr)

Taylor AN, Wasserman RH (1970) Immunofluorescent localization of vitamin D-dependent calcium-binding protein. J Histochem Cytochem 18:107–115

Thomson ABR, Dietschy JM (1977) Derivation of the equations that describe the effects of unstirred water layers on the kinetics parameters of active transport processes in the intestine. J Theor Biol 64:277–294

Toskes PP, Deren JJ (1973) Vitamin B_{12} absorption and malabsorption. Gastroenterology 65:662–683

Troshin AS (ed) (1975) Structure and functions of biological membranes (in Russian). Nauka, Moscow

Tsuboi KK, Schwarts SM, Burill PH, Kwong LK, Sunshine P (1979) Sugar hydrolases of the infant rat intestine and their arrangement on the brush border membrane. Biochim Biophys Acta 554:234–248

Ugolev AM (1960a) On the existence of membrane (contact) digestion (in Russian). Bull Exp Biol Med 49(1):12–17

Ugolev AM (1960b) Influence of the surface of the small intestine on enzymatic hydrolysis of starch by enzymes. Nature 188:588–589

Ugolev AM (1963) Membrane (contact) digestion (in Russian). Izd Akad Nauk SSSR, Moscow

Ugolev AM (1965) Membrane (contact) digestion. Physiol Rev 45:555–595

Ugolev AM (1968) Physiology and pathology of membrane digestion. Plenum, New York

Ugolev AM (1972a) Membrane digestion. Polysubstrate processes, organization and regulation (in Russian). Nauka, Leningrad
Ugolev AM (1972b) Membrane digestion and peptide transport. In: Peptide transport in bacteria and mammalian gut. Ciba Found Symp 4:123–143
Ugolev AM (1974) Membrane (contact) digestion. In: Symth DH (ed) Intestinal absorption. Plenum, London, pp 285–362
Ugolev AM (1975) Chemical and physiological problems of production and use of synthetic food. Carbohydrate nutrition (in Russian). Zinatne, Riga
Ugolev AM (1976) Chemical and physiological problems of production and use of synthetic food: Protein nutrition (in Russian). Zinatne, Riga
Ugolev AM (1977) Structural and functional integration of membrane hydrolysis and transport processes (hypothesis of "permeome") (in Russian). Fiziol Zh SSSR 63: 181–190
Ugolev AM (1978) The integration of enzymic and transport processes at the brush border surface. In: Varro V, Balint GA (eds) Current views of gastroenterology. Hungarian Soc Gastroenterol, Budapest, pp 93–101
Ugolev AM, De Laey P (1973) Membrane digestion. A concept of enzymic hydrolysis on cell membranes. Biochim Biophys Acta 300:105–128
Ugolev AM, Gozitte IK (1972) Digestive functions of the isolated intestinal cells and their regulation. In: Heinz E (ed) Na-linked transport of organic solutes, Int congr physiol sci, Munich. Springer, Berlin Heidelberg New York, p 573
Ugolev AM, Koltushkina GG (1975) Membrane digestion and enzyme apparatus of microvilli (in Russian). In: Structure and functions of biological membranes. Nauka, Moscow, pp 276–306
Ugolev AM, Marauska MK (1964) Data on the physiology of membrane digestion. Comparison of hydrolysis of starch in the intestine and in vitro spectrophotometry of iodine-starch complexes (in Russian). Bull Exp Biol Med 47:16–20
Ugolev AM, Zigure DR, Nurks EE (1970) Accumulating preparation of mucosa – a new method of investigation on initial stages of the transport of substances through intestine cell (in Russian). Fiziol ZH SSSR 56:1638–1641
Ugolev AM, Gredin VG, Gruzdkov AA, De Laey P, Egorova VV, Iezuitova NN, Koltushkina GG, Timofeeva NM, Tuljaganova ECh, Tsvetkova VA, Chernjakhovskaja MYu, Scherbakov GG (1975a) Characterization of multisubstrate processes during digestion. (Data and hypothesis on the interaction and autoregulation of digestive and transport processes). Nahrung 4:299–318
Ugolev AM, Gruzdkov AA, De Laey P, Egorova VV, Iezuitova NN, Koltushkina GG, Timofeeva NM, Tulyaganova ECh, Tsvetkova VA, Chernyakhovskaya MYu, Shcherbakov GG (1975b) Substrate interaction on the intestinal mucosa; a concept for the regulation of intestinal digestion. Br J Nutr 34:205–220
Ugolev AM, Gurman EG, Koltushkina GG (1976a) The influence of the state of glucose transport system on some kinetic characteristics of membrane carbohydrases (γ-amylase and invertase) in the small intestinal mucosa (in Russian) Dokl Akad Nauk SSSR 213:1267–1269
Ugolev AM, Loginov GI, Nurks EE, Smirnova LF (1976b) Interaction of enzyme and transport systems in the digestive membrane. Wiss Z Humboldt Univ Berlin Math Naturwiss 25:45–49
Ugolev AM, Nurks EE, Gurman EG (1976c) Some features of kinetics of accumulation of the free glucose and glucose formed in the hydrolysis of disaccharides in accumulating preparations of rat small intestinal mucosa (in Russian). Dokl Akad Nauk SSSR 231:1018–1020
Ugolev AM, De Laey P, Iezuitova NN (1977a) Absorption of enzymes by cell membrane structure (on the example of enterocytes) under normal and pathological conditions. In: Horejsi J, Kraml J (eds) Enzymology and its clinical use. 19th Scient conf med fac Charles University. University Karlova, Praha, pp 5–19
Ugolev AM, Mityushova NM, Egorova VV (1977b) Regulatory properties of digestive enzymes and biology of polysubstrate digestive processes (in Russian). Zh Evol Biokhim Fiziol 13:589–599

Ugolev AM, Timofeeva NM, Smirnova LF, De Laey P, Gruzdkov AA, Iezuitova NN, Mityushova NM, Roshchina GM, Gurman EG, Gusev VM, Tsvetkova VA, Shcherbakov GG (1977c) Membrane and intracellular hydrolysis of peptides: differentiation, role and interrelations with transport. In: Peptide transport and hydrolysis. Ciba Found Symp 50:221–243

Ugolev AM, Parchkov EM, Egorova VV, Iezuitova NN, Mityushova NM, Smirnova LF, Timofeeva NM, Tsvetkova VA (1978) Distribution of some adsorbed and intrinsic intestinal enzymes between the mucosal cells of the small intestine and the apical glycocalyx separated from them (in Russian). Dokl Akad Nauk SSSR 241:491–494

Ugolev AM, De Laey P, Iezuitova NN, Rakhimov KR, Timofeeva NM, Stepanova AT (1979a) Membrane digestion and nutrient assimilation in early development. In: Development of mammalian absorptive processes. Ciba Found Symp 70:221–246

Ugolev AM, Egorova VV, Iezuitova NN, Mityusova NM (1979b) Die regulatorischen Eigenschaften der Darmenzyme höherer und niederer Tiere als Adaptationsmechanismus der Verdauung und der Resorption. Nahrung 23:371–379

Ugolev AM, Mityushova NM, Egorova VV, Gozite IK, Koltushkina GG (1979c) Catalytic and regulatory properties of the triton and trypsin forms of the brush border hydrolases. Gut 20:737–742

Ugolev AM, Smirnova LF, Iezuitova NN, Timofeeva NM, Mityushova NM, Egorova VV, Parshkov EM (1979d) Distribution of some adsorbed and intrinsic enzymes between the mucosal cells of the rat small intestine and the apical glycocalyx separated from them. FEBS Letters 104:35–38

Ulshen MH, Grand RJ (1979) Site of substrate stimulation of jejunal sucrase in the rat. J Clin Invest 64:1097–1102

Valenkevich LN (1973) Membrane hydrolysis of lipids in elderly and old age (in Russian). Clin Med 51:108–113

Valenkevich LN, Morozov KA, Ugolev AM (1978) A relationship between cavital and membrane digestion in aging (in Russian). Fiziol Chel 4:77–85

Vannier Ch, Louvard D, Maroux S, Desnuelle P (1976) Structural and topological homology between porcine intestinal and renal brush border aminopeptidase. Biochim Biophys Acta 455:185–199

Vasseur M, Ferard G, Pousse A (1978) Rat intestinal brush border enzymes release by deoxycholate in vivo. Pflugers Arch 373:133–138

Volkheimer G (1972) Persorption. Thieme, Stuttgart

Volkheimer G (1974) Passage of particles through the wall of the gastrointestinal tract. Environ Health Perspect 9:215–225

Volkheimer G (1977) Persorption of particles; physiology and pharmacology. Adv Pharmacol Chemother 14:163–187

Volkheimer G (1978) Persorption of carbohydrate particles. In: Varro V, Balint GA (eds) Current views in gastroenterology. Hung Soc Gastroenterol, Budapest, pp 77–91

Wacker H, Semenza G (1977) A brush borderbound peptidase and amino acid transport. In: Peptide transport and hydrolysis. Ciba Found Symp 50:109–116

Wahlqvist ML, Wilmshurst EG, Richardson EN (1978) The effect of chain length on glucose absorption and the related metabolic response. Am J Clin Nutr 31:1998–2001

Walker WA (1979) Gastrointestinal host defence: importance of gut closure in control of macromolecular transport. In: Development of mammalian absorptive processes. Ciba Found Symp 70:201–216

Walker WA, Isselbacher KI (1974) Uptake and transport of macromolecules by the intestine: possible role in clinic disorders. Gastroenterology 67:531–550

Walker WA, Field M, Isselbacher KJ (1974) Specific binding of cholera toxin to isolated intestinal microvillous membranes. Proc Nat Acad Sci USA 71:320–324

Wasserman RH (1974) Calcium absorption and calcium-binding protein synthesis: solanum malacoxylon reverses strontium inhibition. Science 183:1092–1094

Wasserman RH, Taylor AN (1971) Evidence for vitamin D induced calcium-binding protein in New World primates. Proc Soc Exp Biol Med 136:25–28

Wasserman RH, Taylor AN, Kallfelz FA (1966) Vitamin D and transfer of plasma calcium to intestinal lumen in chicks and rats. Am J Physiol 211:419–423

Wells GP, Nicholson JA, Peters TJ (1979) Subcellular localisation of di- and tripeptidases in guinea pig and rat enterocytes. Biochim Biophys Acta 569:82–88
Wilson DB (1978) Cellular transport mechanisms. Annu Rev Biochem 47:933–965
Wilson PA, Dietschy JM (1974) The intestinal unstirred layer: its surface area and effect in active transport kinetics. Biochim Biophys Acta 363:112–126
Wilson PA, Melmed KN, Hampe MMV, Holt SJ (1978) Immunocytochemical study of the interaction of soubean trypsin inhibitor with rat intestinal mucosa. Gut 19:260–266
Wilson TH (1962) Intestinal absorption. Saunders, Philadelphia
Wilson TH, Wiseman G (1954) The use of sacs everted small intestine for the study of the transference of substances from the mucosal to the serosal surface. J Physiol 123:116–125
Winne D (1976) Unstirred layer thickness in perfused rat jejunum in vivo. Experientia 32:1278–1279
Winne D (1977) Correction of the apparent Michaelis constant, biased by an unstirred layer, if a passive transport component is present. Biochim Biophys Acta 464:118–126
Winne D, Kopf S, Ulmer M-L (1979) Role of unstirred layer in intestinal absorption of phenylalanine in vivo. Biochim Biophys Acta 550:120–130
Wiseman G (1964) Absorption from the intestine. Academic, London
Wiseman G (1968) Absorption of amino acids. In: Intestinal absorption. American Physiological Society, Washington, pp 1277–1307 (Handbook of physiology, sec 6. Alimentary canal, vol III
Wiseman G (1974) Absorption of protein digestion products. In: Intestinal absorption. Plenum, London, pp 363–481
Wiseman G (1977) Site of intestinal dipeptide hydrolysis. J Physiol (London) 273:731–743
Wojnarowska F, Gray GM (1975) Intestinal surface peptide hydrolases: identification and characterization of three enzymes from rat brush border. Biochim Biophys Acta 403:147–160
Woodley JF, Kenny AJ (1969) The presence of pancreatic proteases in particulate preparations of rat intestinal mucosa. Biochem J 115:18P
Wright RD, Jennings MA, Florey HW, Lium R (1940) The influence of nerves and drugs on secretion by the small intestine and investigation of the enzymes in intestinal juice. Quart J Exp Physiol 30:73–120
Yamashiro KM, Gray GM (1970) Separation and interrelationship of human intestinal sucrase and isomaltase. Gastroenterology 58:1056
Zaripov BZ, Iezuitova NN, Ugolev AM (1978) Studies on the membrane digestion and transport of carbohydrates in Chronic experiments (in Russian). In: Physiology and pathology of digestion. Comm 2nd bilateral symposium CSSR–USSR. University Palackeho of Olomouci, Olomouc, pp 8–11
Zetterqvist H, Hendrix TR (1960) A preliminary note on an ultrastructural abnormality of the intestinal epithelium in adult celiac disease (nontropical sprue) which is reversed by a gluten free diet. Bull Johns Hopkins Hosp 106:240–249
Zlatkina AR, Misautova AA, Makiyevskaya SE, Kutichkina OA, Lyubchenko PN (1973) Indeces of membrane digestion at gastrointestinal tract diseases (in Russian). In: Membrane digestion. Theoretical and applied aspects. Zinatne, Riga, pp 51–53
Zlatkina AR, Galperin YuM, Makijevskaya SE, Bezzubik KV, Misautova AA, Rybakova GS (1976) Some mechanisms of compensation of membrane digestion disturbances (in Russian). In: Ugolev AM (ed) Digestive enzymes. Comm 1st bilateral symposium USSR–Czechoslovakia. Uzhgorod, pp 40–43
Zwaal RFA (1978) Membrane and lipid involvement in blood coagulation. Biochim Biophys Acta 515:163–205

CHAPTER 20

The Surface pH of the Intestinal Mucosa and its Significance in the Permeability of Organic Anions

M. Lucas

A. Introduction

A general principle of membrane transport which has been extensively investigated is that of the nonionic diffusion of dissociable solutes across membranes. This principle is particularly evident where no specific transport mechanism exists to accelerate their permeation. The pH of a solute-containing phase, by altering the concentration of undissociated solute available for diffusion across a membrane permeable only to the nonionised form, will alter the overall apparent rate of solute transfer. Another expression of this general principle is the pH partition hypothesis based on the central assumption that ionised forms of solutes do not permeate membranes easily, if at all, unless there is a specific transport mechanism in operation. Any pH differences across such a membrane will cause a partition of solute in a predictable manner depending on the pH of the phases and the pK_a of the solute under investigation. This is well known to pharmacologists and has been experimentally substantiated on many occasions by drug elimination studies in the kidney (Milne et al. 1958; Beckett and Rowland 1964), with artificial membrane systems (Doluisio and Swintosky 1964; Samuelov et al. 1979) and in gastrointestinal membranes such as the gastric mucosa, the small bowel, colon and rectum (Shore et al. 1957; Schanker et al. 1957, 1958, Schanker 1959; Hogben et al. 1959). What is perhaps less generally realised is the fact that in the small bowel, especially in the jejunum, although the degree of ionisation and the extent of absorption parallel one another, the two parameters do not coincide. Only in the rectum and colon is there an almost complete correspondence between ionisation and absorption.

In rat jejunum in vivo, there exist what have come to be called "pH shifts" (Koizumi et al. 1964; Kakemi et al. 1969; Morishita et al. 1971; Bridges et al. 1976) or "deviations" from the pH partition hypothesis. The group (Hogben et al. 1959) that first noticed these shifts in the peak of maximum absorption away from the peak of maximum concentration of undissociated solute, proposed that there existed in the jejunum what they termed an "acid microclimate" or "virtual pH". They calculated that the pH immediately juxtaposed to the intestinal wall was some two pH units more acid at a pH of 5.3 when the bulk luminal bathing medium was set at neutral pH. Briefly stated, the microclimate hypothesis (Fig. 1) allows for the conversion of ionised forms at neutral pH into the undissociated form in the more acid pH of the microclimate, if the solute is a weak acid, making more neutral species available for nonionic diffusion into the enterocytes; the converse would be true in the case of weak bases. Although an interposed phase of

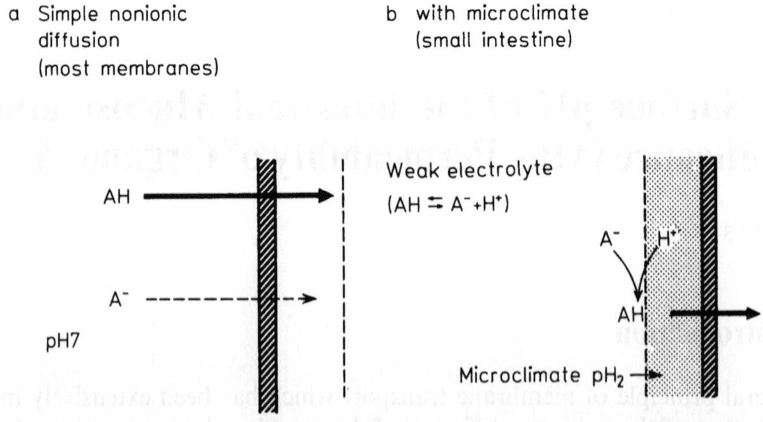

Fig. 1 a, b. Membrane transfer of weak electrolytes. General case (**a**), preferred permeation of undissociated form. Special case for proximal jejunum (**b**), acid region (pH_2) provides a microclimate of hydrogen ions for conversion of ionised forms prior to permeation as undissociated form

altered pH will not affect the final disposition of substance between two end phases, the rate of approach to a steady state will be faster for a weak acid and slower for a weak base where an acid microclimate is involved. If an infinite amount of time were allowable for a substance to cross a membrane, a slow rate of transfer would be of little consequence. In the case of intestinal transport, where nutrient is presented as a bolus passing along the lumen of the gastrointestinal tract, an acid microclimate would have a significant effect on solutes that are presented to the gut wall as acids or as charged groups capable of undergoing dissociation. Transport would be hastened or retarded within the finite amount of time allowed for absorption with possible consequences for the total amounts absorbed.

Deviations from the pH partition hypothesis have been frequently demonstrated using experimental preparations of upper small intestine. Yet the acid microclimate hypothesis has been neglected, either on the grounds of a priori thermodynamic untenability (SMOLEN 1973) or on the grounds that alternative hypotheses are just as valid if not more attractive. Alternative explanations have invoked partial permeability of the upper small bowel to ionised forms, the effects of unstirred layers and lipid extraction; these alternative proposals will be discussed. There is now a growing body of evidence that hydrogen ion secretion occurs in the proximal small bowel both in vivo and in vitro. Since a mucosally directed source of hydrogen ions is arguably a prerequisite for the maintenance of an acid microclimate, the mechanism of hydrogen ion secretion will be discussed. The experimental evidence for the acid microclimate hypothesis and for an alternative alkaline microclimate hypothesis will be considered as well as the possibility of serious derangement in intestinal disease. Particular instances will be reviewed where the microclimate affects absorption and the topic of surface pH will be discussed within the general context of drug absorption in the small bowel.

B. Intestinal pH Measurements

Early measurements of intestinal pH were carried out by investigators who believed that rachitogenic diets were somehow connected with the acid-base state of the small intestine. While the original question connecting rickets and intestinal pH was never resolved, several studies were carried out on rat (REDMAN et al. 1927; MCROBERT 1928; OSER 1928) and dog intestinal pH (GRAYZEL and MILLER 1927; GRAHAM and EMERY 1928) before and after dietary manipulations. These studies showed regional differences in that the pH of washings of luminal content from the proximal small intestine was generally more acid than that of washings from the more distal small intestine. Later work on dog luminal pH showed a similar pattern (ROBINSON 1935; BERK et al. 1942) in that a distally declining gradient of acidity was detected, associated with a high carbon dioxide partial pressure (PCO_2) in the jejunum and a low PCO_2 in the ileum, irrespective of whether the dogs were made acidotic or alkalotic (ROBINSON et al. 1942). At the same time, reports confirmed that human intestinal pH had similar values (ROBINSON et al. 1942; MCGEE and HASTINGS 1942) with intestinal PCO_2 higher than in the plasma.

Later studies with more reliable methods using glass pH electrodes have consistently confirmed these early observations in dog jejunum (ARDISSON et al. 1973; ALDAY and GOLDSMITH 1975) and in human intestinal tract (KRAMER and INGELFINGER 1961; FORDTRAN and LOCKLEAR 1966; SOERGEL 1971; MELDRUM et al. 1972), as well as in the rabbit (CATALA 1975), the pig (BRAUDE et al. 1976) and the sheep (SCOTT 1965). Two alternative mechanisms might be appropriate for causing a distally declining gradient of intraluminal hydrogen ions, ranging from pH 4.5–6.0 in the proximal intestine to pH 6.5–7.5 in the ileum. The gradient could occur by mixing of the gastric secretions with alkaline secretions originating from the pancreas, gallbladder and duodenum. Hence intraluminal pH would simply represent a gradient of the effectiveness of mixing of these acid and alkaline solutions in the lumen. Undoubtedly this is the case for most animals studied so far. An alternative mechanism other than simple mixing would involve the ability of the intestinal mucosa to alter the pH of the luminal contents selectively, either by the continual secretion of a fluid of set pH which is characteristic of a certain region or by the initiation of specific ion movements. The fact that gastric juice neutralisation occurs in the duodenal bulb is well known and will not come under the scope of the present chapter; this process involves backdiffusion of hydrogen ions from the lumen into the bloodstream combined with active bicarbonate secretion (KING and SCHLOERB 1972), originating from the Brunners glands. A distinctly different mechanism also seems to be operative in the jejunum of rat and human.

When solutions of differing pH are instilled into the rat jejunum in vivo, alkaline buffers are acidified until they attain acid values, and where they have been used, acid buffers are progressively neutralised (PONZ and LARRALDE 1950; PARSONS 1956; KOIZUMI et al. 1964; FOERSTER et al. 1967; WALDRON-EDWARD 1971). The same is true in dog (ROBINSON 1935; ARDISSON et al. 1973) and human in vivo (TURNBERG et al. 1970a). These observations have been repeatedly confirmed in the rat in vitro using everted sac preparations where uncertainties as to the amount of systemic influence are excluded. In vitro rat studies have demonstrated that the ability to alter the pH of the bathing fluid is a property of the intestinal mucosa (WILSON 1953, 1956; WILSON and KAZYAK 1957; M.E. SMITH 1971, private communication; BLAIR et al. 1972, 1975; JACKSON et al. 1974; LUCAS 1976; DOLISI et al. 1979). This phenomenon termed "acidification" is considered in greater detail in the following section.

C. Acidification Studies

There have been relatively few studies on the ability of the upper small intestine to acidify the luminal contents, although in recent years the number has been increasing as the relevance to intestinal drug absorption is becoming apparent. Most studies dealing with acidification have concentrated on changes in pH as the measured variable, with relatively few quantifying these pH changes into secretion of hydrogen ion. The pioneering studies of T. Hastings Wilson (WILSON 1953, 1956; WILSON and KAZYAK 1957) using everted sacs from rat jejunum showed that mucosal pH fell and serosal pH rose slightly because of net transport of bicarbonate into the serosal solution. Changes in pH were calculated from the Henderson–Hasselbach equation, knowing the concentrations of bicarbonate and carbon dioxide. Anoxia in vitro reduced the gradient of pH across the tissue, an effect confirmed in latter studies (BLAIR et al. 1972, 1975). WILSON, using bicarbonate buffer solutions in vivo found, that much the same results could be obtained. Essentially, the mucosal pH fell with 85% of this fall being attributed to the mucosal appearance of lactic acid. Although more bicarbonate was lost mucosally than appeared serosally, it was felt that the hydrolysis of phosphates could contribute to the pH differential. WILSON and KAZYAK (1957) proposed that a sodium–hydrogen ion exchange process might occur and that ultimately the source of hydrogen ions could be the hydrolysis of water.

I. The Effect of Mucosal Glucose Concentration

Using glucose-containing buffers and quantifying the amount of secreted hydrogen ion by backtitration of the acidified solution with sodium hydroxide, it can be shown that mucosally appearing lactic acid can account for only about 15% of the hydrogen ions produced and that pyruvate accounts for an even smaller amount (BLAIR et al. 1975). The ability of anoxia to reduce hydrogen ion secretion was also confirmed. A hyperbolic relationship between external glucose concentration and the rate of hydrogen ion secretion was demonstrated (BLAIR et al. 1975). However, the nonmetabolisable sugars galactose and 3-*0*-methylglucose, which are actively transported, did not increase acidification whereas the metabolisable sugars mannose and fructose, which are not actively transported, did increase the rate of acidification, demonstrating that the effect of glucose was at a metabolic level rather than as a consequence of the active transport of hexoses.

II. The Involvement of Carbonic Anhydrase

Parsons and co-workers (PARSONS 1956; MCHARDY and PARSONS 1956), showed in vivo that the fall in pH was most pronounced in the jejunum, less so in the ileum, with a slight alkalinisation occuring in the colon. This occurred whether the lumen was perfused with bicarbonate or phosphate buffer, i.e. the process was not exclusively dependent on the presence of luminal bicarbonate. However, an infusion of 500 μg/ml carbonic anhydrase inhibitor acetazolamide (Diamox) reduced the fall in pH in the jejunum and caused the ileum to acidify. This inhibitory effect of carbonic anhydrase inhibitor was later confirmed in vivo by jejunal perfusion of subjects with pernicious anaemia (TURNBERG et al. 1970a). In these patients PCO_2 rose on acidification of saline solutions, bicarbonate buffer and in combined bicarbonate and phosphate buffers. Bicarbonate transport was found to be saturable with a K_m of approximately 40 m*M*. From a series of "disequilibrium pH" studies, it was concluded that hydrogen ion secretion rather than bicarbonate absorption was the cause of luminal acidification. Although the use of patients with pernicious anaemia might pose the question of whether such subjects had normal jejunal hydrogen ion secretion, other studies in humans have confirmed these observations (WINGATE et al. 1973) and further demonstrated that bicarbonate absorption, i.e. hydrogen ion secretion, was independent of bulk water flow. Contradictory results for acetazolamide were found in rat duodenum in vivo (SCHNELL and MIYA 1970) where little effect on luminal pH was seen. Unbuffered solutions were used and therefore it is difficult to draw firm conclusions from this experiment as to the likely result in bicarbonate buffer. In vitro 10 m*M* acetazolamide had no effect on acidification (BLAIR et al. 1975), although this may have been because sufficient exogenous bicarbonate was present in the buffer to overcome any effects of enzyme inhibition.

III. Sodium Ion Exchange Mechanisms

The original proposal of WILSON that hydrogen ion is exchanged for sodium ion, most probably at the luminal membrane of the enterocyte, has found adherents (TURNBERG et al. 1970) and there is experimental evidence in support of this concept. Reduced luminal bicarbonate concentrations lead to reduced sodium absorption in rat in vivo (HUBEL 1973) and man (SLADEN and DAWSON 1968). Conversely, reduced luminal sodium concentration will reduce both bicarbonate absorption and hydrogen ion secretion in vivo (HUBEL 1973; PODESTA and METTRICK 1977a) and in vitro in rat (LUCAS 1976). Other workers have failed to note a reduction of acidification in vitro in low sodium buffers (JACKSON and MORGAN 1975); in these latter studies, the results were obtained in phosphate buffer containing very low buffering ion concentrations and consequently the measured rates of acidification were very low. Experiments with enterocyte luminal membrane vesicles have shown a close relationship between inwardly directed sodium fluxes and proton fluxes in the reverse direction (MURER et al. 1976). Although in this instance sodium and hydrogen ion movement was coupled, these experiments may not relate to the normal hydrogen ion secretory process which has been shown to have a metabolic input that vesicles cannot provide. One site of interaction for sodium and hydrogen ion may be at the metabolic level since in vitro, low sodium buffers will lead to less glucose uptake (FAUST 962) and a reduction in metabolism (LEVIN and SYME 1975). This would be in agreement with the metabolic dependence of the acidification process. Whether this could explain the in vivo relationship depends on whether sodium-dependent glucose entry is an important source of energy in the in vivo gut.

IV. Hydrogen–Potassium Exchange

A cation not so readily considered is potassium, which might exchange for mucosally directed hydrogen ion (LUCAS 1976). Potassium ion secretion has been shown to change to absorption with increasing luminal bicarbonate concentration (PODESTA and METTRICK 1977a). Nonmetabolisable sugars will cause intracellular potassium levels to be lower than is the case in the presence of metabolisable sugars (BROWN and PARSONS 1962). Potassium influx across the luminal membrane is less in the presence of the nonmetabolisable sugars galactose and methylglucoside, but is increased in the presence of glucose and fructose (REMKE et al. 1975). Stoichiometrically there is a better agreement between potassium flux and hydrogen ion secretion than between acidification and sodium ion movement since far more sodium ion is transported and only a fraction of this could be obligatorily coupled with hydrogen ion movement.

V. Acidification and Electrical Events

Most studies have demonstrated that hydrogen ion secretion is an electroneutral process or at least electrically "silent" since small changes in the transmural potential difference caused by altering the buffering anions in the luminal fluid have little effect on acidification (TURNBERG et al. 1970). Similarly, when chloride ion was replaced with isethionate or other substituent anions, acidification was unchanged in the jejunum (HUBEL 1973; JACKSON and MORGAN 1975; PODESTA and METTRICK 1977a). This is in contrast to the ileum where chloride replacement tends to lead to acidification of the ileal lumen, causing the ileum to resemble the jejunum. There is a chloride–bicarbonate anion exchange mechanism present in the ileum which does not function in the absence of luminal chloride (TURNBERG et al. 1970b; PODESTA and METTRICK 1977b). Since the equilibrium pH for the ileal lumen in chloride-free solutions is 6.6 and clearly below plasma pH, this manoeuvre may unmask an ileal hydrogen ion secretory mechanism.

Substances such as ouabain and aminophylline which reduce short-circuit current also inhibit hydrogen ion secretion (LUCAS 1976), but this may reflect only the common dependence of both on metabolism. As with the ileum, some studies have suggested that the lowering of mucosal sodium ion concentration unmasks a reversed potential difference associated with the hydrogen ion secretory pump (FAELLI and GAROTTA 1971a, b; MCKENNY 1971). It has long been known that Tris substitution reverses the transmural potential difference (LYON and CRANE 1966; BARRY et al. 1967), but this has been previously attributed solely to sodium ion diffusion potential differences (PD) (BARRY and EGGENTON 1972). FAELLI demonstrated (1971a, b) that the sustained reversed or negative transmural potential was inhibited by the presence of acetazolamide and that the sum total of hydrogen ion movements correlated well with the magnitude of the reversed PD (FAELLI and ESPOSITO 1971). The reversed PD can be stabilised and elevated in 30 m*M* sodium-containing Tis buffer and the magnitude altered by mucosal aminophylline and serosal ouabain (LUCAS 1976). This seems to make it unlikely that the reversed PD are solely the result of sodium diffusion PD.

Further experiments in the author's laboratory have shown that the hydrogen ion secretory process may nevertheless be electrically silent. Low sodium buffers reduce the transmural PD in guinea-pig jejunum, which does not acidify its luminal contents, but no reversal of the potential is seen. Similarly, rat jejunum incubated in low sodium buffer with phosphate as the major buffering anion has a lower transmural PD and behaves exactly as guinea-pig jejunum. Only when bicarbonate is present as the dominant buffering anion is a reversal of PD seen in the rat jejunum. This seems to indicate that the PD change is due to an asymmetrical distribution in bicarbonate concentration across the jejunum, dependent on the reduced (LUCAS 1976) but significant hydrogen ion secretion that occurs in low sodium buffer. Hydrogen ions would reduce the concentration of bicarbonate anions at the luminal membrane and, provided that the enterocyte membrane has a finite permeability to bicarbonate anion per se, generate a bicarbonate diffusion PD. Hence on balance it is likely that hydrogen ion secretion is an electrically neutral process.

VI. The Mechanism of Hydrogen Ion Secretion

The detailed mechanism by which jejunal mucosa secretes hydrogen ion is still unclear. It is known that the PCO_2 of luminal solutions in vivo in the rat is significantly higher than the PCO_2 in the mesenteric veins, regardless of whether the animal is breathing air, oxygen or mixtures containing 10% CO_2. Luminal PCO_2 responds to increases in venous PCO_2 but is always 10 mmHg higher (MAGGI et al. 1970). In rat in vivo (PODESTA and METTRICK 1977a) and in human perfusion studies (TURNBERG et al. 1970a), disequilibrium pH experiments in which the initial and final PCO_2 of instilled solutions are monitored seem to favour a hydrogen ion secretory mechanism rather than bicarbonate removal. Since the final equilibrium PCO_2 is higher after acidification, this would seem to indicate generation of hydrogen ions since a removal of bicarbonate would eventually lead to a reduction in PCO_2.

Hydrogen ion secretion implies either secretion of an organic acid or charge separation of hydrogen ions from hydroxyl ions at the secreting membrane with in both instances the formation of an equivalent amount of base somewhere in the system. As the hydrogen ion is mucosally directed it might be argued that the equivalent amount of base is buffered intracellularly. In in vitro experiments in the rat, the serosal compartment as well as the mucosal compartment can acidify (BARRY et al. 1966b; LUCAS and BLAIR 1978) adding support to the concept of intracellular buffering. It is at this point that carbonic anhydrase may be involved, i.e. to provide rapid intracellular buffering rather than participation in the transport step.

The mucosally sited hydrolysis of ATP might be the mechanism for hydrogen ion secretion as has been proposed (WADDELL 1975) since in vitro the largest increase in rate was seen in the presence of external ATP (BLAIR et al. 1975). Although ATP is thought not to enter cells there is some doubt about this (HARMS and STIRLING 1977). It is probable that, in both studies, a considerable amount of hydrolysis of the γ-phosphate group of ATP occurred externally. The most potent inhibitor of hydrogen ion secretion so far studied has been aminophylline, the methylxanthine that prevents the breakdown of cAMP and ultimately of ATP by adenylate cyclase (Blair et al. 1975).

VII. Hormonal Effects

Reports of the effects of hormones on intestinal acidification are sparse. Bethanechol, a compound mimicking the effects of acetylcholine; when given intravenously to rats caused a reduction in the fall in pH normally seen in the jejunum, implying that cholinergic innervation should inhibit ion secretion (Hubel 1977). In accordance with this concept pilocarpine also reduced acidification in the rat, an effect which was blocked by the administration of atropine, which itself slightly stimulated acidification; norepinephrine was without effect (Hubel 1976). Glucagon stimulated (Hubel 1971) and secretin inhibited bicarbonate absorption in in vivo rat jejunum. If it is assumed that alterations in bicarbonate transport automatically mean that hydrogen ion secretion is also altered, then this raises the possibility of enteric hormones being able to affect hydrogen ion secretion. The secretin-induced reduction in bicarbonate transport was unconfirmed in human studies by Hicks and Turnberg (1973), although they noted a 50% reduction which failed to reach significance.

VIII. Infectious Agents

Some work has been done on the effects of infectious agents on the luminal pH changes in the small intestine [1]. Jejunal bicarbonate absorption is reduced in rats with salmonellae enterocolitis caused by *Salmonella typhimurium* (Powell et al. 1971). The mean fall in pH and the rise in PCO_2 were both less in the infected rat. The pattern in the infected ileum resembled the normal jejunum in much the same way that chloride ion replacement causes the ileum to resemble the jejunum. In rats infected with *Vibrio cholerae* toxin, bicarbonate absorption is reduced (Strombeck 1972), and in the golden hamster, the lumen is filled with a clear alkaline fluid (Lepot and Banwell 1976). No human studies have been carried out to date although the concentration of faecal bicarbonate is higher than usual and a metabolic acidosis may occur (Banwell et al. 1970). This is usually attributed to a loss of alkaline secretions because of diarrhoea, although the component due to poor bicarbonate absorption has never been quantified. Similarly, in macaque monkeys infected with *Shigella*, there is a shift to alkalinity in the pH of the small bowel (Takasaka 1978), indicative of inhibition of hydrogen ion secretion. It may be that several diseases that affect the upper small bowel cause a reduction in hydrogen ion secretion as a consequence of damage to the intestinal mucosa. Interesting recent studies on the parasitism of rat small intestine by the tapeworm *Hymenolepsis diminuta* have shed an intriguing light on hydrogen ion secretion. In the parasitised jejunum, hydrogen ion is secreted by the tapeworm while the hydrogen ion secretion of the host is somewhat lower than usual (Podesta and Mettrick 1974). Although one possibility is that the tapeworm acidifies the luminal contents to a pH below that for optimal functioning of the digestive processes of

---

1 See also Chaps. 26 and 27 for the effects of cholera and other bacterial toxins in intestinal permeability

the host, another possibility is the secretion by the tapeworm of a factor that switches off the host hydrogen ion secretory mechanism in much the same way that *Ascaris* secretes a trypsin inhibitory factor (MUKERJI et al. 1977).

D. The Intestinal Acid Microclimate

I. Evidence for the Microclimate Hypothesis

The preceding section on intestinal acidification will have drawn attention to the fact that there is a mechanism in the upper small intestine whereby hydrogen ions appear at the luminal surface, whether by hydrogen ion secretion or by bicarbonate removal is still unclear. Consequently one might expect a gradient of hydrogen ions orthogonal to the intestine as they diffuse away into the bulk bathing medium. Studies on rat jejunum in vitro with Hinke pH microelectrodes have demonstrated the existence of the acid microclimate (LUCAS et al. 1975). Everted and cannulated proximal jejunum was maintained in Krebs bicarbonate buffer containing glucose, with transmural PD measured simultaneously. Adjacent sections were used to demonstrative active glucose transport. As the 60-μm tip electrode was racked down onto the surface of the mucosa, an immediate step change in the recorded pH was measured (Fig. 2) which remained stable for minutes; this observation could be repeated several times. To preclude the possibility of intracellular penetration, the electrode was racked onto the surface at a very oblique angle and the pH change could still be recorded, demonstrating that the measured surface pH was extracellular. Similar results were obtained using slightly larger 80-μm and slightly smaller 45-μm antimony microelectrodes. Parallel experiments using pH indicators failed to show colour changes at the mucosal surface. Because of this, electrode studies became the method of choice (LUCAS et al. 1975).

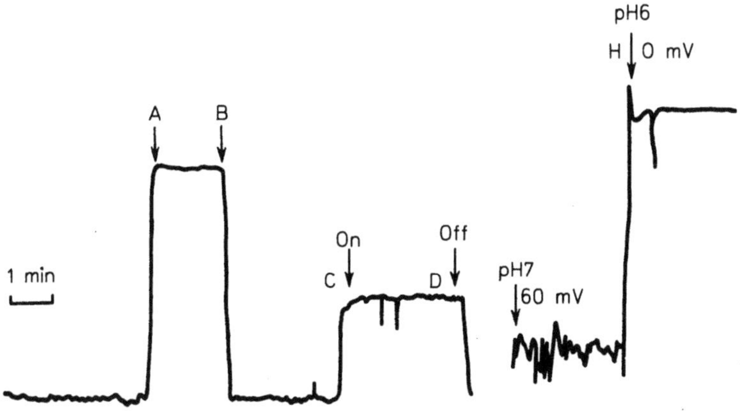

Fig. 2 a–d. Determination of acid microclimate in rat proximal jejunum in vitro. Measurement in everted cannulated preparation (*A*) electrode on surface; (*B*) electrode off surface; (*C*) electrode on surface at oblique angle to prevent intracellular penetration; (*D*) electrode off; (*H*) electrode recalibrated in buffers at pH 6 and 7. Jejunum in bicarbonate buffer gassed with 95.5% O_2/4,5% CO_2 (v/v), at 37 °C containing 10 m*M* glucose. LUCAS et al. (1975)

Using "surface" pH electrodes (PORTNOY 1967) consisting of a convex pH glass membrane sealed onto inert capillary glass which had a sensing "convexity" of approximately 30 µm, these initial studies have been confirmed and extended. The low surface pH, occasionally reaching values as low as 5.3, is dependent on the external glucose concentration, reaching a lowest value in the presence of 10 m*M* external glucose concentration (Fig. 3) and corresponding to the concentration of glucose which gives the maximum rate of acidification (BLAIR et al. 1975; LUCAS and BLAIR 1978). In the absence of glucose, a significantly acid surface pH is still measurable which is lower than the bulk pH (LUCAS and BLAIR 1978). Over a 1-h incubation period, the low surface pH in the presence of glucose remains stable whereas in the absence of glucose the surface pH becomes more alkaline. There is a distally declining gradient of surface pH in that the lowest surface pH recorded was in the proximal jejunum and higher values (Fig. 4) were found in the ileum (LUCAS and BLAIR 1978). Following this trend, the response to external glucose is greatest in the proximal intestine and becomes less on moving distally. This gradient of surface pH is similar to the gradient of luminal pH found, although somewhat lower. This is most probably because in the fasting or interdigestive state, barring changes in luminal pH because of sudden surges of gastric or pancreatic juice, the luminal pH would eventually reflect the surface pH owing to the acidification needed to maintain the surface pH at a characteristically low value.

In the proximal jejunum, the relationship between bulk solution pH and surface pH has been investigated (LUCAS et al. 1976, 1980). Surface pH at the onset of incubation is slightly higher than the bulk pH when the latter is below pH 5.5. Above this value (Fig. 5) the surface pH becomes increasingly independent of bulk pH and remains acid, between pH 5 and 6, in the face of increasing alkalinity of the buffer pH. The surface pH can therefore be maintained when the bulk pH is very alkaline, representing a concentration difference of 3–4 orders of magni-

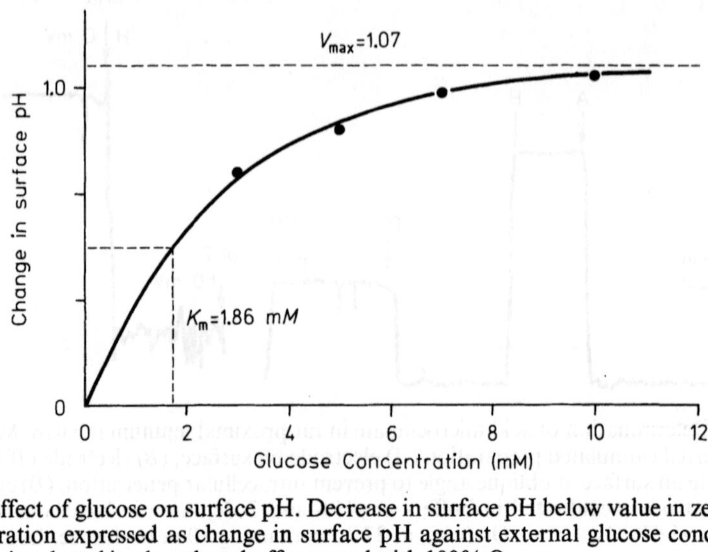

Fig. 3. Effect of glucose on surface pH. Decrease in surface pH below value in zero glucose concentration expressed as change in surface pH against external glucose concentration. Jejunum incubated in phosphate buffer gassed with 100% O_2

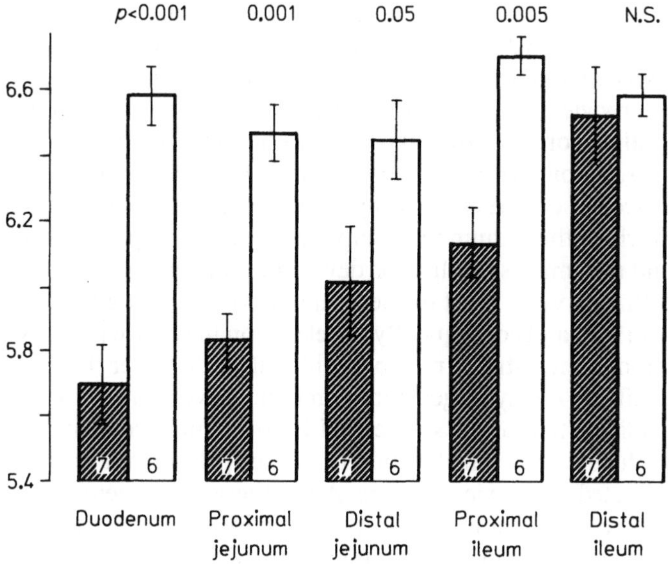

Fig. 4. Distribution of surface pH along the small bowel. Surface pH in rat intestine incubated in bicarbonate buffer with (*hatched columns*) and without (*open columns*) 10 m*M* glucose. Results are expressed as means ± standard error with the number of animals at base of columns. N.S. = not significant

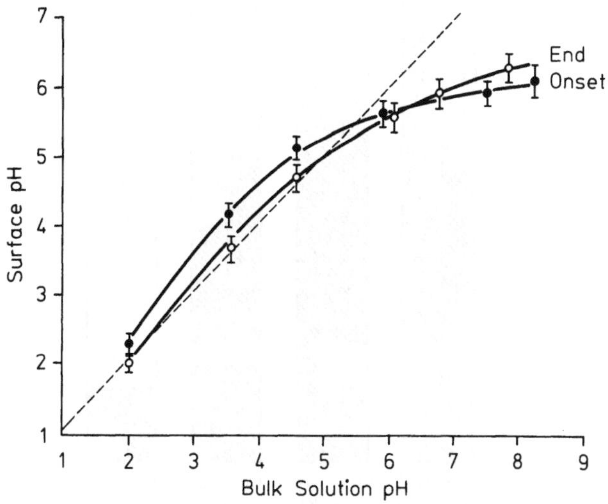

Fig. 5. Relationship between surface pH and bulk solution pH. Surface pH in rat proximal jejunum at the onset (*full circles*) and end (*open circles*) of a 1-h period, incubated in bicarbonate buffer whose bulk pH was altered by increments of HCl or NaOH. Details as for Fig. 4. Six animals per point. *Broken line* is the isohydric line where surface pH equals bulk pH

tude. After 1 h incubation, below a value of 5.5, the bulk pH and the surface pH equalise along an isohydric line. Presumably the bulk hydrogen ions diffuse into the microclimate making it more acid, accumulating because of the impermeability of the enterocyte membrane to hydrogen ion. Above a bulk pH of 5.5, the surface pH remains more acid than the bulk pH because loss from the microclimate into the bulk solutions is replenished by hydrogen ion secretion.

The surface pH can be elevated by anoxia, mucosal ouabain, aminophylline, solutions in which the sodium ion component is largely replaced by potassium or mannitol and also mucosal solutions devoid of potassium (Fig. 6; LEI et al. 1977, LUCAS and BLAIR 1978). Most of these manoeuvres inhibit glucose entry (FAUST 1962; LUCAS 1976) and consequently the elevation in surface pH may relate more to a restriction in the entry of metabolisable substrate under these circumstances than direct effects on hydrogen ion secretion. Nevertheless, these in vitro experiments indicate that a low surface pH is not an in vitro artifact since anoxia and lack of glucose cause an elevation in surface pH and not the lowering which might be expected of anoxic autolysis. All of these experimental conditions also reduce the rate of acidification as discussed previously. Surface pH is also responsive to external sodium ion concentration with an apparent optimum at 120 mM which is just below plasma concentrations (Fig. 7). This effect is again most marked in the proximal jejunum and least so in the ileum (Fig. 8; LUCAS et al. 1980).

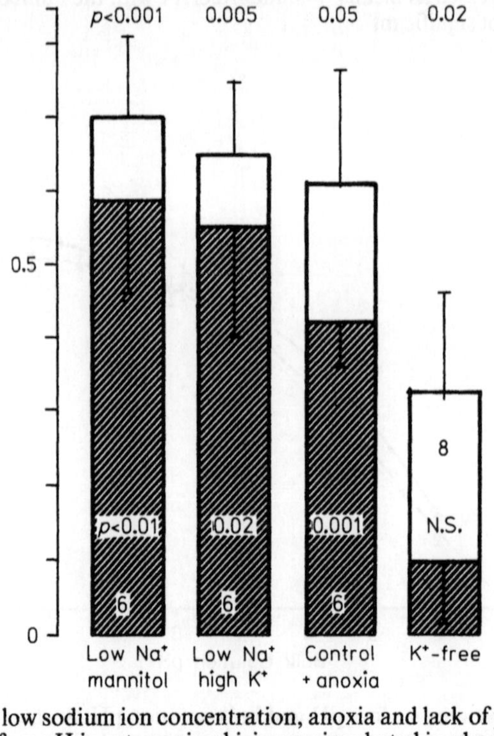

Fig. 6. The effect of low sodium ion concentration, anoxia and lack of potassium on surface pH. Increase in surface pH in rat proximal jejunum incubated in phosphate buffer. Details as for Fig. 4. *Open columns* represent change at onset, *hatched columns* change at end of 1-h incubation period caused by absence of sodium, anoxia and a potassium-free buffer solution. N.S. = not significant

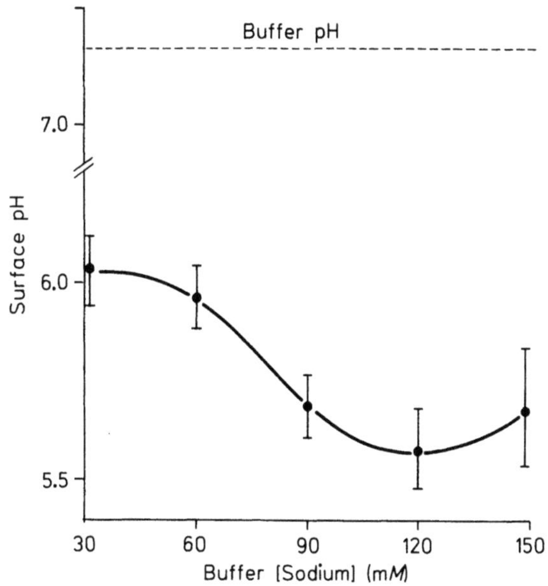

Fig. 7. Effect of buffer sodium ion concentration on surface pH. Surface pH against sodium ion concentration profile for rat proximal jejunum with sodium replaced by mannitol in phosphate buffer. Details as for Fig. 4, six animals per point

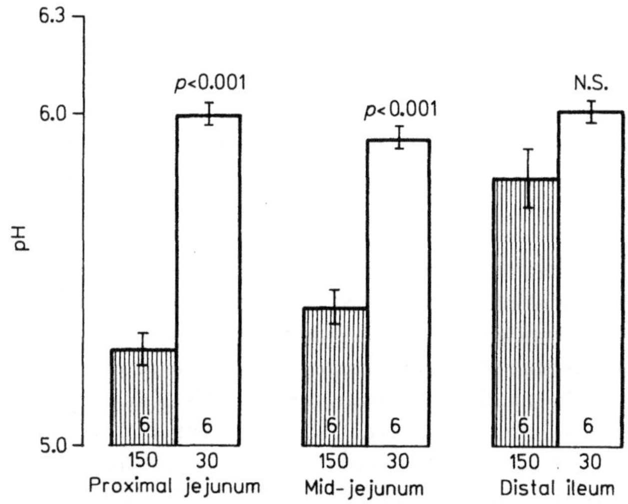

Fig. 8. The effect of sodium ion concentration on surface pH in various regions of rat small intestine. Effect of normal (*hatched columns*) and low (*open columns*) sodium ion concentration in phosphate buffer (sodium replaced by mannitol) in regions of small bowel. Details as for Fig. 4

The striking elevation in surface pH seen on exposure to the methylxanthine, theophylline (an inhibitor of phosphodiesterase) points to an involvement of the cAMP system where presumably elevated cAMP levels are associated with elevations in surface pH. Preliminary and unpublished observations (Table 1)

Table 1. Effect of theophylline, dibutyryl cAMP and cAMP on surface pH in rat proximal jejunum in vitro. Results expressed as mean increase in surface pH with standard error of mean, figures in parentheses indicate number of animals

	Theophylline (10 m*M*) 0.24±0.09 (8)	Dibutyryl cAMP (10 m*M*) 0.23±0.05 (9)	cAMP (10 m*M*) 0.16±0.08 (9)
Significance[a]	0.05	0.05	N.S.
Significance[b]	0.005	0.005	0.05

[a] By Students *t* test
[b] By Wilcoxon matched pairs test. N.S. = not significant

have shown that theophylline produces a transient elevation of surface pH and that external cAMP and the more permeable dibutyryl-cAMP both elevate the surface pH, adding support to the hypothesis that hydrogen ion secretion and intracellular cAMP levels are linked. Phenylalanine, acetazolamide and chloride ion substitution with sulphate are without effect on surface pH, precluding a role for alkaline phosphatase in the hydrogen ion secretory process and a role for carbonic anhydrase-assisted or -mediated bicarbonate–chloride exchange at neutral buffer pH (M. LUCAS et al. 1976, unpublished work).

Since the measuring electrodes have relatively large dimensions, it is probable that surface pH is underestimated. The electrodes could be measuring some of the bulk phase as well as the microclimate if the dimensions of the pH microclimate are less than the sensing length of the electrodes. Also, even if the electrodes are completely in the microclimate it is possible that the electrode measures an average value of a gradient of hydrogen ions and that the pH immediately at the surface is slightly more acid. There are two ways in which estimates of the real surface pH can be obtained. In the steady state, a luminal pH should exist where acidification is at a minimum to maintain an adequately low surface pH. A luminal pH below this value would cause a decrease in the measured surface pH because of diffusion into the microclimate and a luminal pH above this equilibrium value would cause measurable acidification. This approach is similar to that which has been used for turtle bladder acidification studies (STEINMETZ 1974). A plot of acidification against luminal pH (Fig. 9) shows a balance concentration at about pH 4.5. An alternative approach is to plot the measured surface pH against depth of measuring electrode and extrapolate the derived plot for an infinitely small electrode tip (Fig. 10). It can be seen that this also estimates the surface pH to be somewhere between pH 4 and pH 5, depending on whether a linear estimate is made or one based on orthogonal polynomials. Consequently, it seems most likely that the present estimates of the microclimate pH are underestimates and that the true value may be as low as pH 4.5 at the surface of the proximal small intestine. The estimate by HOGBEN et al. (1959) of a "virtual" pH of 5.3 in the jejunum may be an aggregate value over a long section of intestine or an average over an orthogonally directed gradient. There are similar uncertainties about the depth of the microclimate. It cannot extend beyond the unstirred water layer

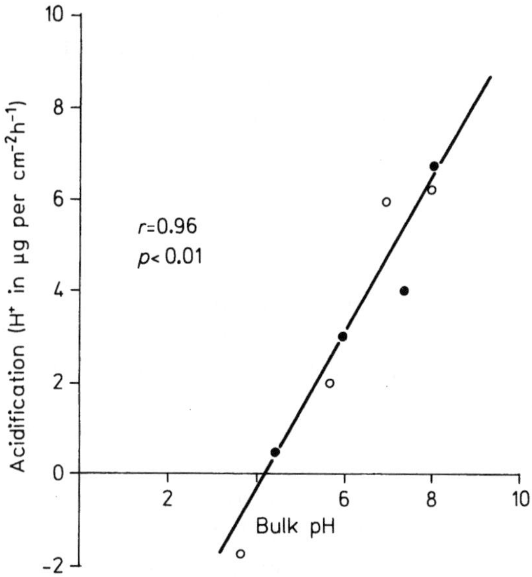

Fig. 9. The dependence of the rate of acidification on luminal pH in rat proximal jejunum. Changes in luminal pH from onset to end of incubation (experimental data recalculated from Fig. 5) expressed as a rate of acidification plotted against luminal pH of phosphate (*full circles*) and bicarbonate (*open circles*) buffers. Details as for Fig. 4. Six animals per point, regression details apply to *upper line*

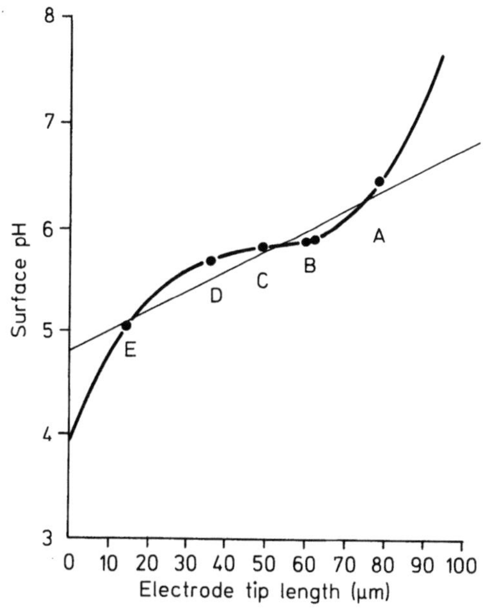

Fig. 10. The dependence of surface pH observations on microelectrode tip length in rat proximal jejunum in vitro. Surface pH plotted against electrode dimensions for (*A*) antimony electrodes; (*B*) Hinke glass electrodes; (*C* antimony electrodes, Giebisch design; (*D*) and (*E*) surface electrode. Intercept approximates microclimate pH immediately next to mucosal membrane by linear or polynomial extrapolation. Experimental details as for Fig. 4

(UWL) because of turbulence, but it is possible that it is considerably smaller than the estimated dimensions of the UWL. From the electrode dimensions and surface pH plot, an outer edge of 80–100 μm might be possible. Resolution of this problem must await studies with smaller electrodes.

II. Clinical Studies

Using human biopsy material obtained during routine clinical investigations on patients with suspected gastrointestinal disease, surface pH studies have been carried out in the same way as those for in vitro rat tissue. Freshly obtained biopsy samples can be maintained in vitro for 1 h at 37 °C in buffer containing 10 m*M* glucose as a metabolisable substrate. A low surface pH has been found for control subjects who were either healthy volunteers or hospital patients with no obvious gastrointestinal disease (LUCAS et al. 1978 a). In two groups of patient with intestinal disease (Fig. 11), Crohn's disease and untreated coeliac disease, the surface pH was, although still lower than the bulk phase, significantly higher than in the normal subjects.

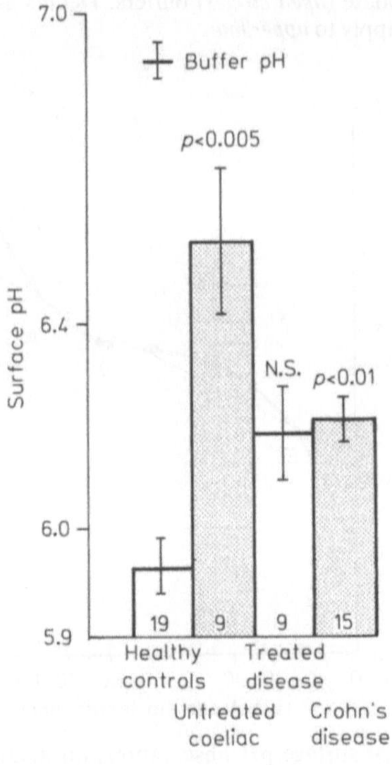

Fig. 11. Surface pH in diseases. Surface pH measured in biopsy samples from human proximal jejunum in vitro, incubated in bicarbonate buffer. Details as for Fig. 4. Data from healthy volunteers, treated and untreated patients with coeliac disease and patients with Crohn's disease

In contrast, treated coeliac patients on a gluten-free diet who were in remission had a surface pH not significantly different from the control subjects. In all subjects, surface pH in the presence of glucose was lower than that in the absence of glucose; the higher the initial surface pH, the smaller was the difference in surface pH between paired tissues incubated with and without glucose. This indicates that the greater the degree of mucosal damage, the less likely the damaged tissue would be able to respond to the presence of added glucose. Surface pH was found to correlate with villous height, the smaller the villi, the higher the surface pH, indicating a morphological component to the maintenance of a low surface pH. Similarly, an inverse correlation was found between measured surface pH and lactase activity (LUCAS et al. 1979). This does not imply that lactase is the enzyme involved with hydrogen ion secretion but rather that surface pH correlated with a sensitive indicator of mucosal damage. This view is partially confirmed by the fact that two subjects with milk allergy who presumably had lactase deficiency, had a normal surface pH. It is interesting to note here the previously discussed putative link between acidification and intracellular cAMP levels. In biopsy material from untreated coeliac patients (TRIPP et al. 1977) Na^+, K^+-ATPase levels were low and intracellular cAMP levels were elevated.

Much the same situation has also been shown to occur in tropical sprue, both in its endemic and epidemic forms (M. L. LUCAS and V. I. MATHAN 1980, unpublished work). About half of the patients with epidemic tropical sprue had a high surface pH compared with hospital controls. The measured surface pH varied directly with 3-day faecal fat excretion and inversely with xylose and vitamin B_{12} absorption. This is not interpreted as a direct involvement of surface pH in xylose and vitamin B_{12} absorption, but that changes in surface pH correlate well with in vivo parameters of intestinal derangement.

III. Related Phenomena

There are many reasons for questioning the concept of a uniform concentration of solute from the bulk phase right up to the membrane face itself. In as simple a system as salt diffusing across artificial membranes, not all the gradient is present solely in the membrane phase, some gradient exists away from the membrane in the unstirred layer, detectable by diffraction techniques (LERCHE 1976). It is known that the interfacial pH at membrane interfaces will differ from bulk solution pH, depending on the zeta potential generated by any fixed negative charges (HARTLEY and ROE 1940). This difference is detectable by fluorescent indicators (VAZ et al. 1978) or by comparing the optimal pH for immobilised and free enzyme and detecting a pH shift (VENKATARAMAN et al. 1977). It is often assumed that this interfacial phenomenon is responsible for the microclimate pH measured at the surface of proximal rat intestine (LEVIN 1979). However, without the ability to replenish protons that are lost to the microclimate on conversion of an anion to the neutral species, it is difficult to see how the fixed negative charge model would facilitate transfer. A basic premise of the microclimate hypothesis (BLAIR and MATTY 1974) is the mucosally directed source of hydrogen ions. A physicochemical model which approximates the conditions at the jejunal mucosa is that of an immobilised hydrolytic enzyme. When papain is immobilised onto a collodion membrane, hydrolysis generates hydrogen ions which are retained in the vicinity of the enzyme. This causes a shift in the optimal pH compared with the free enzyme, comparable with the magnitude of the pH shifts seen in the intestine (GOLDMAN et al. 1965, 1968).

Other ion-selective electrode studies have demonstrated local increased concentrations of hydrogen or other ions in gastrointestinal tissues. In *Amphiuma* small intestine, in the course of experiments designed to measure the intracellular concentration, increased concentrations of potassium and chloride ion have been detected immediately prior to intracellular penetration (WHITE 1976, 1977). Similar local concentrations have been detected in the rabbit ileum in vivo (ZEUTHEN and MONGE 1975) and an acid surface pH was noted in *Necturus* gallbladder (ZEUTHEN 1978). The reverse was found in dog duodenal mucosa (BIRCHER et al. 1965) when bathed in very acid solutions. Here pH electrodes registered a much less acid pH when touched on the surface of dog duodenum bathed in a bulk solution of pH 2 and seemed to demonstrate that the duodenum could secrete locally high concentrations of alkali to protect itself from gastric secretions.

Methods not involving the use of pH electrodes have also been used to yield information on surface pH. In buccal mucosa absorption studies (SCHURMAN and TURNER 1978) pairs of acidic and basic substances were used whose lipid solubility as judged by oil–water partition coefficients was approximately equal. The pH at which equal amounts of undissociated weak acid and base existed was calculated, i.e. at a value approximately equidistant from their respective pK_a values. The authors argued that at this pH, the membrane should not be able to distinguish between acids and bases since the degree of ionisation and lipid solubility was about equal. They found that identical rates of absorption of acid and base did not occur at the calculated pH value and concluded that the surface pH of the human buccal cavity mucosa was about pH 6.6 when the bulk solution is neutral. A similar approach was used in the study of aerosol-borne drug absorption in in vivo lung preparations where uptake of drug was found to be generally in accordance with the pH partition principle (SCHANKER and LESS 1977). The pH absorption profile was studied in buffered and unbuffered solutions and found to be discrepant. In unbuffered solutions, drug absorption at various pH values occurred as in solutions buffered at pH 6.6, leading the authors to conclude that a zone of slightly lower pH existed at the surface of the alveoli.

Therefore, under certain circumstances, several studies have indicated that the pH immediately at the surface of membranes can be more acid than bulk solution bathing media and that ions other than the hydrogen ion may form local accumulations, depending on the nature of the epithelium considered and the ions that are transported across it. These observations serve to illustrate the argument that the concept of a uniform concentration from bulk solution to membrane is probably a very poor approximation. The physiological significance of these local accumulations of ions, as has been proposed for contact digestion (UGOLEV and LAEY 1973), has yet to be fully evaluated (see Chap. 19).

IV. The Role of Mucus

In the microclimate model for folate transfer (BLAIR and MATTY 1974), two requirements were postulated for the maintenance of an acid zone on the surface of intestinal mucosa: (1) a source of mucosally directed hydrogen ions from a secretory mechanism; and (2) the restriction of diffusion within this zone. The second premise was included since without the restriction of diffusion, local gradients of ions accumulating near the membrane would be dissipated rapidly. Although some estimate of the value of the diffusion coefficient might be obtained from a trivial solution of the diffusion equation in the steady state, as some of the parameters (e.g. the thickness of the zone and the hydrogen ion gradient across it) are unknown, such calculations are still speculative. Mathematical modelling (WINNE 1977) seems to indicate that a hindrance of diffusion is necessary since the measured rate of acidification is insufficient if a low surface pH is to be maintained, according to this model. Histological data from the colon shows extracellular mucus to vary from 10 to 180 μm in thickness (W. ENGELHARDT 1979, personal communication). In the jejunum, alterations in the thickness of the mucus coating should increase the dimensions of the acid microclimate. If the second premise is accepted, it allows for manipulation and alteration in the rate of drug absorption by altering the state of intestinal mucus. Histological evidence has shown that in malabsorptive states such as coeliac disease, the mucus coating can be thinner or disrupted in certain areas (SWANSTON et al. 1977).

Some recent studies concerning the effects of mucus on absorption support this second premise. When a dispersion of mucus is added either to a diffusion cell or to rat jejunum in vivo and in vitro (BRAYBROOKS et al. 1975), tetracycline absorption is reduced. Although this might be explicable in terms of the increased morphological resistance caused by extra mucus coating the enterocytes, an alternative explanation is that the added mucus increases the acidity of the microclimate, causing less tetracycline zwitterion to be formed (COLAIZZI and KLINK 1969). In contrast, porcine mucus added to rat everted sac preparations caused an increase in phenylbutazone permeation (LOVERING and BLACK 1974) as would be expected if more of the neutral species of this weak acid, pK_a 4.5 (SEEBALD and FORTH 1975) were formed. It is difficult to reconcile this increase in permeation with mucus simply acting as an additional extracellular morphological barrier. In a similar way, manoeuvres which were assumed to reduce adherent intestinal mucus caused an increase in quinine absorption in the rat everted sac and a reduction in the absorption of the acidic compound phenol red (NAKAMURA et al. 1978). Consequently, there is growing evidence that mucus can modulate the absorption of various drugs and that in vitro this may be via the microclimate.

E. Alternative Concepts

I. The Unstirred Layer Hypothesis

Much attention has focused recently on the possible effects of unstirred layers next to membranes in altering the rate of absorption of compounds, provided the rate of transport across the membrane itself is faster than the rate of movement across the stagnant layer (see also Chap. 21). It will be timely here to draw a distinction between the UWL and the concept of a microclimate as the two terms are often used synonymously (TURNBERG 1977; HORI et al. 1978), which may not be the case. Also the UWL is referred to as a "diffusion barrier" which affects "even small molecules" (SILK 1979). A stagnant or unstirred water layer is a layer of fluid next to a membrane which is unaffected by bulk turbulence except when vigorously stirred and *across which diffusion must take place*, i.e. it is not a barrier to diffusion, but a barrier requiring free diffusion to occur as in aqueous media if the solute is to reach the membrane. The implicit assumption is that free diffusion occurs, a condition which will affect all molecules regardless of size or charge.

In contrast, a further postulate of the microclimate hypothesis (BLAIR and MATTY 1974) is that given the rate of hydrogen ion secretion which occurs mucosally (LUCAS 1976), it is most likely that the diffusion of hydrogen ions away from the surface would have to be restricted if a sufficiently low pH is to be achieved. The surface of the small intestine is covered by a coat of mucous substance both from intestinal goblet cells and from the enterocytes themselves, providing a glycocalyx. According to the Stokes–Einstein equation (MOORE 1965), the diffusion coefficient is related to the reciprocal of the viscosity of the medium in which diffusion is occurring. Clearly, the possibility exists that the diffusion coefficient within any mucus layers on the surface of the intestine is altered by the viscosity of the mucus. Some representative values for mucus viscosity might be similar to that for glycerine which has a value some 600 times that of water. As such, the value of the diffusion coefficient in mucus near the intestinal membranes could be two orders of magnitude smaller than that in free solution. Recent work on gastrointestinal mucus has shown that the viscosity of pig gastric mucus glycoprotein at 40 mg/ml concentration, is at least ten times the viscosity of water (ALLEN 1978). At present there are no estimates of how intestinal mucus affects diffusion coefficients; however, the microclimate hypothesis admits the possibility of restricted diffusion which the UWL hypothesis does not.

Much of the quantitative work done on the UWL depends on calculations from experiments where diffusion potential differences are measured and also the time taken to develop them; this technique was initiated by DIAMOND (1966) who used the half-time for development, t, to estimate the thickness of the unstirred layer, d, according to the equation

$$t = 0.38\frac{d^2}{D}.$$

D being the aqueous diffusion coefficient as used in the studies cited and others (SALLEE and DIETSCHY 1973; LUKIE et al. 1974). It is clear that changes in D will profoundly alter the estimates of unstirred layer thickness. For example, estimates of UWL thickness by NaCl-generated diffusion, PDs are of the order of 200 μm, assuming diffusion coefficients typical of aqueous media (SALLEE and DIETSCHY 1973). A tenfold change in the coefficient used in these calculations reduces the estimate to 70 μm and a change of two orders of magnitude would make this estimate even smaller. The assumption that the mucus or glycocalyx makes no contribution to the extracellular barriers is based (SALLEE and DIETSCHY 1973) on the fact that although the measured half-times to generate diffusion PDs varied threefold over a wide range of solutes, the calculated thickness did not. As there seemed to be little discrimination on the grounds of size or charge, the diffusion barrier was assumed to consist solely of unstirred fluid. However, an increase in medium viscosity will affect all solutes indiscriminately, slowing the diffusion of all solutes to an equal extent. Consequently the lack of discrimination alone does not rule out a contribution of mucus to extracellular permeability properties. Empirical equations (THOMSON and DIETSCHY 1977) have been used to quantify the effects of the UWL on solute absorption, derived from a combination of Fick's first law of diffusion and that for Michaelis–Menten kinetics for solute absorption

$$J = \frac{D}{d}(C_1 - C_2),$$

$$J = \frac{J_{\max} C_2}{K_m + C_2},$$

where J = flux, C_1 = bulk concentration, C_2 = surface concentration.

Since both D and the calculated d (UWL thickness) may be in error and the value of D/d even more so, quantitative conclusions from this equation might be very inaccurate. Models using a linear solution of this equation have been constructed (WINNE 1973; HOYUMPA et al. 1976; THOMPSON and DIETSCHY 1977; READ et al. 1977) without regard to the assumptions in such a model. For example, apparent differences in unstirred layer thickness detected between normal subjects and patients with untreated coeliac disease (READ et al. 1977) may reflect changes in viscosity; furthermore calculations of "real" K_m changes may also be misleading if based on an assumed knowledge of the value of D/d as previously described. The UWL becomes of importance if it is a rate-limiting structure controlling the rate of absorption of solute. Without quantitative knowledge of D and d, it is difficult to assess whether the UWL is genuinely rate limiting. Since it takes 3–6 min to equilibrate unstirred layers fully in rabbit jejunum (LUKIE et al. 1974), accepting provisionally that these are aqueous layers, experiments with short incubation times of 2–3 min (HOYUMPA et al. 1976) will inevitably conclude that the UWL is critical in absorption.

The UWL has been invoked as a possible explanation for the pH shifts seen in drug absorption (WINNE 1977). Clearly, the experimental data point to changes in the rate of absorption of passively and actively absorbed solutes when stirring occurs (SALLEE and DIETSCHY 1973; DUGAS et al. 1975), generally demonstrating an increased uptake of solute such as glucose or octanoate. Vigorous stirring may also be affecting things other than UWL thickness. For example, turbulence may clear away carbon dioxide from the tissues and increase the rate of oxygen delivery, allowing an indirect metabolic site of action of stirring. It is known that stirring shifts the pH absorption profile of xanthone carboxylic acid (CHOWHAN and AMARO 1977) and also that the effects of stirring on absorption can be pH dependent (HO et al. 1976), raising the possibility that stirring itself affects the surface pH of the intestinal mucosa. Such shifts in surface pH if they occur could affect the pH level at which luminal membrane enzymes function, causing changes in the rate of absorption of actively transported substances. Since glucose uptake is affected by pH (BARRY et al. 1966b; CSÁKY and AUTENRIETH 1975), stirring, by altering the surface pH, may affect transport, with the thickness of the UWL having no role at all.

Unstirred layers have been invoked as a possible explanation for the pH shifts seen in drug absorption where, provided that the UWL is rate limiting, the pH at a stage subsequent to diffusion across the UWL should be largely irrelevant. WINNE (1977) proposes a model where in the case of a monovalent dissociable compound, without the UWL, a typical sigmoid absorption curve is seen varying with bulk medium pH. With an UWL the absorption profile is essentially flat because the UWL is rate limiting. Intermediate cases fall between these two extremes with a pH shift occuring because the sigmoid curve is displaced progressively upwards. With a compound with two dissociable groups and a bell-shaped absorption profile (Fig. 12), the UWL hypothesis would predict that on either side of the absorption maximum, the curves should flatten out. However, often the complete bell-shaped absorption profile shifts as with sulphanilamide absorption (KOIZUMI et al. 1964) and this is difficult to explain solely in terms of the UWL as pointed out by WINNE (1977). Since also the rate of absorption changes greatly with luminal pH and this changes the surface pH. it seems unlikely that unstirred

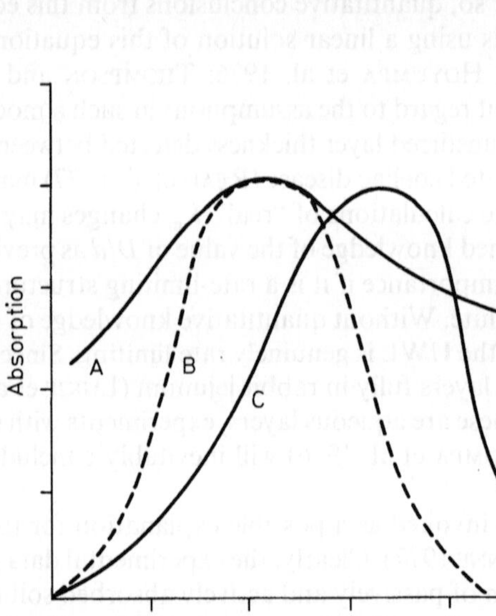

Fig. 12. Deviation from pH partition caused by microclimate and UWL. Curve *B* depicts a typical absorption profile for a compound having two disscociable groups, e.g. sulphonamides, giving maximum absorption near the maximum concentration of zwitterionic form as predicted by the pH partition hypothesis. Curve *C* depicts the pH shifts frequently seen (e.g. KOIZUMI et al. 1964) caused by an acid microclimate. Curve *A* depicts the effects of the UWL (see WINNE 1977) where both ends of the curve are flattened and the inflection points move in opposite directions

layers alone can adequately explain the phenomenon of pH shifts, although they do seem to contribute to the extracellular permeability barriers (WINNE 1978).

II. Permeation of Ionised Forms

As an alternative to the pH microclimate hypothesis to explain pH shifts, permeability of intestinal membrane to the ionised form of drugs is occasionally postulated (NOGAMI and MATSUZAWA 1961; TURNER et al. 1970; CROUTHAMEL et al. 1971; SALLEE and DIETSCHY 1973; BRIDGES et al. 1976). This involves studying the rate of drug absorption over a wide range of luminal pH and partitioning the total transport into the sum of the transport of the ionised and nonionised forms according to the equation

$$\frac{\mathrm{d}Q}{\mathrm{d}t}=(k_n Q_n + k_i Q_i),$$

where n = nonionised; i = ionised, and calculating the values of the nonionised and ionised rate constants from a knowledge of the amounts of ionised and nonionised forms in solution at the given luminal pH (e.g. DIETSCHY and WESTERGAARD 1975). Values between 6:1 and 30:1 have been calculated for the ratio of nonionised to ionised rate constants and are often cited as evidence for deviations from the pH partition hypothesis (CROUTHAMEL et al. 1971; BRIDGES et al. 1976). Implicit in these calculations is the assumption that the surface pH is the same as the luminal pH and hence that transport of ionised forms has taken place. It is of course axiomatic that the reverse is also true; if the surface pH is not the same as the luminal pH, then there is little need to invoke partial permeability to the ionised forms of drugs. Exceptions to this general rule of nonpermeability to ionised forms must be mentioned here: that of quaternary ammonium ion transport, dealt with in detail elsewhere in this volume; and that of ion pair absorption.

Strong evidence exists that ions such as the quaternary ammonium salts which are permanently ionised over a wide range of pH, have special mechanisms involved in their transport (see Chap. 22). In the guinea-pig jejunum such compounds are actively secreted into the lumen (LAUTERBACH 1977) as well as digoxin and naphtholsulphonic acids. As guinea-pig jejunum can alkalinise its luminal contents by the secretion of bicarbonate, the evidence for secretion from the naphthol orange compound studies is perhaps not as strong. However, similar mechanisms may exist in rat and human mucosa and this phenomenon appears not to have been investigated. A second mechanism by which ions may cross the intestinal membrane is by ion pair formation such as is thought to explain the interaction between calcium ion and tetracycline absorption (POIGLER and SCHLATTER 1979) and the interaction between ammonium ion absorption in the lower bowel and bicarbonate (SWALES et al. 1970). In both these instances the positively charged moiety may combine with an anion and cross the intestinal membrane as a loosely bound ion pair resembling a neutral molecule.

Drug absorption studies across artificial membranes have generally upheld the principle of nonionic diffusion, provided compounds are lipid soluble, with the partition between two aqueous phases accurately predicted by the pH partition hypothesis; more or less constant values for the transfer coefficient can be derived, calculated by using the amount of nonionised species in solution (DOLUISIO and SWINTOSKY 1964; CRAMER and PRESTEGARD 1977; SAMUELOV et al. 1979). The permeability properties of the intestinal membranes may be parallelled by artificial lipid membranes only in the most general way, since aqueous channels exist between the enterocytes which may allow permeability of ionised forms (BARNETT et al. 1978). Small charged molecules might pass easily between the paracellular shunt pathways irrespective of the degree of ionisation. Conversely molecules too large to permeate through this pathway may be most affected by surface pH if the lipid route is the sole means by which substances cross the intestinal barrier. Yet even this morphological feature which may accommodate ionic diffusion is open to question as to the pH in the aqueous channels.

Hydrogen ions are secreted mucosally by the enterocyte and it is possible to detect, in vitro in everted sac preparations, a lowering of the serosal pH (BARRY et al. 1966b; LUCAS and BLAIR 1978). This serosal acidification can be caused by as little as 2% backdiffusion of the mucosally directed hydrogen ion through the paracellular pathways, hence the pH in these pathways may be acid. Evidence for this concept comes from studies on pH and cell adhesion in enterocyte populations (MALENKOV and MELIKYANTS 1977), where it was found that cells adhered best at a low pH. Thus it seems that a low pH in the paracellular pathways would favour cell adhesion and would not be incompatible with tissue integrity. Smaller compounds which may diffuse along the intercellular gaps may nevertheless be affected by a low surface pH, although to a lesser extent. In summary, experimental data demonstrating ionic permeation are based on the premise that the bulk pH is representative of the juxtamucosal pH and as such only provide evidence of deviation from the pH partition hypothesis if the effect of a low surface pH is discounted.

III. Extraction Theory

An alternative model for pH shifts has been based on the ability of the membrane to extract solute depending on the lipid solubility of the solute. In this essentially mathematical treatment (WAGNER and SEDMAN 1973) applied to two cases of drug absorption, the uptake of a dissociable acid or base is related to the pH and the pK_a in the usual way, but also to an extraction term, related to the relative volumes of membrane and bulk phase and also to an intrinsic partition coefficient K_u between these two phases. In effect the membrane extracts solute, depending on the value of K_u, into itself such that the fraction extracted f_E is given by

$$f_E = \frac{P_u}{1+P_u} \qquad P_u = \frac{V_m K_u}{V_w},$$

where m = membrane; w = fluid. Hence the pH shift term is related to log (P_u $(1/f_E - 1) - 1$) and examples are given for the buccal absorption of fatty acids and the intestinal absorption of barbital and sulphaethidole. In the model, it is demonstrated that the experimental absorption curves can be approximated well by choosing appropriate numerical values for some of the constants which cannot be measured empirically. Much the same line of argument holds here as for the case of ionic permeation in that the model fits the data only if the possibility of a differing surface pH is discounted. The problems associated with modelling will be dealt with in a later section, but it is relevant to note here that there is little guarantee that the parameter values chosen represent a unique set of values which could not be superseded by another set with equal validity. Also the choice of a partition coefficient term is critical to these calculations and may itself be a reflection of the pH of the aqueous medium next to the enterocytes since oil–water partition coefficients are extremely pH dependent (SCHANKER 1959; JACKSON et al. 1978). Consequently, although lipid extraction may cause some deviations from pH partition, this is as yet a hypothetical case with little empirical evidence to support it.

F. Absorption and the Microclimate Hypothesis: Three Paradigms

I. Folic Acid Absorption

Most attention has focused on the possibility of an acid microclimate being the dominant influence in folic acid and related folate absorption as originally proposed by BLAIR and MATTY (1974). The attractive feature of the acid microclimate hypothesis of folic acid absorption is that it potentially reconciles the evidence for active transport with that for passive transport by providing a compromise position in which the transport step is passive, but dependent on the metabolically determined ability to produce hydrogen ions mucosally.

Evidence for the active transport of folic acid is that: (1) there is a preferred site of absorption in the proximal jejunum where saturation of transport occurs; (2) transport can be inhibited by metabolic inhibitors and is extremely pH dependent; (3) serosal: mucosal and tissue: mucosal concentration ratios greater than unity can be detected in vitro as well as high flux ratios in vivo (BURGEN and GOLDBERG 1962; HERBERT 1967; HEPNER 1969; SMITH et al. 1970; IZAK et al. 1972; OLINGER et al. 1973; SMITH 1973; SELHUB et al. 1973; BLAIR et al. 1974). Since the absorption of folic acid is profoundly influenced by luminal pH (SMITH et al. 1970; BENN et al. 1970; ELSBORG 1974; BLAIR et al. 1976; MACKENZIE and RUSSELL 1976; RUSSEL et al. 1979), the pH partition principle can be expected to apply to folic acid absorption and a low surface pH should modify the rate of folate entry.

In this light, the concentration ratios exceeding unity and indicative of uphill active transport can be explained by pH partition between the external medium and a slightly alkaline intracellular interior; indeed concentration ratios of 2:1 can be caused by a pH difference between these two phases of 0.3. Similarly, a flux ratio above 10:1 (BURGEN and GOLDBERG 1962) can also be explained by the existence of a low surface pH mucosally accelerating the flux from lumen to serosa. A preferred site of absorption would be because the surface pH is lowest in the proximal jejunum; metabolic inhibition of transport would be due to the inhibition of hydrogen ion secretion underlying absorption.

From a consideration of the principle of nonionic diffusion, folic acid, which at neutral pH consists mainly of the dianion, should barely be able to permeate the intestinal wall. An acid microclimate would therefore seem to be of paramount importance if permeation is to be achieved. Some workers have miscalculated the relative amounts of anion, neutral species and cation in solution at a given pH, based on the assumption that the amide ionisation which can occur in the pteridine ring leads to a maximum concentration of the nonionised form of folate around pH 6 (ELSBORG 1974; HALSTED 1979). This is clearly erroneous and it can be calculated from a consideration of all the dissociable groups present in the molecule (POE 1977) that the peak for neutral species formation occurs at the acid pH of between 3.5 and 4. The acid microclimate would allow for formation of the neutral species, but also provides a basis for the saturation phenomenon seen, since folic acid is poorly soluble at low pH. Consequently, after a certain concentration is achieved in the microclimate zone, no more folic acid can dissolve, causing an apparent saturation of the transport mechanism.

Recent studies have involved experiments in which folic acid absorption and surface pH were measured under the same circumstances (LUCAS et al. 1978 b). Substances which reduced folic acid absorption, i.e. methotrexate, low sodium buffers and alcohol were all capable of causing elevations in the surface pH (Table 2). Other studies have examined the possibility that folic acid absorption is microclimate mediated by considering folate transport in abdominal radiation syndromes. It is known that intestinal X-irradiation will drastically inhibit folic acid absorption (KESAVAN and NORONHA 1971). After abdominal irradiation, folic acid absorption could be restored by the addition of external ATP which is known to stimulate acidification (BLAIR et al. 1975). The authors were also able to restore folic acid transport by acidifying the luminal pH to around pH 4. They argued that radiation destroyed the ability to form an acid microclimate, but that sufficient external ATP could restore it. In the absence of a microclimate, an acid luminal pH could carry out the role of the microclimate just as well by providing the correct pH next to the intestinal wall. Taking up the idea of an ATP-dependent hydrogen ion secretion enzyme being involved in acidification, KESAVAN and

Table 2. Alterations in surface pH and mucosal folic acid transport in rat proximal jejunum under various conditions (LUCAS et al. 1978 b). Results expressed as mean values with standard error of mean, figures in parentheses indicate number of animals

Treatment	Folic acid uptake (pmol h^{-1} mg^{-1})	Change in surface pH
20% Alcohol and lib	23.5±1.9 (6)	+0.09 (8)
Phenytoin	20.6±0.9 (6)	+0.06±0.20 (8)
Control	17.0±0.8 (12)	0.0
μ*M* Methotrexate	14.5±1.4 (6)	−0.03±0.09 (6)
3% Alcohol in vitro	13.9±1.5 (6)	−0.33±0.10 (6) [a]
Low Na^+	13.0±1.0 (6) [b]	−0.42±0.10 (12) [c]
Oral methotrexate	10.0±2.1 (6) [c]	−0.39±0.11 (4) [b]

[a] $P<0.05$
[b] $P<0.02$
[c] $P<0.01$
Folic acid transport vs ΔpH $r=0.856$, $P<0.02$

NORONHA (1978) found that brush border Mg-ATPase activity correlated well with folic acid transport and that this could be inhibited by sodium azide (KESAVAN and NORONHA 1978). When the luminal pH was made sufficiently acid to overcome any effects on the microclimate, sodium azide had no effect on folic acid transport. Surface pH is elevated in untreated coeliac disease and Crohn's disease (LUCAS et al. 1978a) where there is folate malabsorption. Consequently, the various features of folic acid transport can be accommodated within the microclimate hypothesis and also provide a model for derangement of intestinal function.

II. Fatty Acid Absorption

The absorption of short- and medium-chain fatty acids which have a pK_a of about 4 typical of the carboxylic acid group should in theory be affected by the surface pH at the luminal membrane. Fatty acid absorption is markedly pH dependent in that decreases in the luminal pH lead to increases in the rate of absorption (BARRY et al. 1966a, b; SALLEE and DIETSCHY 1973; LAMERS and HULSMAN 1975; JACKSON 1975; NAUPERT and ROMMEL 1975) and an acid surface pH should accelerate the absorption of these compounds.

Initial experiments on short-chain fatty acid absorption indicated that compounds of this type were transported against a concentration gradient toward the serosal side in vitro (SMYTH and TAYLOR 1958) which was interpreted as evidence of active transport. Glucose added to the medium stimulated absorption and the nonmetabolisable sugar galactose hindered it. A preferred region of absorption exists in the jejunum (JACKSON 1968; BLOCH et al. 1972) and a dependence on external sodium ion concentration has been detected (JACKSON and SMITH 1968), although found by others to be pH dependent in that, if the luminal pH was 5, sodium dependence could no longer be found (NAUPERT and ROMMEL 1975). Transport could be inhibited by metabolic inhibitors such as dinitrophenol (DNP) and potassium cyanide (BLOCH et al. 1972; NAUPERT and ROMMEL 1975) at high concentrations of fatty acids although not at low concentrations (SALLEE and DIETSCHY 1973). Yet the transport step showed only low values for the temperature coefficient, indicative of passive transport (PORTE and ENTENMAN 1965; LAMERS 1975). Saturation of transport has also been seen in fatty acid absorption in the human ileum in vivo (SCHMITT et al. 1977) and in the rat jejunum (NAUPERT and ROMMEL 1975) although with pH dependent K_m values. The K_m for this process is relatively high at 25 mM compared with other enzymatically controlled processes. Other workers have failed to note saturation (SALLE and DIETSCHY 1973) because of the use of concentrations well below this reported K_m value. Competitive inhibition has also been noted between fatty acids (BLOCH et al. 1972; NAUPERT and ROMMEL 1975) for the transport system in everted sacs and also in isolated epithelial cells (LAMERS and HULSMAN 1975) and on balance the evidence for an active transport system seems strong.

An alternative model for fatty acid absorption based on the acid microclimate hypothesis was first proposed by NAUPERT and ROMMEL (1975) and the present section expands on their arguments. The low temperature coefficient for the transport step coupled with the pH dependence argues strongly for a passive mechanism which is sensitive to the prevailing hydrogen ion concentration and points to nonionic diffusion as the mechanism by which fatty acids enter the epithelial cells.

The effect of providing metabolisable substrate and the ability of a nonmetabolisable sugar to inhibit transport to levels below that in the complete absence of substrate can be explained by alterations in the rate of hydrogen ion secretion (BLAIR et al. 1975). Figure 13 shows that under certain conditions the addition of the nonmetabolisable sugar 3-*O*-methylglucose can cause acidification to be reduced to a level below that occurring in the absence of any added substrate. Similarly, the metabolic dependence of absorption can be explained by inhibition of acidification since DNP will reduce hydrogen ion secretion. Sodium dependence can be reconciled with the properties of an acid microclimate since both hydrogen ion secretion and the maintenance of an acid pH are sodium dependent (LUCAS 1976; LUCAS and BLAIR 1978). Interestingly the sodium dependence was not evident at low pH which could be interpreted to mean that when a sufficiently acid luminal pH overcame the effect of lack of sodium on surface pH, sodium dependence was not seen (NAUPERT and ROMMEL 1975). The ability to show concentration ratios greater than unity varies according to the pH gradient imposed across the intestinal wall and this also resembles that expected from the pH partition hypothesis. Saturation could also be explained by increasing concentrations of fatty acid anions depleting the microclimate of hydrogen ions

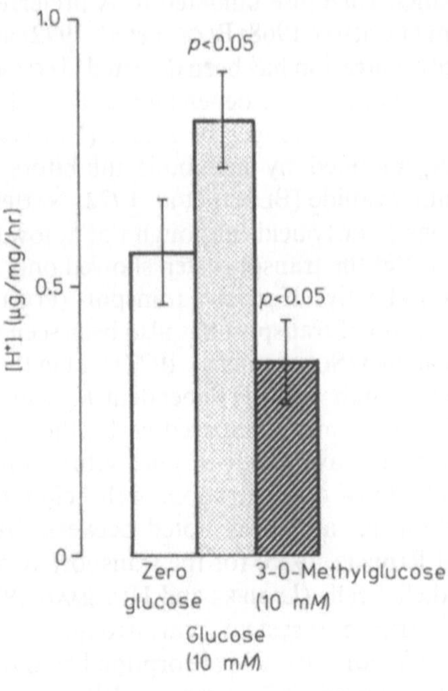

Fig. 13. The effect of glucose (*stippled column*) and 3-*O*-methylglucose (*hatched column*) on acidification by the proximal jejunum in vitro compared with zero glucose (*open column*). LUCAS (1974)

during transport, thus elevating the surface pH and causing a limit on the amount of anion that can be converted to the neutral species. Site specificity can also be referred to the lowest surface pH being found in the jejunum forming an area most favourable to the rapid absorption of weak acids. It will be apparent that the microclimate hypothesis provides a rival explanation for the mechanism for weak acid absorption when there seems to be exceptionally strong evidence for the existence of a specific transport system. Since the acid microclimate takes a relatively long time to dissipate even when inhibited by aminophylline, it is also clear that the failure to see competitive phenomena and the inhibitory effects of anoxia and other compounds [Dietschy, cited by WADDEL (1975) p 44; SALLEE et al. 1972] may be due to the choice of short incubation times.

A radically different model for carboxylic acid uptake into enterocytes has been described (LAMERS and HULSMAN 1975; LAMERS 1975) in which fatty acids and pyruvate enter cells as anions by way of an anion exchange mechanism. A strong piece of evidence for the anion exchange mechanism is that weak acids can elicit the exit of other weak acids from preloaded cells and that this phenomenon decreases as the external pH is lowered when less elicitor anion is available. Whether this exchange mechanism functions in preparations where the membrane asymmetry is preserved is not clear. Isolated cell preparations inevitably present the serosal membrane to the elicitor substance, a circumstance not occurring in other preparations. However, the potential existence of a serosally sited anion exchange mechanism has important consequences for weak acid absorption, particularly with respect to an alternative microclimate model proposed by Jackson and his co-workers.

Experiments on fatty acid and barbiturate absorption have led to the proposal that there is an alkaline microclimate on the surface of rat jejunum exerting a controlling influence on the transport of weak acids and bases (JACKSON et al. 1974; JACKSON 1975, 1977; JACKSON and KUTCHER 1977; JACKSON and AIRALL 1978; JACKSON et al. 1978). Initially, this model was proposed because of the failure to detect luminally directed hydrogen ion secretion in the upper small bowel in weakly buffered solutions (JACKSON and MORGAN 1975). In adequately buffered solutions, benzoic, phenylacetic and pentanoic acid were found to have serosal: mucosal flux ratios greater than unity while benzylamine, hexylamine, and D-amphetamine had ratios less than unity. Both benzoic acid and benzylamine fluxes were pH dependent in a manner predictable by the pH partition hypothesis. Evidence for an alkaline intermediate compartment comes from interactions between weak acid and base transport. Consistent with the *acid* microclimate hypothesis is the observation that pentanoic acid mucosally reduces the absorption rate of benzoic acids and vice versa; this can be interpreted as competition for protons in the acid layer. Acids on the serosal side increase the serosal flux of weak acids, presumably in a manner analagous the way that lowering the serosal pH increases the amount of the nonionised form of any other weak acid present and accelerates its backflux (JACKSON et al. 1974). The evidence for an *alkaline* microclimate seems to rest on the fact that mucosal benzylamine will accelerate the mucosal flux of benzoic acid and retard the serosal–mucosal flux. Serosal benzylamine will cause the exact reverse to occur to the benzoic acid fluxes. However it is possible that benzylamine, even at a low mucosal pH predominantly in the charged form, will have sufficient uncharged form present to diffuse across the luminal membrane. This will cause more of the charged form to become uncharged to restore equilibrium with the resulting deposition of a proton in the acid microclimate. This seems to be an equally acceptable explanation of the accelerated benzoic acid transport, increased by small increments in the hydrogen ion concentration. It is also relevant to stress here that with the existence of a putative anion exchange mechanism probably at the serosal pole of the enterocyte, such interaction studies dealing with the effects of mucosally and serosally applied weak acids and bases may involve different phenomena, the acid microclimate at the mucosal side and the anion exchange mechanism at the serosal side.

Other approaches towards establishing the existence of an alkaline microclimate hypothesis involve mathematical and conceptual modelling which is dealt with later on in this chapter. With the underlying complexity inherent in modelling the system and in the form of the equations as they have been derived, although the alkaline microclimate hypothesis can give a good fit to experimental data, such a model does not represent a *unique* model which rules out all others. Nevertheless the concept of an alkaline intermediate compartment may be an additional feature determining weak acid and base transport although experimental evidence from pH electrode studies seems to rule out the possibility that it is situated on the mucosal surface. Since there is mucosally directed hydrogen ion secretion most probably at the luminal membrane of the enterocyte, it is reasonable to suppose that an equivalent amount of base is formed intracellularly owing to charge separation and that the intracellular pH is alkaline. This may cause an elevated concentration of weak acid anion to exist intracellularly and facilitate the exit of anions via a serosally sited anion exchange mechanism. Clearly, this possibility needs to be investigated and future research may see a convergence of the alternative microclimate hypotheses. For example, the observation that serosal benzylamine reduced the mucosal–serosal flux of benzoic acid might be related to just this point. If the intracellular pH is alkaline and benzylamine has access to the intracellular compartment via a serosally sited anion exchange pump, this will presumably elevate the intracellular pH still further. If mucosal hydrogen ion secretion were sensitive to intracellular pH such that a rise in intracellular pH beyond tolerable limits caused a reduction in further inwardly directed hydroxyl ion formation consequent on the hydrogen ion secretory mechanism, then this would be reflected in an elevation in the acid microclimate pH and a reduction in the benzoic acid flux. However, such speculations must await further experimental data.

III. Propranolol Absorption

A corollary of the microclimate hypothesis is that in disease, a shift in surface pH towards neutrality will cause a change in the rates of weak electrolyte absorption such that weak base transport will be accelerated and weak acid transport will be retarded. In coeliac and Crohn's disease which have been shown to have an elevated surface pH, increased plasma levels of propranolol have been detected after oral administration (SCHNEIDER et al. 1976; PARSONS et al. 1976b). As the buccal absorption of propranolol is pH dependent (SCHUERMAN and TURNER 1978) it is likely that jejunal absorption is similarly pH dependent and potentially affected by these changes in surface pH in these diseases. Consequently, experiments were undertaken to determine whether the elevated levels of propranolol seen after oral administration could be correlated with changes in surface pH and the rate of intestinal absorption.

In a series of control subjects and patients with coeliac disease prior to and after treatment with a gluten-free diet, surface pH was measured using jejunal biopsy samples (KITIS et al. 1979) and differences in surface pH were found as previously reported (LUCAS et al. 1978a). Patients with an erythrocyte sedimentation rate higher than 20 mm/h were excluded from the study as being potentially able to bind more propranolol in the vascular compartment (SCHNEIDER et al. 1979). Absorption studies were then undertaken on the subjects who received, on two separate occasions, an oral dose of propranolol and an oral dose of folic acid for comparison. In the untreated coeliac group with the highest surface pH, folic acid absorption was depressed as judged by plasma levels and propranolol levels were elevated. In contrast, in the healthy group, folic acid absorption was normal and propranolol levels were below the values seen in the patient group (KITIS et al. 1982). Folic acid levels at certain times correlated inversely and propranolol absorption correlated directly with surface pH, as predicted by the acid microclimate hypothesis. Changes in the blood plasma level of drug were modelled by a one-compartment model with an entry and an exit rate process in accordance with the familiar Bateman–Teorell equation (TEORELL 1939).

Drug disposition in the vascular compartment is a composite of absorption and elimination processes, plasma binding and first-pass effects with the additional possibility of an alteration in the fraction of dose absorbed because of unspecified changes in bioavailability. In the group of patients studied, liver function was normal. A kinetic analysis by BMDP iterative nonlinear curve fitting algorithms (JENNICH and RALSTON 1979) showed that although the elimination rate constant in the patient group was diminished and could be a factor in the increased plasma levels seen, the absorption rate constant for propranolol was also elevated in accordance with the microclimate hypothesis (KITIS et al. 1982).

Although there are objections to the use of propranolol as a probe molecule as it is extensively metabolised in the liver, the fact that the absorption rate increases in a disease noted for malabsorption is difficult to explain in terms of a general reduction in surface area or poor intestinal function. As folic acid absorption was depressed, with a diminution in the absorption rate constant, it is difficult to explain these alterations in rate constants in terms other than pH at the luminal membrane or somewhere in the transport sequence of events.

G. Modelling the System

Drug absorption across the intestinal membrane is the result of the complex interplay of several factors, particularly in the case of ionisable molecules capable of dissociating in the physiological pH range. Water and lipid solubility both play a role in absorption as well as the degree of ionisation, itself a dominant factor in determining the relative degree of lipid and water solubility of a solute. If ionised, the direction and magnitude of any prevailing transmural PD can also have an effect on drug absorption. There have been frequent attempts to incorporate all these parameters into a comprehensive mathematical model that would relate flux across the intestine with these parameters. Perhaps the simplest and most familiar models are those which consider only pH differences across membranes, based on the premise that only the undissociated form of the solute can permeate the membrane (SCHANKER et al. 1958; MILNE et al. 1958; HOGBEN et al. 1959). It can be easily shown, starting from the Henderson–Hasselbach equation for a monobasic acid that the disposition across a membrane permeable only to the undissociated form, at equilibrium, is given by

$$\frac{C_2}{C_1} = \frac{1+10^{(\mathrm{pH}_1-\mathrm{p}Ka)}}{1+10^{(\mathrm{pH}_2-\mathrm{p}Ka)}}.$$

This equation is also applicable to two end phases with any number of intermediate phases in between since the interposition of a phase of different pH will not affect the final equilibrium between the two end phases.

Other models have posed the question of how far the ratio of the total concentrations in two end phases will deviate from that predicted by the modification of the Henderson–Hasselbach equation, if there is permeability to the ionised form of drug. This has been done for a single membrane (ROOS 1965) and also for two membranes in series, incorporating the additional complexity that permeation to the ionised species is sensitive to transmembranal PD. Clearly, as the interposition of phases between two end phases does not affect the final equilibrium distribution or steady state ratio, models which accommodate the microclimate hypothesis must concern themselves with the approach to the steady state and consider drug fluxes. A significantly different approach has been to calculate on theoretical grounds the steady state flux ratio J_{ms}/J_{sm}, with an equation similar to Schanker and Hogben's with the important difference that while C_2/C_1 would be related to the pH in the end phases, J_{ms}/J_{sm} should be sensitive to the pH immediately at the membranes across which flux occurs. This and the previous models might be termed "biophysical" models since they concern themselves with the electrochemical variables of the system and ignore lipid solubility. Other models often incorporate a lipid solubility factor but neglect the concept of an acid microclimate on a priori grounds (STEHLE and HIGUCHI 1972; LOVERING and BLACK 1974). Consequently, these models will not be considered here, as sufficient empirical evidence now exists to place them in doubt.

A steady state flux model (JACKSON et al. 1974) elegantly derived from first principles has been proposed which takes into account a two-membrane system with a pH difference somewhere in the system, differing ionised: unionised permeability ratios at the two membranes and an overall transmembranal PD. This model draws attention to the fact, as does the steady state concentration model (STEVENS et al. 1969) that a given pH gradient across one membrane with differential permeability to ionised species at both membranes can cause net transfer to a higher concentration in the *trans* end phase, despite both end phases having equal pH. In effect, solute moves into a central compartment and the difference in permeability coupled with the prevailing PD can cause more to exit through one membrane than the other. A recent modification is a simpler form of the more complex equation with the transmural PD term abandoned, since barbiturate absorption seemed to be little affected by manipulations in the short-circuit current (JACKSON et al. 1978). This equation states that

$$\frac{J_{\text{ms}}}{J_{\text{sm}}}=\frac{(1+a10^{\alpha_1})(1+b10^{\alpha_2})}{(1+b10^{\alpha_1})(1+a10^{\alpha_2})}$$

where $\alpha_1=(\text{pH}_1-\text{p}K_\text{a})$, $\alpha_2=(\text{pH}_2-\text{p}K_\text{a})$, $a=Pi/P_\text{n}$ barrier I and $b=Pi/P_\text{n}$ barrier II; Pi=permeability to ionised, P_n=to nonionised form.

Although the flux ratio is a measurable variable, this equation contains four parameters, some of which have not been directly measured. As yet there is little quantitative information on the relative permeability of the luminal and contraluminal membranes to ionised and nonionised forms of weak electrolytes. The equation has been used to fit flux ratio data for a series of barbiturate compounds (JACKSON et al. 1978) against their appropriate pK_a values in an attempt to estimate all four parameters simultaneously. A satisfactory fit is obtained on assigning values of 7.5 to pH_1 and 8.1 to pH_2 and put forward as evidence for a region of alkaline pH in an intermediate compartment, controlling the rate of drug absorption.

It is clear that best estimates of this equation depend heavily on initial estimates inserted into any iterative procedure and that many possible sets of parameters exist in the four parameter space. To illustrate this point, the empirical data have been fitted (Fig. 14) by one curve which can be generated by very different sets of parameters, all within a "region of indifference" for the residual sum of squares and well within the standard errors of the original data. Using the BMDP (JENNICH and RALSTON 1979) procedure, excellent fits can be obtained with a wide range of values for pH_2 ranging from the alkaline to the acid (Table 3). In particular a good fit can be obtained with pH_1 near neutrality (presumably the bulk phase) and with pH_2 set a the very acid value of 3.5–3.6. These values impose a nondiscriminatory role on the first barrier in that ionised forms are preferred, which may refer to the preferential passage of anions across the UWL because of the prevailing PD and modest discrimination to the second, presumably mucosal, membrane; thus providing equally good evidence for the acid microclimate hypothesis.

This is perhaps arguably a hazard implicit in all attempts at system identification by mathematical modelling where most if not all of the coefficients are unknown or at the present stage of investigation undetermined. Similar difficulties exist in attempts to combine the previous equations with an unstirred layer term. Equations have been based on a combination of Fick's law of diffusion coupled with a Langmuir absorption isotherm in an attempt to define separate resistances to solute permeation due to the unstirred layer and due to the membrane itself. Such a combination has led to the following familiar equation

$$J=\frac{PC_\text{b}}{(1+dP/D)}$$

Table 3. Sets of parameters giving identical fit to date in Fig. 14

Parameters					
	A	*B*	pH_1	pH_2	Residual sum of squares
(1)	2.1792	17.8×10^{-5}	7.50	6.91	0.09494
(2)	2.140	0.538	7.50	3.40	0.08486
(3)	1.752	0.438	7.58	3.50	0.08486
(4)	0.554	0.138	8.08	4.00	0.08486

Data fit[a]	Predicted	Observed	pK_a
	2.93	2.93	4.0
	3.78	3.76	6.1
	2.37	2.50	7.3
	1.63	1.50	7.8
	1.63	1.43	7.8
	1.52	1.62	7.9
	1.43	1.52	8.0
	1.28	1.26	8.2

[a] Data from JACKSON and AIRALL (1978), fit by BMDP from parameter sets (2)–(4)

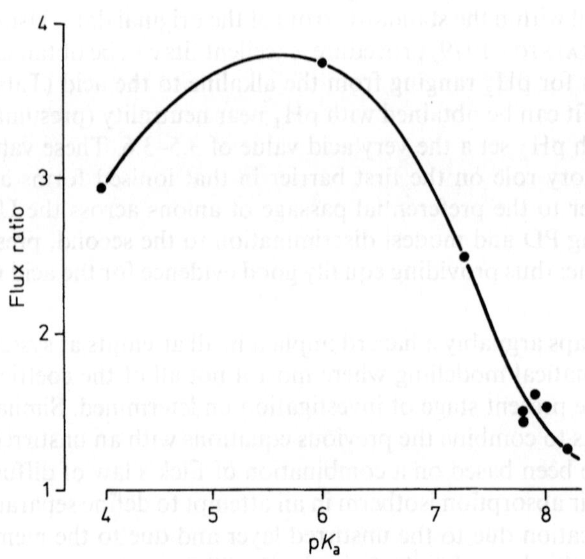

Fig. 14. Modelling the system; dependence of flux ratio of barbiturate permeation in the small intestine on pK_a. Data from JACKSON et al. (1978) for barbiturates fitted by a single curve generated by three sets of parameters (2)–(4) from Table 3, all giving identical fits with identical minimal residual least squares

or rearranged

$$J = \frac{C_b}{(1/P) + (d/D)}$$

where C_b = bulk concentration; P = permeability; D = diffusion coefficient; d = UWL thickness. This equation describes the passive unidirectional flux rate for a solute across the microvillous membrane (DIETSCHY and WESTERGAARD 1975) related to the bulk solution concentration with the permeability term partitioned in a manner analogous to electrical resistance. In much the same way the apparent permeability coefficient has been partitioned into three terms (DAINTY and HOUSE 1966; WINNE 1973) incorporating the permeability contribution of the membrane P_b and terms derived from the UWL on both sides of the membrane.

$$\frac{1}{P_{\text{total}}} = \frac{\delta_1}{D_1} + \frac{1}{P_b} + \frac{\delta_2}{D_2}.$$

While there is no good reason not to do this, it is clear that accurate knowledge of the membrane permeability, the diffusion coefficient and the thickness of the UWL is appropriate for mathematical modelling and that conclusions drawn from numerical assumptions are hazardous. The principle of partition of resistances in combination with weak electrolyte flux equations has been applied to a microclimate model (JACKSON et al. 1978) in an attempt to separate the relative contribution from the unstirred layers and then deduce the pH of an intermediate compartment. Here an equation similar to that proposed by DIETSCHY and WESTERGAARD (1975) has been derived

$$J_{23} = \frac{C}{(1 + 10^{\alpha_2}/P_n) + (d/D)},$$

where P_n is permeability to the nonionised form, $\alpha_2 = (\text{pH}_2 - \text{p}K_a)$ and is used to support the alkaline microclimate hypothesis. Assumptions are made as to the magnitude of the UWL term which as mentioned previously depends heavily on estimates d and D which may be in error. A satisfactory fit is obtained with a particular model, hence allowing the calculation of the pH of the intermediate compartment. Obviously the concept per se is satisfactory, but the numerical value assigned to the pH exponential term must be in dispute. Clearly, inaccurate estimates of the d/D term must be compensated for in the other term. If D becomes smaller in the microclimate zone because of mucus and the ratio becomes larger, the other term must decrease, making the pH in the intermediate compartment just as likely to be acid as alkaline. In summary, modelling the system mathematically tends neither to prove nor disprove assertions about the pH of an intermediate compartment, but shows that a multiplicity of models is possible which can only be restricted by an accurate experimental assessment of the parameters under investigation.

H. Conclusion

In contrast to the alternative hypothesis of an alkaline subepithelial space in the intestine, there is now a growing body of direct evidence demonstrating the presence of an acid microclimate in the proximal jejunum, although in vivo evidence is at present lacking. This acid layer places constraints on the subsequent absorption of weak electrolyte since any substance presented to the mucosa has to be both adequately soluble and significantly undissociated at a low pH, if permeation is to occur by nonionic diffusion. Since many substances of biological and therapeutic interest are capable of dissociation, the acid microclimate should affect a wide variety of compounds for which no specific transport system exists to facilitate absorption. Since also an acid zone can encompass the concepts of saturation, a supposed metabolic input to maintain permeation and a pH differential giving concentration ratios displaced from the expected value of unity, the evidence for supposing that a dissociable compound is actively transported must be scrutinised carefully. Within this area of interest come the water-soluble vitamins whose transport is saturable but thought to be passive, antibiotics and a wide range of pharmaceutical compounds too numerous to cite here.

An attractive aspect of the acid microclimate hypothesis is the ease with which predictions can be made affecting drug absorption because of the physicochemical constraints placed on absorptive phenomena by the acid zone. From the so far determined aspects of hydrogen ion secretion, factors inhibiting acidification should retard the absorption of weak acids and accelerate the absorption of weak bases; N.B. the effect of DNP on the intestinal uptake of passively absorbed sulphonamides (NOGAMI et al. 1966), the effect of acetazolamide on the absorption of amphetamines and salicylic acid (SCHNELL and MIYA 1970). Similarly, the microclimate hypothesis predicts interactions between passive absorption and the mucosal cAMP levels of the kind found with pralidoxime absorption (BRISEID et al. 1977). A further aspect is the possible role of mucus in maintaining the acidity of the surface layer which would lead to interactions between drug absorption and mucus secretion as discussed in Sect. D.IV.

This model for absorption also has the possibility of clarifying how certain kinds of malabsorption occur in small bowel disease and how there can be seemingly paradoxical faster absorption of bases in some of these states. As examples of this, folic acid and propranolol absorption was extensively discussed. There are many examples of malabsorption of passively absorbed weak acids in small bowel disease: penicillin V in childhood coeliac disease (BOLME et al. 1977); phenoxymethylpenicillin in adults with steatorhoea (DAVIS and PIROLA 1968); nalidixic acid which is preferentially absorbed at low pH (TAKASUGI et al. 1968) is malabsorbed in shigellosis (NELSON et al. 1972) in which intestinal acid–base balance is thought to be disturbed (TAKASAKA 1978). Seemingly in contrast, cephalexin (an antibiotic with two dissociable groups of pK_a 5.2 and 7.3) is absorbed to a greater extent in coeliac disease (PARSONS et al. 1976a) because of the increased concentration of zwitterion formed in a less acid microclimate. Fusidic acid is also absorbed to a greater extent in coeliac disease (PARSONS 1977) which at first sight does not accord with the hypothesis since fusidic acid is a weak acid of pK_a

around 5.5. However, fusidic acid is insoluble at low pH and consequently an elevation in surface pH would allow more drug to be available in solution.

Such increases in the amount or rate of absorption in malabsorption syndromes are frequently seen with weak bases; trimethoprim, sulphamethoxazole, propranolol and quinine are all absorbed faster or to a greater extent (MATTILA et al. 1973; PARSONS et al. 1976; PARSONS 1977). It is difficult to reconcile this divergent tendency for bases to be preferred and acids to be retarded in such malabsorption syndromes on grounds other than pH, since general factors such as a reduction in surface area or secretory states should affect weak acids and bases to an equal extent. Some evidence for this divergent tendency also exists in experimental malabsorption syndromes caused by the administration of neomycin (CHENG and WHITE 1962) and triparanol (ROBINSON 1972). Neomycin causes a transient malabsorption of penicillin in humans; triparanol retards the absorption of sulphafurazole but accelerates the transfer of mecamylamine (VENHO 1976). This divergence between acids and bases again points to some pH phenomenon being involved in absorption and emphasises the role that an acid microclimate could play in influencing drug absorption.

In summary, the acid microclimate is an important, if largely unrecognised determinant of weak electrolyte transport in the small bowel, potentially being able to explain several features of drug absorption; whether in vivo drug absorption is similarly affected by a zone of acid pH on the surface of the gut has yet to be determined. An attractive feature of the hypothesis is that it explains quite simply the "pH shifts" and "deviations" from the pH partition hypothesis, clarifies certain aspects of drug absorption in malabsorption syndromes and allows predictions to be made about interactions involving mucus and drug absorption. For didactic reasons sharp distinctions have been drawn in this chapter between the acid microclimate hypothesis and both the alkaline variant and the unstirred layer concept. Ultimately, it may be that the alternative microclimate hypotheses are facets of the acid–base metabolism of intestinal mucosa which together with the unstirred layers in series form a composite extracellular morphological feature having profound effects on the absorption of weak electrolytes.

Acknowledgments. The author is grateful to the Trustees of the Estate of James Watt (1736–1819) and the University of Aston in Birmingham for the provision of a travelling memorial fellowship, during which tenure (1979) this chapter was written.

References

Alday ES, Goldsmith MS (1975) Radiotelemetic monitoring of hydrogen ion levels of small intestine. Surg Gynecol Obstet 141:549–551

Allen A (1978) Structure of gastrointestinal mucus glycoproteins and the viscous and gel-forming properties of mucus. Br Med Bull 34:28–33

Ardisson JL, Dolisi C, Grimand D, Ozon C (1973) Les possibilites d'ajustement du pH au niveau d'une anse jejunal isolee. CR Soc Biol Paris 167:1656–1661

Banwell JG, Gorbach SL, Mitra R, Pierce NF (1970) Fluid and electrolyte changes in the small intestine with acute undifferentiated human diarrhoea. Gastroenterology 58:925

Barnett G, Hui S, Benet LZ (1978) Effects of theophylline on salicylate transport in isolated rat jejunum. Biochim Biophys Acta 507:517–523

Barry RJC, Eggenton J (1972) Ionic basis of membrane potentials of epithelial cells in rat small intestine. J Physiol 227:217–231

Barry RJC, Jackson MJ, Smyth DH (1966a) Handling of glycerides of acetic acid by rat small intestine in vitro. J Physiol 185:667–683

Barry RJC, Jackson MJ, Smyth DH (1966b) Transfer of propionate by a rat small intestine in vitro. J Physiol 182:150–163

Barry RJC, Eggenton J, Smyth DH, Wright EM (1967) Relation between sodium concentration, electrical potential and transfer capacity of rat small intestine. J Physiol 192:647–655

Beckett AH, Rowland M (1964) Urinary excretion kinetics of amphetamine in man. J Pharm Pharmacol 17:628–639

Benn A, Swan CHJ. Cooke WT, Blair JA, Matty AJ, Smith ME (1970) Effect of intraluminal pH on the absorption of pteroylmonoglutamic acid. Br med J i:148–150

Berk JE, Thomas JE, Rehfuss ME (1942) The reaction and neutralising ability of the contents of the first part of the duodenum in normal dogs under fasting conditions. Am J Physiol 136:369–376

Bircher J, Mann V, Carlson HC, Code CF, Rovelstad RA (1965) Intraluminal and juxtamucosal duodenal pH. Gastroenterology 48:472–477

Blair JA, Matty AJ (1974) Acid microclimate in intestinal absorption. Clin Gastroenterol 3:183–197

Blair JA, Lucas ML, Matty AJ (1972) The acidification process of the jejunum. Gut 13:321A

Blair JA, Johnson IT, Matty AJ (1974) Absorption of folic acid by everted sacs of rat jejunum. J Physiol 236:653–661

Blair JA, Lucas ML, Matty AJ (1975) Acidification in the rat proximal jejunum. J Physiol 245:333–350

Blair JA, Johnson IT, Matty AJ (1976) Aspects of intestinal folate transport in the rat. J Physiol 256:197–208

Bloch R, Haberich FJ, Lorenz-Meyer H (1972) Untersuchungen zur Transportkinetik mittelkettiger Fettsäuren am Dünndarm: (in vitro und in vivo Versuche an Ratten). Pflügers Arch 335:198–212

Bolme P, Eriksson M, Stintzing G (1977) The gastrointestinal absorption of penicillin in children with suspected coeliac disease. Acta Paediatr Scand 66:573–578

Braude R, Fulford RJ, Low AG (1976) Studies on digestion and absorption in the intestine of growing pigs. Measurement of digesta and pH. Br J Nutr 36:497–510

Braybrooks MP, Barry BW, Abbs ET (1975) The effect of mucin on the bioavailabilitiy of tetracycline from the gastrointestinal tract; in vivo, in vitro correlations. J Pharm Pharmacol 27:508–515

Bridges JW, Houston JB, Humphrey MJ, Lindup WE, Parke DV, Shillingford JS, Upshall DG (1976) Gastrointestinal absorption of carbenoxolone in the rat determined in vitro and in situ: deviations from the pH-partition hypothesis. J Pharm Pharmacol 28:117–126

Briseid G, Oye I, Briseid K (1977) Increased level of cAMP in the rat intestinal mucosa caused by sodium lauryl sulphate. Naunyn Schmiedebergs Arch Pharmacol 298:263–266

Brown MM, Parsons DS (1962) Observations on the changes in the potassium content of rat jejunal mucosa during absorption. Biochim Biophys Acta 59:249–251

Burgen ASV, Goldberg NJ (1962) Absorption of folic acid from the small intestine of the rat. Br J Pharmacol Chemother 19:313–320

Catala J (1975) Effet de la ligature du canal pancreatique sur le pH intestinal chez la Lapin. CR Acad Sci (Paris) 281:1991–1993

Cheng SH, White A (1962) Effect of orally administered neomycin on the absorption of penicillin-V. N Engl J Med 267:1296–1297

Chowran ZT, Amaro AA (1977) Everted rat intestinal sacs as an in vitro model for assessing absorption of new drugs. J Pharm Sci 66:1249–1253

Colaizzi JL, Klink PR (1969) pH-partition behaviour of teracyclines. J Pharm Sci 58:1184–1189

Cramer JA, Prestegard JH (1977) NMR studies of pH-induced transport of carboxylic acids across phospholipid membrane vesicles. Biochem Biophys Res Commun 75:295–301

Crouthamel WG, Tan GH, Dittert LW, Doluisio JT (1971) Drug absorption IV. Influence of pH on absorption kinetics of weakly acidic drugs. J Pharm Sci 60:1160–1163

Csáky TZ, Autenrieth B (1975) Transcellular and intercellular transport. In: Csáky TZ (ed) Intestinal absorption and malabsorption. Raven, New York, pp 177–185

Dainty J, House CR (1966) "Unstirred layers" in frog skin. J Physiol 182:66–78

Davis AE, Pirola RC (1968) Absorption of phenoxymethyl penicillin in patients with steatorrhoea. Australas Ann Med 17:63–65

Diamond J (1966) A rapid method for determining voltage concentration relation across membranes. J Physiol 183:83–100

Dietschy JM, Westergaard H (1975) The effect of unstirred water layers on various transport processes in the intestine. In: Csáky TZ (ed) Intestinal absorption and malabsorption. Raven, New York, pp 197–207

Dolisi C, Crenesse D, Ardisson JL (1979) Modification des equilibres acido-basiques par le jejunum. Experientia 35:354–357

Doluisio JT, Swintosky JV (1964) Drug partitioning II in vitro model for drug absorption. J Pharm Sci 53:597–601

Dugas MC, Ramaswamy K, Crane RK (1975) An analysis of the D-glucose influx kinetics of in vitro hamster jejunum based on considerations of the mass transfer coefficient. Biochim Biophys Acta 382:576–589

Elsborg L (1974) Folic acid: a new approach to the mechanism of its intestinal absorption. Dan Med Bull 21:1–11

Faelli A, Esposito G (1971) Bicarbonate and transintestinal potential difference of the jejunum of the rat intestine incubated in vitro. In: Broda E, Locker A, Springer-Lederer H (eds) First European biophysics congress, EVIII/29, Wien Med Akad, Vienna, pp 317–321

Faelli A, Garotta G (1971 a) Bicarbonati e potenziale transepitheliale dell'intestino digiuno di ratto incubato in vitro. Nota I. Boll Soc Ital Biol Sper 47:26–29

Faelli A, Garotta G (1971 b) Bicarbonati e potenziale transepitheliale dell'intestino digiuno di ratto incubato in vitro. Nota II. Boll Soc Ital Biol Sper 47:29–32

Faust RG (1962) The effect of anoxia and lithium ions on the absorption of D-glucose by the rat jejunum in vitro. Biochim Biophys Acta 60:604–614

Fordtran JS, Locklear TW (1966) Ionic constituents and osmolarity of gastric and small-intestinal fluids after eating. Am J Dig Dis 11:503–521

Foerster H, Erdlenbruch W, Mehnert H (1967) Untersuchungen über die Beeinflussung der Glukoseresorption durch verschiedene H^+-Ionenkonzentrationen. Z Gesamte Exp Med 144:14–23

Graham WR, Emery ES (1928) The reaction of the intestinal contents of dogs fed on different diets. J Lab Clin Med 13:1097–1108

Grayzel DM, Miller EG (1927) pH concentration of intestinal contents of dog, with special reference to inorganic metabolism. Proc Soc Exp Biol Med 24:668–672

Goldman R, Silman HI, Caplan SR, Kedem O, Katchalski E (1965) Papain membrane on a collodion matrix: preparation and behaviour. Science 150:758–760

Goldman R, Kedem O, Silman HI, Caplan SR, Katchalski E (1968) Papain-collodion membranes. Preparation and properties. Biochemistry 7:486–500

Halsted CH (1979) The intestinal absorption of folates. Am J Clin Nutr 32:846–855

Harms V, Stirling CE (1977) Transport of purine nucleotides and nucleosides by in vitro rabbit ileum. Am J Physiol 233:47–55

Hartley GS, Roe JW (1940) Ionic concentrations at interfaces. Trans Farad Soc 36:101–109

Hepner GW (1969) The absorption of pteroylglutamic (folic) acid in rats. Br J Haematol 16:241–249

Herbert V (1967) Biochemical and hematologic lesions in folic acid deficiency. J Clin Nutr 20:562–569

Hicks J, Turnberg LA (1973) The influence of secretin on ion transport in the human jejunum. Gut 14:485–490

Ho NFH, Park J, Morozowich W, Higuchi WI (1976) A physical model for the simultaneous membrane transport and metabolism of drugs. J Theor Biol 61:185–193
Hogben CAM, Tocco D, Brodie BB, Schanker LS (1959) On the mechanism of intestinal absorption of drugs. J Pharmacol Exp Ther 125:275–282
Hori R, Kagimoto Y, Kamiyama K, Inui KI (1978) Effects of free fatty acids as membrane components on permeability of drugs across bilayer lipid membranes. A mechanism for intestinal absorption of acidic drugs. Biochim Biophys Acta 509:510–518
Hoyumpa AM, Nichols S, Schenker S, Wilson FA (1976) Thiamine transport in thiamine-deficient rats. Role of unstirred water layer. Biochim Biophys Acta 436:438–447
Hubel KA (1971) Effects of secretin and glucagon on intestinal transport of ions and water in the rat. Proc Soc Exp Biol Med 139:656–658
Hubel KA (1973) Effect of luminal sodium concentration on bicarbonate absorption in rat jejunum. J Clin Invest 52:3172–3179
Hubel KA (1976) Intestinal ion transport: effect of norepinephrine, pilocarpine and atropine. Am J Physiol 231:252–257
Hubel KA (1977) Effects of bethanechol on intestinal ion transport in the rat. Proc Soc Exp Biol Med 154:41–44
Izak G, Galevski K, Grossowicz N, Jablonska M, Rachmilewitz M (1972) Studies on folic acid absorption in the rat II. The absorption of crystalline pteroylmonoglutamic acid from selected small intestine segments. Dig Dis Sci 17:599–602
Jackson MJ (1968) Regional variation of propionate transport in rat small intestine. Life Sci 7:517–523
Jackson MJ (1975) Transport of short chain fatty acids. In: Smyth DH (ed) Intestinal absorption: biomembranes. Biomembranes, vol 4B. Plenum, London, pp 673–711
Jackson MJ (1977) Epithelial transport of weak-electrolytes. Properties of a three compartment system. J Theor Biol 64:771–788
Jackson MJ, Airall A (1978) Transport of heterocyclic acids across rat small intestine in vitro. J Membr Biol 38:255–269
Jackson MJ, Kutcher LM (1977) The three compartment system for transport of weak electrolytes in the small intestine. In: Kramer M, Lauterbach F (eds) Intestinal permeation. Excerpta Medica, Amsterdam, pp 65–73
Jackson MJ, Morgan BN (1975) Relations of weak electrolyte transport and acid-base metabolism in rat small intestine in vitro. Am J Physiol 228:482–487
Jackson MJ, Smyth DH (1968) Role of sodium in the intestinal active transport of organic solutes. Nature 219:388–389
Jackson MJ, Shiau YF, Bane S, Fox M (1974) Intestinal transport of weak-electrolytes; evidence in favour of a three compartment system. J Gen Physiol 63:187–213
Jackson MJ, Williamson AM, Dombrowski WA, Garner DE (1978) Intestinal transport of weak electrolytes: determinants of influx at the luminal surface. J Gen Physiol 71:301–327
Jennich RI, Ralston ML (1979) Fitting nonlinear models to data. Annu Rev Biophys Bioeng 8:195–238
Kakemi K, Arita T, Hori R, Konishi R, Nishimura K, Matsui H, Nishimura T (1969) Absorption and excretion of drugs XXXIV. An aspect of drug mechanism of drug absorption from the intestinal tract in rats. Chem Pharm Bull 17:255–261
Kesavan V, Noronha JM (1971) Effect of X-irradiation on the absorption of naturally occurring folates. Int J Radiat Biol 19:205–214
Kesavan V, Noronha JM (1978) An ATPase dependent radiosensitive acidic microclimate essential for intestinal folate transport. J Physiol 280:1–7
King CR, Schloerb PR (1972) Gastric juice neutralisation in the duodenum. Surg Gynecol Obstet 135:22–28
Kitis G, Lucas ML, Schneider RE, Bishop H, Sargent A, Blair JA, Allan RN (1979) Jejunal acid microclimate and its effects on absorption of folic acid and propanolol. Gut 20:438A
Kitis G, Lucas ML, Bishop H, Sargent A, Schneider RE, Blair JA, Allan RN (1982) Surface pH and drug absorption in coeliac disease. Clin Sci Mol Med 63:373–380

Koizumi T, Arita T, Kakemi K (1964) Absorption and excretion of drugs. XX. Some pharmacokinetic aspects of absorption and excretion of sulphonamides (2). Absorption from the small intestine. Chem Pharm Bull 12:421–427

Kramer P, Ingelfinger FJ (1961) The effect of specific foods and water loading on the small intestinal function of ileostomised human subjects. Gastroenterology 40:683A

Lamers JMJ (1975) Some characteristics of monocarboxylic acid transfer across the cell membrane of epithelial cells from rat small intestine. Biochim Biophys Acta 413:265–276

Lamers JMJ, Hulsman WC (1975) Inhibition of pyruvate transport by fatty acids in isolated cells from rat small intestine. Biochim Biophys Acta 394:31–45

Lauterbach F (1977) Intestinal secretion of organic ions and drugs. In: Kramer M, Lauterbach F (eds) Intestinal permeation. Excerpta Medica, Amsterdam, pp 173–166

Lei FH, Lucas ML, Blair JA (1977) The influence of pH low sodium ion concentration and methotrexate on jejunal surface pH: a model for folic acid transfer. Biochem Soc Trans 5:149–152

Lepot A, Banwell JG (1976) The syrian hamster: a reproducible model for studying changes in intestinal fluid secretion in response to enterotoxin challenge. Infect Immun 14:1167–1171

Lerche D (1976) Temporal and local concentration changes in diffusion layers at cellulose membranes due to concentration differences between solutions on both sides of the membrane. J Membr Biol 27:193–205

Levin RJ (1979) Fundamental concepts of structure and function of the intestinal epithelium. In: Duthie HL., Wormsley KG (eds) Scientific basis of gastroenterology. Livingstone, Edinburgh, pp 308–338

Levin RJ, Syme G (1975) Thyroid control of small intestinal oxygen consumption and influence of sodium ions, oxygen tension, glucose and anaesthesia. J Physiol 245:271–287

Lovering EG, Black DB (1974) Drug permeation through membranes III. Effect of pH and various substances on permeation of phenylbutazone through everted rat intestine and polydimethylsiloxane. J Pharm Sci 63:671–676

Lucas ML (1974) Acidification in the rat proximal jejunum. PhD thesis, University of Aston in Birmingham

Lucas ML (1976) The association between acidification and electrogenic events in rat proximal jejunum. J Physiol 257:645–662

Lucas ML, Blair JA (1978) The magnitude and distribution of the acid microclimate in proximal jejunum and its relation to luminal acidification. Proc R Soc Lond, 200:27–41

Lucas ML, Schneider W, Haberich FJ, Blair JA (1975) Direct measurement by pH-microelectrode of the pH-microclimate in rat proximal jejunum. Proc R Soc Lond, 192:39–48

Lucas ML, Blair JA, Cooper BT, Cooke WT (1976) Relationship of the acid microclimate in rat and human intestine to malabsorption. Biochem Soc Trans 4:154–156

Lucas ML, Cooper BT, Lei FH, Holmes GKT, Johnson IT, Blair JA, Cooke WT (1978 a) Surface pH in Crohn's and coeliac disease: a model for folic acid absorption. Gut 19:735–742

Lucas ML, Swanston SK, Leí FH, Mangkornthong P, Blair JA (1978 b) Effect of ethanol, diphenylhydantoin, methotrexate and low sodium ion concentration on jejunal surface pH and folic acid transfer in the rat. Biochem Soc Trans 6:297–298

Lucas ML, Cooper BT, Dunne WT, Cooke WT, Allan RN, Blair JA (1979) IRCS Med Sci 8:181

Lucas ML, Lei FH, Blair JA (1980) The influence of buffer pH, glucose and sodium ion concentration on the acid microclimate in rat proximal jejunum in vitro. Pflügers Archiv 385:137–142

Lukie BE, Westergaard H, Dietschy JM (1974) Validation of a chamber that allows measurements of both tissue uptake rates and unstirred layer thicknesses in the intestine under conditions of controlled stirring. Gastroenterology 67:652–661

Lyon J, Crane RK (1966) Studies on transmural potentials in vitro in relation to intestinal absorption. I. Apparent Michaelis constants for Na^+ dependent sugar transport. Biochim Biophys Acta 112:278–291

MacKenzie JF, Russell RI (1976) The effect of pH on folic acid absorption in man. Clin Sci Mol Med 51:363–368

Maggi P, Brue F, Brousoulle B, Bensimon E, Peres G (1970) Les tensions d'O_2 et de CO_2 au niveau de l'épithelium du Rat au cours d'expériences d'absorption in vivo. Effets del'hyperoxie et de l'hypercapnie. C R Soc Biol Paris 164:2285–2287

Malenkov AG, Melikyants AG (1977) Ion permeability and strength of cell contacts. J Membr Biol 36:97–113

Mattila MJ, Jussila J, Takki S (1973) Drug absorption in patients with intestinal villous atrophy. Arzneim Forsch 23:583–585

McGee L, Hastings AB (1942) The carbon dioxide tension and acid base balance of jejunal secretions in man. J Biol Chem 142:893–904

McHardy GJR, Parsons DS (1956) The absorption of inorganic phosphate from the small intestine of the rat. Q J Exp Physiol 41:399–409

McKenny JR (1971) Electrolyte fluxes and electrical potentials in isolated rat intestine. In: Skoryna SC, Waldron-Edward D (eds) Intestinal absorption of metal ions, trace elements and radionuclides. Pergamon, Oxford, pp 81–100

McRobert GR (1928) Observations on the hydrogen ion concentration of the alimentary canal of the albino rat. Ind J Med Res 16:545–552

Meldrum SJ, Watson BW, Riddle HC, Bown RL, Sladen G (1972) pH-profile of gut as measured by radiotelemetry capsule. Br Med J 8 april:104–106

Milne MD, Scribner BH, Crawford MA (1958) Nonionic diffusion and the excretion of weak acids and bases. Am J Med 24:709–729

Moore WJ (1965) Physical chemistry 4th edn. Longmans, London, p 766

Morishita T, Yata N, Kamada A, Aoki M (1971) Studies on absorption of drugs VI. Effects of buffer component on the absorption of drugs. Chem Pharm Bull 19:1925–1928

Mukerji K, Saxena KC, Misra PK, Ghatak S (1977) Human ascaris – purification of chymotrypsin inhibitor and properties of partially purified chymotrypsin and trypsin inhibitors. Ind J Med Res 66:745–755

Murer H, Hopfer U, Kinne R (1976) Sodium/proton antiport in brush border membrane vesicles isolated from rat small intestine and kidney. Biochem J 154:597–604

Nakamura J, Shima K, Kimura T, Muranishi S, Sezaki H (1978) Role of intestinal mucus in the absorption of quinine and water soluble dyes from the rat small intestine. Chem Pharm Bull 26:857–863

Naupert C, Rommel K (1975) Absorption of short and medium chain fatty acids in the jejunum of the rat. Z Klin Chem Klin Biochem 13:553–562

Nelson JD, Shelton S, Kumiesz HT, Haltalin KC (1972) Absorption of ampicillin and nalidixic acid by infants and children with acute shigellosis. Clin Pharmacol Ther 13:879–886

Nogami H, Hanano M, Aruga M (1966) Studies on absorption and excretion of drugs. VI. Effects of cations and 2,4-dinitrophenol on the transport of sulphonamides through the small intestine of rat. Chem Pharm Bull 14:166–173

Nogami H, Matsuzawa T (1961) Studies on absorption and excretion of drugs. I. Kinetics of penetration of acidic drug, salicylic acid through the intestinal barrier in vitro. Chem Pharm Bull 9:532–540

Olinger EJ, Bertino JR, Binder HJ (1973) Intestinal folate absorption II. J Clin Invest 52:2138–2145

Oser BL (1928) The intestinal pH in experimental rickets. J Biol Chem 80:487–497

Parsons DS (1956) The absorption of bicarbonate saline solutions by the small intestine and colon of the white rat. Q J Exp Physiol 41:411–420

Parsons RL (1977) Drug absorption in gastrointestinal disease with particular reference to malabsorption syndromes. Clin Pharmacokinet 2:45–60

Parsons RL, Jusko WJ, Young JM (1976a) Pharmacokinetics of antibiotic absorption in coeliac disease. J Antimicrob Chemother 2:214–215

Parsons RL, Kaye CM, Raymond K, Trounce JR, Turner P (1976b) Absorption of propranolol and practolol in coeliac disease. Gut 17:139–143

Podesta RB, Mettrick DF (1974) The effect of bicarbonate and acidification on water and electrolyte absorption by the intestine of normal and infected (Hymenolepsis diminuta: Cestoda) rats. Dig Dis Sci 19:725–735
Podesta RB, Mettrick DF (1977a) HCO_3 transport in rat jejunum: relationship to NaCl and H_2O transport in vivo. Am J Physiol 232:62–68
Podesta RB, Mettrick DF (1977b) Bicarbonate and hydrogen ion secretion in rat ileum in vivo. Am J Physiol 232:574–579
Poe M (1977) Acidic dissociation constants of folic acid, dihydrofolic acid and methotrexate. J Biol Chem 252:3724–3728
Poigler H, Schletter Ch (1979) Interactions of cations and chelators with the intestinal absorption of tetracycline. Naunyn Schmiedebergs Arch Pharmacol 306:89–92
Ponz F, Larralde J (1950) La absorcion de azucars en funcion del pH intestinal. Rev Esp Fisiol 6:255–269
Porte D, Entenman C (1965) Fatty acid metabolism in segments of rat intestine. Am J Physiol 208:607–614
Portnoy HD (1967) The construction of glass electrodes. In: Eisenman G (ed) Glass electrodes for hydrogen and other cations. Arnold, London, pp 248–250
Powell DW, Solberg LI, Plotkin GR, Catlin DH, Maenza RM, Formal SB (1971) Experimental diarrhea III. Bicarbonate transport in rat salmonella enterocolitis. Gastroenterology 60:1076–1087
Read NW, Barber DC, Levin RJ, Holdsworth CD (1977) Unstirred layer and kinetics of electrogenic absorption in the human jejunum in situ. Gut 18:865–876
Redman T, Willimot SG, Wokes F (1927) LXXXIII. The pH of the gastrointestinal tract of certain rodents used in feeding experiments and its possible significance in rickets. Biochem J 21:589–605
Remke H, Luppa D, Muller F (1975) Monosaccharidabhängiger K^+-Einfluß über die Mikrovillimembran des Jejunums der Ratte. Acta Biol Med Ger 34:1567–1572
Robinson CS (1935) The hydrogen ion concentration of the contents of the small intestine. J Biol Chem 108:403–408
Robinson CS, Luckey H, Mills H (1942) Factors affecting the hydrogen ion concentration of the contents of the small intestine. J Biol Chem 147:175–181
Robinson JWL (1972) Experimental intestinal malabsorption states and their relation to clinical syndromes. Klin Wochenschr 50:173–185
Roos A (1965) Intracellular pH and intracellular buffering power of the cat brain. Am J Physiol 209:1233–1246
Russell RM, Dhar JG, Dutta SK, Rosenberg IH (1979) Influence of the intraluminal pH on folate absorption: studies in control subjects and in patients with pancreatic insufficiency. J Lab Clin Med 93:428–436
Sallee VL, Dietschy JM (1973) Determinants of intestinal mucosal uptake of short and medium chain fatty acids and alcohols. J Lipid Res 14:475–484
Sallee VL, Wilson FA, Dietschy JM (1972) Determination of unidirectional uptake rates for lipids across the intestinal brush border. J Lipid Res 13:184–192
Samuelov Y, Donbrow M, Friedman M (1979) Effect of pH on salicylic acid permeation through ethyl cellulose PEG 4,000 films. J Pharm Pharmacol 31:120–121
Schanker LS (1959) Absorption of drugs from the rat colon. J Pharm Exp Ther 126:283–290
Schanker LS, Less MJ (1977) Lung pH and pulmonary absorption of nonvolatile drugs in the rat. Drug Metab Dispos 5:174–178
Schanker LS, Shore PA, Brodie BB, Hogben CAM (1957) Absorption of drugs from the stomach. J Pharm Exp Ther 120:528–545
Schanker LS, Tocco D, Brodie BB, Hogben CAM (1958) Absorption of drugs from rat small intestine. J Pharm Exp Ther 123:81–88
Schmitt MG, Soergel KH, Wood CM, Steff JJ (1977) Absorption of short-chain fatty acids from the human ileum. Am J Dig Dis 22:340–347
Schneider RE, Babb J, Bishop H, Mitchard M, Hoare AM, Hawkins CF (1976) Plasma levels of propranolol in treated patients with coeliac disease and patients with Crohn's disease. Br Med J 2 oct: 794–795

Schneider RE, Bishop H, Hawkins CF, Kitis G (1979) Drug binding to α-glycoprotein. Lancet 10 March:554

Schnell RC, Miya T (1970) Altered absorption of drugs from the rat small intestine by carbonic anhydrase inhibition. J Pharm Exp Ther 174:177–184

Schuerman W, Turner P (1978) A membrane model of the human oral mucosa as derived from buccal absorption performance and physicochemical properties of the β-blocking drugs atenolol and propranolol. J Pharm Pharmacol 30:137–147

Scott D (1965) Factors influencing the secretion and absorption of calcium and magnesium in the small intestine of the sheep. Q J Exp Physiol 50:313–329

Seebald H, Forth W (1977) Absorption of ^{14}C-bumadizone – Ca and ^{14}C-phenylbutazone in isolated intestinal segments in vitro and tied off gastrointestinal sections in vivo of rats and guinea pigs. Drug Res 27:624–635

Selhub J, Brin H, Grossowicz N (1973) Uptake and reduction of radioactive folate by everted sacs of rat small intestine. Eur J Biochem 33:433–438

Shore PA, Brodie BB, Hogben CAM (1957) The gastric secretion of drugs: a pH partition hypothesis. J Pharm Exp Ther 120:361–369

Silk DBA (1979) Intestinal absorption of carbohydrate and protein in man. In: Crane RK (ed) Gastrointestinal physiology ed. III. International reviews in physiology. MTP Press, Lancaster, pp 151–204

Sladen G, Dawson AM (1968) Effect of bicarbonate on sodium absorption by the human jejunum. Nature 218:267–268

Smith ME (1973) The uptake of pteroylglutamic acid by the rat jejunum. Biochim Biophys Acta 298:124–129

Smith ME, Matty AJ, Blair JA (1970) The transport of folic acid across the small intestine of the rat. Biochim Biophys Acta 219:37–46

Smolen V (1973) Misconceptions and thermodynamic untenability of deviations from pH-partition hypothesis. J Pharm Sci 62:77–79

Smyth DH, Taylor CB (1958) Intestinal transfer of short chain fatty acids in vitro. J Physiol 141:73–80

Soergel KH (1971) Flow measurements of test meals and fasting contents in the human small intestine. In: Demling L, Ottenjahn R (eds) Gastrointestinal motility. Thieme, Stuttgart, pp 81–96

Stehle RH, Higuchi WI (1972) In vitro model for transport of solutes in a three phase system. I. Theoretical principles. J Pharm Sci 61:1922–1930

Steinmetz PR (1974) Cellular mechanism of urinary acidification. Physiol Rev 54:890–956

Stevens CE, Dobson A, Mammano JH (1969) A transepithelial pump for weak electrolytes. Am J Physiol 216:983–987

Strombeck DR (1972) The production of intestinal fluid by cholera toxin in the rat. Proc Soc Exp Biol Med 140:297–303

Swales JD, Tange JD, Wrong O (1970) The influence of pH, bicarbonate and hypertonicity on the absorption of ammonia from the rat intestine. Clin Sci 39:769–779

Swanston SK, Blair JA, Matty AJ, Cooper BT, Cooke WT (1977) Changes in the jejunal glycocalyx and their relationship to intestinal malabsorption. Trans Biochem Soc 5:152A

Takasaka M (1978) Volatile fatty acids and pH in the gastrointestinal contents of normal and shigella infected monkeys. Jpn J Vet Res 40:343–348

Takasugi N, Nakamura K, Hayashi T, Tsunakawa N, Takeya Y (1968) Studies on gastrointestinal absorption of nalidixic acid. Chem Pharm Bull 16:13–16

Teorell T (1937) Kinetics of distribution of substances administered to the body. I. Extravascular modes of administration. Arch Int Pharmacol 57:205–225

Thomson ABR, Dietschy JM (1977) Derivation of the equations that describe the effects of unstirred water layers on the kinetic parameters of active transport processes in the intestine. J Theor Biol 64:277–294

Tripp JH, Manning JA, Muller DPR, Walker-Smith JA, O'Donoghue DP, Kumar PJ, Harries JT (1977) Mucosal adenylate cyclase and sodium-potassium stimulated adenosine triphosphatase in jejunal biopsies of adults and children with coeliac disease. In: McNichol B, McCarthy CF, Fottrell PF (eds) Perspectives in coeliac disease. MTP Press, London, pp 461–470

Turnberg LA (1977) Intestinal transport of salt and water. Clin Sci Mol Med 54:337–348

Turnberg LA, Fordtran JS, Carter NW, Rector FC (1970a) Mechanism of bicarbonate absorption and its relationship to sodium transport in the human jejunum. J Clin Invest 49:548–556

Turnberg LA, Bieberdorf FA, Morawski SG, Fordtran JS (1970b) Interrelationships of chloride, bicarbonate, sodium and hydrogen ion transport in the human ileum. J Clin Invest 49:557–567

Turner RH, Mehta CS, Benet LZ (1970) Apparent directional permeability coefficients for drug ions: in vitro intestinal perfusion studies. J Pharm Sci 59:590–595

Ugolev AM, Laey P (1973) Membrane digestion: a concept of enzymic hydrolysis on cell membranes. Biochim Biophys Acta 300:105–128

Vaz WLC, Nicksch A, Jaehnig F (1978) Electrostatic interactions at charged lipid membranes. Measurement of surface pH with flourescent lipid pH indicators. Eur J Biochem 83:299–305

Venho VMK (1976) Drug absorption from the small intestine of the triparanol-treated rat in situ. Acta Pharmacol Toxicol 39:321–330

Venkataraman S, Horbett TA, Hoffmann S (1977) The reactivity of α-chymotrypsin immobilised on radiation-grafted hydrogel surfaces. J Biomed Mater Res 8:111–123

Waddell WJ (1975) Role of membrane-bound enzymes in biological transport. In: Csáky TZ (ed) Intestinal absorption and malabsorption. Raven, New York, pp 37–44

Wagner JG, Sedman AJ (1973) Quantitation of rate of gastrointestinal and buccal absorption of acidic and basic drugs based on extraction theory. J Pharmacokinet Biopharm 1:23–50

Waldron-Edward D (1971) Effects of pH and counter-ion on absorption of metal ions. In: Skoryna SC, Waldron-Edward D (eds) Intestinal absorption of metal ions, trace elements and radionuclides. Pergamon, Oxford, pp 373–382

White JF (1976) Intracellular potassium activities in Amphiuma small intestine. Am J Physiol 231:1214–1219

White JF (1977) Activity of chloride in absorptive cells of amphiuma small intestine. Am J Physiol 232:553–559

Wilson TH (1953) Lactate and hydrogen ion gradients developed across rat intestine in vitro. Biochim Biophys Acta 11:448–449

Wilson TH (1956) Concentration gradients of lactate, hydrogen and some other ions across the intestine in vitro. Biochem J 56:521–527

Wilson TH, Kazyak L (1957) Acid base changes across the wall of hamster and rat intestine. Biochim Biophys Acta 24:124–132

Wingate DL, Krag E, Mekhjian JS, Phillips SF (1973) Relationships between ion and water movement in human jejunum, ileum and colon during perfusion with bile acids. Clin Sci Mol Med 45:593–606

Winne D (1973) Unstirred layer, source of biased Michaelis constant in membrane transport. Biochim Biophys Acta 298:27–31

Winne D (1977) Shift of pH-absorption curves. J Pharmacokinet Biopharm 5:53–94

Winne D (1978) Dependence of intestinal absorption in vivo on the unstirred layer. Naunyn Schmiedebergs Arch Pharmacol 304:175–181

Zeuthen T (1978) Intra- and extra-cellular pH of absorptive epithelia measured with microelectrodes. Gastroenterol Clin Biol 3:334A

Zeuthen T, Monge C (1975) Intra- and extra-cellular gradients of electrical potential and ion activities of the epithelial cells of the rabbit ileum in vivo recorded by microelectrodes. Philos Trans R Soc Lond [Biol] 71:277–281

CHAPTER 21

The Role of the Unstirred Water Layer in Intestinal Permeation

A. B. R. THOMSON and J. M. DIETSCHY

A. Unstirred Water Layers: Historical and Conceptual Background

The concept of the unstirred layer (UWL) was originally developed by NOYES and WHITNEY (1897, quoted by DAINTY and HOUSE 1966 a) and later by NERNST (1904, quoted by ANDREOLI and TRAUTMAN 1979), and extended more recently by TEORELL (1936), DAINTY (1963), DAINTY and HOUSE (1966 c), and GINZBURG and KALCHALSKY (1963). These workers called attention to the potential relevance of unstirred layers in regulating the transport of materials across biologic interfaces. The presence of UWLs at solid–liquid interfaces was demonstrated to be a real physical characteristic of such interfaces by direct microscopic examination by GREEN and OTORI (1970). Since it is virtually impossible to stir a solution so that complete mixing occurs right up to the interface (DAINTY 1963), the presence of unstirred layers must be considered in studies of membrane permeation of all but the slowest permeating substances (LORTRUP 1963). The actual thickness of the unstirred layer depends partly on the molecular weight of the probe and partly on the rate of stirring (DAINTY and HOPE 1959 a, b). The fluid in the UWL is not stationary, but is rather a region of slow laminar flow parallel to the membrane in which the only mechanism of transport is by diffusion; the layers are often called "Nernst diffusion layers." The thickness of the layer is not the actual thickness, but rather an operational value.

Whether these unstirred layers play an important part in membrane transport processes depends on the permeability of the membrane to the probe molecule being transported. In considering this question it should be kept in mind that a UWL can be looked upon as a membrane in series with the actual membrane with a permeability coefficient D/d, where D is the diffusion coefficient of the probe in the aqueous solution and d is the effective thickness of the UWL. Since D for many small solutes has the value of approximately 1×10^{-5} cm^2/s, and the value of d varies widely between 100 and 1,000 μm, then the "permeability" of the unstirred layer can be anything between 10^{-4} and 10^{-3} cm/s. Hence the possibility must always be considered that the transport of a rapidly penetrating solute across a membrane may be wholly or partially rate controlled by the UWL and not by the permeability properties of the membrane.

Unstirred layers may modify diffusion processes in a number of systems other than lipid bilayer membranes, including cellulose membranes, plant cells, and epithelial tissues (DAINTY 1963; DAINTY and GINZBURG 1963, 1964 a, b; DAINTY and HOUSE 1966 a, b, c; HAYS 1968; HAYS and FRANKI 1970; HAYS et al. 1971; KEDEM and KALCHALSKY 1961; REDWOOD and HAYDON 1969). Similarly, it has been suggested that this diffusion barrier may retard significantly the dissipative movement of water and solutes into certain cells (LING et al. 1967; DICK 1964, 1966). Furthermore, COLTON (1967) has suggested that the major fraction of the total resistance to diffusion of solutes from blood to bathing medium during hemodialysis may be referable to unstirred layers in the blood phase. The magnitude of the unstirred layers in series with membranes is inversely to the rate of stirring of bulk phases (HAYS 1968, 1972). KAUFMAN and LEONARD (1968) indicated, in terms of fluid mechanics, that the interfacial resistance to diffusion in the aqueous phase adjacent to a membrane includes a region in which convective flow may occur but diminishes progressively, approaching zero at the membrane interface. In this context the thickness of the unstirred layer is an operational term for lamellae which may be partially or completely diffusion limited.

Thus, it is now generally accepted that adjacent to all bilogic membranes there is a layer of relatively unstirred water through which movement of solute molecules is determined only by diffusional forces (COLLANDER 1954; DAINTY 1963). While the effects of unstirred layers on various transport processes have been appreciated for many years (WEDNER and DIAMOND 1969; KIDDER 1970; ANDREOLI and TRAUTMAN 1971; SMULDERS and WRIGHT 1971; SMULDERS et al. 1972; GUTKNECHT and TOSTESON 1973), their profound influence upon absorption across the intestine has only recently been emphasized. Such a UWL exerts a major portion of the total resistance encountered by a probe molecule during its passage from the bulk extracellular water phase in the intestinal lumen into the cell interior (DIAMOND and WRIGHT 1969a, b; WRIGHT and DIAMOND 1969a, b). To correct for unstirred layer effects upon active and passive transport processes so that the permeability characteristic of the limiting lipid membrane may be more precisely described, it is essential, therefore, that the dimensions of the resistance factors by accurately defined. This resistance is determined by three parameters: the effective thickness d, of the UWL, its effective surface area S_w, and the free diffusion coefficient D, of the probe molecule (WESTERGAARD and DIETSCHY 1974a; WILSON and DIETSCHY 1974).. The effective thickness of this layer varies from about 100 to 500 µm in various epithelial surfaces in vitro (HINGSON and DIAMOND 1972; KIDDER 1970), including gallbladder (DIAMOND 1966; DIAMOND and WRIGHT 1969a, b; WEDNER and DIAMOND 1969), choroid plexus (WRIGHT 1972), cornea (GREEN and OTORI 1970), frog skin (DAINTY and HOUSE 1966a, b) and intestine (DIETSCHY 1978a, b; DIETSCHY et al. 1971; WESTERGAARD and DIETSCHY 1974a, b; WILSON and DIETSCHY 1974). The UWL resistance is even greater in the in vivo perfused rat (WINNE 1976) and human jejunum (READ et al. 1976, 1977).

The second characteristic of the UWL is its effective surface area, S_w. For an anatomically simple, flat membrane, the surface of the UWL is equal to that of the underlying membrane (Fig. 1). Because of the presence of villi and microvilli, however, the situation is somewhat more complex for the intestinal mucosa. Here, the UWL lies over and between the intestinal villi. The ratio of the effective surface area of the UWL to that of the underlying brush border membrane is at least 1:500 (WESTERGAARD and DIETSCHY 1974a; WILSON and DIETSCHY 1974). Since solute molecules must first pass through the relatively small area of the UWL before reaching the much greater surface area of the membrane, the UWL becomes

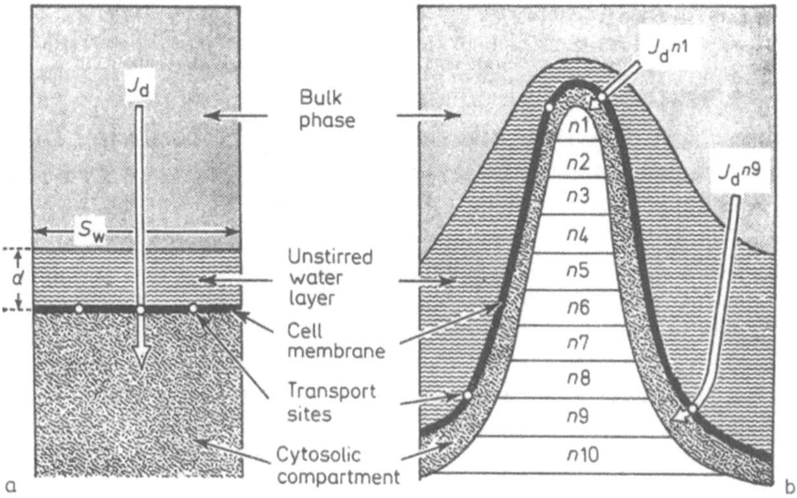

Fig. 1a, b. Diagrammatic representation of the major barriers to active transport. In a flat membrane (**a**) the two major barriers to cell uptake of solute molecules from the bulk phase into the cytosolic compartment are the UWL and the luminal cell membrane. The UWL can be assigned values for an effective thickness *d* and an effective surface area S_w so that the resistance of this layer to molecular diffusion is related to the value of d/S_w. In such a flat membrane it can be assumed that this resistance term has the same value for the UWL overlying all active transport sites on the cell membrane. In contrast, in the case of the intestine (**b**), it is likely that the resistance of the UWL varies over transport sites present at different locations on the villus. For the mathematical presentation of this problem, the villus has been arbitrarily divided into ten segments of equal height, and the active transport sites present at each of these levels have been designated as *n*1 through *n*10. Furthermore, the rate of uptake and the dimensions of the UWL appropriate for the transport sites at each of these levels have been designed as J_d^n, S_w^n and d^n, respectively. THOMSON and DIETSCHY (1977)

an important barrier to intestinal absorption. The importance of this barrier must be considered in relation to active and passive transport processes. Failure to correct for the resistance of the UWL will lead to serious errors in the estimation of the kinetic constants of carrier-mediated transport (DUGAS et al. 1975; LEWIS and FORDTRAN 1975; LUKIE et al. 1974; READ et al. 1976, 1977; REY et al. 1974; THOMSON and DIETSCHY 1977; THOMSON 1979a, b, c, d; WILSON and DIETSCHY 1974; WINNE 1973, 1976, 1977). The UWL also plays a major role in the uptake of passively transported solutes. Numerous studies (DIETSCHY et al. 1971; 1978a, b; LUKIE et al. 1974; THOMSON and DIETSCHY 1980a, b; WESTERGAARD and DIETSCHY 1974, 1976) have clearly demonstrated that a UWL with the dimensions we have described may offer sufficient resistance to constitute the major rate-limiting step for intestinal uptake of a number of passively transported probe molecules. For example, this unstirred diffusion barrier is of major importance in determining the rate of absorption of such physiologically important molecules as long-chain fatty acids, fatty alcoholics, bile acids, cholesterol, and monosaccharides (DIETSCHY and WESTERGAARD 1975; LUKIE et al. 1974; THOMSON and DIETSCHY 1980a, b; WESTERGAARD and DIETSCHY 1974a, 1976; WILSON and DIETSCHY 1972). In previous work with relatively flat membranes, it was usually assumed that the UWL is of uniform thickness and has a surface area equivalent to that of the underlying membrane. It is obvious that such assumptions cannot be applied to a tissue with so complex an anatomy as the intestinal mucosa. Early estimates of the dimensions of the unstirred layer have been obtained in the rat (WILSON and DIETSCHY 1972); the techniques employed were not sufficiently sensitive to allow for precise measurement of solute absorption and thickness of the diffusion barrier while the stirring rate was altered in a systematic and reproducible manner. To obviate these problems, LUKIE et al. (1974) designed a new chamber that allows measurements to be made under more precisely defined conditions. Using this chamber, the effective thickness and surface area of the UWL was quantified (WESTERGAARD and DIETSCHY 1974a) and the effect of this diffusion barrier on solute uptake into biologic system has been further evaluated (THOMSON 1979b, d; THOMSON and DIETSCHY 1980a, b).

The outline of this chapter then will be to consider: the water compartments in and around the intestinal mucosal cell; a comparison of the dimensions of UWL with morphological parameters; the glycocalyx and mucus as diffusion barriers; membrane structure; the general equations for solute movement across diffusion barrier and cell membranes; the relative importance of membrane and diffusion barrier resistance in determining rates of solute movement across a biologic membrane; the estimation of the magnitude of the dimensions of the diffusion and permeation barriers; the potential influence of the constituents of the unstirred layer on membrane permeation; the influence of diffusion barriers on the quantitative and qualitative characteristics of a number of features of molecular movement across diffusion barriers in biologic systems; and the potential applications of the UWL to health and disease in humans.

B. Water Compartments In and Around the Intestinal Mucosal Cell

It is difficult to measure directly the intracellular concentration of water, since the tissue water of the intestinal mucosa is composed of at least three compartments: mucosal extracellular and intracellular fluid, and tissue extracellular water. The mucosal extracellular compartment represents water that is not removed by gentle blotting procedures and remains entrained overlying the villi and between them, and almost certainly is also within the interstices of the glycocalyx. Sometimes this fraction, as measured by markers such as inulin of mannitol placed in the intestinal lumen, may amount to as much as 30%–50% of the total tissue water (JACKSON et al. 1970; SALLEE et al. 1972; SALLEE and DIETSCHY 1973); the exact size however, depends upon the blotting procedure employed.

The second extracellular compartment, the tissue fluid proper, is comprised of the fluid between the cells and deep to them. This water is entirely accessible only from the vascular bed. The third compartment is the intracellular fluid; the concentration of probe molecule in this compartment is not readily measured by examining the tissue concentrations unless the fraction of the total tissue water in each of the three compartments is known, and unless the concentration of the probe in the other compartments is known, or is the same in all compartments of the cellular water. Since the volume of this space and the substrate concentration within it are not easily determined, at present intracellular measurements can be undertaken only by the application of high resolution autoradiography (STIRLING 1967; STIRLING and KINTER 1967; STIRLING et al. 1972) or with observations made upon preparations of isolated mucosal cells (PERRIS 1966; KIMMICH 1970). Indeed, if the mean concentration of a nonmetabolized substrate in the whole tissue water is found to be significantly greater than that in the mucosal fluid, then all that can be said is that the solute is subjected to transport somewhere in the system.

Intracellular water is not a single "well-stirred" aqueous compartment (HECHTER 1965). Instead there are likely distinctive types of aqueous region present in the cells with different structures of water. Water associated with membranes and organelles should be distinguished from the aqueous region between organelles and structural protein filaments.

While the structure of bulk water remains the puzzle it has been for years, water near interfaces is stabilized owing to the presence of the interface itself (DROST-HANSEN 1969; DROST-HANSEN and THORHAUG 1967). Water molecules in the close vicinity of proteins and other biologically important macromolecules appear to exist in a physical state different from that of normal water: the aqueous environment is a major determinant of protein conformation, and the conformation of protein likewise influences the structure of water at the macromolecular surface. Water is a bulk component of membrane systems comprising up to half of the total system, and likely influences therefore the molecular organization of the system (FERNANDEZ-MORAN 1957, 1959; FINEAN 1957). Water in the membrane may be organized in ice-like or crystal hydrate lattices as an integral structural component of the membrane systems serving an essential role for various membrane processes (KLOTZ 1958, 1962). However, there are widely divergent views of the physical state of water in living cells. Several lines of evidence suggest that cell water has different solubility properties for nonelectrolytes, amino acids, and ions than does normal water (LING 1967).

Localized reversible phase changes in ordered water structure might provide the basis for conformational changes in protein layers and concurrently modify the arrangement of the polar lipids from an ordered bimolecular leaflet to a less tightly packed micellar form. Unfortunately, there is no information on the properties of water in the unstirred layer. It is assumed that the value of the free diffusion coefficient D in the unstirred layer on the luminal as well as the cytosolic side of the membrane is the same as the free diffusion coefficient measured in the bulk solution. The fact that the frictional resistances for diffusion between water and water or water and solute in the unstirred layer were altered in direct relationship to bulk aqueous viscosity (ANDREOLI and TRAUTMAN 1971) does not indicate that the magnitude of these resistances in the bulk and unstirred phases is the same. Thus these observations do not exclude the possibility that hydrophobic interactions (KLOTZ 1958, 1962; NEMETHY and SCHERAGA 1962) between the membrane interfaces and adjacent layers of water reduce considerably the values of the free diffusion coefficient of the solute in these regions. Similarly, the diffusive flux through the cytosol is influenced by the presence of obstructions encountered in the cytosol in the form of organelles possessing low or restrictive permeability. The presence of obstacles reduced the total cross-sectional area available for diffusion to a value that is less than in free solutions.

If intracellular organelles do indeed have significantly lower permeabilities to substrates diffusing across the intestinal epithelium, then the obstacles may reduce the value of the effective diffusion coefficient within the cytosol to less than one-half of that for an unobstructed solution of the same viscosity (PARSONS and BOYD 1972).

C. Comparison of Dimensions of the Unstirred Water Layer with Morphological Parameters

As a solute passes from the bulk phase in the intestinal lumen into the cytosolic compartment of the intestinal mucosa cells, it must first pass through the UWL adjacent to the microvillus membrane. The solute penetrates the membrane, and must then diffuse through a further series of unstirred layers both adjacent to the membrane as well as in the cytosolic compartment itself. In order fully to appreciate the functional impact of the UWL, we must briefly review the dimensions and morphological aspects of the villus (Fig. 2). The microvilli tend to be of uniform size and shape, and there are an average of 1,700 microvilli in the brush border of one human jejunal cell (BROWN 1962). The microvilli average 1.0 μm in length and 0.1 μm in width (LUCAS et al. 1978); they increase the epithelial surface 20–40-fold (BROWN 1962; PALAY and KARLIN 1959). The 0.02–0.05-μm spaces between the microvilli constitute narrow channels through which solutes must pass to reach their bases (CREAMER 1974; HAMILTON and MCMICHAEL 1968). The villi project into the lumen and usually range in height from 200 to 500 μm (MOE 1955; LUCAS et al. 1978). Thus, the thickness of the UWL in humans, 532 μm (READ et al. 1977) exceeds the height of the normal human finger-shaped villus (Table 1). It must be stressed, however, that these values for the unstirred layer thickness were obtained in perfusion studies in humans, and may represent an artifact of the intubation procedure that was utilized in these studies.

The microvilli are coated by a loose meshwork of fine intertwining mucopolysaccharide filaments (ITO 1964, 1965, 1969; BENNET 1963) which in humans is between 0.1 and 0.5 μm thick over the absorptive cells and somewhat thinner over the goblet cells (TRIER 1968). The filaments composing the glycocalyx are radially oriented, 25–50 Å in diameter and are seen to be either continuous with the outer leaflet of the plasma membrane (FAWCETT 1965) or continuous through the cell membrane (MUKHERJEE and STACHELIN 1971; MUKHERJEE and WILLIAMS 1967). These structural proteins may bear fixed charges and be responsible for the acid microclimate adjacent to the cell. This enteric or surface coat is of fairly uniform thickness over the columnar cells and is as prominent on cells at the base of the villi as on those near the tips. Goblet cells usually have a less prominent coating and their junction with adjacent absorptive cells may be marked by an abrupt change in the thickness of the fuzzy coat. However, occasional cells have a more prominent surface coat than neighboring cells (MUKHERJEE and WILLIAMS 1967), suggesting that this fuzzy coat is directly related to each individual cell and

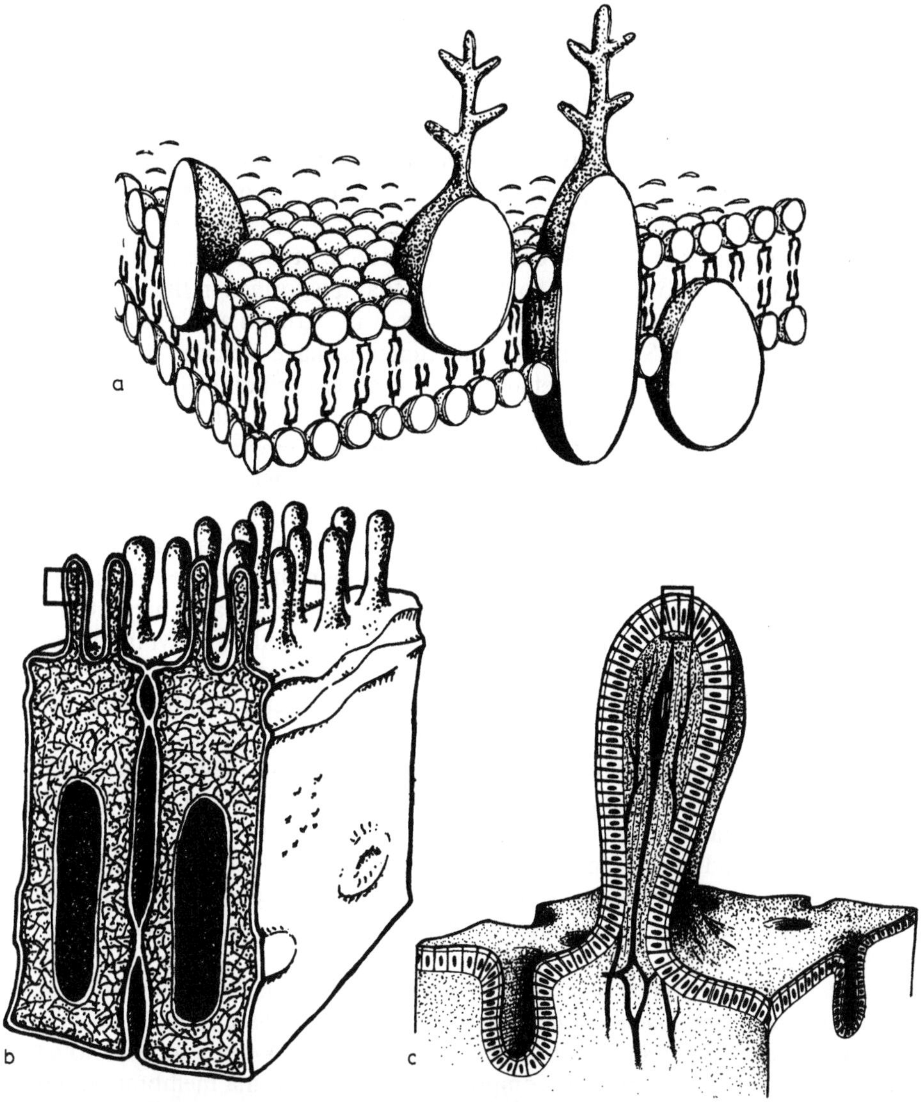

Fig. 2 a–c. Dimensions and morphological aspects of the human villus unit. This is a diagrammatic representation of the surface of the intestine. This figure demonstrates the intestinal villi and crypts, lateral surface of the mucosal cells, and the postulated composition of the brush border membrane

Table 1. Approximate dimensions of human villus unit

Parameter	Thickness of height (μm)
Unstirred water layer	500
Villus	200 –500
Glycocalyx	0.1– 0.5
Microvillus	1.0
Brush border membrane	0.1

is not simply an extraneous layer shared by all the cells of the epithelium. Another indication that the fuzzy coat is specific to each individual cell is the observation (ITO 1965) that the surface coat of cells undergoing extrusion at the villus tips is much less prominent and is all but absent on exfoliated cells. A series of autoradiographic studies also suggests that the enteric coat is synthesized by the columnar cells (ITO 1969). Although the staining characteristics of this fuzzy coat are those of a weakly acidic sulfated mucopolysaccharide, it cannot be removed by various mucolytic or proteolytic enzymes (ITO 1965). Studies of incorporation of labeled precursors into the fuzzy coat suggest that it is formed in the Golgi apparatus and transported to the microvilli, where it is extruded and attached by an unknown mechanism. Speculations on its functions have included protection of the cell against bacteria (RIFAAT et al. 1965) and specific binding of protein before pinocytosis (FAWCETT 1962). It may also be the site of the disaccharidase activity (JOHNSON 1967), and thus the fuzzy coat may play an important role in the digestive function of the brush border (CRANE 1968 a, b; MILLER and CRANE 1961; PARSONS and PRICHARD 1968, 1971; UGOLEV 1965, 1968).

The cells that comprise the sheet of the intestinal mucosa form a heterogeneous population (see also Chap. 2). Of prime importance are the columnar absorbing cells, by far the most numerous cell type. There are also present in the epithelium goblet cells, Paneth cells, enterochromaffin cells, and lymphoid cells (TONER 1968; TRIER 1967). The epithelial cells are packed in a hexagonal array (PARSONS and SUBJECK 1972) with some parts of the lateral membranes in close contact with parts of neighboring membranes. The tight junctions by which cells are attached to each other in lateral apposition extend only a short distance immediately below the brush border (see Fig. 2). The intercellular space existing between the outer faces of individual cells is a region within which local differences of hydrostatic and osmotic pressure may be established (DIAMOND and BOSSERT 1968). Two cell membranes in contact at tight junctions may be sufficiently permeable that molecules and ions move between one cell and its neighbor (LOEWENSTEIN 1966).

There are three types of adherens junctions (see Fig. 2): zonula adherens, fascia adherens, and macula adherens (BRIGHTMAN and REESE 1969; CLAUDE and GOODENOUGH 1973; GOODENOUGH and REVEL 1970; WADE and KARNOVSKY 1974). An adherens junctions is composed of parallel plasma membranes, separated by an interspace of 150–250 Å, and connected at their intercellular side by a thick belt (zonula adherens), sheet (fascia adherens), or disk (macula adherens, or desmosome) of electron-dense protein–aqueous material. These adherens junctions provide regions of strong attachment of adjacent cells. Several basic functional roles have been ascribed to the cell junctions: to stick cells together, to provide a permeability barrier and thereby give rise to a diffusion barrier, and to mediate direct communication between cells via the passage of materials from cell to cell through the cell junctions. A schematic representation of the intercellular junctions found in the intestine is shown in Fig. 2.

The main route of ion permeability in leaky epithelia, such as gallbladder and intestine, is via the tight junctions (BARRY and DIAMOND 1970; BARRY et al. 1971; FROMTER and DIAMOND 1972; WRIGHT et al. 1971, 1972). As a result of the leaky nature of these "tight" junctions, these epithelia have a low electrical resistance, high osmotic permeability, isotonic fluid transport, and only shallow gradients built up by active solute transport. The values of osmotic water permeability measured in the "leaky" intestine may be gross underestimates because of the effect of the UWL; indeed the error in the estimation of the value of the reflection coefficient ϱ of a solute arising from a failure to correct for unstirred layer effects is likely to be much greater in leaky than in tight epithelia. This error in the estimation of ϱ may lead to a number of qualitative errors such as the interpretation of the quantitative aspects of the values of ϱ to signify the presence of "pores" in the underlying membrane. The importance of the UWL in the "pore" theory is discussed in detail in a subsequent section.

D. The Glycocalyx and Mucus as Diffusion Barriers

In addition to the glycocalyx, a layer of mucus lies over the intestinal microvillus membrane, and these two elements could conceivably lead to artifacts in determining rates of absorption. Several lines of evidence suggest that this is not the situation. If some structural element outside the cell membrane contributed significant resistance to free diffusion of the test molecules, then one might reasonably expect that this barrier might discriminate among molecules of different size or charge. This was not the case in the studies of WESTERGAARD and DIETSCHY (1974a): the diffusion barrier did not discriminate between molecules whose molecular weight varied from 26 to 600 and which were either charged or uncharged. Furthermore, UWLs of similar dimensions have been found in other biologic membranes such as gallbladder (SMULDERS and WRIGHT 1971; DIAMOND 1966), which has much less prominent mucus and glycocalyx layers, as well as in artificial membranes that have no mucus or glycocalyx (HOLZ and FINKELSTEIN 1970). In addition, if the mucus or glycocalyx did slow the diffusion of the probe molecule up to the membrane, then this would be reflected in the estimates of unstirred layer resistance using a diffusion-limited probe such as decanol; this was not observed (WESTERGAARD and DIETSCHY 1974a).

This data suggests that the diffusion barrier is in fact principally a layer of unstirred water. It must be appreciated, however, that from a technical point of view the presence of mucus must be recognized: in the presence of mucus a greater portion of the probe molecule will be trapped in the adherent mucosal fluid, and failure to correct for this trapped probe can lead to serious errors in the estimation of rates of uptake. However, even in the presence of mucus, accurate estimates of rates of uptake may be obtained when an extracellular marker is used to estimate the volume of the mucus and other fluid which comprise the adherent mucosal fluid volume. Thus, current knowledge suggests that the intestinal mucus and glycocalyx do not significantly impair the absorption of solutes and do not represent contributing factors to the effective resistance of the UWL (LUKIE et al. 1974; SALLEE and DIETSCHY 1973; WESTERGAARD and DIETSCHY 1974a).

E. Intestinal Membrane Structure

There is an apparent paradox between the specificity and stability of membrane structure on the one hand and its lability and dynamism on the other. There have been many reviews dealing with membrane organization (BRANTON 1969; CRIDDLE 1969; HENDLER 1971; KORN 1969; STOECKENIUS and ENGELMAN 1969). Particular membrane types in cells are specific for their function as well as their composition of protein and lipids (GETZ et al. 1968; SCHNAITMAN 1969). Although all membranes contain protein and lipid, their ratios vary from 0.25:1 for myelin (ASHWORTH and GREEN 1966; COLEMAN and FINEMAN 1966) to 4.6:1 for intestinal microvilli (EICKHOLZ 1967; FORSTNER et al. 1966). Furthermore, the ratio of membrane cholesterol to phospholipids varies from 0 for bacteria and chloroplasts (BISHOP et al. 1967) to about 1:1 to 1:2 for intestinal microvilli of guinea pig, rat, and rabbit (ASHWORTH and GREEN 1966; COLEMAN and FINEAN 1966; EICKHOLZ 1967; FORSTNER et al. 1966; MILLINGTON and FINEAN 1963; PORTEUS and CLARK 1965). The turnover rates of individual proteins isolated from the same membranes differ greatly, (ARIAS et al. 1969; JICK and SHUSTER 1966). Similarly, the lipids of a given membrane are turning over at different rates relative to each other (BAILEY et al. 1967; CUZNER et al. 1966; HOLTZMANN et al. 1970; PASTERNAK and BERGENON 1970). Thus, it would appear that all membrane components are turning over at rates not in concert with one another.

The cell does not loose its identity during the differentiation process; neither do its membranes. As cells arise from cells, so membranes arise from membranes, not as templates but as organizational fields within which occurs the coordinated development of further and more complete membrane structures. While it may be safe to consider the membrane protein as a genetically determined, species-representative component, it is not possible to attribute the same character to the lipids without important reservations. Indeed, very significant alterations in chain length and saturation occur under mere dietary influences in the rabbit and human erythrocyte membrane lipids (MULDER et al. 1963; VAN DEENEN et al. 1963), and those of mitochondrial membranes of sea mammals and birds (RICHARDSON et al. 1962). What is the biologic significance of the lipid composition? Some aspects of its significance may be discerned from a comparison of the differences in composition between species with differences in their biologic activity as, for example, the correlation discovered between composition and permeability (van Deenen et al. 1963). In the sequence rat, rabbit, pig, horse, ox, and sheep, the sphingomyelin : lecithin ratio falls, and, as the oleate content increases, the palmitate and arachidonate content fall (DE GRIER and VAN DEENEN 1961; DAWSON et al. 1960). Remarkably, the permeabilities of the erythrocytes of these species to the four solutes, urea, thiourea, glycerol, and ethylene glycerol, lie in the same sequence, decreasing from rat to sheep. In the intestine, the ratio of cholesterol: phospholipid in the microvillus membrane is 0.5:1 in the rat (MILLINGTON and FINEAN 1963), higher in the rabbit (PORTEUS and CLARK 1965), and 1:1 in the hamster (COLEMAN and FINEAN 1966); this is the same direction as the relative rates of intestinal uptake of a homologous series of saturated fatty acids and cholesterol: hamster > rabbit > rat (THOMSON et al. 1983).

The nature of binding of lipids to the cell membrane is a second chemical characteristic that may influence the permeability of the membrane. The lipid can be fractionated into loosely bound lipid, which is extractable with dry ether; weakly bound lipid, extractable with wet ether; and a strongly bound fraction extracted by alcohol–ether (PARPORT and BALLENTINE 1952). The percentage of loosely bound material varies between species; species with a high permeability to ethylene glycol, glycerol, and thiourea (rabbit, human) contain more of this fraction than species (sheep, ox) with low permeability (ROELOFSEN et al. 1964). The loosely bound fraction contains most of the neutral lipids of the membrane (cholesterol and triglyceride), and a mixture of phospholipids, predominantly lecithin. The phospholipid composition of this fraction isolated from different species is constant, although the total phospholipid content of the red blood cell ghosts of these species varies considerably. Since the strongly bound material, once isolated, is readily soluble in ether, the differential extraction depends on the binding of the lipids rather than on the solubility per se. Possibly, the loosely bound fraction interacts only through van der Waal's forces, while the more tightly bound material is additionally anchored into the membrane by polar forces. ROELOFSEN et al. (1964) have tentatively suggested that a high proportion of loosely bound material is indicative of the presence of the "open" configuration in the membrane and hence the high permeability.

Thus, the chemical composition of the membrane may determine its biologic behavior, or alternatively membrane function may depend upon a particular arrangement of membrane constituents without an apparent change in membrane composition (BERLIN et al. 1975). The approaching horizon in the field of intestinal permeation will be to correlate the changes in the characteristics or composition of the lipid and protein content of the brush border membrane with changes in membrane transport.

F. Movement of Solutes Across Biologic Membranes: General Principles

Solutes may enter the body by one of two basic pathways – transcellular and paracellular. A given substance may permeate across a membrane by diffusion through the lipid portion of the membrane, by passage through polar regions in or between the cell membrane of through aqueous "pores," by vesicular flow (pinocytosis), or by carrier-mediated transport. Conceptually, passive absorption through the lipid membrane may be considered as transport involving an infinite number of sites, whereas all the other processes: carrier-mediated uptake, vesicular flow, and diffusion through polar regions, may be considered as involving a relatively finite number of transport sites. The uptake of lipid substances is influenced more by lipid solubility in the bulk phase and partitioning into the membrane, rather than by molecular size which is an important feature in determining the rate of penetration of polar solute molecules through localized regions of relative high polarity in the membrane.

Diffusion is movement due solely to the kinetic energy and electrical charge of the molecules and to the electrical field in which they exist (TEORELL 1953, 1956, 1958). The equation frequently used to describe diffusion of an uncharged substance across a membrane specifies that its movement at any point within the membrane is proportional to its concentration gradient at that point, and includes several assumptions (CURRAN and SCHULTZ 1968; DIAMOND and WRIGHT 1969a, b) that cannot be verified for biologic systems: these assumptions include no water flow, no chemical reaction, no temperature or pressure gradients, and the constraint that all the differences in observable physical properties are in the direction perpendicular to the membrane; finally, the membrane must be planar. Diffusion of an uncharged molecule exhibits a linear relation between flux and transmembrane concentration difference. However, observation of such a linear relation does not prove diffusion because other transport mechanisms may produce a linear relation (WILBRANDT and ROSENBERG 1961; THOMSON and DIETSCHY 1980b).

With passive transport, molecules must cross the membrane by passage through polar channels within the cell membrane or between adjacent cells, or by passage through the lipid sheet itself. In both types of passive transport net solut movement takes place only in the direction of the prevailing electrochemical gradient; there is no competition between structurally related compounds, and there is usually no inhibition of uptake by metabolic inhibitors, anoxia, or the absence of electrolytes (DIETSCHY 1978a; HOFFMAN and SIMMONDS 1971; SALLEE et al. 1972; SALLEE and DIETSCHY 1973; SIMMONDS 1972; WESTERGAARD and DIETSCHY 1974a, 1976).

The rate of passive movement J of the solute molecule from the outside of the cell across the membrane and into the cytosolic compartment is equal to the product of the difference in the concentration of the molecule between the bulk phase and the cytosol ΔC and the passive permeability coefficient P for the particular solute crossing that particular membrane

$$J = P\Delta C\,. \tag{1}$$

The passive permeability coefficient describes the amount of solute that crosses unit area of the planar cell membrane per unit time per unit concentration of the solute, and has units such as nmol $cm^{-2}\ s^{-1}\ mM^{-1}$, which reduces to the conventional units for P of cm/s.

The molecular mechanisms of passive transfer across biologic membranes are as yet poorly understood. Does passive permeability depend on metabolism, or is the permeability an inherent property of the cell membrane influenced by such factors as fixed positive charges, lipid composition, and calcium? There are as yet no answers to these questions, but it is clear that not all of the passive permeability properties of the brush border membrane reside in the membrane of the mucosal cell. For a leaky epithelium such as the intestine there is a large paracellular shunt pathway which may represent a major route for passive permeation (BOULPAEP and SEELY 1971; FROMTER 1972; HOSHI and SAKA 1967). Leaky epithelia such as the intestine have a smaller range of ion selectivity than single cell membranes (FRIZZELL and SCHULTZ 1972; WRIGHT 1972), and large nonpolar electrolytes move across leaky epithelia with the same ratio of permeabilities as the ratio of their free solution diffusion coefficient (BIBER et al. 1972; WRIGHT and PRATHER 1970). Furthermore, activation energies for the movement of large nonelectrolytes across epithelia are similar to those observed in free solution (SMULDERS and WRIGHT 1971), suggesting that the permeation pathway across the tight junction is highly hydrated.

If a solute crosses a membrane by single-file diffusion (HODGKIN and KEYNES 1955), it flow cannot be described adequately by the equation for simple diffusion.

The basic reason for this departure is that in single-file diffusion, solute molecules interact with one another during passage across the membrane, whereas the equations for simple diffusion are derived on the assumption that there are no such interactions (KEDEM and ESSIG 1965). Other modes of interaction between diffusing solutes are also possible. Thus, formation of uncharged ion pairs may be involved in the transfer of ions across a membrane of low dielectric constant. Association may occur between an ion and a cation at the membrane, and the two may cross the barrier in the form of a neutral salt. A phenomenon known as "nonionic diffusion," involving weak acids or bases in a similar process, occurs in the gastrointestinal tract (HOGBEN 1960; HOGBEN et al. 1959; SCHANKER et al. 1957; SHORE et al. 1957), and its basis may arise from properties related to and influenced by the UWL. The effect of the microenvironment of the UWL on the absorption of weak electrolytes will be discussed in a later section.

The second major type of transport which is important in the movement of solutes across membranes involves the binding of solute to a finite number of sites on the cell membrane, followed by cellular uptake of the solute. The uptake process may involve a "carrier," may be energy dependent ("active") or independent ("facilitative" diffusion), or in the case of lipids may involve an endocytotic process (BROWN et al. 1973; BROWN and GOLDSTEIN 1974) such as the uptake of the chylomicron remnant by the liver and of low density lipoproteins by the human fibroblast (SHERRILL and DIETSCHY 1975; SHERRILL 1978). The specificity of the carrier must be defined quantitatively and qualitatively. Quantitative specificity is established by determining the relative affinities and maximal transport rates for various absorbates. This is usually done by applying Michaelis–Menten kinetics, which is subject to certain limitations and errors arising from the UWL. Qualitative specificity can be expressed in chemical terms as the configuration which can attach to the carrier. Since the interpretation of such data is influenced by accurate measurements of rates of uptake, which in turn may be influenced by the UWL, some reconsideration of the properties of certain carriers is required.

The kinetics of this process may be described by the following relationship

$$J = \frac{J^m C}{K_m + C}, \tag{2}$$

where the J^m is the maximal velocity of transport the system can achieve, and K_m defines the concentration of the solute molecule at the aqueous–membrane interface at which half the value of J^m is achieved. It must be appreciated that J^m, K_m, and P, the maximal transport rate, the Michaelis affinity constant, and the passive permeability coefficient, respectively, represent the "true" values of the kinetic constants of the membrane transport process, and under numerous biologic conditions to be discussed in the next section, may not necessarily be reflected by the experimental estimates of the "apparent" values, J_d^{m*}, K_m^*, and P^*. The major reason for the discrepancy between the true and apparent values is the presence of a diffusion barrier of major dimensions interposed between the bulk solution and the membrane (see Fig. 1).

Biologic transport systems for a number of solutes exhibit substrate specificity, saturation kinetics, and competitive inhibition (CRANE 1968 b). These characteristics have been explained by the carrier hypothesis (WILBRANDT and ROSENBERG 1961) which postulates a cycle in which the transported substance binds reversibly to a carrier at one side of the membrane, and the substrate–carrier complex crosses the membrane and release the substrate at the other side. The carrier then returns to its original side where it can combine with another substrate molecule. When carrier-mediated transport is associated with cellular metabolic processes, it is termed "active transport." Most investigators use the term "active transport" only in a general sense to refer to transport that requires energy and is coupled to cellular metabolism. ROSENBERG (1948, 1954) has defined active transport as a process that results in net movement against an electrochemical potential difference. However, this definition excludes any transport process that is directly coupled to metabolism, but in which net movement is in the same direction as the electrochemical potential difference (BRICKER et al. 1963; JARDETZKY 1957; KLAHR and BRICKER 1964). Furthermore, a transport process would be regarded as active, even though it resulted in net movement against an electrochemical potential difference (PD) only by virtue of being coupled to a second transport process and was not itself directly dependent on metabolic energy. More explicit definitions of active transport have been developed from irreversible thermodynamics, but they have limited applicability in studies of biologic systems because all the necessary variables cannot be measured (JARDETZKY and SNELL 1960; KEDEM 1960).

Facilitated transport refers to a carrier-mediated process that exhibits substrate specificity, competitive inhibition, and countertransport against an electrochemical PD. In contrast to active transport in which the apparent affinity of the carrier for the substrate is greater on one side of the membrane than on the other, facilitated transport requires that the apparent affinity be the same on both sides of the membrane (CRANE 1968 b).

G. Effects of Aqueous Diffusion Barriers on Solute Movement

In most biologic systems under either in vitro or in vivo conditions, the concentration of the solute molecule measured in the bulk phase is not the same as the concentration of the solute molecule which is actually encountered by the cell membrane (Fig. 3). This is true because there is usually a diffusion barrier between the cell surface and the bulk perfusion medium. This diffusion barrier is the UWL. Thus as a molecule moves from the bulk water phase of the intestinal contents into the cell interior it must penetrate at least two barriers, a UWL adjacent to the aqueous–lipid interface, and the cell membrane itself. The UWL consists of a series of water lamellae extending outward from the cell membrane, each progressively more stirred, until they blend imperceptibly with the bulk water phase. Although the boundary between the well-mixed bulk water phase and the UWL is not distinct, it can be assigned a finite functional thickness. This operational value is the equivalent thickness of a single layer in which transport occurs only by diffusion (DAINTY 1963; DIAMOND 1966; WESTERGAARD and DIETSCHY 1974 a; WILSON and DIETSCHY 1974). Since the two "membranes" (the UWL and the

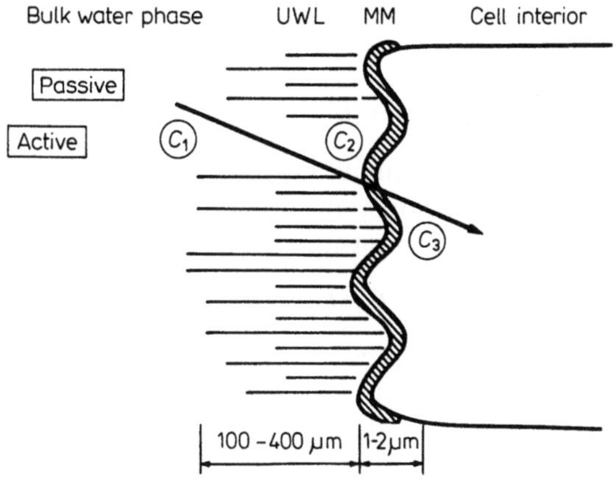

Fig. 3. Diagrammatic representation of the pathway for absorption of a molecule from the bulk water phase in the intestinal lumen into the cell interior across the unstirred water layer (UWL) and through the microvillus membrane (MM) of the mucosal cells. The concentrations of a given probe molecule in the bulk water phase, adjacent to the aqueous–lipid membrane interface, and just beyond the microvillus membrane in the cell interior are given by the terms C_1, C_2, and C_3 respectively. The approximate thickness of the UWL is 100–400 µ*M* or greater, as compared with the relatively small thickness of the MM, 1–2 µm. THOMSON (1978)

brush border) are in series, the rates and characteristics of absorption of solutes are determined by the interaction of these resistances. Movement across the UWL is a simple diffusion process in which the rate of movement is determined by the functional thickness d of the UWL, the aqueous diffusion constant of the molecule D, and the concentration gradient between the bulk water phase and the cell membrane. If C_1 and C_2 represent the concentrations of the molecule in the bulk phase and at the aqueous–membrane interface, respectively (Fig. 3), the rate of flux of the solute across the UWL will be

$$J=(C_1-C_2)\mathrm{D}/\mathrm{d}\,. \tag{3}$$

Thus, in the presence of a UWL, the concentration of the probe molecule at the aqueous–membrane interface C_2 is reduced below the concentration of the probe in the bulk phase C_1. The magnitude of this reduction is obtained by rearranging Eq. (3)

$$C_2=C_1-J(d/D)\,. \tag{4}$$

This is a useful expression since it allows for the calculation of C_2 from the experimentally set or determined value of C_1. Once the solute has diffused through the unstirred layer, at a rate established by Eq. (3), the solute will pass through the membrane at a rate described by Eqs. (1) or (2). In Eq. (1), the velocity of passive flux across the cell surface is determined by the permeability coefficient for the molecule in that membrane, and the concentration gradient of the molecule across the membrane. This gradient is established by the difference in solute concentration between C_2 and C_3, the concentrations of the probe molecule just outside and just inside the membrane, respectively (Fig. 3). The rate of passive flux across the membrane will be given by the formula

$$J=(C_2-C_3)P\,. \tag{5}$$

In a steady state, the rate of passive movement of a molecule across the UWL and the brush border will be equal, and the rate of net movement of the solute from the bulk phase into the cytosol will be given by

$$J=(C_1-C_2)D/d=(C_2-C_3)P\,. \tag{6}$$

In the presence of a UWL, the rate of solute movement across the cell membrane will be determined by C_2 rather than C_1. This applies to passive as well as carrier-mediated mechanisms, so that the concentration term in Eq. (2) must be C_2

$$J=\frac{J^{m}C_2}{K_m+C_2}\,. \tag{7}$$

Since it is usually not possible to measure the value of C_2, Eq. (4) becomes a useful expression since it allows for the calculation of C_2 from the experimentally set or determined value of C_1. By substitution of Eq. (4) into Eq. (7),

$$J=\frac{J^{m}(C_1-J\,d/D)}{K_m+(C_1-J\,d/D)} \tag{8}$$

By rearrangement (THOMSON and DIETSCHY 1977), the following quadratic expression is obtained,

$$J=(0.5)D/d\,\{C_1+K_m+J^{m}(d/D)+[(C_1+K_m+J^{m}(d/D))^2-4C_1J^{m}(d/D)]^{1/2}\}. \tag{9}$$

H. A Consideration of Surface Areas

Equations (6) and (9) describe the rate of passive and carrier-mediated transport across the intestinal membrane. In these equations, the flux term J has the units of mass crossing unit area per unit time. Often the effective areas of the UWL and brush border membrane are unknown, and the experimentally determined flux rate J_d is related to some parameter of tissue mass that is assumed to bear a constant relationship to the surface area of the UWL or membrane. Commonly, J_d is normalized to wet or dry weight of tissue, unit serosal length or surface area, or weight of protein or DNA. The terms S_w and S_m represent the functional area of the UWL and the membrane, respectively, relative to some other parameter such as tissue mass; the units of S_w and S_m must correspond to the appropriate units of J_d. For example, if J_d has the units nmol/100 mg/min, then S_w and S_m will each have the units cm^2/100 mg. Thus, the term

$$J=J_d/S_m \tag{10}$$

corrects the experimentally measured flux to membrane surface area, and the term

$$J=J_d/S_w \tag{11}$$

corrects the experimentally measured flux to the surface area of the UWL overlying a particular membrane. For a simple flat membrane (see Fig. 1), the values of S_w and S_m will be similar, but for the more complex microvillus membrane with its villi and microvilli, S_m will greatly exceed S_w, and Eqs. (10) and (11) need to be considered.

Equation (6) described the rate of flux of a passively transported probe from the bulk phase into the cytosol. Using experimental values of flux J_d and in the steady state, then

$$J_d = (C_1 - C_2)\frac{DS_w}{d} = (C_2 - C_3)P \cdot S_m . \tag{12}$$

Since values of S_m are seldom known for experimental preparations involving the intestine, transport rates are expressed as J_d and the corresponding passive permeability coefficient also must be normalized to the same parameter of tissue mass, and so will not have the conventional units of cm/s. This relationship can be designated as

$$P_d = PS_m \tag{13}$$

and thus Eq. (12) may be expressed entirely in experimental values describing the rate of passive flux of a molecule from the bulk phase into the cytosol in the presence of a UWL

$$J_d = (C_1 - C_2)\frac{DS_w}{d} = (C_2 - C_3)P_d . \tag{14}$$

In order to establish the effect of both the effective thickness d and the effective surface area S_w of the UWL on the discrepancy between C_1 and C_2, Eq. (11) must be substituted into Eq. (4)

$$C_2 = C_1 - \frac{J_d d}{D S_w} . \tag{15}$$

Using experimental values of solute flux J_d, the rate of transport by a carrier-mediated mechanism becomes

$$J_d = (0.5)\frac{DS_w}{d}\left\{C_1 + K_m + \frac{dJ_d^m}{S_w D} + \left[\left(C_1 + K_m + \frac{dJ_d^m}{S_w D}\right)^2 - 4C_1\frac{dJ_d^m}{S_w D}\right]^{\frac{1}{2}}\right\} . \tag{16}$$

Note that the values of the experimentally determined maximal transport rate J_d^m will have the same units as J_d, nmol/100 mg/min. Thus, it is apparent from the equations describing passive and carrier-mediated transport across a membrane, Eqs. (14) and (16), that the rates of uptake of solute molecules into cells may be influenced by the resistance of the UWL, as given by the term (d/DS_w), as well as by the terms that define the membrane transport processes, K_m, J_d^m, and P_d, or P and S_m.

Two extreme conditions may prevail: the permeability of the membrane may be very much larger than the "permeability" of the probe in the UWL ($P \gg DS_w/d$ or $J_d^m/K_m \gg DS_w/d$), in which case the rate of diffusion of the probe across the UWL may limit the rate of cellular uptake. When the "resistance" of the membrane is much greater than the resistance of the UWL, then the other extreme may prevail and the rate of absorption across the cell membrane will become rate limiting to absorption.

Let us consider the extreme where the permeability of the membrane is high, and the "permeability" of the UWL is low. Examples of this special case would be high velocity carrier-mediated transport, or absorption of highly permeant probes such as fatty acids, fatty alcohols, and cholesterol, in tissues with a high resistance of the UWL, such as in the intestine, gallbladder, or choroid plexus

$$J_{\mathrm{d}}=(C_2-C_3)\,PS_{\mathrm{m}} \tag{17}$$

or

$$J_{\mathrm{d}}=(C_2-C_3)\,P_{\mathrm{d}}\,. \tag{18}$$

If the probe is quickly metabolized within the cell, or transported away from the brush border membrane, then $C_2 \gg C_3$, C_2-C_3 approaches C_2, *and*

$$J_{\mathrm{d}}=C_2P_{\mathrm{d}} \tag{19a}$$

or

$$J_{\mathrm{d}}=C_2PS_{\mathrm{m}}\,. \tag{19b}$$

The values of C_2 can be expressed in terms of C_1 by rearranging Eqs. (15) and (19)

$$J_{\mathrm{d}}=\left(C_1-\frac{J_{\mathrm{d}}d}{DS_{\mathrm{w}}}\right)P_{\mathrm{d}} \tag{20a}$$

or

$$J_{\mathrm{d}}=\left(C_1-\frac{J_{\mathrm{d}}d}{DS_{\mathrm{w}}}\right)PS_{\mathrm{m}}\,. \tag{20b}$$

It is essential to emphasize that the transport characteristics of a membrane are described in terms of the passive permeability coefficient (P or P_{d}). In the absence of a UWL

$$P=\frac{J^{\mathrm{d}}/S_{\mathrm{m}}}{C_1} \tag{21a}$$

or

$$P_{\mathrm{d}}=\frac{J_{\mathrm{d}}}{C_1}\,. \tag{22b}$$

However, in the presence of a UWL

$$P=\frac{J_{\mathrm{d}}/S_{\mathrm{m}}}{C_2} \tag{23a}$$

or

$$P_{\mathrm{d}}=\frac{J_{\mathrm{d}}}{C_2}\,. \tag{23b}$$

The value of C_2 can be expressed in terms of C_1 with Eq. (15), and

$$P=\frac{J_{\mathrm{d}}/S_{\mathrm{m}}}{C_1-\left(\dfrac{J_{\mathrm{d}}d}{DS_{\mathrm{w}}}\right)} \tag{24a}$$

or

$$P_{\mathrm{d}}=\frac{J_{\mathrm{d}}}{C_1-\left(\frac{J_{\mathrm{d}}d}{DS_{\mathrm{w}}}\right)}. \tag{24b}$$

The magnitude of the experimentally determined membrane permeability coefficient is given by Eq. (24 b). When the effective resistance of the UWL is zero, this reduces to the simplest form, $P_{\mathrm{d}}=J_{\mathrm{d}}/C_1$, Eq. (22 b).

This situation of zero unstirred layer resistance is rarely encountered in biologic situations, and the magnitude of the error inherent in the failure to account for the resistance of the UWL will be proportional to $J_{\mathrm{d}}d/DS_{\mathrm{w}}$. Thus, for a given membrane with fixed magnitude of s_{m}, and in the presence of a UWL, Eq. (22 b) will underestimate the true permeability coefficient (P or P_{d}) by a magnitude which is directly proportional to J_{d} and d, and inversely proportional to S_{w} and D. These predictions are borne out by experimental data derived from studies in the intestine, to be discussed later (WESTERGAARD and DIETSCHY 1974 a).

The net movement from the bulk phase into the cytosol is given by Eq. (14). The first term $(C_1-C_2)(DS_{\mathrm{w}}/d)$ describes the rate of movement of the solute across the UWL, and the second term $(C_2-C_3)P_{\mathrm{d}}$ gives the net flux of the molecule across the cell membrane. Two extreme situations may be encountered in various membrane systems in which C_2 may assume any value between the limits of C_1 and 0, and J_{d} will be limited by the rate of penetration of either the UWL or the membrane. Consider first the situation in which the rate of movement of the solute molecule across the UWL may be rapid in relation to its rate of movement across the cell membrane, i.e., $DS_{\mathrm{w}}/d \gg P_{\mathrm{d}}$. In this case unstirred layer resistance is negligible, the value of C_2 approaches the value of C_1, and the rate of molecular penetration through the cell membrane becomes totally rate limiting to cellular uptake as described by the following equation formulated by substituting C_1 for C_2 in the right-hand portion of Eq. (14)

$$J_{\mathrm{d}}=(C_1-C_3)P_{\mathrm{d}}\,. \tag{25}$$

This equation predicts that when diffusion is limited by the membrane, then: (a) J_{d} will be proportional to P_{d}, or P and S Eq. (13) for any given concentration gradient; (b) any change in the value of C_3 will greatly influence J_{d}; and (c) J_{d} will be essentially unaffected by the UWL.

The second extreme is the condition in which the rate of penetration of the solute through the membrane is much faster than its rate of diffusion across the UWL ($P_{\mathrm{d}} \gg DS_{\mathrm{w}}/d$). The value of C_2 approaches zero so that $C_1-C_2 \rightarrow C_1$ and

$$J_{\mathrm{d}}=C_1\frac{DS_{\mathrm{w}}}{d}. \tag{26}$$

This equation predicts that when diffusion is limited by the UWL, then: (a) J_{d} will be proportional to D for any given value of C_1, d, and S_{w}; and (b) the value of J_{d}/D will vary inversely with d and directly with S_{w} for any given value of C_1. These predictions have been borne out experimentally (WESTERGAARD and DIETSCHY 1974a), and examples are given in Fig. 4. Here the logarithm of the value

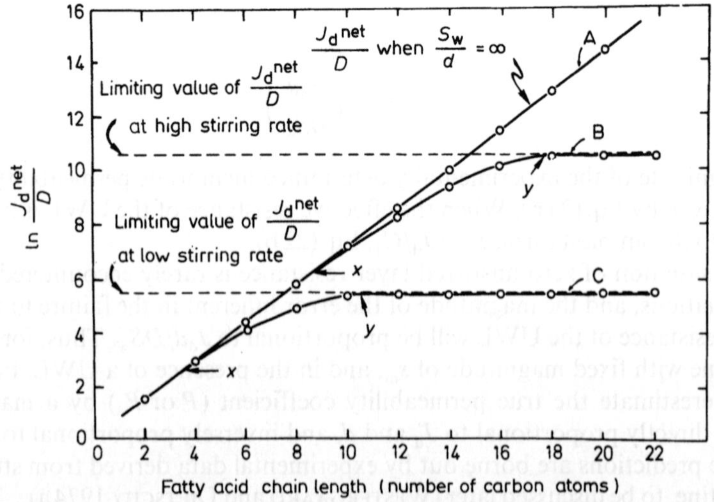

Fig. 4. Diagrammatic representation of the effect of diffusion barriers of varying resistance on the cellular uptake of fatty acids of different chain length. In this example, the concentration gradient across the cell membrane is assumed to be the same for each fatty acid. Under these conditions, the rate of net uptake J_d^{net} will equal the product of the passive permeability coefficient of each fatty acid and its concentration gradient. If no diffusion barrier is present outside the cell membrane, then the uptake rate will be essentially a linear function of the fatty acid chain length (curve *A*). Curve *C* represents the theoretical findings anticipated when the bulk solution is stirred at a very low rate so that the diffusion barrier is relatively thick; curve *B* represents the results anticipated at a higher rate of stirring. For the latter two curves, *x* illustrates the point at which the diffusion barrier begins to exert significant resistance and uptake rates begin to deviate from the linear relationship illustrated by curve *A*. At point *y*, diffusion of fatty acids across the UWL becomes totally rate limiting to cellular uptake so that J_d^{net}/D becomes constant. These theoretical curves are based on actual experimental data derived in several types of epithelial tissues. DIETSCHY (1978b)

J_d/D has been plotted as a function of the fatty acid chain length at several different values for unstirred layer resistance.

In these examples, the concentration gradient between the bulk phase and the cytosol is assumed to be the same for each fatty acid, and the villus is assumed to be homogeneous. Curve A represents the one extreme where unstirred layer resistance is zero, and J_d is determined by the passive permeability coefficient for each fatty acid so that the term $\ln J_d/D$ increases as an essentially linear function of the number of CH_2 groups in each fatty acid (DIAMOND and WRIGHT 1969a, b). However, there is deviation from this linear relationship as soon as the resistance of the UWL assumes a finite value, but the extent of the deviation will depend upon the relative values of the P_d of each fatty acid. In this example, the permeability coefficients of fatty acids C2:0–C8:0 (acetic to octanoic acid) are sufficiently low that membrane penetration is rate limiting (Eq. 26) and the value of $\ln J_d/D$ still falls on the linear portion of the curve. However, the permeability coefficients of the other fatty acids are sufficiently high ($P_d \gg DS_w/d$) that uptake becomes limited by diffusion across the UWL, Eq. (26) prevails, and $\ln J_d/D$

reaches a constant and limiting value dictated by the magnitude of S_w/d (the portion of curve B to the right of point y). The portion of curve B between points x and y delineates those fatty acids where the UWL and the cell membrane both contribute in determining the rate of solute uptake. When the resistance of the UWL is even higher, as is the case in curve C, then this diffusion barrier becomes totally rate limiting to uptake of even the medium-chain fatty acids. It must be emphasized that the greater the passive permeability coefficient for a particular solute, the more likely its rate of uptake will be limited by the UWL rather than by the cell membrane. In vivo, the effective resistance of the UWL is high (READ et al. 1976, 1977; WINNE 1976) and likely limits the uptake of highly membrane-permeant molecules including long-chain fatty acids, various sterols such as cholesterol, bile acids, and steroid hormones (LUKIE et al. 1974; HOLLANDER and MORGAN 1979; HOLLANDER et al. 1977; WESTERGAARD and DIETSCHY 1974a). It therefore follows that the rate-limiting step to the cellular uptake of these biologically important compounds is likely to be diffusion across the various complex diffusion barriers between the bulk phase in the intestinal lumen, blood or extracellular fluid, and the target cell where the solute molecule is absorbed, taken up and utilized, or taken up and triggers a cellular response.

We have dealt with the two major types of intestinal transport processes, those with an infinite and those with a finite number of transport sites in the membrane. Many solutes however may be transported by both a passive and a carrier-mediated process. Examples of such a process would be the absorption of hexoses (THOMSON 1979d; THOMSON and DIETSCHY 1980b) or bile acids (WILSON and TREANOR 1975) in the intestine. The rate of flux of such a solute would be predicted and defined by combining Eqs. (16) and (24b),

$$J_d = (0.5)\frac{DS_w}{d}\left\{C_1 + K_m + \frac{dJ_d^m}{S_w D} + \left[\left(C_1 + K_m + J_d^m \frac{d}{DS_w}\right)^2 - 4C_1 J_d^m \frac{d}{DS_w}\right]^{\frac{1}{2}}\right\} + P_d\left(C_1 - \frac{J_d d}{DS_w}\right). \quad (27)$$

In the event that the contribution of carrier-mediated transport is desired, then the contribution of passive permeation must be appropriately assessed, and subtracted from the experimentally derived uptake rates comprised only of the carrier-mediated component (THOMSON 1979a, b, c, d; THOMSON and DIETSCHY 1980a, b). Failure to correct for the contribution of the passive component will lead to serious errors in the estimation of the kinetic constants J_d^m and K_m, the experimentally measured maximal transport rate and the true Michaelis affinity constant of the membrane process.

J. Consequences of Failure to Correct for the Unstirred Water Layer and Passive Permeation

A number of theoretical and experimental examples are given to stress the point that failure to correct for the contribution of the UWL and passive permeation will lead to serious overestimation in the magnitude of J_d^m and K_m. Once the con-

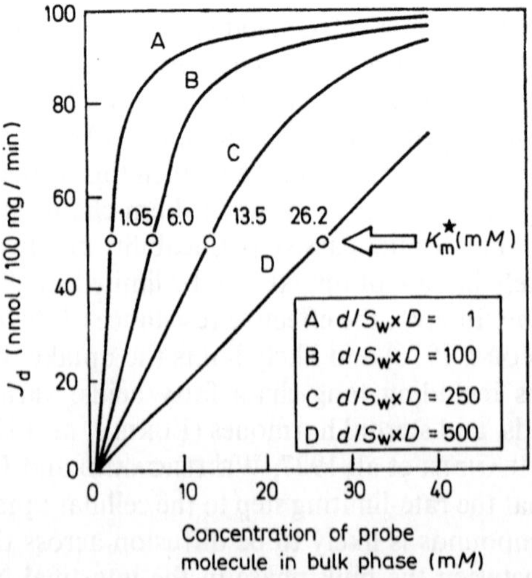

Fig. 5. Estimation of the true Michaelis constant for an active transport process. Four theoretical curves are shown where $d/S_w D$ was varied from 1 to 500 min 100 mg/cm^3. In these calculations, J_d^m was 100 nmol/100 mg/min and K_m was 1 m*M*. THOMSON and DIETSCHY (1977)

tribution of the passive component has been considered and the appropriate corrections made in the value of the experimentally determined flux rate J_d, then it is clear from Eq. (27) that the rate of carrier-mediated transport is dictated by the resistance of the UWL, which is determined by the magnitude of d, S_w, and D, as well as by the values of two membrane-related terms, J_d^m and K_m.

This formulation has a number of important theoretical (THOMSON and DIETSCHY 1977) and practical consequences (THOMSON 1979a, d; WINNE 1976, 1977). First, in the presence of significant UWL resistance, the saturable appearance of the kinetic curve relating J_d to C_1 is lost, and if the resistance of the UWL becomes sufficiently high, then J_d may become a linear function of C_1 (THOMSON and DIETSCHY 1980b). This effect is illustrated by the series of curves derived from Eq. (16) and shown in Fig. 5. When the resistance of the UWL is low (d/DS_w is low), as in curve A, the rate of uptake demonstrates saturation kinetics with a plateau in the relationship between C_1 and J_d at values of C_1 of 10 m*M* and above, and an apparent Michaelis affinity constant K_m^* which is close in value to the true affinity constant ($K_m^* \rightarrow K_m$, and $K_m^* - K_m \rightarrow 0$). As the resistance of the UWL is increased, the line describing the relationship between C_1 and J_d is drawn to the right (Fig. 5). This shift of the curve to the right can be achieved by increasing the value of d, or decreasing the value of D or S_w (THOMSON and DIETSCHY 1977). When the resistance term is increased 500-fold to values which are observed in the intestine in vivo, then J_d increases in essentially a linear fashion with respect to the concentration of the solute molecule in the bulk solution (Fig. 5, curve D). Thus, in the presence of a major UWL diffusion barrier such linear kinetics are to be anticipated and should not be construed as evidence against the possibility that the uptake process involves translocation by a finite number of transport sites.

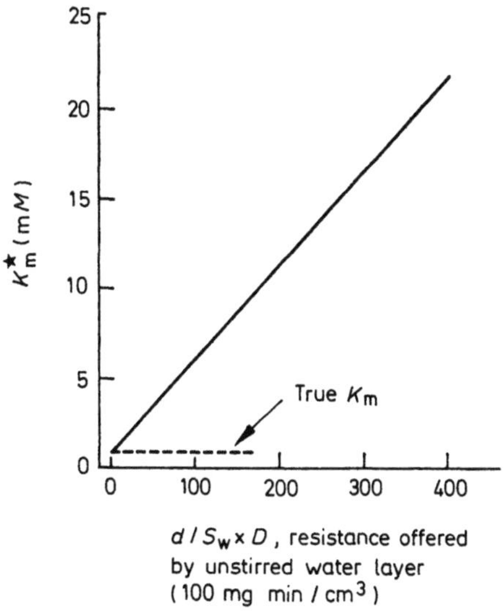

Fig. 6. Estimation of the true Michaelis constant for an active transport process. The values of K_m^* shown in Fig. 5 were plotted as a function of the effective resistance offered by the UWL, d/S_wD. It is evident from this plot that when d/S_wD equals zero, K_m^* equals K_m. Thus, by experimentally determining K_m^* at various values of d/S_wD, it becomes possible to extrapolate to zero resistance and thereby obtain an estimate of the true Michaelis constant of the transport process. THOMSON and DIETSCHY (1977)

Second, the presence of a UWL of significant dimensions leads to gross overestimation of the true Michaelis affinity constant K_m. By referring once again to Fig. 5, the true affinity constant K_m has been assigned a value of 1.0 mM, and as the resistance of the UWL is increased and the curve is shifted to the right, the discrepancy between the true and apparent values, K_m and K_m^*, respectively, increases. Indeed, the value of K_m^* increases linearly with the resistance of the UWL (Fig. 6) as given by the equation (DIETSCHY 1978 b; THOMSON and DIETSCHY 1977; WINNE 1973)

$$K_m^* = K_m + 0.5 \frac{dJ_d^m}{S_wD}. \tag{28}$$

This is a particularly useful equation since it provides a means to calculate the magnitude of K_m from values which may be experimentally measured, K_m^*, d, J_d^m, D, and S_w. This theoretical prediction has been borne out experimentally (THOMSON and DIETSCHY 1980 b), and it is now apparent that major discrepancies exist between the true and apparent values of K_m (THOMSON and DIETSCHY 1980 b). As seen in the example in Fig. 6, increasing the resistance of the UWL over a 500-fold range leads to an increase in the value of the affinity constant from an assigned value of 1.0 mM to an anticipated value of 26.2 mM. This provides for the first time a plausible explanation for part of the difference in the values of affinity constants estimated in vivo and in vitro: the value of the affinity constant for a given solute and in a given species is usually at least an order of magnitude higher in vivo than in vitro, and the thickness of the UWL is generally much higher in vivo (READ et al. 1976, 1977; WINNE 1976).

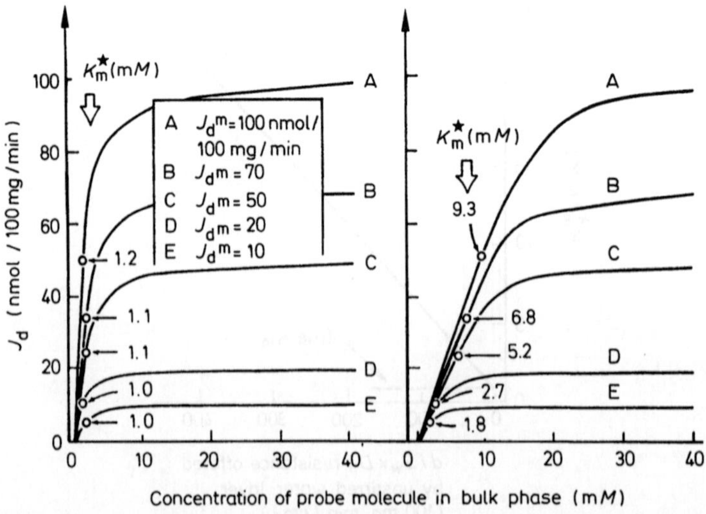

Fig. 7. Theoretical relationship between the kinetics of active transport and variations in the maximal transport rate. This diagram illustrates the manner in which the apparent Michaelis constant is altered by changes in J_d^m, from 10 to 100 nmol/100 mg/min, under conditions where the resistance offered by the unstirred layer was either low or high. In these calculations, K_m was 1 mM and D was 30×10^{-5} cm^2/min. Thomson and Dietschy (1977)

Third, in the presence of a significant diffusion resistance, K_m^* becomes a dependent variable of J_d^m. This effect is illustrated by the series of curves shown in Fig. 7, where the true K_m value is set equal to 1.0 mM. When the resistance of the UWL is low, increasing the value of J_d^m tenfold has only a minimal effect in increasing the value of K_m^* to 1.2 mM (Fig. 7a). However, a similar increase in J_d^m under circumstances where the resistance of the UWL is high results in an increase in K_m^* to 9.3 mM (Fig. 7b). In fact, at a given value of the resistance of the UWL, there is a linear relationship between J_d^m and K_m^* (Fig. 8), and as expected from Eq. (28), K_m^* will approach K_m as J_d^m approaches zero. Unfortunately, there are no experimental models available which will allow for a systematic change in J_d^m, without a concurrent change in d/DS_w, and it has not proven practical to estimate the true affinity constant by this means.

We must now consider the use and limitations of the so-called linear transformation plots of the Michaelis–Menten equation. First, the presence of a diffusion barrier will lead to overestimation of the maximal transport rate J_d^m if the value of this kinetic constant is estimated from so-called linear transformations of the Lineweaver–Burk equation (Thomson 1979b, c; Winne 1973). When the resistance of the UWL is zero, the relationship between J_d and C_1 is described by Eq. (2), and takes the form of a rectangular hyperbola. When replotted in the double-reciprocal from such a curve becomes linear and has an intercept on the vertical axis that equals $1/J_d^m$ (Fig. 9b, curve A). However, when the diffusion barrier is present over the transport sites, then Eq. (16) describes the relationship between J_d and C_1; this does not take the form of a rectangular hyperbola, and the double-

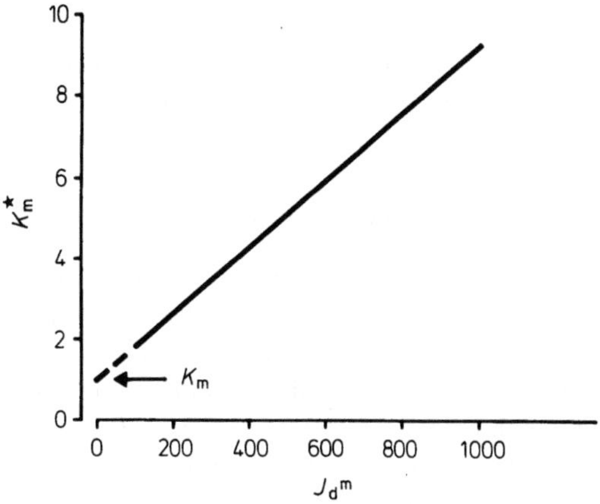

Fig. 8. Influence of maximal transport rate on the estimation of the apparent affinity constant. This diagram illustrates the manner in which the apparent Michaelis constant K_m^* is altered by changes in J_d^m. By experimentally determining K_m^* at various values of J_d^m, it becomes possible to extrapolate to zero J_d^m and thereby obtain an estimate of the true Michaelis constant of the transport process. The slope of this line is d/S_wD, and thus the influence of J_d^m upon K_m^* is influenced by the effective resistance of the UWL

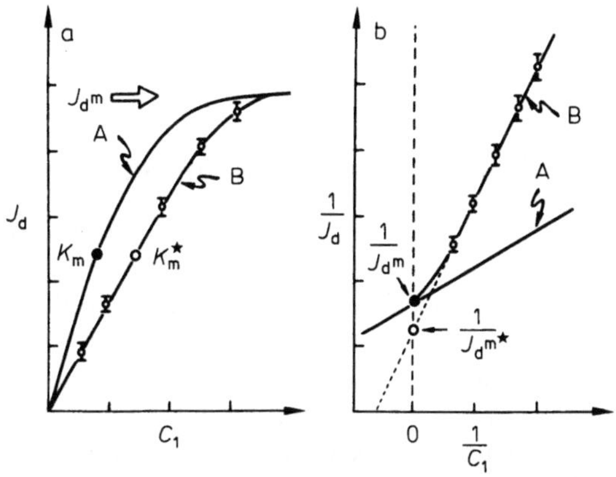

Fig. 9 a, b. Effect of diffusion barriers on determination of maximum transport velocities J_d^m by use of double-reciprocal plots. **a** two kinetic curves for uptake of a solute molecule in the absence (*A*) and presence (*B*) of a significant diffusion barrier. In the presence of the diffusion barrier K_m is shifted to the right, but both curves achieve the same value of J_d^m, **b** the same curves replotted as the reciprocals of these two variables. Linear extrapolation of the data points in curve *B* gives a value for J_d^m much higher than the true maximal transport rate, i.e., $1/J_d^{m*}$ is artifactually lower than $1/J_d^m$. DIETSCHY (1978 a)

reciprocal form does not transform into a straight line, but rather turns sharply upward as it approaches the vertical axis to intercept at $1/J_d^m$ (Fig. 9b, curve B). However, if as is commonly done, the experimental points are used to construct a linear regression curve and this curve is extrapolated to the vertical axis, then an artifactually high value for J_d^m will be obtained (WILSON and DIETSCHY 1974; WINNE 1973). Furthermore, any error in the estimation of J_d^m will also result in an error in the estimation of K_m (see Fig. 7b). These theoretical considerations have recently been confirmed experimentally (THOMSON 1979d; THOMSON and DIETSCHY 1980b) and are discussed in detail in a later section.

K. Diffusion Barriers of Greater Complexity

Consider the more complex situation where the solute molecule must pass from the bulk perfusate to a target cell, such as from the serum to an adipocyte. There will be a series of tissue spaces and cell membranes. The total resistance encountered during this diffusion process equals the sum of the resistances encountered in diffusion through each membrane in series, i.e., $1/P_{d1} + 1/P_{d2} + 1/P_{d3} + \ldots$, plus the sum of the resistances encountered in duffusing through each aqueous space, i.e., $(d/DS_w)_1 + (d/DS_w)_2 + (d/DS_w)_3 + \ldots$ Therefore, the determination of the dimensions and permeability characteristics of any one of these series of diffusion barriers to passive mucosal uptake may be experimentally difficult and theoretically complex. Furthermore, in vivo one must consider the potential effect of variations of blood flow and the solubility of the probe molecule in the bulk phase of the blood; thus, the rate of cellular uptake will ultimately be determined by the rate of passage through a variety of cell membranes, the rate of blood flow to a particular organ, the solubility of the solute in the blood, and the rate of metabolism of the solute before it reaches its final destination.

L. Possible Functional Heterogeneity of the Villus

It should be emphasized that Eqs. (16) and (24b) are derived on the basis of three assumptions: (a) that the diffusion barrier has a homogeneous structure in which the values of d, S_w, and D are uniform along the villus; (b) that the intestinal membrane is a homogeneous structure in which each portion is equally avid in transporting solute; and (c) that the same area of the villus is used for the absorption of closely related compounds. There is no basis for these tacit assumptions, and indeed there is some early theoretical and experimental evidence that these assumptions may be invalid (THOMSON and DIETSCHY 1977; THOMSON 1979b, c).

Heterogeneity of the villus may influence the uptake of passively absorbed solutes. By examining Eqs. (20a) and (20b), it is apparent that J_d will be enhanced by increasing S_m and S_w. For a flat membrane $S_w = S_m$ (see Fig. 1), and the value of S_w/S_m will approach unity. The intestinal villi and microvilli greatly increase the value of S_m, but the value of S_w is only increased sixfold by reducing the effective resistance of the UWL (WESTERGAARD and DIETSCHY 1974a). Because $S_m \gg S_w$, then large changes in S_m will have relatively less effect on J_d than small changes in S_w. First consider the special situation where S_w/S_m is uniform for a series of probe molecules, and P is similar at each site along the villus (see Fig. 1). Varying the value of d and S_w will influence J_d in accordance with Eqs. (20a) and (20b), and no difference will exist in the J_d of a solute into the first as compared with the tenth villus segment. On the other hand, if the resistance of the UWL is lower over the tip of the villus than from the more basal portions, changes in the surface area of the membrane will have relatively little effect on J_d. In contrast, for a poorly permeant probe molecule ($DS_w/d \gg P$), differences in d between the tip and crypt of the villus will have comparatively little effect on J_d, but the uptake of the probe molecule will be much more readily affected by changes in S_m.

These considerations have been examined in detail by WINNE (1978). The equations used thus far to correct the permeability coefficient for the unstirred layer's influence are valid only for flat membranes. WINNE (1978) has derived equations for membranes with a villous surface. These equations take into account the possible nonlinear concentration gradient in the intervillous part of the unstirred layer, but the application of these considerations is limited by the lack of quantitative information about the geometry of the villous surface and the unstirred layer thickness. The concentration of highly permeant substances likely drops sharply in the upper part of the intervillous space, so that the tips of the villi function as an effective absorbing area. The intervillous concentration gradient of a substance with a low permeability coefficient is so small that such a substance is absorbed by the total surface area of the villous membrane. The effective absorbing area of substances with intermediate permeability coefficient lies between these two extremes. If a substance is absorbed exclusively by the tips of the villi, P^* equals the permeability coefficient of the wall of the tips and the area of S_w will almost equal S_m, assuming the intervillous space is narrow, a reasonable assumption since the width to depth ratio of the intervillous space is small (CREAMER 1974).

WINNE (1978) has developed the following equation to describe the uptake of solutes absorbed from different positions along the villus

$$J_d = P_d^* S_w (C_1 - C_c) = \left(\frac{d_{UL}}{DS_w} + \frac{1}{PS_{aff}} \right)^{-1} (C_1 - C_c) . \tag{29}$$

P_d^* is an experimentally determined apparent permeability coefficient of the membrane wall, including the unstirred layer. To determine the permeability coefficient of the wall of a membrane with a villous surface the following quantities are needed: the permeation rate J_d, the concentration difference $(C_1 - C_c)$ between the well-mixed bulk phase and the core of the villus, the unstirred layer area S_w, the effective thickness d_{UL} of the supravillous part of the unstirred layer, the diffusion constants D_{UL} and D_{IV} of the substance in the supra- and intervillous part of the unstirred layer, and a value for S_{aff}. The value of S_{aff} is represented by the expression

$$S_{aff} = AL + A_L B , \tag{30}$$

where AL is the area of the tip of the villi, A_L is the area of the lateral surface of the villi, and B is the width of the intervillous space divided by its depth. This equation assumes: that the membrane is not cylindrical, that only the concentration gradient normal to the main plane is important, i.e., the concentration gradient in a section parallel to the main plane may be neglected; that the lateral surface of the villus is normal to the main plane of the membrane; that the permeability constant is similar at each portion of the villus; and finally, that there is a uniform concentration in the villus core. This latter assumption may not be valid if there is an effective countercurrent exchange in the villus (WINNE 1975).

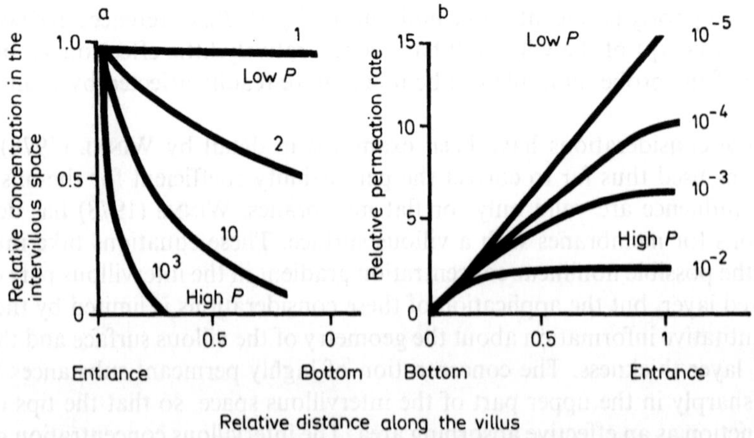

Fig. 10 a, b. The permeability coefficient of the wall of a villus membrane. **a** the dependence of the concentration profile in the intervillous space on the permeability of the villus wall. Permeation through the intervillous bottom is ignored, and the concentration of the probe molecule in the villus core is assumed to be zero. The value of the permeability coefficient P is shown; **b** the effect of intervillous depth on the relative permeation rate. The permeation rate is related to the rate obtained with closed intervillous space. Once again, permeation through the bottom of the intervillous space is ignored, and the concentration of the probe in the villus core is assumed to be zero. Adapted from WINNE (1978)

Granting these assumptions, a number of predictions are possible. When the permeability coefficient of the solute is low, or when the intervillous space is wide relative to its depth, there is only a small drop in the concentration of the solute at different positions along the villus (Fig. 10 a). With highly permeant solutes, or when the intervillous space is narrow relative to its depth, the concentration of the solute drops abruptly (Fig. 10 a) so that only the tips of the villi function as the absorbing surface. For intermediate conditions, the concentration of the solute drops in a curvilinear fashion between the top and the bottom of the villus (Fig. 10 a). If the permeability of the solute is high, then the solute will be absorbed largely from the tip of the villus, so that changing the intervillous depth will have little effect on the relative permeation rate (Fig. 10 b). In contrast, solutes with a low permeability coefficient are absorbed along the entire length of the villus, and any change in the intervillous depth, or of the membrane surface area, will have a profound effect on the relative permeation rate (Fig. 10 b). The calculation of true membrane coefficients requires an estimation of membrane surface area, S_m. However, the value of S_m cannot be obtained simply from histologic measurements, since different portions of the membrane may be contributing to the functional value of S_m for different solutes. For highly permeant solutes, the villus tips will be largely responsible for absorption, and the membrane surface area will approach the value of the surface area of the UWL. In contrast, for poorly permeant probes, the entire surface area of the membrane is functionally important, and under this special condition it may be valid to use the entire villus surface area to calculate permeability coeficients. However, for most solutes the exact surface area of the villus over which absorption occurs will be unknown, and the values of their permeability coefficient on the one hand may be grossly underestimated if the effect of the UWL is not taken into account, but on the other hand the value of the P may be grossly overestimated if the surface area of the entire villus is used for the calculation of permeability coefficients.

M. Effect of Carrier Molecules, Solubility of Probe, and Metabolism in the Cytosolic Compartment

The rate of passive movement of a solute into the cell will be determined by the overall concentration gradient between the bulk phase and the cytosolic compartment. As the concentration of the solute in the cytosol C_3 increases, the gradient $C_1 - C_3$ or $C_2 - C_3$ becomes significantly influenced by the magnitude of C_3. This has two profound effects. First, the rate of uptake will slow and will deviate from the expected linear relationship between substrate concentration and the rate of uptake. Second, solute may begin to move out of the cell at a rate determined by $C_2 - C_3$. It is a reasonable assumption that the cell membrane behaves symmetrically with respect to passive permeability so that the same value of P can be utilized regardless of the direction of molecular diffusion. If the solute is not bound within the cytosol, not metabolized, and not transported rapidly out of the cell, then C_3 will eventually equal C_2 and net flux will cease. If however the solute is rapidly bound, metabolized, or transported, the value of C_3 will never become of importance, and for all practical purposes can be ignored.

It must be further appreciated that if the solute in question is actually synthesized within the cell, then the value of C_3 may rise and reduce the concentration gradient available for uptake across the cell membrane. This transport of solute out of the cell will, of course, also be influenced by unstirred layers. The length of the diffusion pathway within the cell might, on first reflection, be considered to be short because of the relatively small size of cells such as those of the intestinal mucosa, but the length of the diffusion pathway might be considerably longer if the probe must diffuse around organelles. Furthermore, the value of the diffusion coefficient within the cytosol may be considerably greater than in the bulk aqueous phase owing to the viscosity of the cytosol. While there is no experimental data on this point, it is likely that unstirred layers are important for the release of solute from the cell into extracellular spaces.

The relative dimensions of the UWL or membrane resistances ($1/P$ versus d/DS_w) will also influence the exit of solute from the cell into an extracellular compartment. Consider a highly permeant solute which accumulates within the intestinal mucosal cell. As the value of C_3 increases, net uptake into the cell will fall as the rate of flux increases back into the UWL. At the luminal side of the microvillus membrane, the probe may either reenter the cell at a rate determined by $C_2 - C_3$, or the probe may diffuse across the UWL and into the bulk phase in the intestinal lumen. Because $P \gg DS_w/d$, and because the resistance of the UWL is high, the highly permeant probe will tend to remain in the microenvironment adjacent to the luminal surface of the membrane, awaiting reentry into the cell as soon as the concentration gradient becomes more favorable to further uptake. However, the rate of backflux from the membrane into the bulk phase is influenced by the UWL.

Because $C_1 > C_2$, and $P_d > DS_w/d$, then there will be little tendency for the highly permeant solute to pass from the cell, back across the UWL, and into the bulk phase. In contrast, relatively more of a poorly permeant solute may pass back across the UWL: when $P \ll DS_w/d$, the membrane rather than the UWL becomes rate limiting to uptake. Assuming that the membrane behaves symmetrically with respect to P, then once the solute is in the cytosol, its tendency to leave the cell will be low, even if $C_3 \gg C_2$. Any solute which does reach the luminal surface of the microvillus membrane, however, will be in a situation in which once again $P \ll DS_w/d$, and the molecule will have a greater tendency to diffuse back across the UWL than back across the membrane. Thus for highly permeant molecules, the UWL becomes rate limiting to uptake, but serves to discourage subsequent passage of the probe back into the bulk phase. For a relatively impermeable solute the membrane becomes rate limiting for uptake, but also discourage subsequent passage of the solute back out of the cell.

In the equations thus far we have assumed infinite solubility of the probe molecule in the bulk phase. However, interactions do occur between the solute molecules in the bulk phase and various "carrier" molecules, thereby influencing the rate of both unidirectional and net solute movement. Consider the examples of long-chain fatty acids and cholesterol bound to or solubilized by the bile acid micelle, or steroid hormones and fatty acids bound to carrier proteins such as albumin in the plasma. The rate of movement of the probe molecule across the membrane will be determined by the concentration gradient multiplied by the permeability coefficient. The concentration of the poorly soluble probe in the aqueous milieu of the intestinal lumen will itself be limited by its maximum solubility in water. Although the total amount of solute dispersed in the aqueous phase may be high, the actual amount of the solute in true solution and therefore available for penetration of the membrane may still be exceedingly small. Consider the example of cholesterol which is virtually insoluble in water, and which is "solubilized" by use of bile salts which form a mixed micelle with the cholesterol. The ratio of the concentration of the solute in the micelle C_m and in the aqueous phase near the membrane C_2 can be defined in terms of a partition coefficient, K

$$K = C_m/C_2 \,. \tag{31}$$

The concentrations may be expressed in terms of the masses of the solute molecule in the water and micellar phases, M_w and M_m respectively, and in terms of the volumes of the aqueous and micellar phases, V_w and V_m respectively

$$C_m = M_m/V_m \tag{32a}$$

and

$$C_2 = M_w/V_w \,. \tag{32b}$$

Equation (31) may be rewritten, substituting values for C_m and C_w from Eqs. (32 a) and (32 b).

$$K\left(\frac{M_w}{V_w}\right) = \left(\frac{M_m}{V_m}\right). \tag{33}$$

The total mass of solute in the system M_T, represents the total of M_w and M_m

$$M_T = M_w + M_m \tag{34}$$

and therefore

$$M_m = M_T - M_w . \tag{35}$$

This value of M_m can be substituted in Eq. (33), and after rearranging the terms the following expression is obtained

$$\frac{M_w}{V_w} = \frac{M_T}{KV_m + V_w} . \tag{36}$$

Since J_d is proportional to C_2, which in turn is proportional to M_w/V_w (Eq. 32b), then the rate of uptake can be calculated from the total mass of solute in the system M_T from the volume of the micellar phase V_m which in turn is calculated from the concentration of the solubilizing agent in the perfusate and its appropriate partial specific volume. The value of the partition coefficient K is unknown for most solutes in the intestine, but for the purposes of theoretical consideration, arbitrarily low and high values may be substituted into Eq. (36).

At least three different mechanisms may explain events which occur during the uptake of solutes from a solubilizing or binding agent, such as a micelle. The first possibility is that the micelle might be taken up into the cell intact. This seems unlikely since the various constituent molecules in the mixed micelle are absorbed at essentially independent rates, and the ratio for uptake of any two lipid solutes does not necessarily agree with the ratio in the micelle, and therefore there is no evidence that the uptake step occurs through a process akin to pinocytosis (SIMMONDS 1972; SIMMONDS et al. 1968; THORNTON et al. 1968; WILLIX 1970; WILSON and DIETSCHY 1972).

The second possibility is that the micelle interacts with or binds to the microvillus membrane during a direct "collision" between the micelle and the cell membrane. The micelle and membrane would presumably interact in such a way that water is excluded from the interface, after which the molecule solubilized in the micelle would move directly into the cell, leaving the micelle to return to the bulk phase, available once again to solubilize more probe solute. In this model, the rate of absorption would be proportional to C_m, the concentration of the probe in the micelle. This model does not fit experimentally derived data (WESTERGAARD and DIETSCHY 1976).

In the third model, the absorption of the probe molecule solubilized in the micelle would occur from an aqueous phase, with partitioning of the solute from the micelle into the aqueous phase, and thence into the lipid phase of the membrane. As the solute is taken into the cell, more solute would quickly partition from the micelle and become available for permeation into and through the microvillus membrane. Thus, the micelle would act only as a solubilizer to convey the relatively insoluble probe molecule across the UWL and up to the cell surface, where the maximum monomer concentration might be maintained and the full potential of membrane uptake could be achieved. The curves shown in Fig. 11 have been derived from this equation and represent experimentally confirmed results (WESTERGAARD and DIETSCHY 1976). As the concentration of the detergent

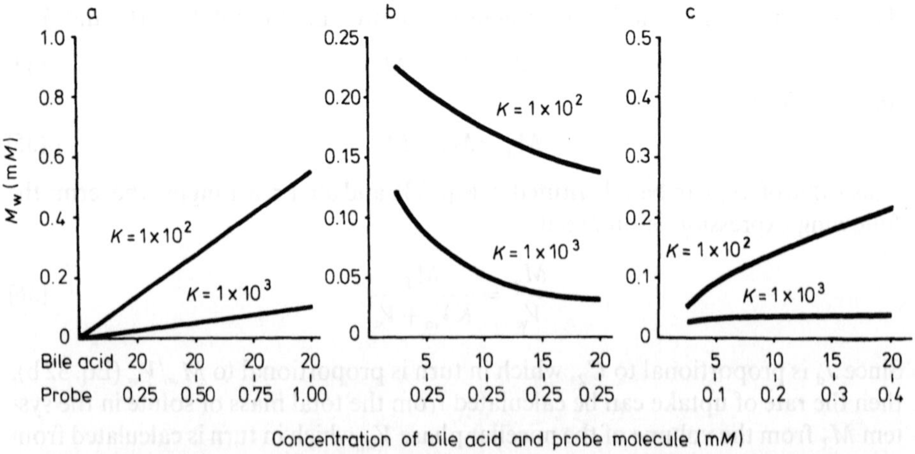

Fig. 11 a–c. Theoretical curves illustrating the manner in which the mass of a probe molecule in the water phase M_w varies under different experimental circumstances. M_w, as well as the mass in the lipid phase M_L, and therefore J_d should increase linearly when the concentration of the lipid probe molecule is increased while the concentration of the micellar solvent is kept constant; this was found to be the case for the probes C12:0, C16:0, and C18:0 (**a**). When the concentration of the bile acid is increased, but that of the lipid probe molecule is kept constant, there should be a reciprocal decrease in M_m, as was observed experimentally for C16:0 (**b**); if the second model were correct (lipid–protein phase), then there should be a curvilinear increase in M_L, which did not occur. This decrease in J_d with increasing concentration of bile acids may be explained by the decreased monomolecular concentration in equilibrium with the micelles, since the excess of micellar solution renders the micelles relatively unsaturated with lipid. For C18:0, M_w showed only a slight initial rise and then remained essentially constant (**c**), as predicted for uptake from an obligatory aqueous rather than lipid phase. Accurate partition coefficients K for the long-chain fatty acids are unknown, and these curves were generated using two values of K. The derivation of these curves is given in WESTERGAARD and DIETSCHY (1976)

is kept constant while that of the solute is increased, J_d increases in a linear relationship to the total concentration of the solute (Fig. 11 a). Two points warrant emphasis: first, the magnitude of J_d is markedly influenced by the value of K; and second, this relationship is compatible with either model, uptake from a lipid–lipid phase, or uptake from an aqueous–lipid phase.

In Fig. 11 b, the concentration of the solute is kept constant while the concentration of the detergent is increased. Note that experimentally the uptake of cholesterol solubilized with bile acids follows this shape: the rate of uptake declines in a curvilinear fashion. The actual shape of the curve depends upon the value of K; this model is consistent with uptake from an aqueous phase. Indeed, if uptake were from lipid–lipid phase (micelle to membrane), then J_d would increase as the concentration of the detergent is increased.

Further evidence for uptake from an aqueous phase is provided in Fig. 11 c, where the concentrations of both the solute and the detergent are increased in parallel (increased C_w and C_m, but C_m/C_w constant). The J_d initially increases, and then approaches a plateau. If uptake of solute were from micelle to membrane, then J_d would increase in a linear fashion as the concentrations of both detergent and solute were increased. Once again the shape of the curve depends upon the magnitude of K, but this type of experimental result clearly allows for separation between the different possible mechanisms of uptake from a carrier substance. In vitro experiments in animals have confirmed the shape of the curves shown in Figs. 11 a, b, c, and provide strong evidence for uptake of solute from the micelle into the membrane through an obligatory aqueous phase (WESTERGAARD and DIETSCHY 1976). Similar results have been obtained in different intestinal sites, animals of different ages, different species, in diabetic rats, as well as different in vitro techniques (THOMSON 1980 a, b, c; THOMSON et al. 1983).

It must therefore be emphasized that when the rate of uptake of a solute is measured from a solution which contains other molecules with which the solute can interact, such as in the case for cholesterol and bile acid micelles, then the observed rates of J_d may be determined both by the properties of the microvillus membrane, as well as by events which occur in the bulk phase. Unless the value of the partition coefficient K is known, or unless appropriate mathematical or experimental corrections can be made to establish C_2, then it will be impossible to determine the relative contribution to uptake of the interaction of the solute with the carrier, or with the membrane.

It must also be emphasized that simple inspection of the curve relating uptake to concentration does not by itself permit comment on the kinetic nature of the absorption process (infinite or finite number of carriers, i.e., passive or carrier-mediated transport). Recall that when the resistance of the UWL is high, the relationship between the concentration and uptake of an actively transported molecule such as D-glucose (see Fig. 5) may be linear, rather than curvilinear as expected for carrier-mediated absorption. On the other hand, a curvilinear relationship between solute concentration and uptake does not necessarily signify carrier-mediated transport. This arises from the fact that as solute accumulates in or is added to the cytosolic compartment, the concentration gradient responsible for passive uptake ($C_2 - C_3$) declines, and the relationship between J_d and C_2 will deviate from linearity. Furthermore, as shown in Fig. 11 c, the relationship between J_d and the total concentration of solute will superficially resemble a "saturable" kinetic curve, particularly if the value of K is low (WESTERGAARD and DIETSCHY 1976) or if the resistance of the UWL is high.

N. Effect of Membrane Polarity on Penetration of Passively Transported Molecules

The rate of diffusion of a solute through a membrane is influenced by the diffusion coefficient of the molecule in the membrane D_m and the thickness of the membrane itself d_m. Note that the value of D_m may vary from the value of the free diffusion coefficient of the solute D and that the value of d_m will be very much less than the effective thickness d of the UWL ($d \gg d_m$). The value of the passive permeability coefficient for the solute P is unique for each membrane and each solute, and is determined by the polar characteristics of both the solute and the membrane. We have previously considered the determination of the value of the membrane permeability coefficient from J_d, S_m, and C_2 (Eq. 23); in addition, the value of P for a particular solute can be described by the expression (DIAMOND and WRIGHT 1969a, b; LIEB and STEIN 1969, 1971; WRIGHT and BINDSLEV 1976)

$$P = {}^{\mathrm{m}}K\left(\frac{D_{\mathrm{m}}}{d_{\mathrm{m}}}\right), \tag{37}$$

where ${}^{\mathrm{m}}K$ represents the partition coefficient for the solute molecules between the aqueous phase adjacent to the membrane, and the lipid phase of the cell membrane; D_{m} represents the diffusion coefficient of the solute in the membrane; and d_{m} is the thickness of the membrane. The value of ${}^{\mathrm{m}}K$ may vary over a very wide range (DIAMOND and WRIGHT 1969a, b; WRIGHT and BINDSLEV 1976), whereas the values of d_{m} and D_{m} are likely to vary much less (DIETSCHY 1978b).

The recognition of the importance of the partition coefficient of the solute has underscored a useful way of assessing and comparing the "functional" polarity of membranes from different biologic systems, and determining the potential mechanisms responsible for changes in the permeability properties of the membrane. The relative polarity of the membrane may be assessed by comparing the natural logarithm of the passive permeability coefficient of a series of solutes, such as a homologous series of saturated fatty acids, with the natural logarithms of the partition coefficients of these same fatty acids into a variety of different bulk organic solvents (Fig. 12). If the values of P were obtained after appropriate correction for the effects of the UWL, then a close relationship between $\ln P$ and $\ln K$ suggests that the "effective" polarity of the solvent and the cell membrane must be approximately the same. Studies of this nature have been performed in a number of mammalian cell preparations, and most mammalian membranes are relatively polar structures, behaving more like the bulk solvent isobutanol, than very nonpolar solvents such as triglyceride, olive oil, or diethyl ether (DIAMOND and WRIGHT 1969a, b; SMULDERS and WRIGHT 1971).

An easier approach to the determination of the relative polarity of a membrane includes the determination of the manner in which the addition of a particular substituent group to a series of solute molecules alters the rate of movement of the solute across a given membrane (DIAMOND and WRIGHT 1969a, b; SHERRILL and DIETSCHY 1975; WRIGHT and BINDSLEV 1976). The relationship between the partitioning of a solute between the aqueous phase and the cell membrane, ${}^{\mathrm{m}}K$, and several thermodynamic parameters can be described by the following relationship

$${}^{\mathrm{m}}K = \exp(-\Delta F_{\mathrm{w}\to 1}/RT), \tag{38}$$

where $\Delta F_{\mathrm{w}\to 1}$ is the free energy change associated with the movement of 1 mol solute from the bulk phase to the membrane, R is the gas constant, and T is the absolute temperature. For a complete discussion and detailed consideration of the intermolecular forces that provide the thermodynamic explanation for the effect of various substituent groups or permeability and partition coefficients, the interested reader is directed to the work of DIAMOND and WRIGHT (1969a, b), and WRIGHT and BINDSLEV (1976). It is difficult to obtain absolute values of $\Delta F_{\mathrm{w}\to 1}$ for a solute, but the change in $\delta\Delta F_{\mathrm{w}\to 1}$, i.e., the incremental free energy change, brought about by the addition of the substituent group to the solute is given by

$$\delta\Delta F_{\mathrm{w}\to 1} = -RT \ln P^{+}/P^{0} \tag{39}$$

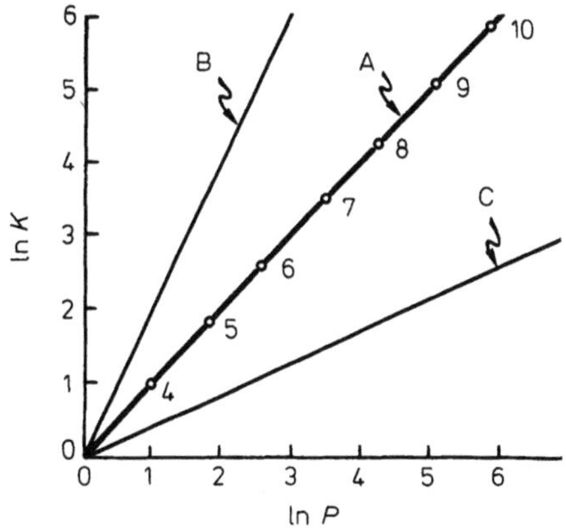

Fig. 12. Comparison of passive permeability coefficients *P* for a series of fatty acids with the partition coefficients of these same molecules between bulk buffer solution and bulk organic solvent. Logarithm of *K* is plotted in arbitrary units on the vertical axis; logarithm of *P* is shown on the horizontal axis. Line *A* represents the situation in which the polarity of the bulk solvent and membrane lipids is identical, line *B* represents the situation where the organic solvent is less polar, and line *C* represents the situation where the solvent is more polar than the membrane. The number beside each data point represents a fatty acid containing the number of carbon atoms noted. DIETSCHY (1978 a)

in which P^+ represents the membrane permeability coefficient for the solute with and P^0 represents the permeability coefficient for the solute without the substituent group. A similar formula may be used to calculate the value of the incremental free energy change based on measurements of the effect of this substituent group on the partitioning of the solute into a bulk phase. In general, the addition of a polar group such as hydroxyl (OH) increases the value of $\delta\Delta F_{w\rightarrow 1}$, and represents a reduction in the passive permeability of the membrane toward the solute; the addition of a nonpolar substituent group such methylene (CH_2) reduces the value of $\delta\Delta F_{w\rightarrow 1}$ (it becomes more negative), indicating a greater membrane permeability towards the probe molecule. The addition of a methylene group has an unexpectedly small effect on increasing the passive permeability coefficients, suggesting that membranes such as human erythrocytes, the gallbladder of rabbits, and the jejunum of rats, rabbits, guinea pig, hamsters, and humans behave as relatively polar structures (DIAMOND and KATZ 1974; SAVITZ and SOLOMON 1971; SHERRILL and DIETSCHY 1975; SMULDERS and WRIGHT 1971; THOMSON 1980 a, b, c, d; WESTERGAARD and DIETSCHY 1974 a).

This type of plot (see Fig. 4) has allowed for the full recognition that many biologic membranes behave as relatively polar structures. We must consider the implications of the interrelationship between membrane polarity and molecular aqueous solubility, the use of this type of plot to make certain interpretations of the possible membrane-related mechanisms responsible for variation in the rate of solute uptake, and finally we must examine possible explanation for the anomalous behavior of certain polar, low molecular weight solutes.

The maximal rates of monomolecular diffusion depend on the polarity of the cell membrane and the solubility of the probe molecule. Let us examine a specific

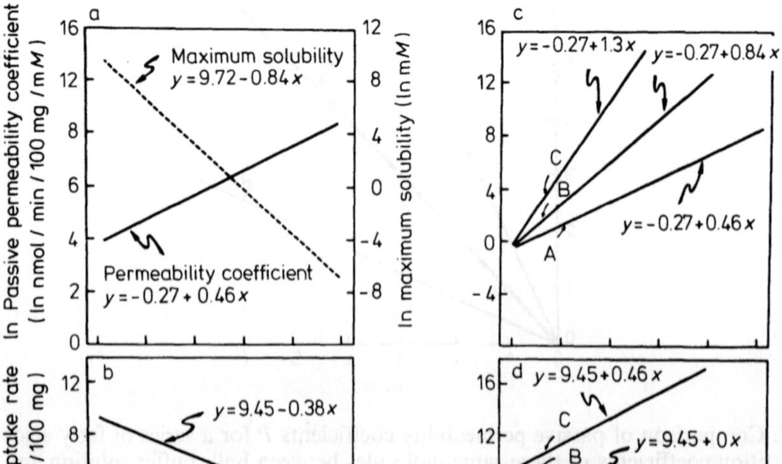

Fig. 13a–d. Effect of relative polarity of a solute molecule on its maximum rate of transmembrane movement. **a, b** actual experimental data obtained on uptake of fatty acids of various chain lengths into the intestinal mucosal cell (WESTERGAARD and DIETSCHY 1976). **a** logarithm of passive permeability coefficients and maximum aqueous solubilities of the homologous series of saturated fatty acids; **b** logarithm of the maximum uptake rate, which equals the passive permeability coefficient multiplied by the maximum sulobility for each individual fatty acid. **c, d** effect of altering polarity of the biologic membrane. Curves *A*, *B*, and *C* show theoretical results obtained where the membrane is made progressively less polar so that the addition of each CH_2 group to the fatty acid chain increases the passive permeability coefficient by a factor of 1.58 (*A*), 2.32 (*B*), and 3.67 (*C*). These values correspond to $\delta \Delta F_{w \to 1}$ values of −283, −517, and −801 cal/mol for the CH_2 group in these three situations. Results are based on experimental data in which the permeability coefficients and uptake rates were normalized to 100 mg dry weight of intestinal tissues. DIETSCHY (1978a, b)

set of data taken from the literature (WESTERGAARD and DIETSCHY 1974, 1976), and shown diagrammatically in Fig. 13. The passive permeability coefficients P_d were calculated from J_d/C_2, and the natural logarithm of P_d for a homologous series of saturated fatty acids was plotted against the number of carbon atoms in the fatty acid chain. The actual experimental line demonstrated some deviation at the shorter fatty acid chain lengths, and the line shown in Fig. 13 represents an extrapolation of the linear component of the experimental curve. The value of P_d increased by a factor of 1.58 (slope of the semilogarithmic plot of 0.46 shown in Fig. 13a, *full line*) for each methylene group added to the fatty acid chain. In the same study, the maximum solubility of each fatty acid decreased by a factor of 0.43 (slope of the semilogarithmic plot of −0.84, shown in Fig. 13a, *broken line*). The maximal rate of intestinal uptake of any passively absorbed probe molecule will be given by the product of its concentration in the perfusate and the passive permeability coefficient. The maximum rate of uptake will be limited by the maximal solubility of the probe. When the permeability coefficient for each fatty acid is multiplied by its maximum solubility, the maximum rate of uptake decreases by a factor of 0.68 (slope of the semilogarithmic plot of -0.38, Fig. 13b) for each CH_2 group added to the fatty acid chain. Thus, when the concentration of each fatty acid is elevated to the limit of its solubility, the highest relative rates of uptake are seen within the less polar probe molecules, and the relative rate of uptake declines with decreasing polarity and solubility.

Certain experimental manipulations may give rise to a greater passive permeability of the membrane (THOMSON 1980a, b, c, d). Under these circumstances, the value of $\delta\Delta F_{w\to 1}$ is decreased ($\delta\Delta F_{w\to 1}$ becomes more negative), signifying that the membrane has become less polar. With falling polarity of the membrane, the slope of the relationship between the logarithm of maximal uptake rate and fatty acid chain length will rise (Fig. 13d, curves B and C). In the special circumstance where the addition of a methylene group results in an exactly equal incremental increase in P and decrement in solubility (curve B), the maximal uptake rate will become independent of chain length. As the membrane becomes even less polar, the maximal uptake rate will actually begin to rise with decreasing solute polarity and solubility (curve C).

Most biologic membranes examined to date in this manner have been shown to be relatively polar, and this is certainly true for the intestine. Indeed, the polarity of the intestine may have been underestimated in the past (SALLEE 1979), making these considerations even more pertinent. Figure 14 demonstrates the manner in which the relative polarity and solubility of the probe molecule influence both the interaction between the solute and its detergent, and the relative influence of the UWL on relative rates of mucosal absorption. The *full line* illustrates the situation where there is no UWL, and it is clear (DIETSCHY 1978b; THOMSON 1978; WESTERGAARD and DIETSCHY 1974b) that the relative rate of mucosal absorption of the passively transported solute declines with decreasing polarity and solubility. For each group of lipids the term ϱ defines the degree to which the presence of bile acid micelles facilitates absorption. The value of ϱ is close to 1 for short- and medium-chain fatty acids, which signifies that bile acid micelles do not significantly enhance mucosal uptake of these compounds. It progressively increases, however, with long-chain saturated or unsaturated fatty acids and steroids so that the presence of bile acid significantly enhances the uptake of the fatty acids and becomes obligatory for the absorption of cholesterol (FERNANDES et al. 1962; PORTER et al. 1971; SALLEE 1979; SIPERSTEIN et al. 1952; TREADWELL and VAHOUNY 1968; WESTERGAARD and DIETSCHY 1976).

In the intestine, however, there is a UWL of significant dimensions, and the maximum uptake is reduced to the extent that this diffusion barrier exerts an additional resistance to the molecular uptake. Thus, under conditions of constant resistance of the UWL, uptake will vary as a function of both the passive permeability and free diffusion coefficients for the particular probe molecule, as well as a function of the maximum aqueous solute concentration and the membrane partition coefficient. Consequently, the maximum uptake observed in the presence of a UWL will be considerably less for the more hydrophobic, less polar mole-

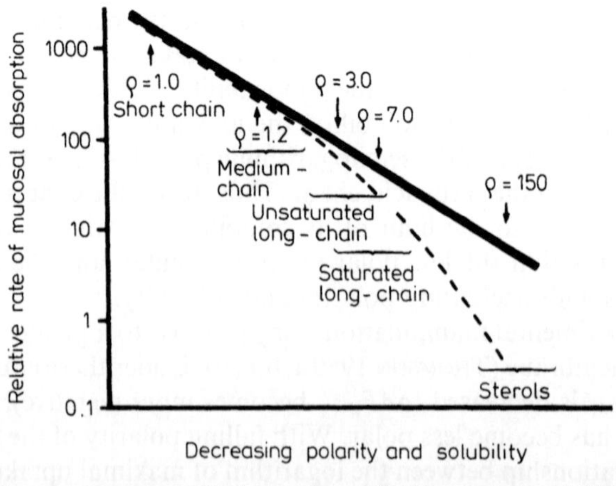

Fig. 14. The relative rates of mucosal absorption of lipid molecules of different polarity in the presence and absence of bile acid micelles. The *full line* shows the relative rate of intestinal mucosal cell uptake for compounds of differing polarity and solubility in the presence of bile acid micelles while the *broken line* shows the rates expected in the absence of bile acid. For each group of lipids the ratio ϱ defines the degree to which the presence of bile acid micelles facilitates absorption. The value of ϱ is close to unity for the short- and medium-chain fatty acids, i.e., bile acid micelles do not significantly enhance mucosal uptake of these compounds. The value of ϱ progressively increases, however, with fatty acids of longer chain length and sterols so that the presence of bile acid micelles significantly enhances the uptake of these particular compounds into the intestinal mucosal cell. WESTERGAARD and DIETSCHY (1974 b, 1976)

cules, than would be predicted if no UWL were present. Thus, in the presence of a UWL, the maximum rate of absorption will be described by a line below the theoretical line and the deviation between the theoretical and experimental lines (see Fig. 14, curve A versus curves B and C) represents a manifestation of the effect of the resistance of the UWL. The important point to make from this figure is the appreciation that the effect of the UWL will be quantitatively much less for polar molecules such as the short-chain fatty acids, but quantitatively very important for less polar molecules such as long-chain fatty acids and cholesterol.

O. Anomalous Behavior of Diffusion of Certain Solutes Across the Intestine

In Fig. 12 the incremental change in free energy $\delta\Delta F_{w\rightarrow 1}$ was calculated from the linear portion of the curve between fatty acids C 6:0 (hexanoic) to C 12:0 (lauric acid). When this linear component is extrapolated towards the short-chain fatty acids, it becomes clear that there are anomalously high permeability coefficients for the lower molecular weight, more polar solutes in the series, such as acetic and butyric acid (WESTERGAARD and DIETSCHY 1974 a). Similar results have been reported in a variety of other membranes, including those of the intestine, gallbladder, fat cell, and muscle cell (SALLEE and DIETSCHY 1973; SALLEE 1979; SHERRILL and DIETSCHY 1975; THOMSON 1980 a, b, c, d; WESTERGAARD and DIETSCHY 1974),

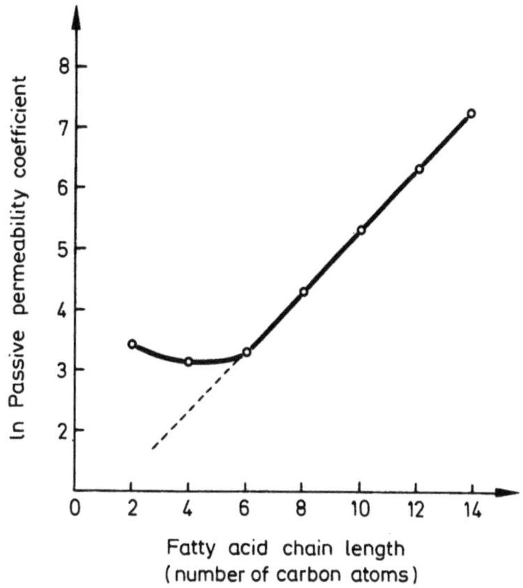

Fig. 15. Relationship of the passive permeability coefficient to the chain length of various saturated fatty acids. This diagram illustrates that the shorter, more polar members of this homologous series have higher passive permeability coefficients than would be expected from the linear extrapolation of the results obtained with fatty acids containing six or more carbon atoms. DIETSCHY (1978)

and for other low molecular weight molecules (DIAMOND and WRIGHT 1969a, b; NACCACHE and SHA'AFI 1973; SALLEE and DIETSCHY 1973; SHERRILL and DIETSCHY 1975; SMULDERS and WRIGHT 1971; WRIGHT and DIAMOND 1969a, b). The etiology of this unexpectedly higher uptake is unknown, and suggestions have included carrier-mediated diffusion, or the presence of "aqueous" pores. There is no firm data to support either of these suggestions (SALLEE 1979). It has recently been suggested that the anomalously high permeability coefficients may be due to an inherent property of the membrane (SALLEE 1979a, b; WRIGHT and BINDSLEV 1976), although this in itself is not a mechanistic explanation. If the short-chain fatty acids are absorbed from a different portion of the villus, or over a larger surface area, then perhaps the higher uptake may be explained on this basis (WINNE 1978). Furthermore, the observation that this higher uptake of short-chain fatty acids in the intestine is not observed with all in vitro preparations (THOMSON and O'BRIEN 1980) or in all species (THOMSON et al. 1983) raises the possibility that this may not necessarily be a universal phenomenon. Furthermore, when the chain length of the homologous series of saturated fatty acids is extended beyond 12 carbon atoms (SALLEE 1979), the slope of the line is even steeper. The solubilization of the long-chain fatty acid is achieved with bile acids, and such studies (SALLEE 1979) raise the possibility that the intestinal brush border membrane is even more nonpolar than previously appreciated. However, if the linear component of the curve between C 12:0 and C 18:0 is extrapolated, then the passive permeability coefficients of C 6:0–C 10:0 now appear to be anomalously high (Fig. 15). Therefore, it would appear that any consideration of the apparently anomalous behavior of the short-chain fatty acids must also include an explanation of the phenomenon of unexpectedly higher uptake of the medium-chain fatty acids.

P. Methods Available for the Measurement of the Dimensions of the Unstirred Water Layer

I. Effective Thickness of the Unstirred Water Layer

1. Change in Transmembrane Potential Difference

The method of DIAMOND (1966) was originally used to measure the effective thickness of the UWL in the rabbit gallbladder, and has been applied to the measurement of the effective thickness of the UWL of the intestine, both in vivo and in vitro. Briefly, the technique consists of measuring the change in the transmural PD caused when the mucosal surface of the membrane is suddenly exposed to a hypertonic solution. As solute diffuses from the well-stirred bulk solution through the unstirred layer, its concentration immediately adjacent to the gallbladder wall gradually builds up, and it is this "wall" concentration rather than the bulk concentration which is related to the development of the PD.

The effect in the case of streaming potentials is that water flow across a membrane separating solutions of identical ionic composition will concentrate the solution in the boundary layer on one side of the membrane and dilute the solution in the opposite boundary layer. The slow buildup of the streaming potential probably reflects the time required for the solute to reach its final concentration in the unstirred layer adjacent to the surface of the membrane. The time required to achieve half the new steady state PD, $t_{1/2}$, is a function of the thickness of the unstirred water layer d and the diffusivity of the molecule used to induce the change in potential difference D (Fig. 16). Thus, the thickness of the UWL can be calcu-

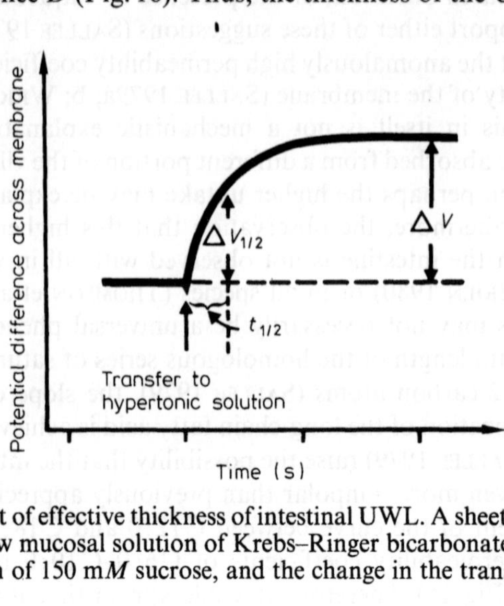

Fig. 16. Measurement of effective thickness of intestinal UWL. A sheet of intestine was rapidly transferred a new mucosal solution of Krebs–Ringer bicarbonate buffer made hypertonic by the addition of 150 mM sucrose, and the change in the transmural potential difference was recorded

lated from the formula derived by DIAMOND (1966) as well as from the work of CRANK (1957), DAINTY and HOUSE (1966 a), and OLSON and SCHULTZ (1942)

$$d = \left(\frac{Dt^{\frac{1}{2}}}{0.38}\right)^{\frac{1}{2}}. \tag{40}$$

In the derivation of this equation, DIAMOND (1966) emphasized that the applicability of this method for measurement of the functional thickness of the unstirred layer depends critically upon the validity of several assumptions with respect to the characteristics of this barrier in the intestine:

1. The properties of the UWL must not change with alterations in the composition of the bulk perfusate, i.e., the properties of the mucosal unstirred layer must be unaffected by the changes in osmolarity, salt concentration, and water flow occurring during the development of the electrical transients. This appears to be the case, since the estimated values of d were essentially constant under all circumstances tested (WESTERGAARD and DIETSCHY 1974 a).

2. The value of D for the probe molecule used to induce the change in PD must be essentially constant throughout the concentration range used. The small change in the value of D between infinite dilution and the hypertonic solutions used by several groups (READ et al. 1976, 1977; WESTERGAARD and DIETSCHY 1974 a) would not introduce a significant error into the calculation of d (SHERRILL et al. 1973). While it is probably true that the value of D in the UWL on the luminal side of the cell is similar to the free diffusion coefficient, this may not be the case in the cytosol and submucosal layers where diffusion through the muscle and connective tissue may be lower than in free solution.

3. Any permeability changes in the membrane induced by the buildup of the concentration of the probe molecule at the interface must occur very rapidly relative to the time course of the electrical transient. The fact that d measured under isotonic conditions from the electrical transient of the diffusion potential generated from a NaCl gradient was nearly the same as the values obtained with all the other probe molecules suggests that this condition was met in the intestine. It must be noted that in one in vivo assessment of the value of d in the human intestine (READ et al. 1977), there was a significant difference in the values of d estimated from osmotic and diffusion potentials. It must be challenged therefore whether this criteria has been adequately satisfied in this human perfusion study; nonetheless, these estimates of d likely represent an acceptable approximation of the effective thickness of the UWL.

4. The fourth assumption inherent in the derivation of Eq. (42) is that the probe molecule diffuses from the bulk solution up to a flat membrane, considered for practical purposes to be an infinite plane. This condition is not met when the intervillus spaces are open, but at least when using intestinal sheets in vitro after 30 min of incubation in Krebs–Ringer bicarbonate (KRB), the intervillus spaces are fully occluded (WESTERGAARD and DIETSCHY 1974 a). What are the lines of evidence to suggest that the intestinal mucosal surface could be considered as an essentially flat plane? As seen in Fig. 17 a, after only 5 min of incubation at 37 °C the unstirred layer had an apparent thickness d of 230 ± 18 µm at a stirring rate of 500 rpm. However, with more prolonged incubation in KRB, d became pro-

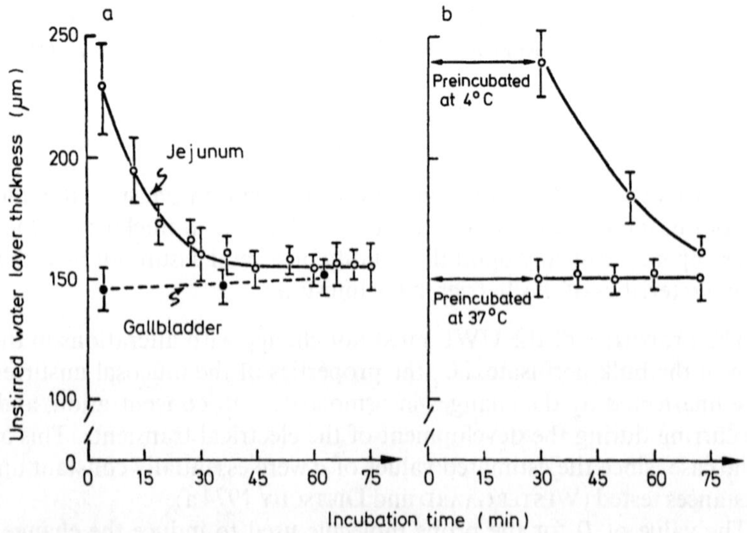

Fig. 17 a, b. The effect of duration of incubation on the effective thickness of the instirred layer, determined in rabbit jejunum and gallbladder incubated in Krebs–Ringer bicarbonate (KRB) buffer. In these studies, the effective thickness of the unstirred layer *d* was measured by rapidly transferring each tissue specimen from KRB buffer to buffer made hypertonic by the addition of 150 m*M* sucrose. The stirring rate of the bulk phase was 500 rpm. After the development of the electrical transient, (Fig. 16), $t_{1/2}$ was determined, and the tissue was returned to isotonic KRB buffer until the next measurement was made. **a** measurements of *d* repeated in jejunum and gallbladder incubated in KRB at 37 °C from the time the tissue was mounted in the chambers; **b** paired jejunal specimens from the same animal preincubated in KRB buffer at either 4° or 37 °C for 30 min, at which time the specimen preincubated at 4 °C was transferred to buffer at 37 °C. WESTERGAARD and DIETSCHY (1974 a)

gressively smaller until a constant value of approximately 155 µm was achieved at 30 min of incubation. This finding was in contrast to measurements made simultaneously in the rabbit gallbladder where, at the same stirring rate, *d* remained constant at about 150 µm throughout the period of observation. Furthermore, the morphology of the electrical transients was altered after 30 min of incubation (Fig. 18): the electrical transient rapidly reached a maximum value ($t_{1/2} = 9$ s) and remained constant thereafter. In contrast, in intestine incubated for only 5 min, the transient had an initial rapidly rising phase followed by a very prolonged linear upsweep until a constant steady state PD was finally achieved at about 5 min. Again, this contrasted with the findings in the gallbladder, where the electrical transients at any time during the incubation were of the type seen in intestine after 30 min of incubation (Fig. 17 a).

This gradual decrease in *d* seen during the incubation of the jejunum (Fig. 17 a) was very likely the result of obliteration of the deep components of the unstirred layer as the villi swelled, and was not related to other nonspecific effects of prolonged incubation, since unstirred layer thicknesses measured simultaneously in the gallbladder were unchanged throughout this period of observation. Gallblad-

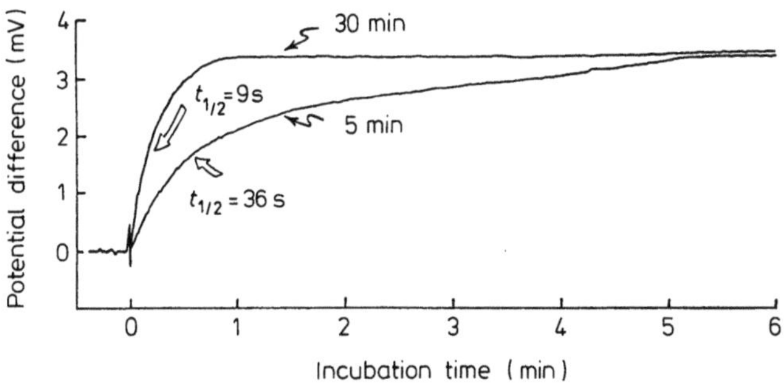

Fig. 18. The effect of preincubation for 5 or 30 min at 37 °C on the morphology of the electrical transients. As is apparent, the same maximum change in potential difference was achieved, but the two curves have markedly different $t_{1/2}$ values of 9 and 36 s. WESTERGAARD and DIETSCHY (1974)

der epithelium lacks villi: thus, in contrast to the situation in the intestine, even though submucosal edema developed in these specimens, essentially no change should occur in the dimensions of the overlying diffusion barrier. Furthermore, beyond 30 min of incubation, *d* approached a constant value essentially the same as that measured under the same conditions in the gallbladder (Fig. 17a). These findings suggested that some structural alterations might be taking place in the intestinal specimens during prolonged incubation in KRB, that indirectly were influencing the morphology of the unstirred layer. It was repeatedly demonstrated that after 5 min of incubation the central lacteals were barely visible and the individual villi were separated by wide intervillous spaces (WESTERGAARD and DIETSCHY 1974). After 30 min of incubation, however, the central lacteals were widely dilated, causing the villi to swell laterally and to obliterate the intervillous spaces. In this manner, the highly convulated jejunal mucosa was in essence transformed into an essentially flat surface similar in morphology to that of the gallbladder. This morphological change likely resulted from solute transport into the tightly clamped piece of intestine; when samples of jejunum were preincubated in KRB for 30 min at a stirring rate of 500 rpm at 4 °C, the intervillous spaces were open and *d* equalled approximately 240 μm (Fig. 17b). With continued incubation at 37 °C, *d* fell to 160 μm as histologic examination revealed progressive swelling of the villi (WESTERGAARD and DIETSCHY 1974a). These findings were consistent with the view that the value of *d* measured in intestine incubated at 37 °C for 30 min represented the effective thickness of a superficial layer of unstirred water overlying the upper villi, whereas the value measured in tissue incubated for only 5 min represented a mean value of a very complex unstirred layer, consisting of the superficial component plus a deep component interdigitated between the lateral surfaces of the villi.

A further line of evidence that the jejunum preincubated for 30 min could be considered to behave as a flat membrane is derived from the similarity between the effect of stirring on the values of *d* obtained in the intestine and gallbladder. The thickness of the diffusion barrier overlying jejunum preincubated for 30 min diminished in response to increased stirring of the bulk mucosal solution, as in

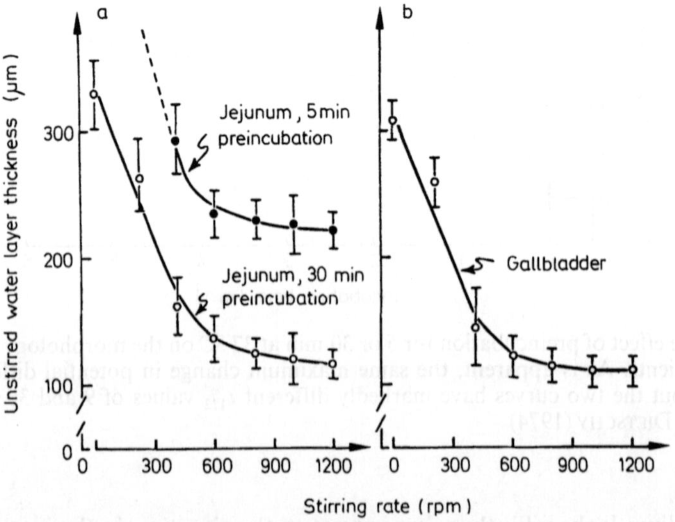

Fig. 19 a, b. The effect of the stirring rate of the bulk mucosal solution on the effective thickness of the unstirred layer. The effective thickness of the unstirred layer *d* was measured in the rabbit jejunum and gallbladder at stirring rates that varied from 0 to 1,200 rpm. **a** Values of *d* obtained in jejunum preincubated 5 or 30 min; **b** values of *d* obtained in the rabbit gallbladder. WESTERGAARD and DIETSCHY (1974 a)

the gallbladder (Fig. 19 a). This was true in terms of both the profile of the curves relating *d* to stirring rate and the absolute values of *d* at any particular rate of mixing. In contrast, in specimens incubated 5 min and subjected to stirring rate of less than 400 rpm, so much time was required to reach a new steady state potential difference that accurate values of $t_{1/2}$ could not be obtained (Fig. 19 a). At higher stirring rates, however, the apparent mean thickness of the total unstirred layer decreased from approximately 300 to 200 µm. In the jejunal samples preincubated for 30 min, *d* was 334 µm in the unstirred condition, and this value decreased in a nearly linear fashion to 160 µm as the stirring rate was increased to 400 rpm; at higher rates of mixing, however, *d* approached an essentially constant value of approximately 110 µm. Therefore, it is concluded that the intestinal membrane, under the very special condition of preincubation for 30 min in vitro, resembles an infinite plane, and it is valid to apply the method of DIAMOND (1966) to the measurement of the effective thickness of the intestinal UWL. Such a rigid validation of Diamond's technique has not always been possible to achieve (READ et al. 1976, 1977). WINNE (1976) has suggested that in most intestinal preparations the application of Diamond's equation derived for planar surfaces may lead to the underestimation of the thickness of the UWL in the intestine by as much as 28%. This error may not be important in the assessment of rates of uptake of those probe molecules such as medium-chain fatty acids and hexoses (WESTERGAARD and DIETSCHY 1974 a; KINTER and WILSON 1965) which are absorbed predominantly from the tips of the villi.

2. Equilibration of Nonabsorbable Probe

The effective thickness of the UWL may also be estimated from the $t_{1/}{}^{2}$ required for equilibration of a nonabsorbable marker in the adherent mucosal fluid volume. With knowledge of the value of the free diffusion coefficient D of the nonabsorbable probe molecule, it is possible to calculate the value of d from Eq. (40). The same assumptions are of course inherent in this technique as in the method of estimating d from the $t_{1/2}$ required for the generation of electrical transients. This method is of limited application in vivo because it is during the early mixing period required to achieve steady state conditions that distribution of a nonabsorbable marker occurs in this space.

3. Varying Rate of Intestinal Perfusion

The relative change in the effective thickness of the UWL can be estimated from the effect of varying the rate of intestinal perfusion on the rate of disappearance of a probe molecule from the intestinal lumen (WINNE 1976)

$$\Delta d = d_1 - d_2 = C_1 D S_w \left(\frac{1}{J d_1} - \frac{1}{J d_2} \right). \tag{41}$$

Where Δd is the change in the effective thickness of the unstirred layer, d_1 and D_2 are the values of the thickness of the UWL at two rates of perfusion which give rise to two different rates of uptake, J_1 and J_2. Using this maneuver, WINNE (1976) has estimated the change in the effective thickness of the UWL in the rat jejunum perfused at different rates to be about 530 µm. This value represents the lower limit of d in this experimental setting since the mixing of the solution in the lumen by air bubbles is presumably not complete and does not reach into the intervillous spaces. WINNE estimated tha value of S_w from the outer circumference of the intestine multiplied by the length of the loop; this gives the area of the cylinder touching the tops of the villi. This area was considered the average area of the UWL in vitro; the same approach to measure S_w was used by WILSON and DIETSCHY (1974). However, Eq. (43) requires a measurement of S_w, and the granting of the assumption that the value of S_w does not itself change with varying rates of perfusion. In vitro studies have suggested that the value of S_w increases 4-fold as the dimension of d declines 12-fold (WESTERGAARD and DIETSCHY 1974a). Thus, this formulation leads to an underestimation of the value of Δd, and Eq. (41) must be rewritten to take into account the changes in S_w at different rates of perfusion

$$\Delta R_e = R_1 - R_2 = (C_1 - C_2)(1/J_1 - 1/J_2)\,, \tag{42}$$

where ΔR_e represents the change in the effective resistance of the UWL ($R_e = d/S_w D$), R_1 and R_2 are the values of the effective resistance of the UWL corresponding to the two rates of uptake, J_1 and J_2. While this formulation does not provide a quantitative assessment of the components of $R_e(d, S_w, D)$, it does provide an assessment of the resistance of the diffusion barrier which takes into account the different rates of change of d and S_w at varying rates of intestinal perfusion. This formulation is most useful for the application of values of R_e under conditions where the UWL rather than the membrane limit uptake ($P \gg DS_w/d$) or $V_m/K_m \gg DS_w/d$), since under these conditions $C_1 - C_1 \rightarrow C_1$, and the values D, C_1, J_1, and J_2 are known.

4. Direct Visual Observation

The unstirred layer of fluid bounding the outer surface of the rabbit cornea fitted with a contact lens has been directly measured using a pachymeter and polystyrene latex spheres. With the bulk solution unstirred the layer was 350 μm thick on the cornea and 150 μm thick on the contact lens. Following vigorous stirring, the layer was reduced to 65 μm on the cornea and to less than 20 μm on the contact lens (GREEN and OTORI 1970).

The permeability coefficient of any substance is dependent upon the rate of stirring of the ambient solution (DAINTY and HOPE 1959a, b; DAINTY and HOUSE 1966a–c). As stirring is increased, the magnitude of the apparent permeability coefficient rises until additional stirring does not facilitate a more rapid transfer of the probe. This phenomenon has been explained by the presence of a layer adherent to the membrane which is both stagnant and of considerable thickness. The damaged cornea swells, and during this rapid swelling there was rapid uptake of water into the tissue and the value of d fell. Thus, any net movement of water into or across the tissue appears to reduce the UWL at the surface from which the water is flowing (GREEN and OTORI 1970). Why is d less for contact lens than for cornea? Is this related to the relative smoothness of the artificial compared with the biologic membrane? The answer is not forthcoming, nor is it known why there are differences in the value of d in different membranes.

5. Rate of Uptake of Diffusion-Limited Molecules

As discussed in Sect. P.II, the value of d/S_w may be calculated from the permeability coefficient of a highly permeant solution (WILSON and DIETSCHY 1974; WESTERGAARD and DIETSCHY 1974a, VAN OS and SLEGERS 1973).

6. Examples of Thickness of Unstirred Layers in Various Tissues

Table 2 shows the values of d obtained in a variety of tissues. For isolated cells such as erythrocytes, d is small, and indeed in isolated intestinal mucosal cells no unstirred layer effect can be demonstrated (WILSON and TREANOR 1975). The values of d in everted sacs tend to be lower than in sheets of intestine, but it is apparent that varying the stirring rate did not necessarily cause a proportionate or reproducible change in the thickness of the aqueous diffusion barrier, since the everted segments would commonly occupy different positions in the vortex of the stirred bulk solution. In addition, in order to measure the mean thickness of the unstirred layer, it was necessary to fix the intestinal segments at the end of a catheter so that these pieces of tissue were subjected to different shearing forces than those in which tissue uptake was determined – a situation which might introduce significant errors into the calculation of UWL effects.

Table 2. Measurements of thickness of unstirred layers in the intestine and other membrane preparations

Membrane		Preparation	Species	Thickness of UWL (µm)	Stirring	Reference
1. Intestine,	in vitro	Everted jejunal sac	Rat	180–220	1,800 rpm	Wilson and Dietschy (1972, 1974)
		Everted jejunal sac	Control rat	213	Unstirred	Hoyumpa et al. (1976)
				159	Vigorous	
			Thiamine deficient rat	198–217	Unstirred	
				141–159	Vigorous	
		Everted jejunal sac	Rat	160	Vigorous	Jackson et al. (1978)
		Ileal sac		150		
		Jejunal sheet	Rabbit	330	Unstirred	Westergaard and Dietschy (1974a)
				110	800 rpm	
				150	500 rpm	Lukie et al. (1974)
	in vivo	Jejunum	Rat	530	Bubbling	Winne (1976) Debman and Levin (1975b)
				410–420		
		Jejunum	Human, control	632		Read et al. (1976, 1977)
			Human, untreated sprue	442		
2. Gallbladder,	in vitro	Sheets, mucosa	Rabbit	113		Diamond (1966)
		Serosa		300		
		Sacs, serosa	Rabbit	875		Smulders and Wright (1971) Wright et al. (1972)
3. Choroid plexus		Ventricular side	Frog	330		Wright and Prather (1970)
4. Eye		Cornea	Rabbit	350		Green and Otori (1970)
		Contact lens		150		
5. Isolated cells		Erythrocyte		5–10		Miller (1972); Sha'afi et al. (1967)

Table 2 (continued)

Membrane	Preparation	Species	Thickness of UWL (μm)	Stirring	Reference
6. Skin	Outer surface	Frog	40– 60	120 rpm	DAINTY and HOUSE (1966a, b)
			30– 50	300 rpm	
			30– 40	500 rpm	
	Inner surface		150–230	120 rpm	
			120–200	300 rpm	
			100–170	500 rpm	
7. Urinary bladder		Toad	200	Stirred	WRIGHT and PIETRAS (1974)
8. Artificial lipid bilayer			100–120		ANDREOLI et al. (1969); BECK and SCHULTZ (1972); CASS and FINKELSTEIN (1967); GUTKNECHT and TOSTESON (1973)

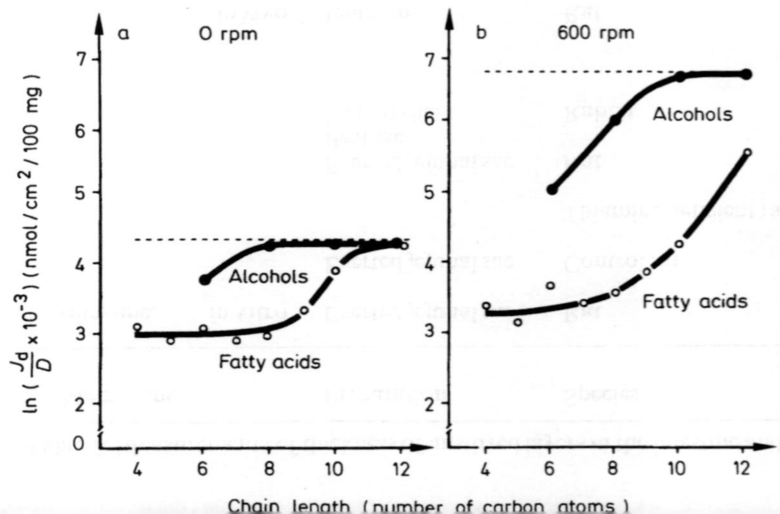

Fig. 20a, b. The relationship between the rates of uptake of a homologous series of fatty acids and alcohols and the number of carbon atoms in each compound. The logarithm of the quantity $(J_d/D)\times 10^{-3}$ determined for a series of fatty acids and alcohols is plotted as a function of the chain length of each compound; data in **(a)** the unstirred and **(b)** stirred (600 rpm) situations, respectively. In addition, the two limiting values have been calculated which denote the maximum rates of passive uptake at the two stirring rates that any compound can achieve: at these rates the UWL becomes absolutely rate limiting to absorption. WESTERGAARD and DIETSCHY (1974a)

II. Effective Surface Area of the Unstirred Water Layer

The next major problem of importance is to arrive at values of the effective surface area S_w of the UWL. In the special circumstance where J_d is measured for a probe molecule whose uptake is totally limited by the UWL, then C_2 becomes essentially equal to zero ($C_1 - C_2 \rightarrow C_1$) and the C_2 term can be deleted from the equation. Hence

$$S_w = \frac{J_d d}{C_1 D}. \tag{43}$$

This equation, then, allows for the calculation of S_w in terms of the known quantities, J_d, d, C_1, and D. Experimentally (Fig. 20) it has been shown that decanol and dodecanol are probe molecules that penetrate the microvillus membrane very much faster than they move across the UWL (i.e., $P \gg D/d$). J_d of decanol was then measured at a variety of stirring rates, and these values of J_d were plotted against the mean value of d for the superficial unstirred layer appropriate for the degree of stirring at which each uptake rate was measured. As shown in Fig. 21, there was an exponential decrease in J_d of decanol as d increased.

Now, if the effective surface area of the UWL remained constant at all stirring rates, then the uptake of decanol should vary in an inverse linear manner with d (Fig. 21). It is apparent, however, that the experimentally determined values progressively deviated from the theoretical values as the stirring rate was increased and the effective thickness of the unstirred layer decreased (Figs. 21 and 22). This indicates that both S_w and d vary with the rate of stirring. When the rate of stirring of the bulk phase was increased there was an exponential decline in the mag-

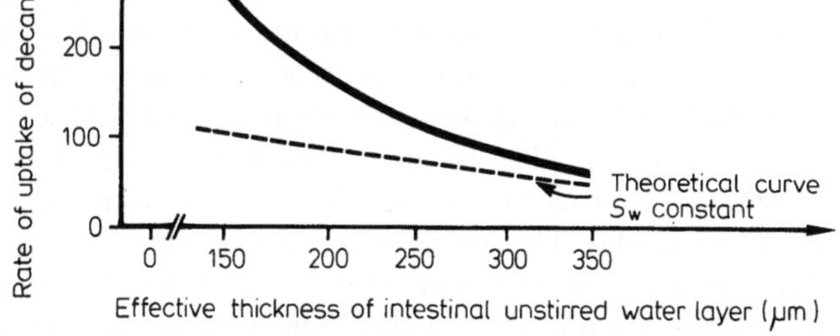

Fig. 21. The effect of varying the effective thickness of the unstirred layer on the rate of uptake of decanol into the jejunum. The bulk phase was stirred at 0–800 rpm to vary the effective thickness of the unstirred layer d. The rate of uptake of decanol J_d was plotted against the d value appropriate for each particular rate of stirring. The *broken line* shows the theoretical values of J_d as a function of d, if the effective surface area of the unstirred layer S_w remained constant at all degrees of stirring. As shown in Fig. 22b, the values of S_w varied with different rates of stirring of the bulk phase

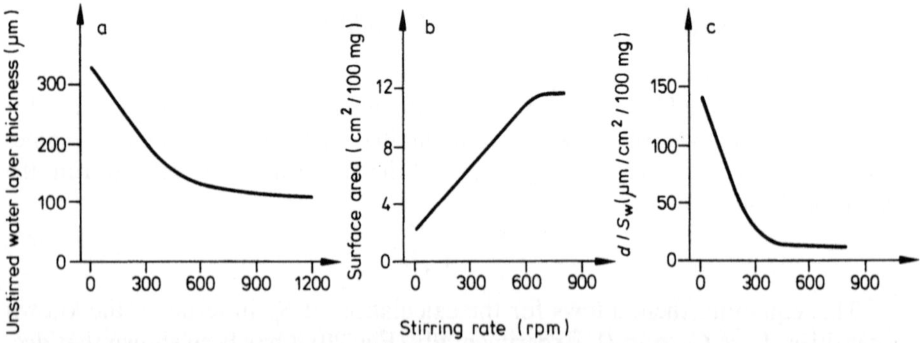

Fig. 22 a–c. The effect of the rate of stirring of the bulk mucosal solution on the effective thickness, effective surface area, and effective resistance of the intestinal UWL. The rate of stirring of the bulk phase was varied from 0 to over 800 rpm, and the values of d, S_w, and d/S_w were plotted as a function of the rate of stirring. **a** Effect of varying the rate of stirring on the values of d; **b** effect of changing the rate of stirring on the values of S_w; **c** effect of varying the rate of stirring of the bulk mucosal solution on the value of d/S_w. In order to calculate the effective resistance of the UWL, d/S_w must be divided by the value of D of the probe molecule

nitude of d (Fig. 22a). In contrast, the effective surface area of the UWL increased as a linear function of stirring rate between 0 and 500 rpm, and achieved a plateau only at 600 rpm and beyond (Fig. 22b). When the bulk phase was unstirred, the resistance of the UWL was higher. As the rate of stirring of the bulk phase was increased, there was an initial abrupt decline in the value of d/S_w (Fig. 22c). Increasing the rate of stirring of the bulk phase from 0 to 300 rpm was associated with an almost tenfold reduction in d/S_w, but further stirring between 400 and 800 rpm was associated with only a further 10% decline.

As a molecule is passively absorbed from the bulk aqueous solution of the intestinal contents into the cytosol of the mucosal cell, it must cross two major diffusion barriers: the UWL external to the cell and the protein–lipid membrane of the microvilli. The first surface area encountered by the probe molecule then is S_w, the effective surface area of the UWL, and it is only after passage through this major diffusion barrier that the prove encounters the much greater surface area of the membrane, S_m. The minimum value of S_w occurs when the UWL resistance is high (0 rpm), but even vigorous stirring of the bulk phase increases the value of S_w only fivefold (Fig. 22b). In the unstirred condition, the estimates of the value of S_w (Table 3) approach the value of the serosal surface area (2.4 versus 3.2 cm^2/100 mg, respectively). This value of the serosal area is equivalent to the minimum surface area of the intestinal membrane if there were no villi or microvilli present on the minimum flat surface area overlying the villus tips. Using the method of FISHER and PARSONS (1950), it can be calculated that the villi increase the mucosal surface area by a factor of over 24, and the microvilli increase this by a further factor of 20–40 (BROWN 1962; PALAY and KARLIN 1959). Thus, when the resistance of the UWL was high, S_w and the minimum membrane surface area given by the villus tips were almost identical. With thinning of the UWL, S_w increased to fe fourfold greater than the area of the villus tips, but only 15%

Table 3. Dimensions of the surface area of the barriers to diffusion in the intestine

	S_w or S_m (cm^2/100 mg)
1. Unstirred water layer	
High resistance (0 rpm)	2.4
Low resistance (800 rpm)	11.3
2. Intestinal membrane	
Serosal surface area	3.2
Villus surface area	79
Microvillus surface area	1,894

of the villus surface area, and less than 1% of the microvillus surface area (Table 3).

The estimation of the passive permeability coefficient of a probe molecule towards a given membrane may be calculated from the values of the unidirectional flux rate J_d and the concentration of the probe molecule at the aqueous–membrane interface (Eq. 23 b). In order to obtain values of the passive permeability coefficient normalized to the area of the microvillus membrane, a value for S_m is required (Eq. 23 a). However, there are several words of caution. The calculation of values of P from P_d and S_m assumes that all of the microvillus membrane participates in the absorptive process. As emphasized by WINNE (1978), different probes may use different areas of the villus. For the more permeant probes, such as dodecanol, most of the uptake would occur from the villus tips; indeed there is experimental evidence to suggest that this is in fact the case (WESTERGAARD and DIETSCHY 1974 a). In this instance the value of S_m would be much smaller; indeed, for these highly permeant probes $S_m \rightarrow S_w$, and the calculated values of $P(P=P_d/S_m)$ would represent minimum values.

There is a second area of caution necessary in calculating values of $P_d(P_d=J_d/C_2)$. The values of d and S_w apply to the specific situation where $P \gg D/d$ and $C_1-C_2 \rightarrow C$. It does not necessarily follow, however, that these values are appropriate for molecules whose uptake is primarily membrane limited such as is the case for the short-chain fatty acids. In this case $P \ll D/d$, the difference between C_1 and C_2 will be small, and the value of S_w may be different from those shown in Table 3. The resistance of the UWL depends upon the value of d/S_w. If a larger surface area of the UWL (and therefore of the membrane) is involved in the absorption of these less permeant compounds, then it is likely that the mean value of d would also increase as the molecules move further down the villus (see Figs. 1 and 10). Indeed, if the value of d/S_w is doubled for these less permeant probes, $\ln J_d/D$ will not be linear with respect to chain length, but rather the curve will turn sharply upward, indicating an inappropriate overcorrection for chain length. On the other hand, if the value of d/S_w is halved from the values used in Fig. 22, the calculated permeability coefficients P_d are reduced only slightly. Thus, there is some uncertainty as to the values of d and S_w that are appropriate for passively absorbed molecules of low permeability. Furthermore, the calculation of P

requires knowledge of S_m, and this potential error may be further magnified because S_w/S_m may vary for different probes, and a change in S_m/S_w would profoundly influence estimates of P. Therefore, while the estimation of P may be reasonably ascertained when uptake is largely from the tips of the villi, the situation is much less clear for less permeant molecules, for which the estimates of P may be significantly in error.

Q. Examples of the Effect of Unstirred Water Layers on Intestinal Transport

The recognition that the diffusion barriers outside of the cell rather than the cell membrane may be rate limiting to the uptake of various solute molecules has important implications with respect to a number of passive and active transport processes; several examples follow.

I. Estimates of the Temperature Coefficient

The passive monomolecular diffusion of a solute across a biologic membrane has been assumed to have a low temperature coefficient and a correspondingly low activation energy. In some instances an abrupt change in activation energy has been found when the temperature is lowered. Figure 23 shows a diagrammatic representation of the effect of diffusion barriers on the apparent "transition temperatures" and activation energies for solute molecules with various permeability coefficients. In this figure the natural logarithm of the apparent permeability coefficient has been plotted against the reciprocal of the absolute temperature. For a molecule with a low passive permeability coefficient a linear relationship is obtained between $\ln P^*$ and $1/T$ (Fig. 23a, curve A). For a solute which more readily penetrates the membrane, the curve has two components: at high temperatures the slope of the line is shallow (Fig. 23a, curve D, part y). As the temperature is lowered, a "transition" point is reached below which the line acquires a steeper slope that corresponds to a larger temperature coefficient and a higher activation energy (Fig. 23a, curve D, part x). When such a curve is corrected for unstirred layer effects (Fig. 23b, curve B), the transition point largely disappears and a single linear regression curve is produced that has a steep slope over the entire curve (BINDSLEV and WRIGHT 1976; WRIGHT and BINDSLEV 1976).

It warrants emphasis therefore that the demonstration of an inflection depends in part upon the passive permeability coefficient of the solute, and in part on the effective resistance of the UWL, and raises the question whether the apparent transition points reported for passive solute uptake across biologic membranes might be partially a function of the UWL: thus the low temperature coefficient simply reflects the low activation energy for the diffusion of the solute through the aqueous environment of the UWL. As the temperature is decreased, a point is reached at which penetration through the cell membrane, rather than through the diffusion barrier, becomes rate limiting and the apparent activation energy increases. Thus, it is possible that the breaks in the Arrhenius plot which

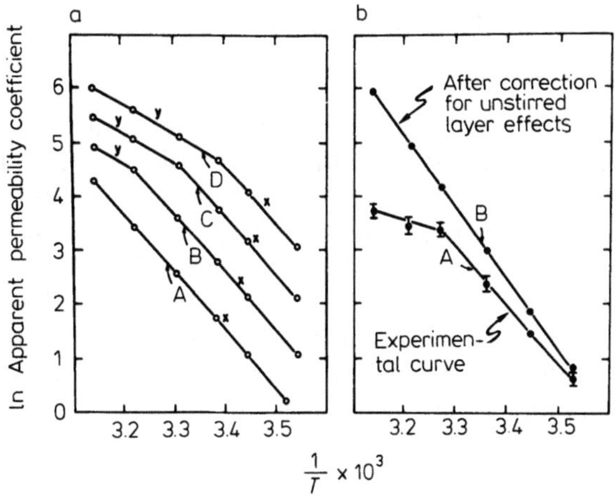

Fig. 23. a Diagrammatic representation of the effect of diffusion barriers on apparent "transition temperatures" and on activation energies for solute molecules with various permeability coefficients. Logarithm of the apparent permeability coefficient P^* plotted against the reciprocal of the absolute temperature. Results that might be obtained with four different solute molecules that penetrate a biologic membrane at different rates. Curve *A* represents a molecule with the lowest passive permeability coefficient; curve *D* represent a molecule with a much higher *P* value. In this diagram, the segment of each curve labeled *x* has a relatively steep slope and therefore yields a high value for the activation energy; the segments labeled *y* have lower slopes and correspondingly lower values for activation energies. These theoretical relationships are based on actual experimental data. DIETSCHY (1978). **b** The effect of pH and the UWL on the permeation rate of a weak acid. The permeation rate of a weak electrolyte is plotted against the bulk phase pH. When the effective resistance of the unstirred layer is low, a sigmoid curve is obtained and the inflection point of the pH absorption curve is situated at the pH value equal to the pK_a of the permeating substance. With increasing effective resistance of the unstirred layer, the rate of uptake declines and the inflection point is shifted, to the right for a weak acid and to the left for a weak base. Curve *A* shows the theoretical predictions, and curve *B* shows experimental data for the effect of varying the rate of stirring of the bulk phase on the permeation of phenylbutazone through a polydimethylsiloxane membrane. WINNE (1977)

occur in tissues with a large UWL actually correspond to the point where the major resistance to molecular uptake of the solute shifts from the UWL to the cell membrane (BINDSLEV and WRIGHT 1976). For solutes with a low value of *P* ($P \ll D/d$), the rate of uptake will be limited by the membrane, and there will be little unstirred layer effect. Note also that there is no apparent transition point. But, when the solute readily penetrates the membrane ($P \gg D/d$), then the unstirred layer may become rate limiting to uptake, and it is in this instance that the curve deviates from linearity. Other authors (DIETSCHY 1978a, b; BINDSLEV and WRIGHT 1976) have even questioned whether the low activation energies previously reported for such processes simply reflect failure to make appropriate corrections for unstirred layer effects. Furthermore, it must be asked whether the transition point is an artifact, resulting from the failure to correct for the UWL, rather than representing a phase transition in the lipid structure of the cell membrane.

II. Estimates of Kinetic Constants of Carrier-Mediated Transport

1. Theoretical Considerations

The use and limitation of the other so-called linear transformations of the Michaelis–Menten equation have recently been considered in detail. Let us first examine the limitations of the Eadie–Hofstee plot to estimate kinetic parameters of intestinal transport in the presence of UWL. A series of curves was produced by substituting biologically relevant values for each of the variables in Eq. (16). These values of J_d at different values of C_1 were then plotted according to the Eadie–Hofstee derivation of the Michaelis–Menten equation. In this manner it is possible to illustrate the way in which variation in each variable influences the estimate of the magnitude of the kinetic constants K_m and J_d^m from the plot of J_d vs J_d/C.

a) Varying the Effective Resistance of the Unstirred Water Layer

When the effective resistance of the unstirred layer is zero, there is a linear relationship between J_d and J_d/C_1 (Fig. 24, curve A). In this example, the slope is -1, which represents the assigned value of the K_m of 1 mM. As the resistance of the unstirred layer is increased, the relationship between J_d and J_d/C_1 deviates from the ideal linear relationship. The curvilinearity is produced regardless of the manner by which the magnitude of the resistance of the unstirred layer is increased: by increasing the effective thickness of the unstirred layer, by decreasing the effective surface area of the unstirred layer, or by decreasing the value of the free diffusion coefficient. Since this relationship is curvilinear over a wide range of values of J_d/C_1, and therefore of C_1, it is not possible to identify a linear portion from which extrapolation of the y-axis would be possible. Therefore, this plot has little use in the identification of the maximal transport rate, even when the resistance of the unstirred layer is low.

Using the Eadie–Hofstee plot, the magnitude of the Michaelis constant K_m is normally derived from the slope of J_d versus J_d/C_1. Clearly, this is not possible in the presence of an unstirred layer because of the curvilinearity of the relationship (Fig. 24). When the resistance of the unstirred layer is zero, $J_d = J_d^m/2$ when $C_2 = K_m$. As the resistance is varied, $J_d = J_d^m/2$ when J_d/C_1 approaches J_d/K_m. Thus, an estimate of the magnitude of the deviation of the apparent affinity constant K_m^* from the true Michaelis constant K_m can be approximated from the difference between the value of J_d/C_1 at $J_d = J_d^m/2$ when the effective resistance of the unstirred layer is zero, compared with the corresponding value of J_d/C_1 at different magnitudes of unstirred layer resistance. These values of $(J_d/C_1) - (J_d/C_1)^*$ are derived from Fig. 24 and are shown in Fig. 25 as a function of the effective resistance of the unstirred layer. It must be stressed that since the relationship between J_d and J_d/C_1 is linear only under the special condition of zero unstirred layer resistance (Fig. 24, curve A), the K_m cannot be estimated from this plot when UWL resistance is greater than zero. For this reason, the K_m^* of curves B–H, Fig. 22 cannot be determined. The value $(J_d/C_1) - (J_d/C_1)^*$ at $J_d/2$ simply reflects the deviation of the value of J_d/C_1 for curves B–H at $J_d^m/2$ from the value of J_d/C_1 for zero UWL resistance, and as such indirectly reflects the deviation between the true and apparent values of the Michaelis constant. When the resistance ap-

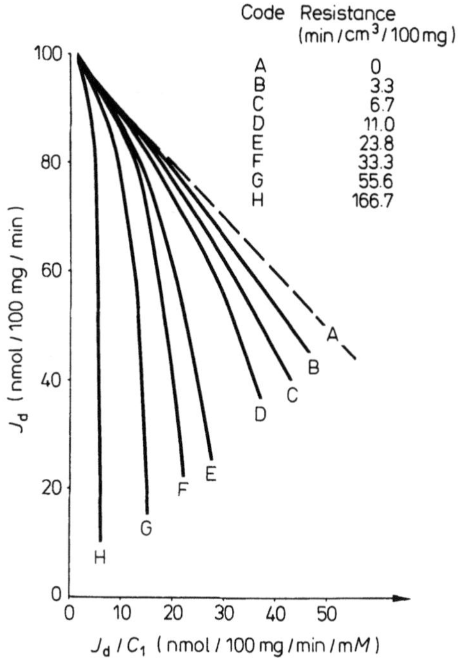

Fig. 24. Estimation of affinity constant K_m and maximal transport rate J_d^m from the relationship between J_d and J_d/C_1, derived from the Michaelis-Menten equation. J_d is the unidirectional flux rate, and C_1 is the concentration of the probe molecule in the bulk phase. Extrapolation of this linear relationship to the y-axis gives the value of the maximal transport rate J_d^m and extrapolation to the x-axis gives the value J_d^m/K_m, where K_m is the true Michaelis affinity constant. The slope has the value $-K_m$. The *broken line* in this figure represents the relationship between J_d and J_d/C_1 when the effective resistance of the UWL is zero. This diagram illustrates the manner in which the kinetics of carrier-mediated intestinal transport are altered by changes in the effective resistance of the UWL from 3.3 to 166.7 min 100 mg/cm^3; the different values for the resistance were obtained by changing the effective thickness of the UWL d from 10^{-2} to 10^{-1} cm, by varying the effective surface area of the UWL S_w from 1 to 10 cm^3/100 mg, and by altering the free diffusion coefficient of the probe molecule D from 10^{-4} to 5×10^{-4} cm^2/min. In these calculations, J_d^m was 100 nmol/100 mg/min, and K_m was 1 mM. These assigned values for J_d^m, K_m, d, S_w, and D were substituted into a newly derived equation (Thomson and Dietschy 1977) describing intestinal carrier-mediated transport in the presence of a UWL. Thomson (1979a)

proaches zero (Fig. 25), K_m^* equals K_m and the value of K_m can accurately be determined from the slope of the relationship between J_d and J_d/C_1. With increasing values of unstirred layer resistance the deviation between (J_d/C_1) and $(J_d/C_1)^*$ increases markedly. For a given change in the value of the resistance, the deviation is greater for lower rather than for higher magnitudes of resistance. Thus, it would be anticipated that the experimental demonstration of variations in K_m^* under conditions selected to yield different values of unstirred layer resistance would be easier to demonstrate when the resistance was initially relatively low, rather than high. The failure of a given experimental manipulation to produce a change in K_m^* may be due to the presence of a very high unstirred layer resistance: the manipu-

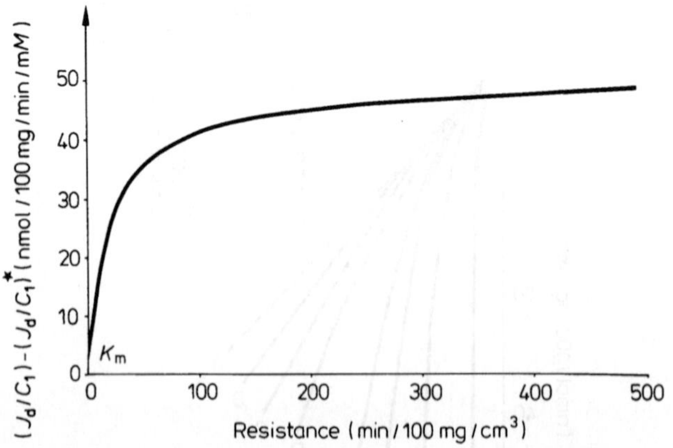

Fig. 25. Theoretical relationship between the effective resistance of the intestinal and the deviation of J_d/C_1 (when the resistance of the unstirred layer was zero) from the value of $(J_d/C_1)^*$ at $J_d^m/2$ at different values of unstirred layer resistance. The effective resistance of the UWL was varied by altering the values of each variable (d, S_w, and D). K_m is estimated from the slope of the relationship between J_d and J_d/C_1 (THOMSON 1979c). Thus, when $J_d = J_d^m/2$, $J_d/C_1 = J_d/K_m$. For example, in this diagram, $J_d^m = 100$ nmol/100 mg/min, J_d at $J_d^m/2$ is 50 nmol/100 mg/min. When the resistance of the UWL was zero, the value of J_d/C_1 at $J_d = 50$ nmol/100 mg/min was 50 nmol/100 mg/min/mM; therefore, the negative value of the slope was 1 mM, the assigned value of the true Michaelis constant. The value of J_d/C_1 at $J_d = J_d^m/2$ was arbitrarily chosen, and the deviation between the value of J_d/C_1 at $J_d^m/2$ at zero UWL resistance and J_d/C_1 at $J_d^m/2$ at the varying UWL resistances was plotted as a function of $d/S_w d$, the effective resistance of the UWL. Similar curves were obtained when different values of J_d were arbitrarily chosen, e.g., $J_d^m/3$, $J_d^m/4$. As an additional example, when the resistance of the UWL was 55.6 min/100 mg/cm^3 (Fig. 24, curve 6), J_d/C_1 at $J_d^m/2$ for UWL resistance of 55.6 min 100 mg/cm^3 was 50–17 = 33 nmol/100 mg/min/mM. This value was then plotted as a function of $d/S_w D$. Note that initially small increases in the effective resistance of the UWL were associated with marked increases in the magnitude of the difference between the values of J_d/C_1 for zero unstirred layer resistance and the value of J_d/C_1 for curves drawn in the presence of an unstirred layer; but as the value of the UWL resistance increased further, there was relatively less change in the deviation between J_d/C_1 at zero UWL resistance, and J_d/C_1 at high values of resistance. In addition, half of the maximum deviation was achieved at a UWL resistance of only 20 min 100 mg/cm^3. It must be further stressed that, since the relationship between J_d and J_d/C_1 was curvilinear except under the special circumstance when UWL resistance was zero (Fig. 24), the multitude of K_m^* values could not be accurately assessed from the relationship between J_d and J_d/C_1 in the presence of a UWL. The value $(J_d/C_1)-(J_d/C_1)^*$ is not equal to $K_m - K_m^*$, though it is related to it, and in this figure the value $(J_d/C_1)-(J_d/C_1)^*$ simply reflects the deviation of curves $B-H$ in (THOMSON 1979c) from the value of J_d/C_1 at $J_d^m/2$ when UWL resistance is zero, as in curve A

lation may have greatly reduced the resistance, but its magnitude may have remained sufficiently large to obscure the demonstration of changes in the apparent affinity constant K_m^*.

b) Varying the True Michaelis Constant

The theoretical relationship between J_d and J_d/C_1 in the presence of an unstirred layer of zero resistance is shown by the *broken line* in Fig. 26. When the resistance

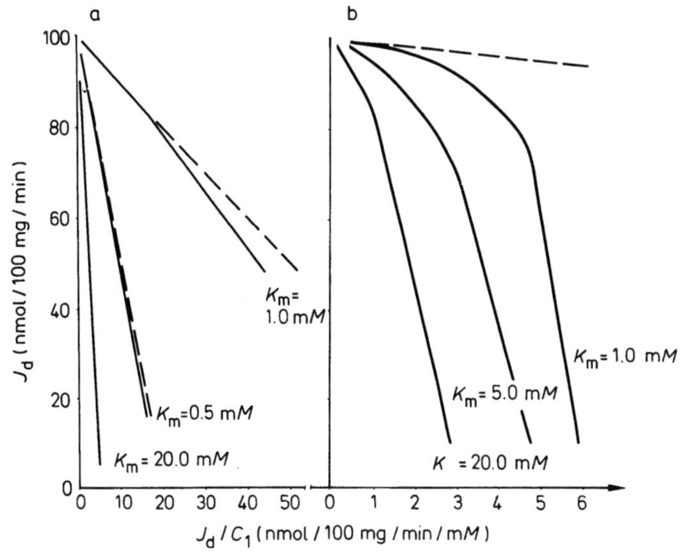

Fig. 26a, b. Theoretical effect of varying K_m, on K_m^* (apparent affinity constant) and J_d^{m*} (apparent maximal transport rate), estimated from the relationship between J_d and J_d/C_1. This diagram illustrates the manner in which transport kinetics are altered by changes in the K_m of the transport carrier from 1 to 20 m*M* under conditions where the resistance offered by the UWL was neither low (**a**) or high (**b**). In these calculations J_d^m was 100 nmol/100 mg/min and *D* was 30×10^{-5} cm²/min. The *broken lines* represent the relationship between J_d and J_d/C_1 when the effective resistance of the UWL was zero. In **b** only one *broken line* is drawn: the scale of the *x*-axis in **b** is much less than in **a**, and the three separate *broken lines* for $K_m - 1.0$ m*M*, $K_m - 5.0$ m*M*, and $K_m = 20$ m*M* very closely approximate the *single line* shown. When the effective resistance of the UWL was low (**a**, 3.3 min 100 mg/cm³), there was a close similarity between the true K_m and apparent K_m^* affinity constants, and the discrepancy between K_m and K_m^* was smaller when K_m was high (20 or 5 m*M*) than low (2 m*M*). When the effective resistance of the UWL was high (**b**, 166.7 min 100 mg/cm³), there was a curvilinear relationship between J_d and J_d/C_1; also note that there was a gross discrepancy between K_m and K_m^* and between J_d^m and J_d^{m*}, both when K_m was low and high. THOMSON (1979c)

of the unstirred layer is low, K_m^* approaches K_m; for a given value of unstirred water resistance, there is less deviation between K_m and K_m^* when K_m is large than when small (Fig. 26). In contrast, when the resistance of the unstirred layer is large, there is a greater deviation between K_m and K_m^* when K_m is larger.

c) Varying the Maximal Transport Rate

The theoretical relationship between J_d and J_d/C_1 in the presence of an unstirred layer of zero resistance is shown by the *broken line* in Fig. 27. When the resistance of the unstirred layer is low, there is less deviation between K_m and K_m^* when J_d^m is low (Fig. 27, curves C and D), than when high (curves A and B). When the resistance of the unstirred layer is high, there is gross deviation of the relationship between J_d and J_d/C_1 from linearity, and no approximation of J_d^m or K_m is possible (Fig. 27).

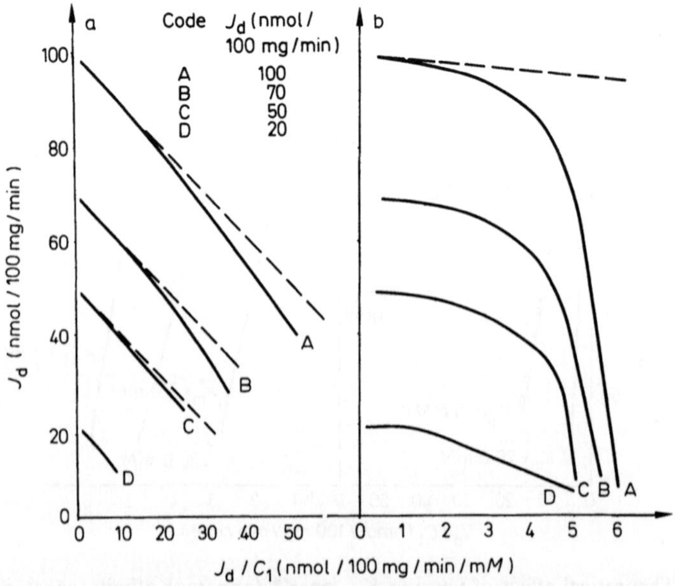

Fig. 27a, b. Theoretical effect of varying the J_d^m on K_m^* and J_d^{m*} estimated from the relationship between J_d and J_d/C_1. This diagram illustrates the manner in which the apparent Michaelis constant and the apparent maximal transport rate are altered by changes in J_d^m from 10 to 100 nmol/100 mg/min, under conditions where the resistance offered by the UWL was either low (**a**, 3.3 min/100 mg/cm^3) or high (**b**, 166.7 min 100 mg/cm^3). In these calculations, K_m was 1 mM and D was 30×10^{-5} cm^2/min. The *broken lines* represent the relationship between J_d and J_d/C_1 when the effective resistance of the UWL was zero. In **b**, only one *broken line* is drawn; the scale of the x-axis in **b** is much less than in **a**, and the separate dashed lines for $J_d^m = 100$, 70, 50, and 20 very closely approximate the *single line* drawn. When the resistance of the UWL was low (**a**), there was only a small discrepancy between K_m and K_m^*, and this difference became less as the value of J_d^m declined. Similarly, the discrepancy between J_d^{m*} and J_d^m was less for lower than for higher values of J_d^m (curves C and D, as contrasted with curves A and B). When the resistance of the UWL was high (**b**), there was a gross discrepancy between K_m and K_m^*, and J_d^m could not be estimated owing to the curvilinear relationship between J_d and J_d/C_1. THOMSON (1979)

Thus, both quantitative and qualitative errors arise from the use of the Eadie–Hofstee plot to estimate the values of K_m and J_d^m. The necessary provision of a linear relationship between J_d and J_d/C_1 was apparent only under the following special circumstances:

1. low resistance of the unstirred layer (Fig. 24);
2. high numerical value of the Michaelis constant (Fig. 26 a);
3. low maximal transport rate (Fig. 27 a).

Under these special circumstances the y-axis intercept gives a reasonable approximation of J_d^m, and the slope yields an approximate value of K_m. Under all other conditions, there is gross overestimation of the values of both J_d^m and K_m.

Similar limitations have been recently described using the plot of C_1/J_d versus C_1 to estimate the kinetic constants of carrier-mediated transport in the presence of a UWL (THOMSON 1979 b): only by the assessment of uptake rates under experimental conditions in which the effective resistance of the unstirred layer is known or can be varied in a systematic and reproducible manner, will it be possible to obtain valid estimates of kinetic constants of carrier-mediated transport. A number of examples follow.

d) Varying the Effective Resistance of the Intestinal Unstirred Water Layer

When the resistance of the intestinal unstirred layer is low, there is a nearly linear relationship between C_1/J_d and C_1, with a y-axis intercept of K_m/J_d^m, an x-axis intercept of $-K_m$, and a slope of $-J_d^m$ (Fig. 28, curves A, B). With increasing UWL

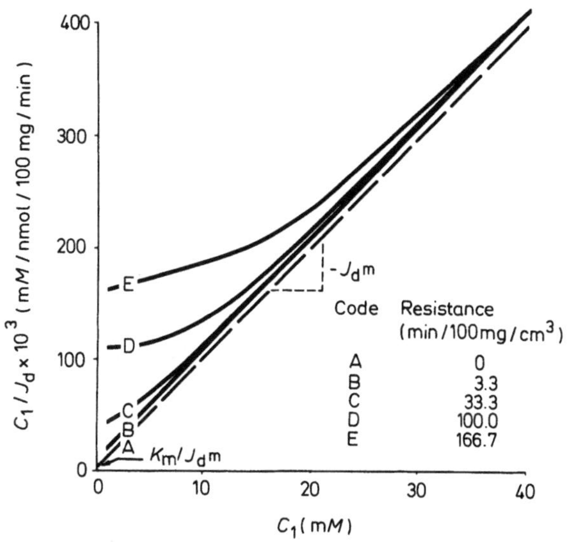

Fig. 28. Theoretical effect of varying effective resistance offered by UWL on estimation of apparent affinity constant K_m^* and maximal transport rate J_d^{m*}, using plot of C_1/J_d versus C_1. C_1 represents concentration of probe molecule in bulk phase, and J_d represents unidirectional flux rate of probe molecule from bulk phase into mucosal cell. Extrapolation of linear transformation of Michaelis-Menten equation to y-axis gives K_m/J_d^m, where K_m is the true Michaelis affinity constant, and J_d^m is true maximal transport rate. Note that this relationship remains linear only when resistance offered by UWL is zero (curve *A*). Slope of this straight line is $-J_d^m$. This diagram illustrates manner in which kinetics of carrier-mediated transport are altered by changes in effective thickness and surface area of UWL and by changes in free diffusion coefficient of probe molecule. Effective thickness of unstirred layer D was varied from 1×10^{-2} to 5×10^{-2} cm, effective surface area of unstirred layer S_w was varied from 1 to 10 cm^2/100 mg, and free diffusion coefficient was 30×10^{-5} cm^2/min. All active transport sites were considered to be at tip of villus ($f_n = 1.0$). In this and all subsequent figures, concentration of probe molecule in bulk phase C_1 is shown on horizontal axis, and ratio of C_1/J_d is given on vertical axis. Maximal transport rate J_d^m was set equal to 100 nmol/100 mg/min, and true Michaelis constant K_m was assigned a value of 1 mM. These assigned values for J_d^m, K_m, d, S_w, D, and f_n were substituted into a newly derived equation, which describes unidirectional flux rate J_d in presence of a UWL. Concentration of probe molecule in bulk phase was varied from 0.5 to 40 mM and equation was solved for J_d at various values of C_1. These values of J_d at the various C_1 values were then plotted as a function of C_1($C_1 J_d$ versus C_1). Note that there was much less discrepancy between true J_d^m and apparent maximal transport rates J_d^{m*} than between true K_m and apparent affinity constant K_m^*. Also note marked upward displacement of y-axis intercept with increasing values of resistance of unstirred layer. THOMSON (1979b)

resistance, there is a progressive upward displacement of the y-axis intercept, with relatively less effect on the slope (Fig. 28). Thus J_d^m may be estimated with reasonable accuracy over a wide range of values of UWL resistance and over a wide range of values of J_d^m. For example, even when the effective resistance of the UWL is high (as in Fig. 28, Curve E), the apparent maximal transport rate J_d^{m*} is 114 nmol/100 mg/min, whereas the assigned value of the true maximal transport rate J_d^m was 100 nmol/100 mg/min. The discrepancy between J_d^m and J_d^{m*} is even less for lower values of UWL resistance. In contrast, unless the UWL resistance is small, K_m cannot be assessed accurately from extrapolation, regardless of the value of K_m or J_d^m.

e) Effect of Varying the Effective Resistance of the Unstirred Water Layer and True Maximal Transport Rate on the Apparent Affinity Constant

As the value of the effective resistance of the unstirred layer is increased, the discrepancy between the true and apparent Michaelis affinity constant, K_m and K_m^*, respectively, also increases. The relationship between increasing resistance of the unstirred layer and K_m^* is linear between 3.3 and 166.7 min/100 mg/cm³ (Fig. 29), and a change in the resistance of the UWL of 11 min/100 mg/cm³ is associated with a 1 mM increase in K_m^*.

The discrepancy between the true and apparent affinity constants K_m and K_m^* is also influenced by the magnitude of J_d^m. As J_d^m increases, the value of the apparent affinity constant falls, and the discrepancy between K_m and K_m^* lessens. The relationship between K_m^* and J_d^m is curvilinear (Fig. 29). When the value of J_d^m is initially low, a small increase in the value of J_d^m is associated with a precipitous fall in the value of K_m^*; when the value of J_d^m is initially higher, increasing J_d^m has relatively less effect on K_m^* (see Fig. 27). Thus, any change in J_d^m is associated with an obligatory change in K_m^* (Fig. 29; THOMSON and DIETSCHY 1977).

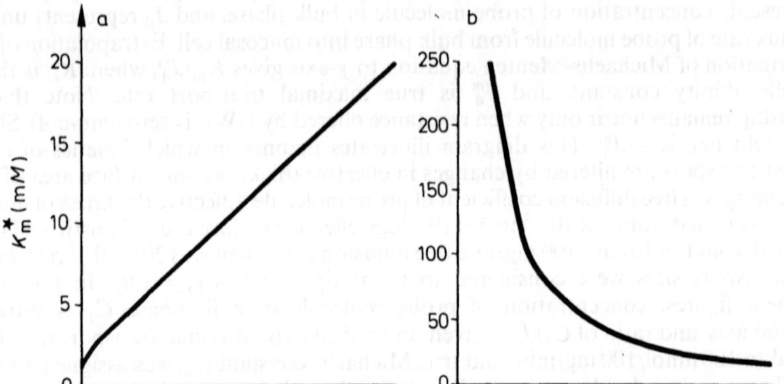

Fig. 29a, b. Factors influencing theoretical discrepancy between K_m and K_m^*, estimated using plot of C_1/J_d versus C_1. This diagram illustrates effect of increasing UWL resistance on discrepancy between K_m and K_m^* (**a**) and shows as well effect of increasing assigned value of true maximal transport rate J_d^m on difference between K_m and K_m^* (**b**) THOMSON (1979b)

2. Experimental Confirmation

The theoretical predictions related to the effect of the UWL have been confirmed experimentally (THOMSON 1979a, b, c, d; THOMSON and DIETSCHY 1980a, b) and will be considered in some detail.

a) Influence of Type of Transport Preparation on Rate Constants

Numerous in vitro methods are available for the study of intestinal transport, but it remains unknown whether it is valid to compare the results obtained with different techniques. Three in vitro tissue preparations were used to derive rate constants for the transport of D-glucose in rabbit jejunum. The resistance of the UWL was varied by altering the rate of stirring of the bulk phase. Marked quantitative differences in the rate of glucose uptake were noted with each technique (Fig. 30). The apparent permeability coefficient P^* of the rabbit jejunum for D-glucose was much higher from everted sacs and full-thickness biopsies than from discs, and P^* was further increased by a reduction in UWL (Table 4). Failure to adjust the experimentally determined flux J_d for the contribution of the passive component led to errors in the estimation of the maximal transport rate, J_d^m, and therefore in the apparent affinity constant, K_m^*, as well (Fig. 31). After correction of J_d for passive permeation, major differences in J_d^m were observed: J_d^m was 3–5 times higher in biopsies than in everted sacs or discs (Fig. 30). K_m^* was also higher in biopsies. With each tissue, K_m^* but not J_d^m, was markedly reduced by stirring the bulk phase (Table 4). The results indicate that failure to account for the effect of the passive component and the UWL leads to major errors in the estimation of K_m^* and J_d^m. Furthermore, the magnitude of P^*, K_m^*, and J_d^m are each influenced by the type of in vitro system used to derive these constants, and it is therefore invalid to extrapolate the results obtained using one preparation to those utilizing another preparation, or to the in vivo situation (THOMSON and DIETSCHY 1980b).

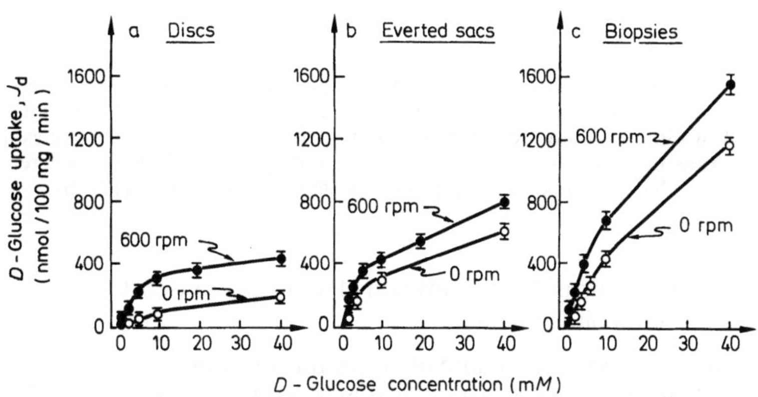

Fig. 30a-c. The effect of stirring of the bulk phase on D-glucose uptake. Jejunal tissue from the same animal was used to prepare (**a**) discs, (**b**) everted sacs, and (**c**) full-thickness biopsies; these were preincubated 4 min in oxygenated Krebs-Ringer bicarbonate buffer at 37 °C, and then transferred to beakers containing varying concentrations of ratiolabeled D-glucose. After an 8-min incubation period the tissue was removed and prepared for counting. THOMSON and DIETSCHY (1980b)

Table 4. Estimation of the apparent passive permeability coefficient P^*, Michaelis constant K_m^* and maximal transport rate J_d^m of D-glucose in the jejunum of rabbits in different in vitro tissue preparations under stirred and unstirred conditions. The values of P^* represent the mean of values obtained by two methods: from the slope of the glucose uptake curve between 10 and 40 mM (Fig. 29), and from the slope of the relationship between the concentration and uptake of L-glucose (THOMSON and DIETSCHY 1980 b)

Jejunal tissue preparation	Rate of stirring (rpm)	P^* (nmol/100 mg/min/mM)	K_m (mM)	J^m (nmol/100 mg/min)
Discs	600	3.9±0.3	3.3	210±19
	0	3.0±0.2	60	
Everted sacs	600	11.0±1.0	1.3	300±27
	0	6.8±0.7	4.9	
Biopsies	600	14.1±1.6	10	1,000±98
	0	11.9±1.1	20	

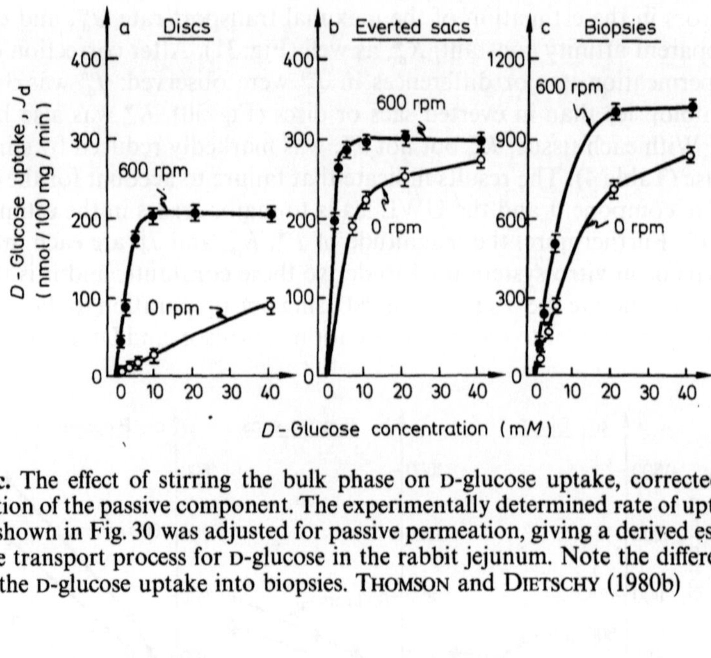

Fig. 31a-c. The effect of stirring the bulk phase on D-glucose uptake, corrected for the contribution of the passive component. The experimentally determined rate of uptake of D-glucose, shown in Fig. 30 was adjusted for passive permeation, giving a derived estimate of the active transport process for D-glucose in the rabbit jejunum. Note the different scales used for the D-glucose uptake into biopsies. THOMSON and DIETSCHY (1980b)

b) Effect of the Unstirred Water Layer on Membrane Transport of D-Glucose in Rabbit Jejunum

It is now appreciated that the rate of active transport of a probe molecule into the intestinal mucosal cells is determined by the rate of movement of the solute molecule across two barriers, the UWL and the microvillus membrane of the epithelial cell. Previously, a theoretical equation (THOMSON and DIETSCHY 1977) has been derived which described J_d, the velocity of unidirectional flux, as a function of the characteristics of the transport carrier in the membrane and of the resistance of the overlying UWL. The predictions of these equations have been tested

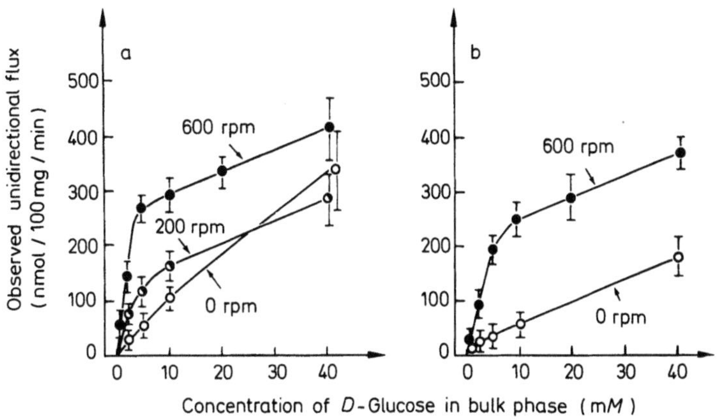

Fig. 32a, b. Effect of stirring of the bulk phase on the unidirectional flux of D-glucose. Jejunal discs were preincubated for either 30 min (**a**) or 4 min (**b**), while being stirred at 600, 200, or 0 rpm. The samples were then incubated for 8 min in ^{14}C-labeled solutions of D-glucose concentrations varying from 1 to 40 mM. During this time the same rate of stirring was maintained for each specimen. THOMSON and DIETSCHY (1980a)

Table 5. Esimation of the kinetic constants K_m^* and J_d^m of the active transport process for D-glucose in the rabbit jejunum under different conditions of preincubation and stirring (THOMSON and DIETSCHY 1980 a)

Type of plot of experimental data	Preincubation 30 min Rate of stirring		Preincubation 4 min Rate of stirring	
	0 rpm	600 rpm	0 rpm	600 rpm
Apparent Michaelis constant, K_m^* (mM)				
1. C_1 versus J_d, Fig. 3 and 5	17.7	1.9	60	3.3
2. $1/C_1$ versus $1/J_d$, with correction for passive permeation	33	2.4	14.3	5.0
3. $1/C_1$ versus $1/J_d$, without correction for passive permeation	100	4.3	63	4.5
Maximal transport rate, J_d^m (nmol/100 mg/min)				
1. C_1 versus J_d, Fig. 3 and 5	230	230	210	210
2. $1/C_1$ versus $1/J_d$, with correction for passive permeation	400	280	400	280
3. $1/C_1$ versus $1/J_d$, without correction for passive permeation	1,000	400	1,000	400

experimentally (THOMSON and DIETSCHY 1980 a) by studying the effect of the rate of stirring of the bulk phase on the in vitro uptake of D-glucose by rabbit jejunum (Fig. 32). These studies demonstrated that alterations in the UWL have a profound effect on the magnitude of the apparent affinity constant, K_m^*, of the active transport process (Table 5; Fig. 33). Second, at bulk phase concentrations in excess of K_m, the passive component of the experimentally determined flux rate be-

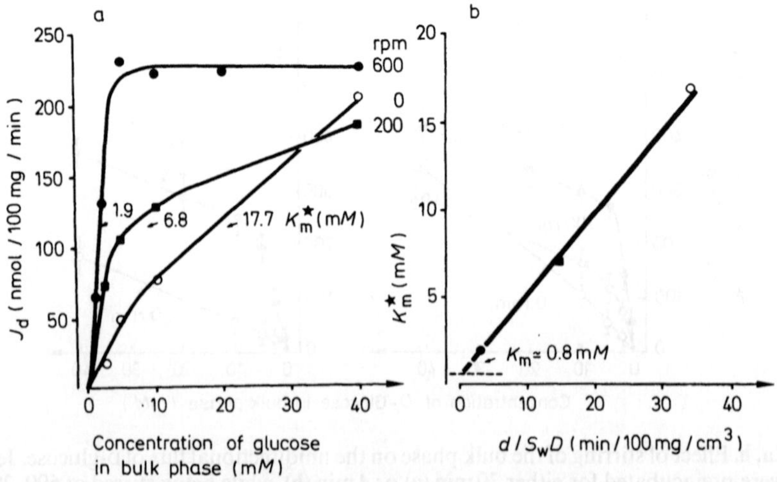

Fig. 33a, b. Effect of stirring the bulk phase on the kinetic constants of the active transport for D-glucose in jejunal tissue preincubated 30 min. The experimentally determined unidirectional flux (Fig. 32) was corrected for passive permeation in order to obtain an accurate assessment of the kinetic constants of the active transport process. In **a** increasing the rate of stirring of the bulk phase from 0 to 200 to 600 rpm was associated with a marked decline in the magnitude of the apparent affinity constant, K_m^* from 17.7 to 6.8 to 1.9 m*M*, respectively; **b** relationship between the effective resistance of the UWL, $d/S_w \cdot D$, and the apparent affinity constant, K_m^*. The magnitude of the effective thickness *d* and effective surface area S_w of the UWL, as well as the free diffusion coefficient of D-glucose, have been reported previously. When these values at each stirring rate were substituted into the formula d/S_wD, a measure of the effective resistance of the UWL was obtained. Note that when $d/S_wD=0$, $K_m^*=K_m$. Thus, from extrapolation, the true affinity constant K_m is predicted to be approximately 0.8 m*M*. THOMSON and DIETSCHY (1980a)

comes of such magnitude as to introduce significant error into the estimate of both the maximal transport rate J_d^m and the true K_m. Third, as a result of the UWL, the use of double-reciprocal plots to determine J_d^m and K_m leads to the overestimation of these constants (Table 5). Fourth, it is possible experimentally to determine the true affinity constant of the membrane carrier for glucose by plotting the values of K_m^* versus the effective resistance of the unstirred layer, and extrapolating back to zero resistance (Fig. 33). Finally, failure to account for the UWL leads to important quantitative errors describing the number of characteristics of the transport process: these include an underestimation of the temperature coefficient (Fig. 34) and the effect of sodium ion on the active transport of glucose in the jejunum (Fig. 35). The results confirm that the kinetic characteristics of the uptake of an actively transported molecule are a complex function of the resistance of both the UWL and the mucosal cell membrane, and this transport process can be adequately described by a newly derived equation. It is apparent that there are serious limitations in the interpretation of much of the previously published data dealing with active transport processes in the intestine, since these studies failed to account for the effect of the UWL.

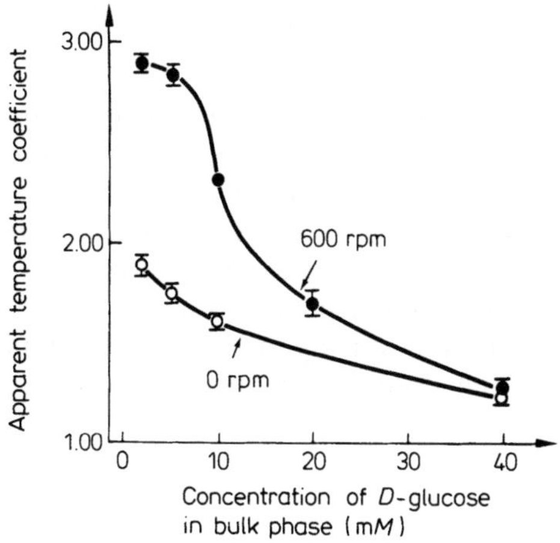

Fig. 34. Effect of stirring of the bulk phase on the estimation of the apparent temperature coefficient of the intestinal transport process for D-glucose in jejunal tissue preincubated for 30 min. The unidirectional flux of varying concentrations of glucose in the bulk phase C_1 was determined at 37° and 4 °C in tissue preincubated for 30 min and stirred at either 600 or 0 rpm. The values of the apparent temperature coefficient at the two different rates of stirring were then plotted as a function of C_1. THOMSON and DIETSCHY (1980a)

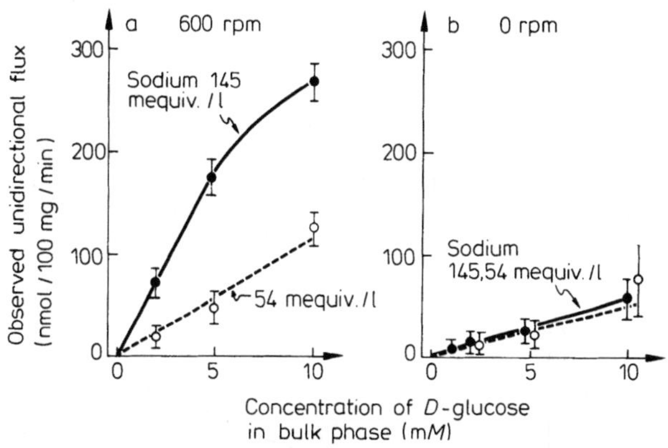

Fig. 35a, b. Effect of stirring the bulk phase on the undirectional flux of D-glucose in jejunal tissue preincubated for 4 min with normal (145 mM) and low (54 mM) concentrations of sodium chloride in the bulk phase. The low sodium concentration was achieved by substituting D-mannitol for an isotonic amount of sodium chloride. **a** bulk phase stirred at 600 rpm to minimize the effective resistance of the unstirred layer; lowering the concentration of sodium chloride in the bulk phase was associated with a fall in unidirectional flux rate J_d and a rise in the magnitude of the apparent affinity constant, K_m^*; **b** bulk phase unstirred and high unstirred layer resistance; varying the sodium concentration had no effect on J_d or K_m^*. THOMSON and DIETSCHY (1980a)

c) Unstirred Water Layer and Age-Dependent Changes in Rabbit Jejunal D-Glucose Transport

The rate of glucose absorption increases in a varity of species shortly after birth, but there are conflicting reports as to the kinetic basis for this change. However, the influence of age on intestinal absorption is influenced by the effect of the resistance of the UWL (Fig. 36): then the resistance of the UWL was high, the uptake from high concentrations of glucose increased as the animals grew older; this change with aging was not seen from low concentrations of glucose. When UWL resistance was minimized by stirring the bulk phase, similar amounts of glucose were absorbed from high doses, but uptake from low doses was greater in young

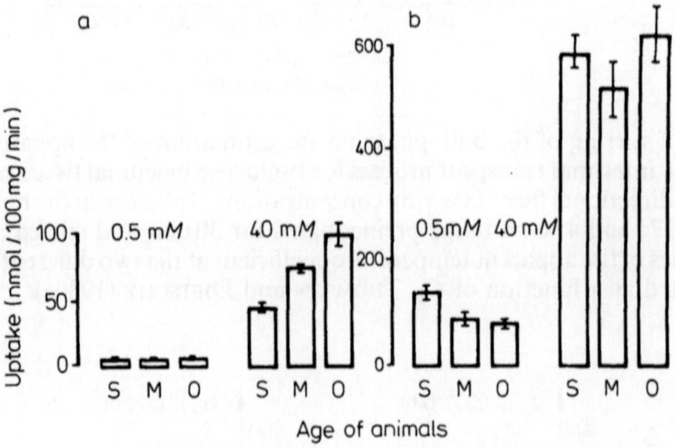

Fig. 36a, b. Effect of age, dose, and UWL resistance on unidirectional flux of D-glucose. Jejunal discs from suckling (*S*), mature (*M*), and old (*O*) animals were incubated in vitro in radiolabeled solutions containing 0.5 or 40 m*M* D-glucose. Effective resistance of UWL was varied by stirring bulk phase. High resistance of UWL was obtained by leaving bulk phase unstirred (**a**), and a low resistance (**b**) was achieved by stirring bulk phase at 600 rpm. Height of bars represents mean uptake of at least eight animals; the standard error is also shown. THOMSON (1979a)

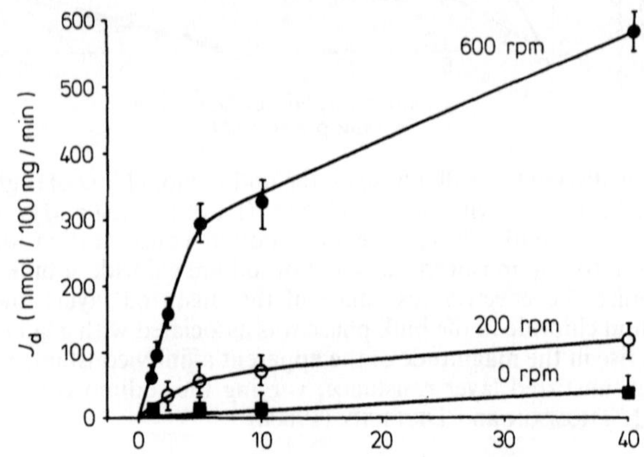

Fig. 37. Effect of stirring bulk phase on unidirectional flux of D-glucose in suckling rabbits (2- to 3-week-old). Resistance of UWL was varied by stirring bulk phase at 600, 200, or 0 rpm. Kinetic constants derived from these have been published. THOMSON (1979a)

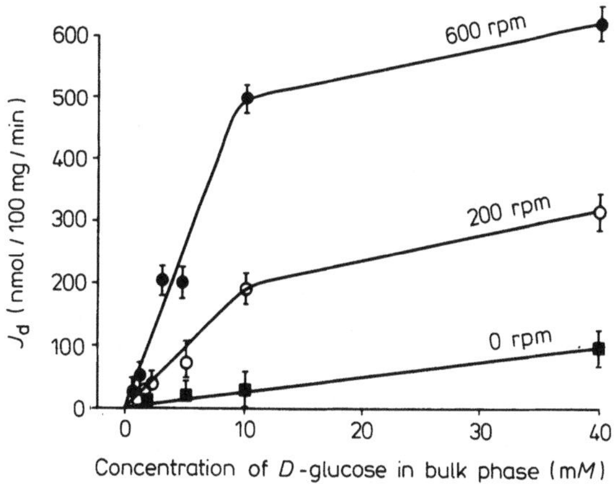

Fig. 38. Effect of stirring bulk phase on unidirectional flux of D-glucose on old rabbits (11- to 12-month-old). Each point represents mean ±standard error of at least eight animals. Resistance of UWL was varied by stirring bulk phase at 600, 200, or 0 rpm. Kinetic constants derived from these curves are given in Table 6. THOMSON (1979a)

Table 6. Kinetic constants for unidirectional flux of D-glucose into jejunum of suckling, mature, and old rabbits. Values are means ± standard error of observations on at least eight animals. J_d^m, maximal transport rate; K_m^*, apparent affinity constant; P^*, apparent passive permeability coefficient. The values of the K_m^* and P^* at 200 rpm are not shown, but for the three groups of animals the values lie between those obtained at 600 and 0 rpm. The values of P^* were obtained from the slope of the pateau portion of the kinetic curve of D-glucose at concentrations between 10 and 40 m*M* (plateau, D-glucose), from the slope of the linear portion of the kinetic curve of L-glucose, and from the slope of the linear portion of the kinetic curve for D-glucose at 4 °C, corrected to the predicted value at 37 °C using the temperature coefficient of the process (THOMSON and DIETSCHY 1980b). The apparent affinity constants were derived from experiments in which the bulk phase was stirred at 600 rpm; when the bulk phase was unstirred (0 rpm), the relationship between the uptake and concentration was linear, thereby preventing calculation of K_m^*. However, this value exceeded 40 m*M* in the suckling, mature, and old animals (THOMSON 1979a)

Age	J_d^m (nmol/ 100 mg/min)	K_m^* (m*M*)	P^* (nmol/100 mg/m*M*)					
			Plateau, D-glucose		L-glucose		4 °C, D-glucose	
			600 rpm	0 rpm	600 rpm	0 rpm	600 rpm	0 rpm
Suckling, 1 week	220	0.5	8.1 ±0.4					
Suckling, 2–3 weeks	210	0.6	8.3 ±0.5	1.0 ±0.1	7.4 ±0.5	2.0 ±0.2	7.2 ±0.6	3.0 ±0.3
Mature, 6–8 weeks	215	1.2	5.2 ±0.2	1.6 ±0.2	4.1 ±0.5	1.0 ±0.4	5.8 ±0.5	1.0 ±0.1
Old, 11–12 months	440	4.0	3.9 ±0.3	1.4 ±0.1	2.3 ±0.2	1.5 ±0.2	3.0 ±0.3	1.9 ±0.2

than in old animals (THOMSON 1979a). Studies undertaken to determine the kinetic basis of these age-related changes showed that there was a profound effect of stirring the bulk phase on the absorption of D-glucose from each age group of rabbits (Figs. 37 and 38), and that with increasing age: (a) the apparent passive permeability coefficient P^* of glucose fell; (b) the maximum transport rate J_d^m rose; and (c) the apparent affinity constant K_m^* increased (Table 6). These differences were not observed when the resistance of the UWL was high: P^* and K_m^* were similar in suckling, mature, and old animals, and the increase in glucose uptake with age was due to the greater J_d^m. Thus, the potential benefit of the high affinity, high permeability transport system of young animals may be obscured by high resistance of the UWL.

d) Transport Kinetics of D-Glucose in Human Small Intestinal Mucosa: Histologically Normal and Abnormal Biopsies

Using D-glucose as the probe molecule, we analyzed conditions which must be fulfilled in mucosal biopsy studies before the kinetic nature of the transport process can be established. Mucosal biopsies were obtained from the region of the ligament of Treitz from 4 healthy volunteers and from 46 patients: 29 of the 47 had histologically normal mucosa; 7 had mild abnormalities; and 11 had moderate or severe, "flat" abnormalities in villus architecture (THOMSON and WEINSTEIN 1979). The rate of uptake of 40 mM glucose was constant only between 4 and 10 min, extrapolating through zero uptake at zero time with a constant adherent mucosal fluid volume (Fig. 39). Incubation for shorter or longer periods was associated with over- or underestimation of the rate of uptake. Failure to use a nonabsorb-

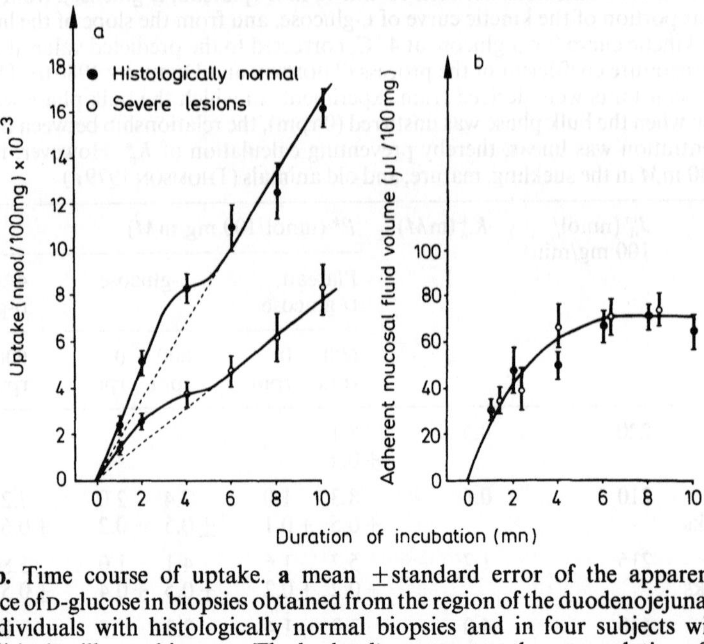

Fig. 39a, b. Time course of uptake. **a** mean ±standard error of the apparent rate of appearance of D-glucose in biopsies obtained from the region of the duodenojejunal junction in ten individuals with histologically normal biopsies and in four subjects with severe abnormalities in villus architecture. The *broken lines* represent the extrapolation of the linear portion of the uptake curves at zero uptake at zero time; **b** shows the rate of equilibration of the nonabsorbable marker in the normal and abnormal biopsies. THOMSON and WEINSTEIN (1979)

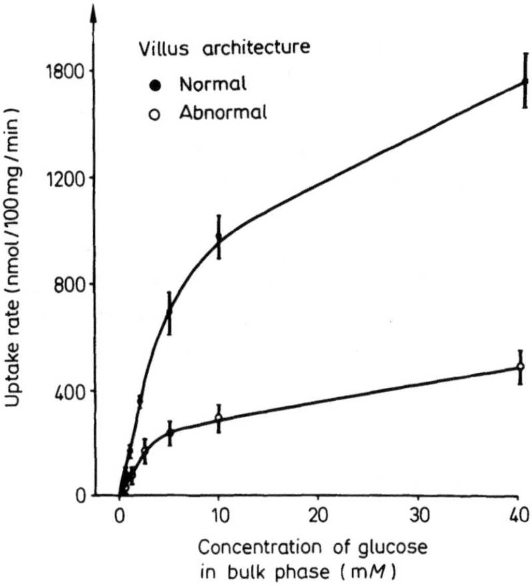

Fig. 40. Concentration study. Mean ± standard error of the rate of uptake of D-glucose in histologically normal and abnormal biopsies obtained from the region of the duodenojejunal junctions. Histologically normal biopsies were obtained from 18 subjects. The abnormal biopsy group consisted of 7 patients with severe (flat) lesions and 4 with moderate changes. THOMSON and WEINSTEIN (1979)

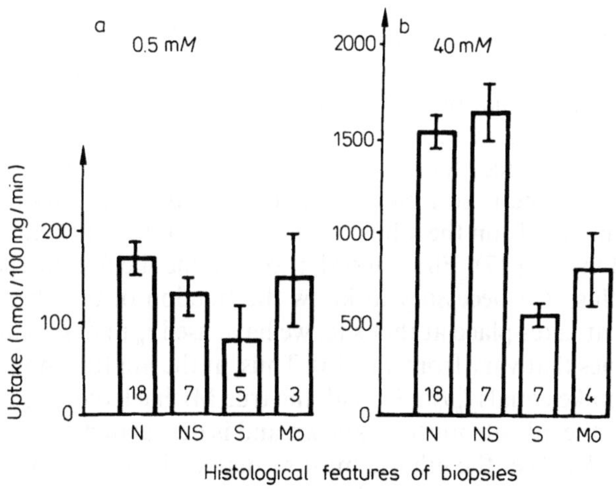

Fig. 41a, b. Glucose uptake and morphology. Comparison of glucose uptake into biopsies showing varying degrees of histologic abnormalities. Mean ± standard error of unidirectional flux of D-glucose into biopsies obtained from the region of the duodenojejunal junction. Biopsies were graded as normal (*N*) or as showing mild (*M*), moderate (*Mo*), or severe (*S*) changes in villus architecture. The number of patients in each group is shown. Glucose uptake was compared between 0.5 m*M* (**a**) and 40 m*M* (**b**) glucose. THOMSON and WEINSTEIN (1979)

able marker was also associated with overestimation of the rate of uptake. When biopsies were incubated for 6 min, a curvilinear relationship was observed between uptake rate and concentrations (Fig. 40). In biopsies with moderate and severe abnormalities, there was a marked reduction in the magnitude of the maximal transport rate and the apparent passive permeability coefficient, with little change in the magnitude of the apparent affinity constant. Thus, differences in glucose uptake between histologically normal and abnormal biopsies were best demonstrated using high substrate concentrations (Fig. 41), conditions best suited to reflect the differences in J_d^m and P^* in the different patient groups. Thus, when human mucosal biopsies are used to study nutrient absorption, certain criteria must be fulfilled to establish valid rate constants and to make comparison between normal and abnormal mucosa.

e) Unstirred Water Layer and Functional Heterogeneity of the Villus

We have already examined the possible influence of heterogeneity of the villus on passive transport. Heterogeneity of the villus is also a consideration for carrier-mediated transport. When the villus is arbitrarily divided into segments and the values of d, S_w, and K_m of each segment are varied, then the potential role of the UWL may be more fully appreciated (THOMSON and DIETSCHY 1977). Although there are limitations in the use of the transformation plots of the Michaelis–Menten equation (THOMSON 1979 b, c; THOMSON and DIETSCHY 1980 b), these plots do provide the opportunity of qualitatively assessing whether the distribution of transport sites along the villus is similar for solutes absorbed by a common transport mechanism. Let us examine the theoretical and experimental basis for the potential influence of the heterogeneity of the villus on carrier-mediated transport.

α) Theoretical Considerations. Distribution of Transport Sites Along the Villus. All data presented thus far have been based on Eq. (7) which is appropriate for an experimental situation such as that shown in Fig. 1 a where all membrane transport sites are assumed to have the same K_m and are all subject to the same unstirred layer resistance. As shown in Fig. 1 b, however, it is likely that the situation in the intestine is still more complex in that the transport sites are distributed at many levels on the villus. In this circumstance, additional terms must be introduced into Eq. (7). First, in order to describe the flux rate at a particular site on the villus, it is necessary to know the fraction of the observed maximal uptake rate that takes place at that site: we have used f_n to designate this fraction and it has values that vary from 0 to 1.0. Thus, at the nth transport site the maximal rate of uptake equals $f_n J_d^m$. Second, the true Michaelis constant for the transport carrier at the nth site must be known and is designated K_m^n. Third, the resistance of the UWL over the nth site must be defined in terms of values for the effective surface area and thickness of this diffusion barrier that are appropriate for the nth site, i.e., S_w^n and d_d^n. Substituting these various new items into Eq. (7), the observed rate of transport at the nth site, J_d^n, on the villus is given by the expression

$$J_d^n = 0.5\,D\left(\frac{S_w^n}{d^n}\right)\left\{C_1 + K_m^n + \frac{f_n d^n J_d^m}{S_w^n D} \pm \left[\left(C_1 + K_m^n + \frac{f_n d^n J_d^m}{S_w^n D}\right)^2 - 4C_1\left(\frac{f_n d^n J_d^m}{S_w^n D}\right)\right]^{\frac{1}{2}}\right\}. \quad (44)$$

The overall observed rate of active transport obviously must equal the sum of the rates of transport at all *n*th sites so that

$$J_d = \Sigma J_d . \tag{45}$$

Using Eqs. (44) and (45), it is now possible to examine the effect of varying the distribution of transport sites on the villus upon the relationship of J_d to C_1 (THOMSON and DIETSCHY 1977).

1. The effect of varying the distribution of transport sites on the villus, f_n. In order to make these calculations, the villus was arbitrarily divided into ten segments of equal length designated *n* 1 to *n* 10 as seen in Fig. 1 b. Figure 42 illustrates the effect of altering the distribution of transport sites from the situation where all uptake occurs at one site ($f_n = 1.0$) to the situation where uptake is assumed to occur equally at 10 different sites ($f_n = 0.1$). When the resistance of the unstirred

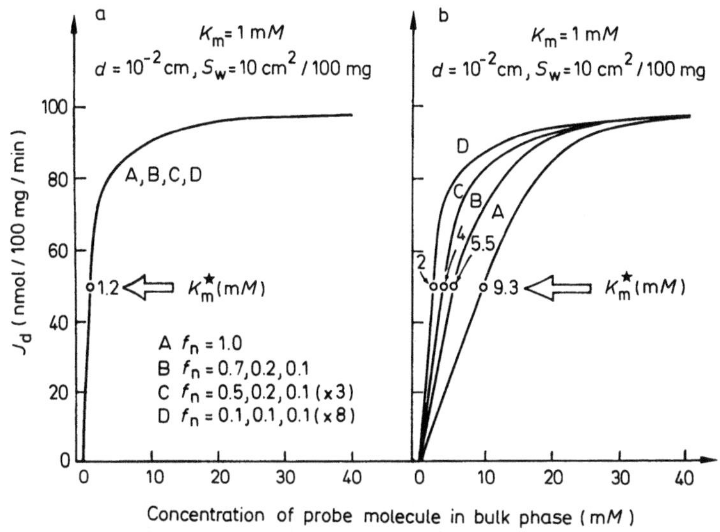

Fig. 42a, b. Theoretical relationship between the kinetics of active transport and variations in the distribution of the active transport sites along the villus. This diagram illustrates the manner in which active transport kinetics are altered by changes in f_n. **a** low resistance of the UWL; **b** high resistance. The perpendicular height of the villus was divided into ten equal segments numbered $n1 - n10$. The proportion of the total active transport sites present on each segment is indicated as f_n. Curve *A* shows the kinetics of active transport when all the active transport sites were in the first of the ten equal segments ($f_{n1} = 1.0$). In curve *B*, 70% of the total active transport sites were located in the first segment ($f_{n1} = 0.7$); 20% were in the second segment ($f_{n2} = 0.2$), and 10% were in the third segment ($f_{n3} = 0.1$). The total active transport J_d is given by the sum of the individual fluxes contributed by each nth segment J_d^n. In curve *C*, 50% of the active transport sites were located in the first segment ($f_{n1} = 0.5$), 20% in the second segment ($f_{n2} = 0.2$), and 10% in the third, fourth and fifth segments ($f_{n3} = 0.1$, $f_{n4} = 0.1$, $f_{n5} = 0.1$), and the total flux was given by the sum of the fluxes occurring over these five segments. In curve *D*, 10% of the active transport sites were located in each of the ten segments ($f_{n1} = 0.1$, $f_{n2} = 0.1, \ldots, f_{n10} = 0.1$) and the total flux was obtained from the sum of the fluxes occurring over these ten segments. In these calculations J_d^m was 100 nmol/100 mg/min, *D* was 30×10^{-5} cm^2/min, and K_m was 1 m*M*. THOMSON and DIETSCHY (1977)

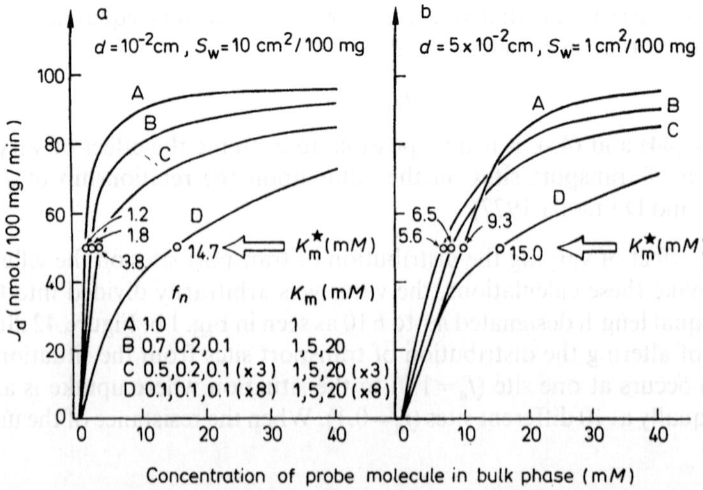

Fig. 43a, b. Theoretical relationship between the kinetics of active transport and variations in both the distribution of the active transport sites along the villus and the true Michaelis constant. This diagram illustrates the manner in which the kinetics of active transport are affected by changes in both f_n and K_m^n. **a** low resistance of the UWL; **b** high resistance. In curve *A*, all the active transport sites were located on the first intestinal segment and K_m for these sites was 1 m*M*. In curve *B*, 70%, 20%, and 10% of the active transport sites were located in the first, second, and third villus segments, and $K_m^{n1} = 1$, $K_m^{n2} = 5$, and $K_m^{n3} = 20$ m*M*; the total flux was obtained from the sum of the individual fluxes at each segment. In curve *C*, 50% of the total active transport sites were located in the first villus segment, 20% in the second segment, and 10% in the third, fourth, and fifth segments; their Michaelis constants were $K_m^{n1} = 1$ m*M*, $K_m^{n2} = 5$ m*M*, and $K_m^{n3,4,5} = 20$ *M*, respectively. Curve *D* was constructed in a similar manner. In these calculations J_d^m was 100 nmol/100 mg/min and *D* was 30×10^{-5} cm²/min. THOMSON and DIETSCHY (1977)

layer is low, changes in the distribution of transport sites along the villus have no appreciable effect on K_m^* of the active transport process (Fig. 42a). This is in contrast to the striking effect of manipulations of f_n on K_m^* when the unstirred layer resistance is high: changing f_n from 1.0 to 0.1 is associated with a marked decrease in K_m^* from 9.3 to 2.0 m*M* (Fig. 42b). In this illustration, it should be emphasized that the K_m and the resistance of the UWL were considered to be the same at all transport sites.

2. The effect of varying both the distribution f_n and Michaelis constant K_m of the transport sites. The special circumstance can now be examined where K_m varies at different transport sites. In curve D, for example, in Fig. 43a, the resistance of the unstirred layer was low and the same over all transport sites, 10% of J_d^m occurred at each villus segment ($f_{n1} = 0.1$) and K_m of the first segment was 1.0 m*M* ($K_m^{n1} = 1.0$ m*M*), K_m of the second segment was 5.0 m*M* ($K_m^{n2} = 5.0$ m*M*) and K_m of the third through tenth segments equaled 20.0 m*M* ($K_m^{n3-10} = 20.0$ m*M*). Under these conditions, the apparent Michaelis constant equaled 14.7 m*M*. Progressively increasing the proportion of the total transport taking place in the first segment (Fig. 43a, curves B and C) shifted the curves to the left, causing a reduction in K_m^*. When all active transport occurred at the first villus segment, and

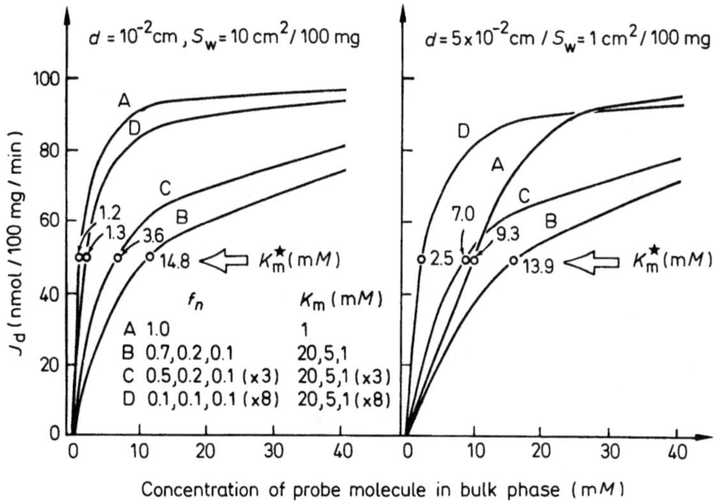

Fig. 44a, b. Theoretical relationship between the kinetics of active transport and changes in both the distribution of the active transport sites and the true Michaelis constant. This diagram illustrates the manner in which the kinetics of active transport are affected by changes in both f_n and K_m^n. **a** low resistance of the UWL, **b** high resistance. The designation of f_n and K_m^n used in each curve is as noted. The total flux was derived from the sum of the individual fluxes at each segment. In these calculations J_d^m was 100 nmol/100 mg/min, and D was 30×10^{-5} cm²/min. THOMSON and DIETSCHY (1977)

K_m^{n1} equaled 1.0 mM, K_m^* was 1.2 mM (Fig. 43a, curve A). Thus, when unstirred layer resistance is low, changes in K_m override the influence of f_n, and a reduction in K_m is associated with a decline in K_m^*. This is in contrast to the situation shown in Fig. 43b, where the resistance of the unstirred layer is high. When f_{n1} equaled 0.1, K_m^* was 15.0 mM (Fig. 43b, curve D). Increasing f_{n1} to 0.5 (Fig. 43b, curve C) or to 0.7 (Fig. 43b, curve B) shifted the curves to the left and reduced K_m^*. However, when all active transport occurred at the villus tip ($f_{n1} = 1.0$), the curve was shifted back to the right and K_m^* was increased (Fig. 43b, curve A). Thus, when unstirred layer resistance is high, both K_m and f_n have an important influence on K_m^*.

We must also consider the situation where the K_m at the tip of the villus is higher than the K_m for transport sites lower on the villus. When the unstirred layer resistance was low (Fig. 44a, curve A) and the highest K_m was at the tip ($K_m^{n1} =$ 20.0 mM), then reducing the proportion of J_d^m contributed by the n 1 segment had the effect of shifting the curve to the left (Fig. 44a, curves Band D). In contrast, when the diffusion barrier was large, changing f_n as well as K_m shifted the curve either to the right or to the left (Fig. 44b).

3. The effect of varying f_n, K_m, d, and S_w. Thus, from the foregoing discussion one can summarize how changes in the characteristics of the transport carrier are influenced by manipulations in the resistance of the UWL. An alteration in the unstirred layer resistance would be expected to produce a very significant change in the kinetic curves of active transport under conditions where the transport sites were localized to a relatively small region of the villus and where the K_m of these

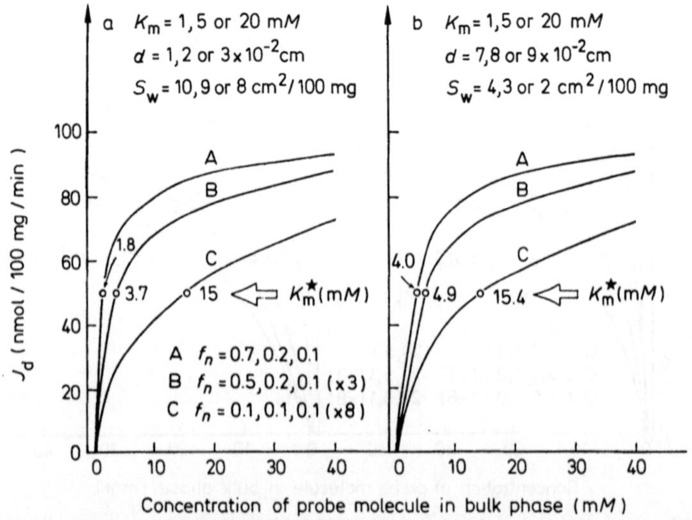

Fig. 45a, b. Theoretical relationship between the kinetics of active transport and change in the distribution of the active transport sites, the true Michaelis constant at each site, and the dimensions of the UWL overlying each site. This diagram illustrates the manner in which the kinetics of active transport are affected by changes in f_n, K_m^n, d^n, and S_w^n. **a** low resistance of the UWL; **b** high resistance. In curve *A* of **a**, $f_{n1}=0.7$, $f_{n2}=0.2$, $f_{n3}=0.1$, $K_m^{n1}=1$, $K_m^{n2}=5$, $K_m^{n3}=20$ m*M*; $d^{n1}=1\times10^{-2}$, $d^{n2}=2\times10^{-2}$, $d^{n3}=3\times10^{-2}$ cm; and $S_w^{n1}=10$, $S_w^{n2}=9$, $S_w^{n3}=8\,\mathrm{cm}^2/100$ mg. In curves *B* and *C* $K_m=20$ m*M*, $d=3\times10^{-2}$ cm, and $S_w=8\,\mathrm{cm}^2/100$ mg for $f_{n3}-f_{n5}$ and $f_{n3}-f_{n10}$, respectively. In these calculations J_d^m was 100 nmol/100 mg/min and *D* was $30\times10^{-5}\,\mathrm{cm}^2$/min. THOMSON and DIETSCHY (1977)

sites was low. In contrast, an identical alteration in unstirred layer resistance would be expected to have relatively little effect on the kinetics of active transport if the transport sites were more widely distributed on the villus and if K_m of these sites was higher. These two possibilities are illustrated in Fig. 45. When the transport sites were distributed over only three villus segments with relatively low K_m values, as shown in curve A, then changing the unstirred layer resistance from a low to a high value (Fig. 45a to Fig. 45b, respectively) increased K_m^* by 122%, from 1.8 to 4.0 m*M*. In contrast, when the transport sites were widely distributed and had relatively higher K_m values, a comparable change in unstirred layer resistance shifted the K_m^* less than 3%, from 15 to 15.4 m*M*. Thus, the magnitude of the experimentally measured kinetic constant K_m^* may be influenced by the distribution of transport sites along the villus as well as by the J_d^m and the effective resistance of the unstirred layer, d/S_wD.

β) Use of Transformation Plots to Establish the Functional Heterogeneity of the Villus for Carrier-Mediated Transport. In the calculations thus far, the characteristics of the carrier have been assumed to be similar at each location along the villus and the resistance of the unstirred layer has been assumed to be similar at each locus. However, there is no experimental justification for this concept. Indeed, it is possible that the transport characteristics of the crypt cells differ from those near the villus tip. Therefore, the villus was arbitrarily divided into ten equal

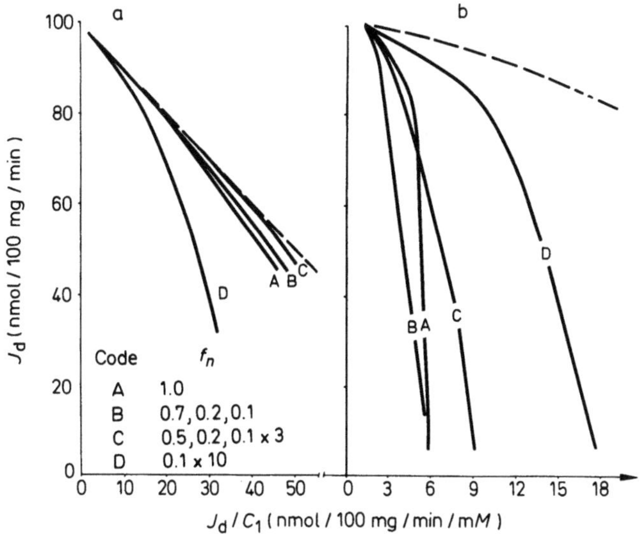

Fig. 46a, b. Theoretical effect of varying the distribution of transport sites along the villus f_n on K_m^* and J_d^{m*}, estimated for the relationship between J_d and J_d/C_1. This diagram illustrates the manner in which carrier-mediated transport kinetics are altered by changes in f_n (K_m) and effective resistance of the UWL over each carrier being similar). **a** low effective resistance of the UWL (3.3 min 100 mg/cm³); **b** high resistance (166.7 min 100 mg/cm³). The *broken line* represents the theoretical relationship between J_d and J_d/C_1 when the effective resistance of the UWL was zero. Curve *A* shows the kinetics of transport when all the transport carriers were in the first of ten equal villus segments ($f_{n1}=0.1$). In curve *B*, 70% of the total active transport sites were located in the first segment ($f_{n1}=0.7$); 20% were in the second segment ($f_{n2}=0.2$), and 10% were in the third segment ($f_{n3}=0.1$). The total flux J_d is given by the sum of the individual fluxes contributed by each nth segment J_d^n. In curve *C*, 50% of the active transport sites were located in the first segment ($f_{n1}=0.5$), 20% in the second segment ($f_{n2}=0.2$) and 10% in the third, fourth, and fifth segments ($f_{n3}=0.1$, $f_{n4}=0.1$, $f_{n5}=0.1$) and the total flux was given by the sum of the fluxes occurring over these five segments. In curve *D*, 10% of the active transport sites were located in each of the ten segments ($f_{n1}=0.1$, $f_{n2}=0.1, \ldots, f_{n10}=0.1$) and the total flux was obtained from the sum of the fluxes occurring over these ten segments. In these calculations J_d^m was 100 nmol/100 mg/min. Note that when the effective resistance of the UWL was low (**a**), changing the distribution of transport sites from the tip of the villus ($f_n=1.0$, curve *A*) to the upper half of the villus ($f_n=0.7$, 0.2, 0.1, curve *B*; and $f_n=0.5$, 0.2, 0.1 × 3, curve *C*), shifted the relationship between J_d and J_d/C_1 towards the theoretical line of zero UWL resistance (*broken line*), but that the equal distribution of transport sites along the villus ($f_n=0.1\times 10$, curve *D*) was associated with a further deviation away from the theoretical line. In contrast, when UWL resistance was high (**b**), relocating the carrier sites from the tip towards the base of the villus was initially associated with increased (curve *B*) and then decreased (curves *C* and *D*) deviation from the theoretical line. THOMSON and DIETSCHY (1977)

segments, and the characteristics of transport at each site is varied (see Fig. 1); thus, the rate of uptake and the dimensions of the UWL appropriate for the transport sites present in the ten equal segments have been designated as J_d^m, S_w^m, and d^m, respectively. When the resistance of the unstirred layer is low, there is little difference in the Eadie–Hofstee plot (Fig. 46a) when all transport occurs at one segment ($f_n=1.0$, Fig. 46a, curve A), as compared with 70% of the total maximal

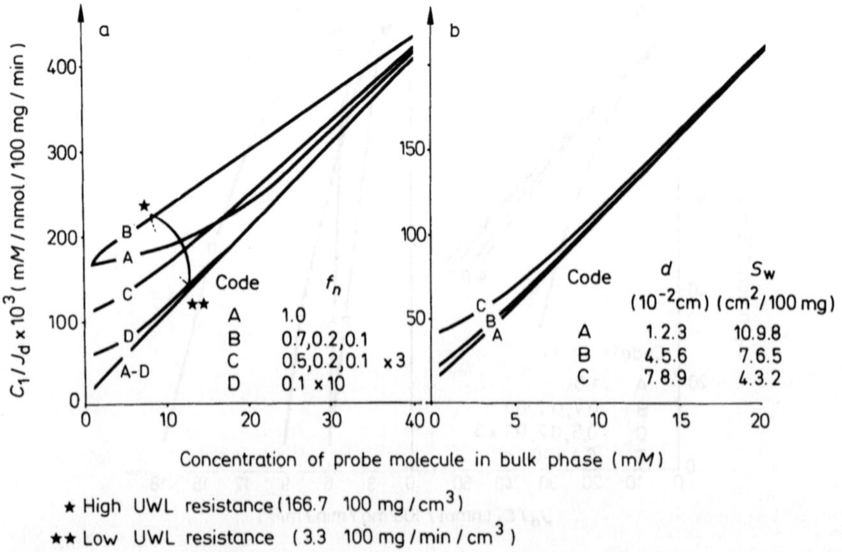

Fig. 47a, b. Theoretical effect of varying distribution of transport sites along villus on K_m^* and J_d^m, estimated using plot of C_1/J_d versus C_1. This diagram illustrates manner in which carrier-mediated transport kinetics are altered by changes in f_n, distribution of transport sites along villus. Perpendicular height of villus was divided into ten equal segments numbered $n1$–$n10$. Proportion of total carrier transport sites present on each segment is indicated as f_n. **a** Curve *A* shows kinetics of transport when all transport carriers were in first of ten equal segments ($f_{n1}=1.0$). In curve *B*, 70% of total active transport sites were located in first segment ($f_{n1}=0.7$); 20% were in second segment ($f_{n2}=0.2$), and 10% were in third segment ($f_{n3}=0.1$). Total flux J_d is given by sum of individual fluxes contributed by each nth segment J_d^n. In curve *C*, 50% of active transport sites were located in first segment ($f_{n1}=0.5$), 20% in second segment ($f_{n2}=0.2$), and 10% in third, fourth, and fifth segments ($f_{n3}=0.1$, $f_{n4}=0.1$, $f_{n5}=0.1$), and total flux was given by sum of fluxes occurring over these five segments. In curve *D*, 10% of active transport sites were located in each of ten segments ($f_{n1}=0.1, f_{n2}=0.1, \ldots, f_{n10}=0.1$), and total flux was obtained from sum of fluxes occurring over these ten segments. Effective resistance of unstirred layer was either low (3.3 min 100 mg/cm^3) or high (166.7 min 100 mg/cm^3); **b** 70% of total active transport sites were located in first segment ($f_{n1}=0.7$); 20% were in second segment ($f_{n2}=0.2$); and 10% were in third segment ($f_{n3}=0.1$). Total flux J_d is given by sum of individual fluxes contributed by each nth segment. However, in contrast to Fig. 48a, the effective thickness and surface area of unstirred layer varied over villus sites; in curve *A*, $d^{n1}=10^{-2}$, $d^{n2}=2\times10^{-2}$, and $d^{n3}=3\times10^{-2}$ cm; $S_w^{n1}=10$, $S_w^{n2}=9$, and $S_w^{n3}=8$ cm^2/100 mg. In curve *B*, $d^{n1}=4\times10^{-2}$, $d^{n2}=5\times10^{-2}$, and $d^{n3}=6\times10^{-2}$ cm; $S_w^{n1}=7$, $S_w^{n2}=6$, and $S_w^{n3}=5$ cm^2/100 mg. In curve *C*, $d^{n1}=7\times10^{-2}$, $d^{n2}=8\times10^{-2}$, and $d^{n3}=9\times10^{-2}$ cm; $S_w^{n1}=4$, $S_w^{n2}=3$, and $S_w^{n3}=2$ cm^2/100 mg. K_m of each villus segment was similar and assigned a value of 1.0 m*M*; J_d^m was 100 nmol/100 mg/min, and *D* was 30×10^{-5} cm^2/min. THOMSON (1979)

transport occurring at the first segment ($n=1$), 20% from the second segment ($n=2$), and the remaining 10% from the third segment ($n=3$), as is shown in Fig. 46a, curve B. The line of $f_n=0.5$, 0.2, and 0.1×3 approaches the ideal line even more closely (Fig. 46a, curve C), and the discrepancy between K_m and K_m^* increases further (Fig. 46 , curve D) when the transport sites are evenly distributed along the villus ($f_n=0.1\times10$). When the resistance of the unstirred layer is high (Fig. 46b), there is a curvilinear relationship between J_d and J_d/C_1, and once

Table 7. Theoretical effect of varying f_n on J_d^m and K_m^* estimated using plot of C_1/J_d versus C_1 under high UWL resistance conditions. This distribution of transport sites along the villus f_n was varied as described in the legend of Fig. 28. The apparent maximal transport site (J_d^{m*}) was calculated from the slope of this relationship; where the line was curvilinear, the slope was calculated from the linear portion at high values of C_1. The true maximal transport rate J_d^m was assigned a value of 100 nmol/100 mg/min. The apparent affinity constant K_m^*) was calculated from the y-axis intercept K_m/J_d^m, using J_d^m. The true affinity constant K_m had an assigned value of 1.0 mM. Note that the values reported in this table were obtained in the presence of high (166.7 min/100 mg/cm^3) UWL resistance, as shown in the upper portion of Fig. 47. Also note that the resistance of the UWL was similar over each villus site and that the true affinity of all carriers was identical (THOMSON 1979 d)

f_n	J_d^{m*} (nmol/100 mg/min)	K_m^* (mM)
1.0	114	16.7
0.7, 0.2, 0.1	154	16.7
0.5, 0.2, 0.1 × 3	114	11.0
0.1 × 10	100	6.0

again neither J_d^m nor K_m can be estimated with any degree of confidence, regardless of the distribution of the transport sites along the villus.

Similar limitations are apparent in the use of the plot of C_1/J_d versus C_1 when the transport sites are distributed along the villus (THOMSON 1979 d). When the UWL resistance and K_m are similar over each villus site and when the resistance of the unstirred layer is low, varying the distribution of the transport sites along the villus has little effect on either the slope or the intercept (Fig. 47). When the resistance of the unstirred layer is high, redistributing the transport sites from the tip of the villus (f_n=0.7, 0.2, 0.1) was associated with an upward displacement of the line, with a marked change in the slope (154 compared with 118 nmol/100 mg/min), but with little change in the y-axis intercept (Fig. 47 a, curves A and B, high UWL resistance). However, when the sites were distributed more distally along the villus (F_n=0.5, 0.2, 0.1 × 3 and f_n=0.1 × 10), the line was displaced downwards (Fig. 47 a, curves C and D, high UWL resistance), and the apparent maximal transport rates were 114 and 100 nmol/100 g/min, respectively (Table 7), close to the assigned value of 100 nmol/100 mg/min. The change in the distribution of transport sites from the upper portion of the villus (f_n=1 and f_n=0.7, 0.2, 0.1) to a distribution along the entire villus (f_n=0.1 × 10) was associated with a decline in K_m^* from 16.7 to 6.0 mM (Table 7) and a diminution of the discrepancy between K_m^* and K_m. Thus, shifting the distribution of transport sites towards the base of the villus has no effect on the estimate of J_d^{m*} and K_m^* when the resistance of the UWL is low. However, when UWL resistance is high, J_d^{m*} initially increases and then decreases to approach the value of the true J_d^m; as the transport sites became distributed more evenly towards the base of the villus, the value of K_m^* falls and approaches the value of K_m.

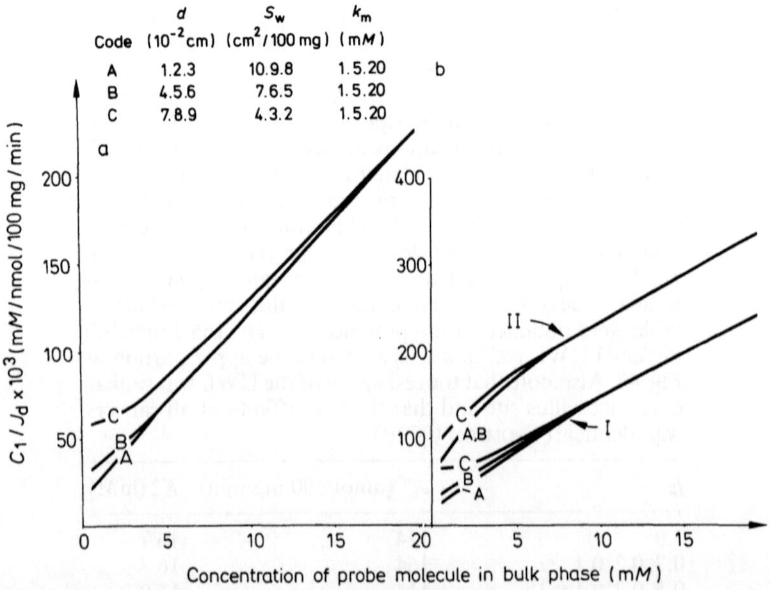

Fig. 48a, b. Theoretical effect of varying distribution of transport sites along villus f_n, effective resistance offered by UWL, and K_m of carriers in different segments of villus, on K_m^* and J_d^{m*}, estimated using the plot of C_1/J_d versus C_1. This diagram illustrates manner in which kinetics of active transport are affected by changes in f_n, K_m^n, d^n, and S_w^n. **a** 70% of total carrier transport sites were located in first villus segment ($f_{n1}=0.7$), 20% were in second segment ($f_{n2}=0.2$), and 10% were in third segment ($f_{n3}=0.1$); **b I** (lower curves) 50% of active transport sites were located in first segment ($f_{n1}=0.5$), 20% in second segment ($f_{n2}=0.2$), and 10% in third, fourth, and fifth segments ($f_{n3}=0.1$, $f_{n4}=0.1$, $f_{n5}=0.1$); **b II** (upper curves) 10% of carrier transport sites were located in each of 10 segments ($f_{n1}=0.1$, $f_{n2}=0.1, \ldots, f_{n10}=0.1$), and total flux was obtained from sum of fluxes occurring over each segment of villus. In curve *A*, $K_m^{n1}=1$, $K_m^{n2}=5$, and $K_m^{n3-10}=20$ m*M*; $d^{n1}=10^{-2}$, $d^{n2}=2 \times 10^{-2}$, and $d^{n3-10}=3 \times 10^{-2}$ cm; $S_w^{n1}=10$, $S_w^{n2}=9$, and $S_w^{n3-10}=8$ cm^2/100 mg. In curves *B*, $K_m^{n1}=1$, $K_m^{n2}=5$, and $K_m^{n3-10}=20$ m*M*; $d^{n1}=4 \times 10^{-2}$, $d^{n2}=5 \times 10^{-2}$, and $d^{n3-10}=6 \times 10^{-2}$ cm; $S_w^{n1}=7$, $S_w^{n2}=6$, $S_w^{n3}=5$ cm^2/100 mg. In curves *C*, $K_m^{n1}=1$, $K_m^{n2}=5$, and $K_m^{n3-10}=20$ m*M*; $d^{n1}=7 \times 10^{-2}$, $d^{n2}=8 \times 10^{-2}$, and $d^{n3}=9 \times 10^{-2}$ cm; $S_w^{n1}=4$, $S_w^{n2}=3$ and $S^{n3-10m}=2$ cm^2/100 mg. In these calculations, J_d^m was 100 nmol/100 mg/min and *D* was 30 $\times 10^{-5}$ cm^2/min. THOMSON (1979b)

If the resistance of the unstirred layer overlying each transport site is varied with increasing resistance towards the base of the villus and the least resistance at the tip of the villus, the slope of the linear portion of the relationship of C_1/J_d and C_1 is relatively unchanged, but the *y*-axis intercept is drawn upward (Fig. 48). Thus, the *y*-axis intercept was displaced upward with increasing resistance of the UWL, both when the transport sites were located at the tip of the villus (Fig. 48 a) and when they were distributed more evenly toward the crypt (Fig. 48 b).

In contrast, when the transport sites are distributed over the upper 30% of the villus ($f_n=0.7$, 0.2, 0.1), when the K_m is less for transport sites over the tip compared with those closer to the crypt and when the resistance of the unstirred layer overlying the distal sites is greater than over the tip, then the slope of the relation

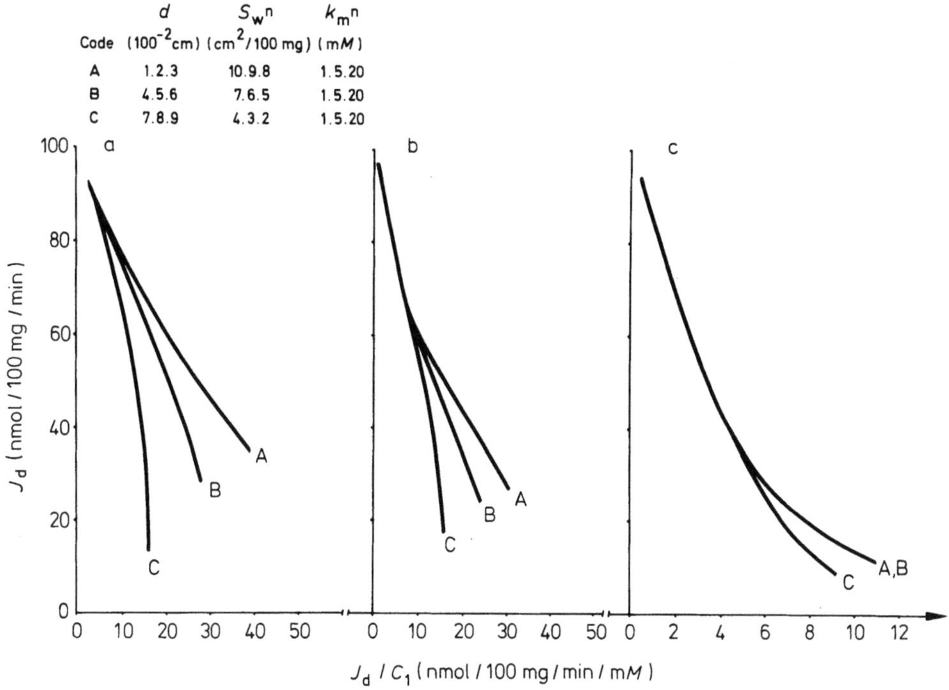

Fig. 49a-c. Theoretical effect of varying the distribution of transport sites along the villus, the effective resistance offered by the UWL, and K_m of the carriers in the difference segments of the villus, on K_m^* and J_d^{m*}, estimated from the relationship between J_d and J_d/C_1. This diagram illustrates the manner in which the kinetics of active transport are affected by changes in f_n, K_m^n, d^n, and S_w^n. In contrast with Fig. 46, the value of both K_m and the effective thickness and surface area of the UWL overlying the different villus segments was varied. **a** 70% of the total carrier transport sites were located in the first villus segment ($f_{n1}=0.7$); 20% were in the second segment ($f_{n2}=0.2$), and 10% were in the third segment ($f_{n3}=0.1$); **b** 50% of the transport sites were located in the first segment ($f_{n1}=0.5$), 20% in the second segment ($f_{n2}=0.2$), and 10% in the third, fourth, and fifth segments ($f_{n3}=0.1$, $f_{n4}=0.1$, $f_{n5}=0.1$); **c** 10% of the carrier transport sites were located in each of the ten segments ($f_{n1}=0.1$, $f_{n2}=0.1, \ldots, f_{n10}=0.1$) and the total flux was obtained from the sum of the fluxes occurring over each segment of the villus. In curves *A*, $K_m^{n1}=1$, $K_m^{n2}=5$, and $K_m^{n3-10}=20\,mM$; $d^{n1}=10^{-2}$, $d^{n2}=2\times10^{-2}$, and $d^{n3-10}=3\times10^{-2}$cm; $S_w^{n1}=10$, $S_w^{n2}=9$, and $S_w^{n3-10}=8\,cm^2/100\,mg$. In curves *B*, $K_m^{n1}=1$, $K_m^{n2}=5$, and $K_m^{n3-10}=20\,mM$; $d^{n1}=4\times10^{-2}$, $d^{n2}=5\times10^{-2}$, and $d^{n3-10}=6\times10^{-2}$cm; $S_w^{n1}=7$, $S_w^{n2}=6$, and $S_w^{n3-10}=5\,cm^2/100\,mg$. In curves *C*, $K_m^{n1}=1$, $K_m^{n2}=5$, and $K_m^{n3-10}=20\,mM$; $d^{n1}=7\times10^{-2}$, $d^{n2}=8\times10^{-2}$, and $d^{n3}=9\times10^{-2}$cm; $S_w^{n1}=4$, $S_w^{n2}=3$, and $S_w^{n3-10}=2\,cm^2/100\,mg$. In these calculations J_d^m was 100 nmol/100 mg/min. Note that the relationship between J_d and J_d/C_1 was linear (**a**, curve *B*), curvilinear downwards (**a**, curves *B* and *C*; **b**, curve *C*), or curvilinear upwards (**b**, curves *A* and *B*; **c**, curves *A–C*), depending upon the values assigned to f_n, d^n and S_w^n. THOMSON (1979c)

between C_1/J_d and C_1 is influenced, and the *y*-axis is drawn sharply upwards (Fig. 48 a, curve C).

The shape of the line indicating the relationship between C_1/J_d and C_1 is influenced by the distribution of the transport sites. Changing the distribution of the transport sites and the resistance of the unstirred layer over the different villus sites causes an upward displacement of this relationship from linearity (Fig. 47a and b), but concurrent change in K_m^n as well as f_n, d^n, and S_w^n may be associated with a downward displacement of this relationship from linearity (Fig. 48b, curves A and B). Thus, the finding of a downward deviation from linearity suggests: the transport sites are distributed along the villus, the affinity constant of the carrier changes at the different villus sites, and the resistance of the UWL changes over the different villus sites, becoming greater towards the base of the villus.

If specific conditions are chosen when the resistance of the unstirred layer is known to be low, then the shape of the relationship between J_d and J_d/C_1 or C_1/J_d may provide useful information as to the characteristics of the membrane carriers at different sites along the villus. Assuming first that the appropriate corrections have been made for the passive component, then an upward deviation of the relationship between J_d and J_d/C_1 (Fig. 49a, b, c, curves A) or a downward displacement of the y-axis intercept of C_1/J_d versus C_1 (Fig. 48b), occurs only when the value of the true affinity constant varies at different sites along the villus, and when the resistance of the unstirred layers over each villus segment also varies. This relationship is never seen when just the distribution of the transport sites along the villus is changed or when the resistance of the unstirred layer overlying each villus segment is altered.

γ) Experimental Demonstration of the Functional Heterogeneity of the Villus. A previously validated in vitro technique was employed to determine the unidirectional flux rate of glucose, galactose, 3-*O*-methylglucose, and fructose into the rabbit jejunum under carefully defined conditions of stirring of the bulk phase known to yield different values for the effective resistance of the UWL. For each monosaccharide, uptake is much greater when the resistance of the UWL is low than when high (Fig. 50). The maximal transport rate J_d^m of glucose was half as large as J_d^m of galactose and 3-*O*-methylglucose, and was twice as great as the J_d^m of fructose (Fig. 51). The apparent affinity constant, K_m^*, of glucose is less than that of fructose, which was lower than the K_m^* of galactose and 3-*O*-methylglucose (see Fig. 51). The use of the Lineweaver–Burk double-reciprocal plot is associated with an overestimation of both J_d^m and K_m^* (Table 8). This discrepancy between the true and apparent values of the kinetic constants is much greater for lower than for higher values of J_d^m and K_m^*; variations in the resistance of the unstirred layer influence the magnitude and direction of the discrepancy. The apparent passive permeability coefficient is similar for each sugar, but because of the different values of J_d^m, passive permeation contributes relatively more to the uptake of glucose and fructose than of galactose or 3-*O*-methylglucose. Under conditions of high unstirred layer resistance, differences in uptake rates of the sugars are due to differences in their J_d^m rather than their K_m^*.

Despite the serious limitations of the use of the three "linear" transformations of the Michaelis–Menten equation to estimate the quantity of the kinetic constants, they do provide the means to assign certain qualitative interpretations to transport processes. For example, when the resistance of the UWL is high and adequate corrections have been made for the contribution of passive permeation, the relationship between C_1/J_d and C_1 is linear over a wide range of values of C_1,

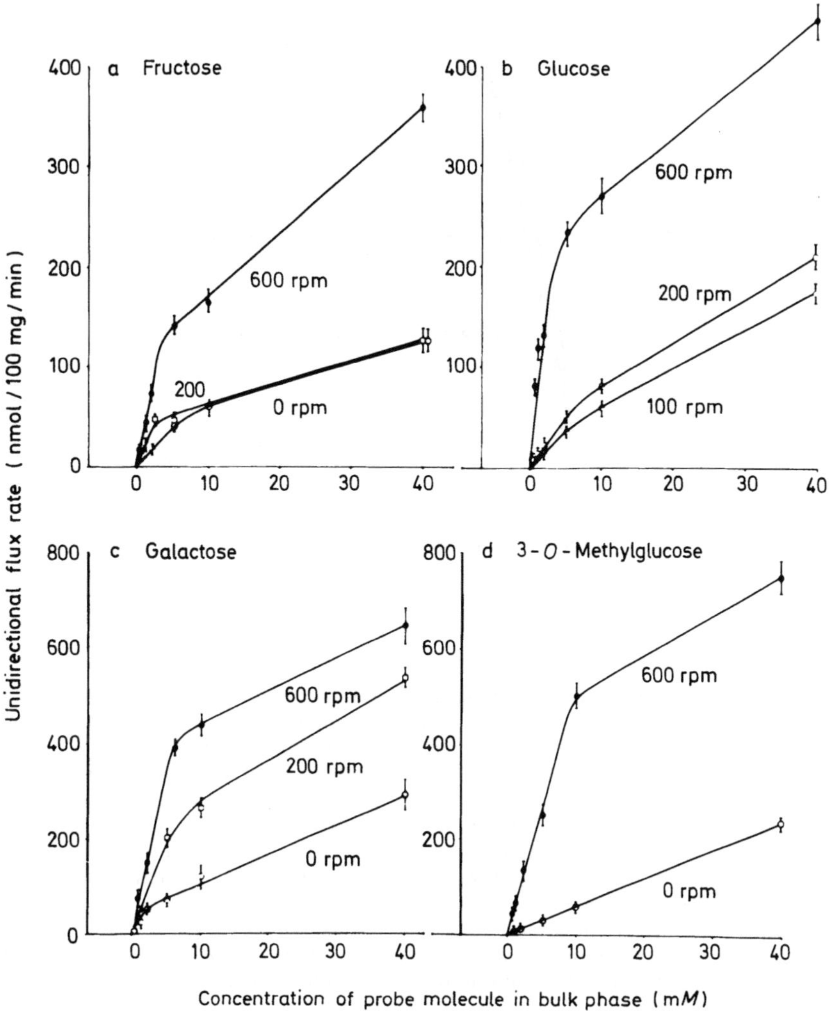

Fig. 50a-d. Unidirectional flux rates of four monosaccharides into rabbit jejunum under conditions selected to yield low, intermediate, and high effective resistance of the UWL. THOMSON (1979d)

(see Fig. 47a). At lower values of C_1, however, the relationship deviates either upward or downward from an extension of the linear portion of the line obtained at higher values C_1. Upward deviation, with a higher value of the y-axis intercept, is provided by several conditions, including increasing resistance of the unstirred layer, increasing values of K_m, decreasing values of J_d^m, or distribution of most of the transport sites along the upper portion of the villus. For theoretical purposes, the villus is not considered as a homogeneous unit, since the effective resistance of the unstirred layer may vary at different sites along the villus, and since the transport characteristics of the mucosal cells at different points along the villus may in fact vary. Downward displacement of the relationship between C_1/J_d and

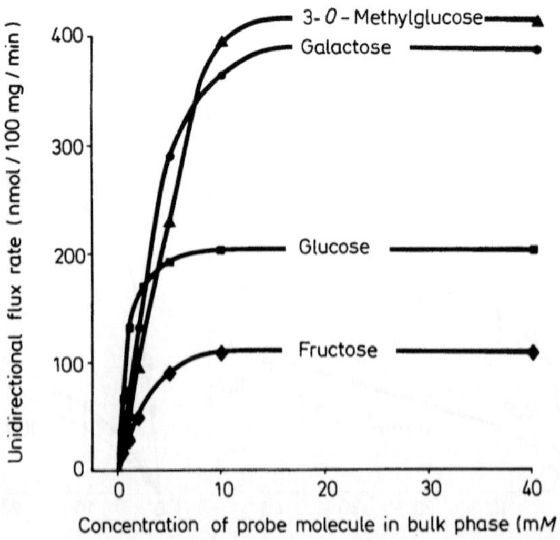

Fig. 51. Comparison of unidirectional flux rates of four monosaccharides into rabbit jejunum under conditions selected to yield low effective resistance of the UWL with correction of the experimental data for the contribution of the passive component. THOMSON (1979d)

Table 8. Kinetic constants for the in vitro unidirectional flux rate of glucose, galactose, 3-*O*-methylglucose, and fructose into rabbit jejunum; mean values ± standard error. The bulk phase containing the monosaccharide probe molecules was stirred at 600, 200, or 0 rpm; the magnitude of the apparent passive permeability coefficient P^*, maximal transport rate J_d^m and apparent Michaelis affinity constant K_m for the 200 rpm group are not shown in this table, but their values are intermediate between those obtained at 600 and 0 rpm. The experimental data used to obtain these results are shown in Fig. 51. The values for the maximal transport rate were obtained at 600 rpm, and were assumed to represent an acceptable approximation of the true maximal transport rate of the appropriate hexose carrier (THOMSON 1979d)

Monosaccharide probe	Apparent passive permeability coefficient P^* (nmol/100 mg/min/m*M*)		Maximal transport rate, J_d^m (nmol/100 mg/min)	Apparent Michaelis affinity constant K_m^* (m*M*)	
	600 rpm	0 rpm		600 rpm	0 rpm
Glucose	5.9±0.5	3.7±0.3	206±20	0.8±0.1	>40
Galactose	6.6±0.4	5.7±0.5	388±39	3.0±0.2	>40
3-*O*-Methylglucose	7.0±0.6	5.6±0.5	417±40	4.3±0.3	>40
Fructose	6.7±0.5	2.5±0.3	107±11	1.7±0.2	>40

C_1 can only be achieved when three conditions prevail together: when the transport sites are distributed along the villus, when the effective unstirred layer resistance varies along the villus, and when the affinity constant of the transport sites near the base of the villus is higher than the transport sites at the villus tip (Fig. 48b). It must be emphasized that the relationship between C_1/J_d and C_1 at high values of unstirred layer resistance (0 rpm) is clearly different for glucose on the one hand, and galactose and 3-*O*-methylglucose on the other (Fig. 52): there is up-

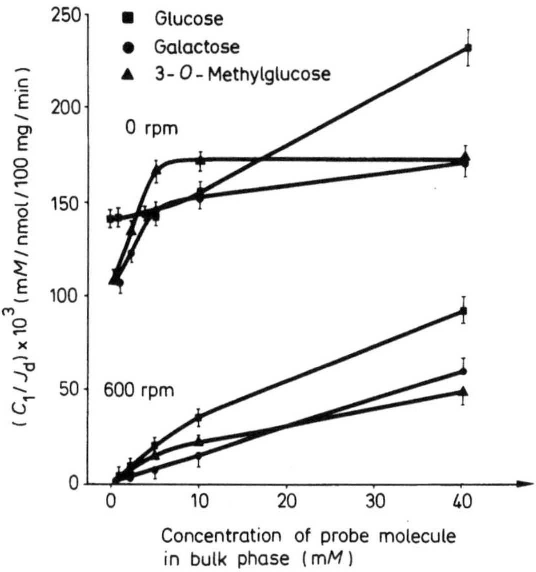

Fig. 52. Estimation of kinetic constants of intestinal transport of three monosaccharides, using the Eadie-Hofstee plot, under conditions selected to yield variable effective resistance of the UWL. The experimental data shown in Fig. 51 are redrawn according to the plot of C_1/J_d versus C_1, where C_1 is the concentration of the monosaccharide probe molecule in the bulk phase, and J_d is the unidirectional flux rate. THOMSON (1979d)

ward deviation from the extension of the linear portion of the relationship between C_1/J_d and C_1 for glucose obtained at higher values of C_1, and downward deviation for galactose and 3-*O*-methylglucose. Theoretical considerations have suggested that, assuming adequate correction for the contribution of passive permeation, this qualitative relationship between C_1/J_d and C_1 is compatible with the suggestion that the distribution of transport sites along the villus is different for glucose than for galactose and 3-*O*-methylglucose: glucose transport is likely to occur near the tips of the villus, whereas the transport of galactose and 3-*O*-methylglucose is likely to occur along the length of the villus, and the affinity constants are likely to be lower at the tip of the villus than towards the base.

Thus, it is proposed that there are multiple or heterogeneous intestinal carriers for glucose, galactose, and 3-*O*-methylglucose in the jejunum of the rabbit, and that the glucose carriers are predominantly near the tip of the villus, whereas those for galactose and 3-*O*-methylglucose are located along the entire villus and k_m of their carriers at the tip of the villus is lower than K_m towards the base of the villus.

f) The Importance of the Assessment of the Contribution of Passive Permeation to Carrier-Mediated Transport

To assess the magnitude of the kinetic constants of carrier-mediated transport, it is first necessary to assess the magnitude of passive permeation. The apparent passive permeability coefficient of glucose may be estimated using a number of techniques such as: the slope of the glucose concentration curve at high values of C_1, the rate of uptake J_d of L-glucose, or J_d of D-glucose at 4 °C. These values closely agree and were assumed to represent the passive permeation of glucose into the rabbit jejunum. However, these values are likely to be less than the true permeability coefficient of the intestine to glucose, since passive permeation is also influenced by the effective resistance of the unstirred layer. This arises from the difference in the concentration of the probe molecule in the bulk phase in the intestinal lumen C_1, and the concentration at the aqueous–membrane interface C_2. The value of C_2 can be estimated from Eq. (15).

Substituting the appropriate values of C_1, J_d, D, and the published values of d and S_w for rabbit jejunum stirred at 600 rpm, the value of C_2 for glucose may be shown to be 0.9 mM, when C_1 is 1 mM. Thus, the true value of the passive permeability coefficient of glucose is greater than the apparent value of 5.9 nmol/100 mg/mM (P^*/C_1), and is estimated to be 6.6 nmol/100 mg/min (P^*/C_2). The apparent passive permeability coefficients of galactose, 3-O-methylglucose, and fructose were estimated from the slope of the linear portion of the concentration curve at high values of substrate concentration (see Fig. 50). The rationale and validity of this approach is as follows: the total rate of absorption of a probe molecule which is transported by both active and passive processes is

$$J = \frac{J^m C_2}{K_m + C_2} + PC_2 . \qquad (46)$$

When $C_2 \gg K_m$, J becomes approximately proportional to J^m. For values of C_2 several times greater than K_m, the value of J/J^m approaches unity, i.e., further increases in C_2 produce further increases in J by a factor PC_2, the contribution of passive permeation. The estimated values of the apparent affinity constants of glucose, galactose, and 3-O-methylglucose were 0.8, 3.0, and 4.3 mM, respectively (Table 8). Although these K_m^* values were estimated under conditions selected to minimize the effect of the unstirred layer, the resistance of the unstirred layer was still of sufficient magnitude to allow for a small overestimation of the true affinity constants. Thus the true affinity constants of these hexoses is less than the values given in Table 8, and at the bulk phase concentrations of 10–40 mM, the value of C_2 would indeed be much greater than the value of K_m ($C_2 \gg K_m$), further uptake would be approximately proportional to J_d^m, and the slope of the concentration curves between 10 and 40 mM would therefore represent a valid estimate of passive permeation PC_2.

An assessment of the adequacy of the correction for passive permeation can be made from inspection of the slope of the relationship between J_d and J_d/C_1 obtained under conditions of low unstirred layer resistance (Fig. 53). Theoretical considerations have shown that this complex curvilinear relationship is achieved only when the experimental values contain a passive component. After correction for this component the shape of the relationship changes (Fig. 53b). This new form is compatible with adequate correction for passive permeation. Although small variations are present between the mean values of the apparent passive permeability coefficients for the four hexoses obtained when the bulk phase was stirred at 600 rpm (Table 8), these differences are small and statistically insignificant ($P > 0.05$), and it is likely that these values represent a reasonable approximation

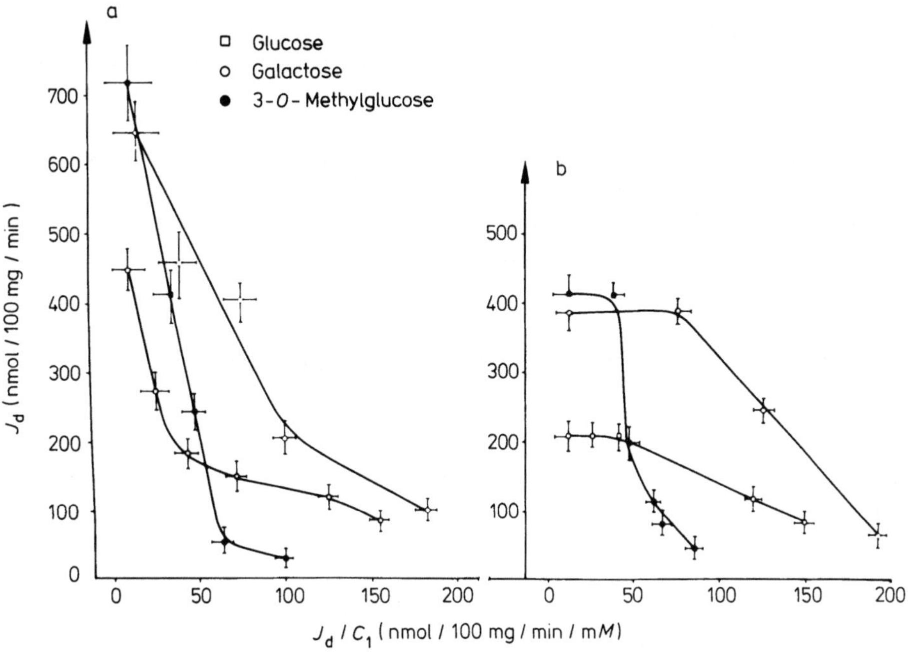

Fig. 53a, b. Estimation of kinetic constants of intestinal transport of three monosaccharides using the plot of J_d versus J_d/C_1, both uncorrected (**a**) and corrected (**b**) for passive permeation, under conditions selected to yield low effective resistance of the UWL. The unidirectional flux rate is represented by J_d, and C_1 is the concentration of the probe molecule in the bulk phase. The experimental data shown in Fig. 50 are redrawn according to the plot of J_d versus J_d/C_1. THOMSON (1979d)

of the true passive permeability coefficient and therefore of the contribution of passive permeation under conditions of low unstirred layer resistance.

The apparent passive permeability coefficients of the hexoses were lower when the bulk phase was instirred (see Table 8). The estimated K_m^* of each monosaccharide obtained when unstirred layer resistance was high exceeded 40 m*M*, and thus the slope of the line between 10 and 40 m*M* at 0 rpm does not represent passive permeation alone, but a combination of passive and carrier-mediated transport. Thus, these apparent passive permeability coefficients for the four monosaccharides obtained at 0 rpm reflect neither the quantitative nor qualitative aspects of passive membrane permeability towards the sugars. What is the explanation for the lower values for the apparent permeability coefficients of glucose and fructose than of galactose and 3-*O*-methylglucose, under conditions of high unstirred layer reistance? When the bulk phase is unstirred, the value of the apparent affinity constant of each hexose is greatly increased (Table 8), and uptake becomes more dependent upon the values of J_d^m and P (Eq. 49). Since the value of the apparent permeability coefficient of the hexoses is similar when unstirred layer resistance is low (Table 8), the most likely explanation for the higher rates of uptake of galactose and 3-*O*-methylglucose than of glucose and fructose under conditions of high unstirred layer resistance is the much larger values of their maximal transport rates (388 and 417 versus 206 and 107 nmol/100 mg/min, respectively, Table 8). Thus, the values of the apparent passive permeability coefficients estimated under conditions of high unstirred layer resistance reflect the effective resistance of the unstirred layer, the maximal transport rate, as well as the true passive permeability coefficient.

In summary, the apparent passive permeability coefficients of hexoses cannot be accurately estimated in the presence of a UWL of significant dimensions, and the magnitudes of K_m^* and J_d^m cannot be estimated until adequate correction has been made for the contribution of the passive permeation.

III. Permeation of Weak Electrolytes: Acid Microclimate

Nonionic diffusion was proposed to explain ionic fluxes that were neither exclusively determined by electrochemical PD nor directly coupled to cellular metabolism. According to this hypothesis, the membrane is essentially impermeable to the dissociated from of certain weak acids and bases (HOGBEN 1970, 1959; SCHANKER 1962; SCHANKER et al. 1957, 1958; SHORE et al. 1957) such as drugs, and they cross the membrane in their undissociated form. This mechanism postulates the association between an anion and a cation in the external solution on one side of the membrane. The resulting complex then crosses the membrane, enters the solution on the opposite side and dissociates to the original anion and cation. The net effect of nonionic diffusion is eventual transfer of ionized compounds from one side of a membrane to the other; however, it is the undissociated form, and not the ionic, that actually crosses the membrane. Thus, nonionic diffusion accounts for the situation in which movement of a charged species is not dependent on the electrical PD, but is highly dependent on the hydrogen ion concentration. The transported substances crosses the membrane as a complex, but the complex is formed in the external solution.

The acid–base metabolism of the jejunum is characterized by luminal acidification, but in the ileal region the secretion of bicarbonate is associated with luminal alkalinization (BLAIR et al. 1972, 1975; BLAIR and MATTY 1974; JACKSON 1972; JACKSON et al. 1970, 1978; JACKSON and MORGAN 1975). This would favor the absorption of weak acids in the jejunum, and weak bases in the ileum. It has been proposed that this process of luminal acidification maintains the surface of the proximal jejunum at a pH not in equilibrium with the pH of the incubation medium in vitro and the luminal pH in vivo (see also Chap. 20). This acid microclimate was invoked to explain the fact that the pH for maximum drug absorption often did not correspond with the pH for maximum concentration of the respective nonionized form (HOGBEN et al. 1959; LUCAS et al. 1978) as calculated by using the pH of the incubation buffer. These workers argued that weak electrolytes must be confronted with a region of acid pH lower than the measurable luminal pH if transfer were to be explained solely by nonionic diffusion. Experiments with pH microelectrodes (BLAIR et al. 1972, 1975; BLAIR and MATTY 1974; LUCAS et al. 1975, 1976, 1978; LUCAS and BLAIR 1978) have demonstrated that such a region of acid pH exists, having a value of at least 5.5 when the bulk phase pH is 7.4. Other studies have shown a low surface pH in humans by means of biopsy samples from the proximal jejunum (LUCAS et al. 1978) and alterations in the pH of this microclimate have been reported in celiac and Crohn's disease (LUCAS et al. 1978).

It is suggested that a weak electrolyte penetrates the cellular compartment in the nonionized form, and that the influx of a weak electrolyte is proportional to the concentration of its nonionized form in the surface fluid layer. Weak acids and weak bases behave oppositely with respect to the influence of pH on the distribution between ionized and nonionized forms. If the pH in the surface fluid layers is lower than that in the bulk phase, the distribution of a weak acid will be shifted towards the nonionized form and the influx will be enhanced, but the distribution of a weak base will favor the ionized form and depress influx. This means that permeability values calculated from observed influxes and nonionized concentration in the bulk phase will be exaggerated in the case of a weak acid and underestimated in the case of a weak base. Conversely, if the pH in the surface fluid layer is greater than that of the bulk phase, the permeabilities of weak bases will be overestimated and those of weak acids will be depressed. With a microclimate pH of 5.0, accelerated transfer of weak acids can be envisaged without carriers or specific biochemical pathways other than that of a hydrogen ion gradient cross the luminal cell wall. The production of hydrogen ions at the luminal enterocyte membrane causes a decreased pH to be found at the gut surface, allowing electrolytes that form neutral species at this pH to diffuse across the membrane as the neutral form.

The mechanism responsible for this acid microclimate is unknown. The lower surface pH in the rat jejunum becomes more neutral in the ileum and is less acidic in the presence of 10 m*M* mucosal aminophylline or ouabain and in the absence of added 10 m*M* glucose. Acidification is not a product of the submucosal layers, but of structurally intact mucosal cells and was unaccounted for by lactic acid and pyruvic acid appearance. The surface pH was altered by removal of sodium, or transiently by the removal of potassium and was dependent on aerobic conditions (LUCAS et al. 1978).

However, the studies of JACKSON et al. (1978) do not support the concept of a microclimate of distinctive pH at the epithelial surface; indeed, the UWL may be responsible for the deviations from the pH partition hypothesis, as applied to weak electrolyte transfer in the intestine. Their experiments suggested that the intestinal transport of weak electrolytes is influenced by a region of distinctive pH at the luminal surface of the epithelium. The determinations of weak electrolyte permeation in the intestine included the resistance of the UWL, the degree of ionization of the weak electrolyte at the cell surface, and the cellular permeability to the nonionized weak electrolyte. A uniform set of permeability data, including both weak acids and weak bases was obtained only when it was assumed that the pH in the surface fluid layer was equal to that in the bulk phase, and these studies did not support the concept of a microclimate of distinctive pH at the epithelial surface as a determinant of weak electrolyte transport.

The need to postulate the existence of an acid microclimate in the jejunum is no longer necessary once the effect of the UWL on the uptake of weak electrolytes has been taken into account. JACKSON et al. (1978) have shown that:

$$J_{\mathrm{d}} = \frac{P_{\mathrm{d}} C_2}{1 + 10^{\sigma^2}}, \tag{47}$$

where σ^2 reflects the distribution of the weak electrolyte between the ionized and nonionized forms at the aqueous–membrane interface.

$$\sigma^2 = \mathrm{pH}_2 - \mathrm{p}K_\mathrm{a} \tag{48}$$

for a weak acid, and for a weak base

$$\sigma^2 = \mathrm{p}K_\mathrm{a} - \mathrm{pH}_2 \,. \tag{49}$$

In these expressions, pH_2 refers to the pH value of the fluid layer at the epithelial surface and $\mathrm{p}K_\mathrm{a}$ is the logarithm of the reciprocal of the dissociation constant for the weak electrolyte. C_2 is the total concentration (ionized and nonionized) of the weak electrolyte at the aqueous–membrane interface. When a surface area term for the UWL is included, then

$$C_2 = \frac{C_1}{1 + \left[\dfrac{P_\mathrm{d} d}{DS_\mathrm{w}(1+10^{\sigma^2})}\right]} \tag{50}$$

and

$$J_\mathrm{d} = \frac{C_1}{\left[\dfrac{(1+10^{\sigma^2})}{P_\mathrm{d}} + \dfrac{d}{DS_\mathrm{w}}\right]} \tag{51}$$

When σ^2 is positive and greater than unity, the weak electrolyte exists mainly in the ionized form, and small or negative values of σ^2 indicate small degrees of ionization. Thus, the term $(1+10^{\sigma^2})/P_\mathrm{d}$ reflects the interaction between the permeability of the epithelial cells to the nonionized form of the weak electrolyte and the degree of ionization of the compound at the epithelial surface as determinants of the movement of weak electrolyte through the epithelial cell membrane. The component of d/DS_w represents the influence of the UWL and the second component $(1+10^{\sigma^2})/P_\mathrm{d}$ is concerned with the movement of weak electrolytes into the epithelial cells.

When $(1+10^{\sigma^2})Pd \gg d/DS_\mathrm{w}$, the rate-limiting step in the influx process is the movement of the weak electrolyte from the surface fluid layer into the epithelial cells. The characteristics of weak electrolyte molecules that may contribute to this situation include poorly permeant nonionized forms (low values of P_d) and high degrees of ionization in the surface fluid layer (large, positive values of σ^2). In the second extreme case the rate-limiting step is the diffusion of weak electrolyte through the UWL. This situation is described by the relation $(1+10^{\sigma^2})P_\mathrm{d} \ll d/DS_\mathrm{w}$ which indicates that the influx of weak electrolytes may be limited by the UWL when the nonionized forms are highly permeant (high values of P_d), or are poorly ionized in the surface fluid layer (small or negative values of σ^2). Values of σ^2 will be larger for acids of low $\mathrm{p}K_\mathrm{a}$, such as fatty acids C2:0–C10:0, with a $\mathrm{p}K_\mathrm{a}$ of 4.75–4.90 respectively. This means that the term $(1+10^{\sigma^2})/P_\mathrm{d}$ may change by several orders of magnitude with variations in acidic strength, and that the influxes of highly ionized weak electrolytes are less likely to be restricted by diffusion in the surface fluid layer than are the influxes of poorly ionized compounds.

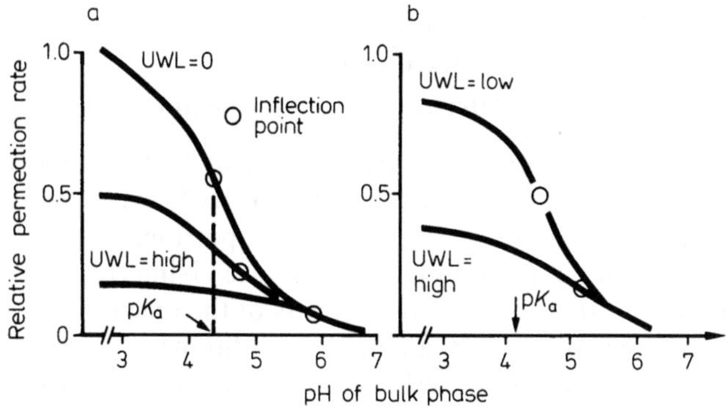

Fig. 54a, b. Permeation of weak acid and unstirred layer. **a** theoretical curves for the dependence of the relative permeation rate on the pH of the bulk phase, and on the effective resistance of the UWL. When the effective resistance of the UWL is zero, the inflection point coincides with the pK_a value, but with increasing effective resistance of the UWL, the inflection point is shifted to the right; **b** experimental results for the permeation of phenylbutazone through a polydimethylsiloxane membrane at different stirring rates WINNE (1978)

The inflection point of a pH absorption curve may be affected by the resistance of the UWL. When the permeation rate of a weak electrolyte is plotted versus the bulk phase pH, usually a sigmoidal curve is obtained (Fig. 54). In the absence of an effective unstirred layer the inflection point of the so-called ph absorption curve is situated at the pH value equal to the pK_a of the permeating substance in agreement with the pH partition theory. According to WINNE (1976)

$$pH_{IP} = pK_a + \log_{10}(1 + P/P_{UL}) \quad (52)$$

where pH_{IP} is the pH of the inflection point, P is the permeability of the membrane, and P_{UL} is the permeability of the UWL; the sign will be positive for weak acids, and negative for weak bases. Several experimental studies have confirmed these theoretical predictions: when the resistance of the UWL is increased, permeation rate is reduced and the inflection point is shifted to the right for an acid and to the left for a base (KAKEMIE et al. 1969; Lôvering and BLACK 1974; SUZUKI et al. 1970a, b; WINNE 1977; WINNE et al. 1979). An example of the curve shift is shown in Fig. 54b.

Thus, the apparent failure of the pH partition theory to explain the rates of permeation of weak electrolytes through the intestinal membrane may be due to the effect of the UWL. While it is not necessary further to invoke the explanation of an acid microclimate to explain the permeation rates of these solutes, direct measurements of the surface pH of the intestine of animals and humans have demonstrated a pH differential between the bulk phase and the membrane surface. It is possible that the more acid pH is arising from the intervillous spaces which are probably unnecessary for the absorption of the highly permeant weak electrolytes, thereby providing a potential explanation for the presence of the lower pH, but its relative lack of functional importance.

IV. Effect of Volume Flow, "Sweeping Away" Effects, and Unstirred Layers on the Estimation of Effective Osmotic Pressure Across a Membrane

NERNST 1904, quoted by ANDREOLI and TRAUTMAN 1979) assumed that d was a constant for a given fluid motion, but current theory (LEVICH 1962) predicts that the thickness of a diffusion layer is inversely proportional to the square root of the velocity at which liquid flows past the surface giving rise to the UWL. This raises the possibility that the effective tickness of the unstirred layer may not be identical for different substances, and under conditions of varying rates of water flow. Even in the absence of a UWL, the absorption of water from the intestine may facilitate the movement of solutes across the intestinal mucosa. With "solvent drag" the solutes are in effect caught in the moving stream of water and swept through the pores of the intestinal cells. The extent to which solvent flow across a membrane will promote the net movement of a given solute is directly related to the reflection coefficient of that solute, (KEDEM 1961; KEDEM and KATCHALSKY 1961; KEDEM and ESSIG 1965)

$$J_{ds} = J_v C_2 (1-\sigma), \tag{53}$$

where J_{ds} is the rate of movement of solute due to solvent drag; J_v is the rate of movement of the solvent, which is usually water in biologic systems; C_2 is the concentration of the solute at the aqueous–membrane interface; and σ is the reflection coefficient of the solute. Equation (53) applies when there is no UWL. In the presence of a UWL the value of C_2 is substituted from Eq. (15), and

$$J_{ds} = J_v \left(C_1 - \frac{J_{ds} d}{D S_w} \right) (1-\sigma). \tag{54}$$

If the reflection coefficient is low, or if the resistance of the UWL is small, then the movement of solvent will have a large solvent drag effect on the movement of solute, whereas if σ is large, solvent drag will have little effect; if the resistance of the UWL is high, then the magnitude of solvent drag will be greatly underestimated. Similarly, in the presence of a high resistance of the UWL, experimental estimates of σ will be grossly underestimated.

An additional unstirred layer effect that must concern us is the so-called sweeping away effect: water flow across a membrane tends to concentrate solute on one side of the membrane, and to dilute the solution on the other side. Consider the example (Fig. 55) in which sucrose in a NaCl-containing buffer has been added to the mucosal side of the membrane: osmotic water flow towards the mucosal solution will be proportional to the effective osmotic pressure exerted by the sucrose. The magnitude of the osmotic pressure exerted by sucrose will be less than the value in the bulk phase, because of the drop in the concentration of sucrose across the UWL. The osmotic pressure gradient across the membrane due to sucrose will be given by $\Delta\Pi_2$ (sucrose), the osmotic pressure of sucrose at the aqueous–membrane interface, rather than by the osmotic pressure of sucrose in the bulk phase. However, another factor which affects the magnitude of the effective concentration gradient across the membrane is the flow of water across the membrane. Water flow tends to reduce the solute concentration gradient by con-

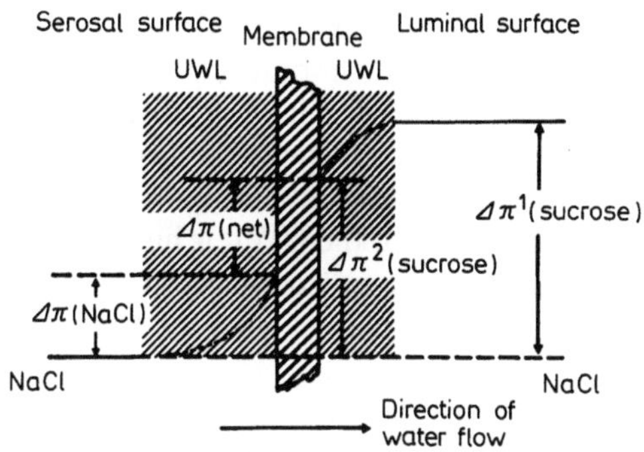

$\Delta\pi(\text{net}) = \Delta\pi^2(\text{sucrose} - \Delta\pi(\text{NaCl}))$

Fig. 55. Effect of volume flow, "sweeping away" effects, and unstirred layers on the estimation of effective osmotic pressure across a membrane

vectively enhancing the solute concentration in the unstirred layer on one side of the membrane and by depleting the solute concentration on the other side. The solute concentration adjacent to the membrane C_2 is related to the velocity of the water flow J_v by the equation

$$C_2 = C_2 \exp(\pm J_v d/DS_w), \tag{55}$$

where C_1 is the bulk phase concentration, d the unstirred layer thickness, and D the free diffusion coefficient. Thus in a leaky tissue where J_v is large, or where the resistance of the UWL is small, water flow could produce a large difference between C_2 and C_1. In this example (Fig. 55) the flow of water across the epithelium J_v will tend further to reduce the concentration of sucrose and NaCl concentration at the mucosal surface of the epithelial cell by the factor $\exp(-J_v d/DS_w)$, and this water flow will tend to enhance the solute concentration at the serosal face of the cell by a factor $\exp(J_v d/DS_w)$ (WRIGHT et al. 1972; WRIGHT and PRATHER 1970). This local salt concentration gradient across the epithelium $\Delta\Pi$(NaCl) will tend to produce a backflow of water across the epithelium, further reducing the osmotic pressure gradient across the mucosa. An unstirred layer of significant dimensions is present on the serosal surface (DIAMOND 1966; SMULDERS and WRIGHT 1971) and this will further retard the dissipation of the solute concentration gradient at the serosal surface which has been produced by water flow. Thus, in the steady state the effective osmotic pressure across the membrane, $\Delta\Pi$(Net) will be given by $\Delta\Pi_2$ (sucrose) $-\Delta\Pi$(NaCl) and will be very considerably less than the osmotic pressure of the sucrose added to the bulk phase, $\Delta\Pi_1$ (sucrose).

V. Membrane "Pores"

The net effect then of these unstirred layers and the sweeping away effect is markedly to reduce the effective osmotic pressure across the membrane. It has long been recognized that the osmotic pressure generated by a given solute across a membrane may be less than the calculated theoretical pressure (in Fig. 55, $\Delta\Pi$(Net) versus $\Delta\Pi_1$(Sucrose). The ratio of the observed osmotic pressure to the theoretical osmotic pressure is known as the reflection coefficient σ (STAVERMAN 1951). The reflection coefficient of membranes can range from unity for an impermeant solute to zero for a membrane unable to distinguish between solute and solvent. Thus, the value of σ reflects the permeability of the membrane to a given solute, as well as the two other major determinants, the effect of the UWL and of water flow; when the resistance of the UWL is high, σ will be low. Thus, in the presence of UWLs and water flow, a reflection coefficient less than unity does not necessarily accurately reflect the permeability of the membrane towards the solute.

Lipid-soluble solutes are absorbed in proportion to their lipid solubility. Since water-soluble molecules cannot readily dissolve in the lipid portion of the membrane, since they are absorbed in proportion to their molecular radius, and since their reflection coefficient is often greater than zero, the presence of water-filled "pores" in the membrane has been postulated. Indeed, the value of the reflection coefficient σ has been used to estimate the size of pores in membranes, including the intestine (LINDEMAN and SOLOMON 1962; SOLOMON 1960, 1968). For a solute that is as large as or larger than the water-filled pores, the effective and theoretical osmotic pressures will be equal, and the reflection coefficient will be unity. For solutes that are smaller than the "pore", the effective osmotic pressure will be less than the theoretical value and σ will fall between zero and unity. Similar measurements of the reflection coefficient σ, a parameter that characterizes the movement of a solute during bulk flow, suggest for erythrocyte membranes that certain nonelectrolyte substances may permeate through pores (GOLDSTEIN and SOLOMON 1960; RICH et al. 1967). However, the reflection coefficient data for the rabbit gallbladder do not require the assumption of pores (DIAMOND and WRIGHT 1969a, b). Similarly, DAINTY and GINZBURG (1963, 1964a, b) have concluded that there is nothing in their reflection coefficient data for the algal cells *Chara australis* and *Nitella translucens* that makes it necessary to assume pores. LIEB and STEIN (1969) concluded that there was no need to postulate the existence of aqueous pores in biologic membranes if their "sieve-like" properties could be explained by treating the membranes as a homologous polymer network. Indeed, DAINTY (1963) suggested that the demonstration of a reflection coefficient less than unity is not adequate evidence for the existence of pores. The complexity and potential pitfalls of explaining values of σ less than unity on the basis of membrane pores must be further emphasized to be appreciated (SMULDERS et al. 1972)

$$\sigma = 1 - \frac{w\bar{V}_s}{L_p} - f, \tag{56}$$

where w is the permeability coefficient, V_s is the partial molar volume of the solute, L_p is the hydraulic conductivity of the membrane, and f is the frictional interaction between solutes and water in the membrane. The value f is assumed to be zero. The value of w is related to the experimentally measured permeability of the solute

$$P = wRT \tag{57}$$

and

$$L_p = \frac{P_{H_2O} \cdot \bar{V}_{H_2O}}{RT}, \tag{58}$$

where P_{H_2O} is the measured permeability to water. By substitution into and rearrangement of Eqs. (56), (57), and (58)

$$\sigma = 1 - \frac{P_s \bar{V}_s}{P_{H_2O} \bar{V}_{H_2O}}. \tag{59}$$

Since the experimentally measured values P_s and P_{H_2O} are affected by the UWL on each side of the membrane, then

$$\frac{1}{P_s} = \frac{1}{P_{sm}} + \frac{d_1/D_1 S_{w_1}}{D_1 H_2 O S_{w_1}} + \frac{d_2/D_2 S_{w_2}}{D_2 H_2 O S_{w_2}} \tag{60}$$

and

$$\frac{1}{PH_2O} = \frac{1}{PH_2O_m} + \frac{d_1/D_1 S_{w_1}}{D_{1+s} S_{w_1}} + \frac{d_2/D_2 S_{w_2}}{D_{2+s} S_{w_2}} \tag{61}$$

where P_{sm} is the permeability of the membrane to solute, P_{H_2Om} is the permeability of the membrane to water, d_1 and d_2 are the values of the thickness of the UWL on the luminal and cytosol side of the membrane corresponding to outside and inside values of effective thickness of the UWL, S_{w_1} and S_{w_2}, respectively; D_{1S} is the diffusion coefficient of the solute in the UWL on the luminal side of the membrane, and D_2H is the diffusion coefficient of the solute on the cytosol side of the membrane. D_{1H_2O} and D_{2H_2O} are the diffusion coefficients of water on each side of the membrane. It can then be shown, from a modification of an equation developed by SMULDERS et al. (1972) that

$$\sigma^1 = 1 - \frac{\left[\bar{V}_s\left(\frac{1}{P_{H_2O}} + \frac{S_1}{D_{1H_2O}} + \frac{S_2}{D_{2H_2O}}\right)\right.}{\left.\bar{V}_{H_2O}\left(\frac{1}{P_s} + \frac{S_1}{D_{1S}} + \frac{S_2}{D_{2S}}\right)\right]} \tag{62}$$

This equation allows for the calculation of values of σ corrected for unstirred layer effects. Only after such corrections have been applied will values of σ adequately reflect P_{sm}, the permeability of the membrane to the solute. Thus, extreme caution is required in the interpretation of reflection coefficients obtained from different membranes in the presence of unstirred layers, and the presence of pores in the membrane can be deduced only when it is assumed that the solute does not interact with water, when the appropriate corrections have been made for the UWL, and when sweeping away effects have been taken into account. It has been proposed that these apparent pores might be important for the transport of solutes in the presence of bulk flow. Thus, it is often found (CURRAN 1960; DURBIN 1960; DURBIN et al. 1956; HANNAI et al. 1965, 1966; MAURO 1957; PAGANELLI and SOLOMON 1957; PRESCOTT and ZEUTHEN 1953; VILLEGAS et al. 1958) that the bulk movement of water under a hydrostatic force P_{os} is greater than the exchange flow of water under an equivalent chemical gradient of labeled water P_{dH_2O} (DICK 1964, 1966). This has usually been interpreted to mean that water is passing through pores, although the same behavior has been observed in nonporous synthetic membranes (THAU et al. 1966). DAINTY (1963) has suggested that P_{os}/P_{dH_2O} values in excess of unity ($P_{os} > P_{dH_2O}$) could depend on unstirred layers rather than on quasilaminar osmotic water flow through aqueous membrane channels (MAURO 1957; PAPPENHEIMER et al. 1951), since the unstirred layers may impede isotopic diffusion to a greater degree than hydrostatic water flux. In this connection DAINTY and HOUSE (1966a, b, c) observed in frog skin that the values of P_{dH_2O}) were affected to a considerably greater extent than those of P_{os} by the magnitude of the unstirred layers. GINZBURG and KATCHALSKY (1963) noted that the values of P_{dH_2O} in artificial cellulose membranes were directly related to the rate of stirring in the aqueous phase. Similarly, HAYS (1968, 1972) demonstrated that the vasopressin-dependent increment in P_{dH_2O} for the toad urinary bladder could be raised from less than twofold to approximately fivefold when the aqueous phases were stirred vigorously. In the case of unmodified, or native, lipid bilayer membranes, there is reasonable experimental evidence from a number of laboratories (REDWOOD and HAYDON 1969) which supports the view that the primary mode of water transport through the membranes during osmosis is by diffusion, and that differences between P_{os} and P_{dH_2O} depend on the thickness of the unstirred layers. Furthermore, it has been demonstrated that the results of estimates of water permeabilities using isotope diffusion experiments gave results that were almost independent of whether the membrane was of lipid, cellophane, or glass mesh (HANAI et al. 1966), and these authorities have suggested that the discrepancy between the osmotic and diffusion permeabilities was probably attributable to the presence of effectively stagnant layers of solution adjacent to the membrane surfaces. Convincing evidence in support of this suggestion has been provided by CASS and FINKELSTEIN (1967) who have shown that by decreasing the thickness of the wall that supports the membrane, an isotope diffusion permeability may be obtained that is approximately the same as the corresponding osmotic value. Since most measurements of P_d have failed to account for unstirred layers inside and outside the cell, so the value of P_{dH_2O} has been underestimated and $P_{dH_2O} \rightarrow P_{os}$. Cell membranes are very permeable to water and so even a small UWL would have a profound effect on measuring P_{dH_2O}. A UWL would have little effect on the measurement of P_{os}; because the net water flow J_v has a significant velocity, the impermeable solute is swept away from the face of the membrane by this water flow. This outward, connective movement of the solute is opposed, within the unstirred layer, by inward diffusion down the concentration gradient formed (see Fig. 53).

Thus, the existence of pores has not been unequivocally demonstrated for biologic membranes. The pathway for water flow and low molecular weight water-soluble molecular absorption may occur through relatively polar regions in the membrane; alternatively, this pathway may represent paracellular rather than transcellular transport.

VI. Potential Role of the Intestinal Unstirred Water Layer in Disease

The precise mechanism for the decrease in the thickness of the UWL in thiamine deficiency remains to be established (HOYUMPA et al. 1976). The change in the thickness of the UWL does not appear to be related to the height of the villi, since this morphological pattern changed in different directions in sprue and in diabetes. There does, however, appear to be a teleological role of the reduction in the UWL: this reduced UWL thickness in thiamine deficiency may be viewed as a possible adaptive mechanism which allows the affected animal to absorb more efficiently whatever meager supply of thiamine may be available. The same adaptive mechanisms may hold true in sprue (Read et al. 1976, 1977), as well as in the other conditions associated with thinning of the UWL, such as drug-induced diabetes mellitus, or aging (Thomson 1980b, c).

Change in the acid microclimate may be affected in disease. For example (Lucas et al. 1978), the surface pH of human proximal jejunum is 5.93 ± 0.05 in biopsy samples from healthy control individuals, 6.21 ± 0.04 in patients with Crohn's disease, and 6.56 ± 0.14 in a group of untreated celiac patients, falling to 6.19 in those treated with a gluten-free diet (Lucas et al. 1978). This may serve partially to explain the frequently observed development of folate deficiency in these conditions. Clearly, much future consideration must be given not just to the possible role of the UWL in the aggravation or diminution of malabsorption in diesease, but also to the definition of those factors which influence the dimensions of the UWL in health and disease.

References

Andreoli TE, Trautmann SL (1971) An analysis of unstirred layers in series with "tight" and "porous" lipid bilayer membranes. J Gen Physiol 57:464–478

Andreoli TE, Dennis VW, Weigl AM (1969) The effect of amphotericin B on the water and nonelectrolyte permeability of their lipid membranes. J Gen Physiol 53:133–156

Arias IM, Doyle D, Schimke RT (1969) Studies on the synthesis and degradation of protein of the endoplasmic reticulum of rat liver. J Biol Chem 244:3303–3315

Ashworth LAE, Green C (1966) Plasma membranes; phospholipid and sterol content. Science 151:210–211

Bailey E, Taylor CB, Bartley W (1967) Turnover of mitochondrial components of normal and essential fatty acid-deficient rats. Biochem J 104:1026–1032

Barry PH, Diamond JM (1970) Junction potentials, electrode standard potentials, and other problems in interpreting electrical properties of membranes. J Membr Biol 3:93–122

Barry PH, Diamond JM, Wright EM (1971) The mechanism of cation permeation in rabbit gallbladder. Dilution potentials and biionic potentials. J Membr Biol 4:358–394

Beck RE, Schultz JS (1972) Hindrance of solute diffusion within membranes as measured with microporous membranes of known pore geometry. Biochim Biophys Acta 255:273–303

Bennett HS (1963) Morphological aspects of extracellular polysaccharides. J Histochem Cytochem 11:14–23

Berlin RD, Oliver JM, Ukena TE, Yin HH (1975) The cell surface. N Engl J Med 292:515–520

Biber TUL, Aceves J, Mandel LJ (1972) Potassium uptake across serosal surface of isolated frog skin epithelium. Am J Physiol 222:1366–1373

Bindslev N, Wright EM (1976) Effect of temperature on nonelectrolyte permeation across the toad urinary bladder. J Membr Biol 29:265–288

Blair JA, Matty AJ (1974) Acid microclimate in intestinal absorption. Clin Gastroenterol 3:183–198

Blair JA, Lucas ML, Matty AJ (1972) The acidification process in the jejunum. Gut 13:321

Blair JA, Lucas ML, Matty AJ (1975) Acidification in the rat proximal jejunum. J Physiol 245:333–350

Boulpaep EL, Seely JF (1971) Electrophysiology of proximal and distal tubules in the autoperfused dog kidney. Am J Physiol 221:1084–1096
Branton D (1969) Membrane structure. Annu Rev Plant Physiol 20:209–238
Bricker NS, Biber T, Ussing HH (1963) Exposure of the isolated frog skin to high potassium concentrations at the internal surface. I. Bioelectric phenomena and sodium transport. J Clin Invest 42:88–99
Brightman WM, Reese TS (1969) Junctions between intimately apposed cell membranes in the vertebrate brain. J Cell Biol 40:648–677
Brown AC Jr (1962) Microvilli of the human jejunal epithelial cell. J Cell Biol 12:623–627
Brown MS, Goldstein JL (1974) Familial hypercholesterolemia: defective binding of lipoproteins to cultured fibroblasts associated with impaired regulation of 3-hydroxy-3-methylglutaryl coenzyme A reductase activity. Proc Natl Acad Sci USA 71:788–792
Brown MS, Dana SE, Goldstein JL (1973) Regulation of 3-hydroxy-3-methylglutaryl coenzyme A reductase activity in human fibroblasts by lipoproteins. Proc Natl Acad Sci USA 70:2162–2166
Cass A, Finkelstein A (1967) Water permeability of thin lipid membranes. J Gen Physiol 50:1765–1784
Chapman D, Williams RM, Ladbrooke BD (1967) Physical studies of phospholipids. VI. Thermotropic and lyotropic mesomorphism of some 1,2-diacylphosphatidylcholines. Chem Phys Lipids 1:445–475
Chapman D, Keough KM, Urbina J (1974) Biomembrane phase transitions. Studies of lipid-water systems using differential scanning calorimetry. J Biol Chem 249:2512–2521
Claude P, Goodenough DA (1973) Fracture faces of zonula occludentes from "tight" and "leaky" epithelia. J Cell Biol 58:390–400
Coleman R, Finean JB (1966) Preparation and properties of isolated plasma membranes from guinea-pig tissues. Biochim Biophys Acta 125:197–206
Collander R (1954) The permeability of nitella cells to non-electrolytes. Physiol Plant 7:420–445
Colton CK (1967) Artificial Kidney – Chronic Uremia Program, National Institute of Arthritis and Metabolic Disease. National Institutes of Health, USPHS Federal Clearinghouse Accession No PB 182–281
Crane RK (1968a) Digestive-absorptive surface of the small bowel mucosa. Annu Rev Med 19:57–68
Crane RK (1968b) Absorption of sugars. In Code CF (ed) Handbook of physiology, sect 6, vol III, Am Physiol Soc, Washington, DC pp 1323–1351
Crank J (1957) The Mathematics of Diffusion. Oxford University Press, London
Creamer B (1974) Intestinal structure in relation to absorption. Biomembranes 4A:1–42
Criddle RS (1969) Structural protein of chloroplasts and mitochondria. Annu Rev Plant Physiol 20:239–252
Curran PF (1960) Na, Cl, and water transport by rat ileum in vitro. J Gen Physiol 43:1137–1148
Curran PF, Schultz SG (1968) Transport across membranes: general principles. In: Code CF (ed) Handbook of physiology, section 6, alimentary canal. Vol 3 intestinal absorption. American Physiological Society, Washington, DC, pp 1217–1243
Cuzner ML, Davison AN, Gregson NA (1966) Turnover of brain mitochondrial membrane lipids. Biochem J 101:618–626
Dainty J (1963) Water relations of plant cells. Adv Bot Res 1:279–326
Dainty J, Ginzburg B (1963) Irreversible thermodynamics and frictional models of membrane processes, with particular reference to the cell membrane. J Theor Biol 5:256–265
Dainty J, Ginzburg BZ (1964a) The permeability of the cell membranes of Nitella translucens to urea, and the effect of high concentrations of sucrose on this permeability. Biochim Biophys Acta 79:112–128
Dainty J, Ginzberg BZ (1964b) The permeability of the protoplasts of chara australis and nitella translucens to methanol, ethanol, and isopropanol. Biochim Biophys Acta 79:122–128
Dainty J, Hope AB (1959a) The water permeability of cells of chara australis. Aust J Biol Sci 12:136–145

Dainty J, Hope AB (1959 b) Ionic relations of cells of Chara australis. I. Ion exchange in the cell wall. Aust J Biol Sci 12:395–411
Dainty J, House CR (1966 a) "Unstirred layers" in frog skin. J Physiol 182:66–78
Dainty J, House CR (1966 b) An examination of the evidence for membrane pores in frog skin. J Physiol 185:172–184
Dainty J, House CR (1966 c) Unstirred layers in frog skin. J Physiol 182:66–78
Dawson RMC, Hemington N, Lindsay DB (1960) The phospholipids of the erythrocyte "ghosts" of various species. Biochem J 77:226–230
Debman ES, Levin RJ (1975 a) An experimental method of identifying and quantifying the active transfer electrogenic component from the diffusive component during sugar absorption measured in vivo. J Physiol 246:181–196
Debman ES, Levin RJ (1975 b) Effects of fasting and semistarvation on the kinetics of active and passive sugar absorption across the small intestine in vivo. J Physiol 252:681–700
De Grier J, Van Deenen LLM (1961) Some lipid characteristics of red cell membranes of various animal species. Biochim Biophys Acta 49:286–296
Diamond JM (1966) A rapid method for determining voltage-concentration relations across membranes. J Physiol 183:83–100
Diamond JM, Bossert WH (1968) Functional consequences of ultrastructural geometry in "backwards" fluids-transporting epithelia. J Cell Biol 37:694–702
Diamond JM, Katz Y (1974) Interpretation of nonelectrolyte partition coefficients between dimyristoyl lecithin and water. J Membr Biol 17:121–154
Diamond JM, Wright EM (1969 a) Biological membranes: the physical basis of ion and nonelectrolyte selectivity. Annu Rev Physiol 31:581–646
Diamond JM, Wright EM (1969 b) Molecular forces governing nonelectrolyte permeation through cell membranes. Proc R Soc Lond [Biol] 172:273–316
Dick DAT (1964) The permeability coefficient of water in the cell membrane and the diffusion coefficient in the cell interior. J Theor Biol 7:504–531
Dietschy JM (1970) Difficulties in determining valid rate constants for transport and metabolic processes. Gastroenterology 58:863–874
Dietschy JM (1978 a) Effect of diffusion barriers on solute uptake into biological systems. In: Snere PA, Eastabrook RW (eds) Microenvironments and metabolic compartmentation. Academic, New York, pp 401–418
Dietschy JM (1978 b) General principles governing movement of lipids across biological membranes. In: Dietschy JM, Gotto AM, Ontko JA (eds) Disturbances in lipid and lipoprotein metabolism. Am Physiol Soc, Bethesda, pp 1-28
Dietschy JM, Westergaard H (1975) The effect of unstirred water layers on various transport processes in the intestine. In: Csaky TZ (ed) Intestinal absorption and malabsorption. Raven, New York, pp 197–207
Dietschy JM, Sallee VL, Wilson FA (1971) Unstirred water layers and absorption across the intestinal mucosa. Gastroenterology 61:932–934
Drost-Hansen W (1969) Structure of water near solid interfaces. Ind Eng Chem 61:10–47
Drost-Hansen W, Thorhaug AK (1967) Temperature effects in membrane phenomena. Nature 215:506–508
Dugas MC, Ramaswamy K, Crane RK (1975) An analysis of the D-glucose influx kinetics of in vitro hamster jejunum based on considerations of the mass-transfer coefficient. Biochim Biophys Acta 382:576–589
Durbin RP (1960) Osmotic flow of water across permeable cellulose membranes. J Gen Physiol 44:315–326
Durbin RP, Frank H, Solomon AK (1956) Water flow through frog gastric mucosa. J Gen Physiol 39:535–551
Eickholz A (1967) Structural and functional organization of the brush border of intestinal epithelial cells. III. Enzymatic activities and chemical composition of various fractions of trisdisrupted brush borders. Biochim Biophys Acta 135:475–482
Fawcett DW (1962) Physiologically significant specializations of the cell surface. Circulation 26:1105–1125

Fawcett DW (1965) Surface specializations of absorbing cells. J Histochem Cytochem 13:75–91
Fernandes J, Van de Kamer JH, Weijers HA (1962) Differences in absorption of the various fatty acids studied in children with steatorrhea. J Clin Invest 41:488–494
Fernandez-Moran H (1957) In: Richter D (ed) Metabolism of nervous tissue. Pergamon, London pp 1
Fernandez-Moran H (1959) In: Ondey JL (ed) Biophysical science – a study program. Wiley, New York, p 319
Finean JB (1957) The role of water in the structure of peripheral nerve myelin. J Biochim Biophys Cytol 3:95–102
Fisher RB, Parsons DS (1950) The gradient of mucosal surface area in the small intestine of the rat. J Anat 84:272–282
Forstner GG, Sabesin SM, Isselbacher KJ (1966) Biochemical and ultrastructural characterization of isolated intestinal microvillar membranes. J Cell Biol 31:35A
Frizzell RA, Schultz SG (1972) Ionic conductances of extracellular shunt pathway in rabbit ileum: influence of shunt on transmural Na transport and electrical potential differences. J Gen Physiol 59:318–346
Fromter E (1972) The rate of passive ion movement through the epithelium of Necturus gallbladder. J Membr Biol 8:259–301
Fromter E, Diamond JM (1972) Route of passive ion permeation in epithelia. Nature 235:9–13
Getz GS, Bartley W, Lurie D, Nolton BM (1968) Phospholipids of various sheep organs, rat liver and their subcellular fractions. Biochim Biophys Acta 152:325–339
Ginzburg BZ, Katchalsky A (1963) The frictional coefficients of the flows of electrolytes through artificial membranes. J Gen Physiol 47:403–418
Goldstein DA, Solomon AK (1960) Determination of equivalent pore radius for human red cells by osmotic pressure measurements. J Gen Physiol 44:1–17
Goodenough DA, Revel JP (1970) A fine structural analysis of intercellular junctions in the mouse liver. J Cell Biol 45:272–290
Green K, Otori T (1970) Direct measurements of membrane unstirred layers. J Physiol 207:93–102
Gutknecht J, Tostøson DC (1973) Diffusion of weak acids across lipid bilayer membranes: effects of chemical reactions in the unstirred layers. Science 182:1258–1261
Hamilton JD, McMichael HB (1968) Role of the microvillus in the absorption of disaccharides. Lancet 2:154–157
Hanai T, Haydon DA, Taylor J (1965) Some further experiments on bimolecular lipid membranes. J Gen Physiol 48:59–63
Hanai T, Haydon DA, Redwood WR (1966) The water of bimolecular lipid membranes. Ann NY Acad Sci 137:731–739
Hays RM (1968) A new proposal for the action of vasopressin, based on studies of a complex synthetic membrane. J Gen Physiol 51:385–398
Hays RM (1972) The movements of water across vasopressin-sensitive epithelia. In: Bronner F, Kleinziller A (eds) Current topics in membranes and transport. Academic, New York, pp 339–366
Hays RM, Franki N (1970) The role of water diffusion in the action of vasopressin. J Membr Biol 2:263–276
Hays RM, Franki N, Soberman R (1971) Activation energy for water diffusion across the toad bladder: evidence against the pore enlargement hypothesis. J Clin Invest 50:1016–1018
Hechter O (1965) Role of water structure in the molecular organization of cell membranes. Fed Proc 24:5–91
Hendler RW (1971) Biological membrane ultrastructure. Physiol Rev 51:66–97
Hingson DJ, Diamond JM (1972) Comparison of nonelectrolyte permeability patterns in several epithelia. J Membr Biol 10:93–135
Hodgkin AL, Keynes RD (1955) The potassium permeability of a giant nerve fibre. J Physiol 128:61–88

Hoffman NE, Simmonds WJ (1971) The intestinal uptake and esterification in vitro, of fatty acid as a diffusion limited process. Biochim Biophys Acta 241:331–333

Hogben CA (1960) The alimentary tract. Annu Rev Physiol 22:381–406

Hogben CAM, Tocco DJ, Brodie BB, Schanker LS (1959) On mechanism of intestinal absorption of drugs. J Pharmacol Exp Ther 125:275–282

Hollander D, Morgan D (1979) Aging: its influence on vitamin A intestinal absorption in vivo by the rat. Exp Gerontol 14:301–305

Hollander D, Rim E, Morgan D (1979) Intestinal absorption of 25-hydroxyvitamin D_3 in unanesthetized rat. Am J Physiol 236:E441–E445

Holz R, Finkelstein A (1970) The water and nonelectrolyte permeability induced in thin lipid membranes by the polyene antibiotics nystatin and amphotericin. J Gen Physiol 56:125–145

Holtzman JC, Gram TE, Gillette JR (1970) The kinetics of ^{32}P incorporation into the phospholipids of hepatic rough and smooth microsomal membranes of male and female rats. Arch Biochem Biophys 138:199–207

Hoshi T, Sakai F (1967) A comparison of the electrical resistance of the surface cell membrane and cellular wall in the proximal tubule of the newt kidney. Jpn J Physiol 17:627–637

Hoyumpa AM Jr, Middleton HM III, Wilson FA, Schenker S (1975) Thiamine transport across the rat intestine. I. Normal characteristics. Gastroenterology 68:1218–1227

Hoyumpa AM Jr, Nichols S, Schenker S, Wilson FA (1976) Thiamine transport in thiamine-deficient rats: role of the unstirred water layer. Biochim Biophys Acta 436:438–447

Ito S (1964) The surface coating of enteric microvilli. Anat Rec 148:294

Ito S (1965) The enteric surface coat of cat-intestinal microvilli. J Cell Biol 27:475–491

Ito S (1969) Structure and function of the glycocalyx. Fed Proc 28:12–25

Jackson MJ (1972) Transport of short chain fatty acid. In: Smyth DH (ed) Intestinal absorption. Plenum, London

Jackson MJ, Morgan BN (1975) Relations of weak electrolyte transport and acid-base metabolism in rat small intestine in vitro. Am J Physiol 228:482–487

Jackson MJ, Cassidy MM, Weller RS (1970) Studies on intestinal fluid transport. I. Estimation of the extracellular space of everted sacs of rat small intestine. Biochim Biophys Acta 211:425–435

Jackson MJ, Williamson AM, Dombrowski WA, Garner DE (1978) Intestinal transport of weak electrolytes: determinants of influx at the luminal surface. J Gen Physiol 71:301–327

Jardetzky O (1957) On the distinction between the effects of agents on active and passive transport of ions. Science 125:931–932

Jardetzky O, Snell FM (1960) Theoretical analysis of transport processes in living systems. Proc Natl Acad Sci USA 46:616–622

Jick H, Shuster L (1966) The turnover of reduced nicotinamide adenine dinucleatide phosphate-cytochrome c reductase in the livers of mice treated with phenobarbital. J Biol Chem 241:5366–5369

Johnson CF (1967) Disaccharidase: localization in hamster intestine brush borders. Science 155:1670–1672

Kakemi K, Arita T, Hori R, Konishi R, Nishimura K, Matsui H, Nishimura T (1969) Absorption and excretion of drugs. XXXIV. An aspect of the mechanism of drug absorption from the intestinal tract in rats. Chem Pharm Bull (Tokyo) 17:255–261

Kaufmann TG, Leonard EF (1968) Mechanisms of interfacial mass transfer in membrane transport. J Am Inst Chem Eng 14:421

Kedem O (1961) Criteria of active transport. In: Kleinzeller A, Kotyk A (eds) Membrane transport in metabolism: proceedings of a symposium held in Prague, August 22–27, 1960. Academic, New York, pp 87–93

Kedem O, Essig A (1965) Isotope flows and flux ratios in biological membranes. J Gen Physiol 48:1047–1070

Kedem O, Katchalsky A (1961) A physical interpretation of the phenomeno-logical coefficients of membrane permeability. J Gen Physiol 45:143–179

Kidder GW (1970) Unstirred layers in tissue respiration: application to studies of frog gastric mucosa. Am J Physiol 219:1789–1795
Kimmich GA (1970) Preparation and properties of mucosal epithelial cells isolated from small intestine of the chicken. Biochemistry 9:3659–3668
Kinter WB, Wilson TH (1965) Autoradiographic study of sugar and amino acid absorption by everted sacs of hamster intestine. J Cell Biol 25:19–39
Klahr S, Bricker NS (1964) On the electrogenic nature of active sodium transport across the isolated frog skin. J Clin Invest 43:922–930
Klotz IM (1958) Protein hydration and behavior. Science 128:815–822
Klotz IM (1962) Water. In: Kasha M, Pullman B (eds) Horizons in biochemistry. Academic, New York, pp 523
Korn ED (1969) Biological membranes. Theor Exp Biophys 2:1–65
Levich VG (1962) Physiochemical Hydrodynamics. Prentice-Hall, Englewood Cliffs
Lewis LD, Fordtran JS (1975) Effect of perfusion rate on absorption, surface area, unstirred water layer thickness, permeability, and intraluminal pressure in the rat ileum in vivo. Gastroenterology 68:1509–1516
Lieb WR, Stein WD (1969) Biological membranes behave as nonporous polymeric sheets with respect to the diffusion of nonelectrolytes. Nature 224:240–243
Lieb WR, Stein WD (1971) The molecular basis of simple diffusion within biological membranes. In: Bronner F, Kleinzeller A (eds) Current topics in membranes of transport, vol 2. Academic, New York, 2:1–39
Lieb WR, Stein WD (1972) The influence of unstirred layers on the kinetics of carrier-mediated transport. J Theor Biol 36:641–645
Lindemann B, Solomon AK (1962) Permeability of luminal surfaces of intestinal mucosal cells. J Gen Physiol 45:801–810
Ling GN (1965) The physical state of water in living cell and model systems. Ann NY Acad Sci 125:401–417
Ling GN, Ochsenfeld MM, Karreman G (1967) Is the cell membrane a universal rate-limiting barrier to the movement of water between the living cell and its surrounding medium? J Gen Physiol 50:1807–1820
Loewenstein WR (1966) Permeability of membrane junctions. Ann NY Acad Sci 137:441–472
Lortrup S (1963) On the rate of water exchange across the surface of animal cells. J Theor Biol 5:341–359
Lovering EG, Black DB (1974) Diffusion layer effects on permeation of phenylbutazone through polydimethylsiloxane. J Pharm Sci 63:1399–1402
Lucas ML, Blair JA (1978) The magnitude and distribution of the acid microclimate in proximal jejunum and its relation to luminal acidification. Proc R Soc Lond [Biol] 200:27–41
Lucas ML, Schneider W, Haberich FJ, Blair JA (1975) Direct measurement by pH-microelectrode of the pH-microclimate in rat proximal jejunum. Proc R Soc Lond [Biol] 192:39–48
Lucas ML, Blair JA, Cooper BT, Cooke WT (1976) Relationship of the acid microclimate in rat and human intestine to malabsorption. Biochem Soc Trans 4:154–156
Lucas ML, Cooper BT, Lei FH, Johnson IT, Holmes GKT, Blair JA, Cooke WT (1978) Acid microclimate in coeliac and Crohn's disease: a model for folate malabsorption. Gut 19:735–742
Lukie BE, Westergaard H, Dietschy JM (1974) Validation of a chamber that allows measurement of both tissue uptake rates and unstirred layer thickness in the intestine under conditions of controlled stirring. Gastroenterology 67:652–661
Mauro A (1957) Nature of solvent transfer in osmosis. Science 126:252–253
Miller D, Crane RK (1961) The digestive function of the epithelium of the small intestine. II. Localization of disaccharide hydrolysis in the isolated brush border portion of intestinal epithelial cells. Biochim Biophys Acta 52:293–298
Miller DM (1972) The effect of unstirred layers on the measurement of transport rates in individual cells. Biochim Biophys Acta 266:85–90

Millington PF, Finean JB (1969) In: Frazer AC (ed) Biochemical problems of lipids. Elsevier, Amsterdam, pp 116
Moe H (1955) On goblet cells, especially of intestine of some mammalian species. Int Rev Cytol 4:299–334
Mukherjee TM, Williams AW (1967) A comparative study of the ultrastructure of microvilli in the epithelium of small & large intestine of mice. J Cell Biol 34:447–461
Mukherjee TM, Stachelin LA (1971) The fine structural organization of the brush border of intestinal epithelial cells. J Cell Sci 8:573–599
Mulder E, DeGrier J, Van Deener LLM (1963) Selective incorporation of fatty acids into phospholipids of mature red cells. Biochim Biophys Acta 70:94–96
Naccache P, Sha'afi RI (1973) Patterns of nonelectrolyte permeability in human red blood cell membrane. J Gen Physiol 62:714–736
Nemethy G, Scheraga HA (1962) The structure of water and hydrophobic bonding in proteins. III. The thermodynamic properties of hydrophobic bonds in proteins. J Chem Phys 36:3382–3400
Nernst W (1904) Theorie der Reaktionsgeschwindigkeit in heterogenen Systemen. Z Phys Chem 47:52–55. Quoted by Andreoli TE, Trautman SL (1971) J Gen Physiol 57:464–478
Noyes AA, Whitney WR (1897) Über die Auflösungsgeschwindigkeit von festen Stoffen in ihren eigenen Lösungen. Z phys Chem 23:689–692. Quoted by Dainty J, House CR (1966) J Physiol 182:66–78
Olson FCW, Schultz OT (1942) Temperatures in solids during heating or cooling. Int Eng Chem 34:874–877
Paganelli CV, Solomon AK (1957) The rate of exchange of tritiated water across the human red cell membrane. J Gen Physiol 41:259–277
Palay SL, Karlin LJ (1959) An electron microscopic study of the intestinal villus. II. The pathway of fat absorption. J Biophys Biochem Cytol 5:373–383
Pappenheimer JR, Renkin EM, Borrero LM (1951) Filtration, diffusion and molecular sieving through peripheral capillary membranes. A contribution to the pore theory of capillary permeability. Am J Physiol 167:13–46
Parport AK, Ballentine R (1952) In: Barron ESG (ed) Modern trends in physiology and biochemistry. Academic, New York, p 135
Parsons DS, Boyd CAR (1972) Transport across the intestinal mucosal cell: hierarchies of function. Int Rev Cytol, 32:209–255
Parsons DS, Prichard JS (1968) Disaccharide absorption by amphibian small intestine in vitro. J Physiol 199:137–150
Parsons DS, Prichard JS (1971) Relationships between disaccharide hydrolysis and sugar transport in amphibian small intestine. J Physiol 212:299–319
Parsons DF, Subjeck JR (1972) The morphology of the polysaccharide coat of mammalian cells. Biochim Biophys Acta 265:85–113
Pasternak CA, Bergeron JJM (1970) Turnover of mammalian phospholipids. Stable and unstable components in neoplastic mast cells. Biochem J 119:473–480
Perris AD (1966) Isolation of the epithelial cells of the rat small intestine. Can J Biochem 44:687–693
Peterson MA, Gregorl HP (1959) Diffusion-exchange of exchange ions and nonexchange electrolyte in ion-exchange membrane systems. J Electrochem Soc 106:1051
Porter HP, Saunders DR, Tytgat G, Brunser O, Rubin CE (1971) Fat absorption in the bile fistula man. A morphological and biochemical study. Gastroenterology 60:1008–1019
Porteus JW, Clark B (1965) The isolation and characterization of subcellular components of the epithelial cells of rabbit small intestine. Biochem J 96:159–171
Prescott DM, Zeuthen E (1953) Comparison of water diffusion and water filtration across cell surfaces. Acta Physiol Scand 28:77–94
Read NW, Levin RJ, Holdworth CD (1976) Electrogenic glucose absorption in untreated and treated coeliac disease. Gut 17:444–449
Read NW, Barber DC, Levin RJ, Holdworth CD (1977) Unstirred layer and kinetics of electrogenic glucose absorption in the human jejunum in situ. Gut 18:865–876

Redwood WR, Haydon DA (1969) Influence of temperature and membrane composition on the water permeability of lipid bilayers. J Theor Biol 22:1–8
Rey F, Drillet F, Schmidt J, Rey J (1974) Influence of flow rate on the kinetics of the intestinal absorption of glucose and lysine in children. Gastroenterology 66:79–85
Rich GT, Sha'afi RI, Barton TC, Solomon AK (1967) Permeability studies on red cell membranes of dog, cat and beef. J Gen Physiol 50:2391–2405
Richardson T, Tappel AL, Smith LM, Houle ER (1962) Polyunsaturated fatty acids in mitochondria. J Lipid Res 3:344–350
Rifaat MK, Iseri OA, Gottlieb LS (1965) An ultrastructural study of the "extraneous coat" of human colonic mucosa. Gastroenterology. 48:593–601
Roelofsen B, De Gier J, Van Deenen LLM (1964) Binding of lipids in the red cell membrane. J Cell Physiol 63:233–243
Rosenberg T (1948) On accumulation and active transport in biological systems. I. Thermodynamic considerations. Acta Chem Scand 2:14–33
Rosenberg T (1954) The concept and definition of active transport. Symp Soc Exp Biol 8:27–41
Sallee VL (1979) Permeation of long-chain fatty acids and alcohols in rat intestine. Am J Physiol 236:E721–727
Sallee VL, Dietschy JM (1973) Determinants of intestinal mucosal uptake of short and medium chain fatty acids and alcohols. J Lipid Res 14:475–484
Sallee VL, Wilson FA, Dietschy JM (1972) Determination of unidirectional uptake rates for lipids across the intestinal brush border. J Lipid Res 13:184–192
Savitz D, Solomon AK (1971) Tracer determinations of human red cell membrane permeability to small nonelectrolytes. J Gen Physiol 58:259–266
Schanker LS (1962) Passage of drugs across body membranes. Pharmacol Rev 14:501–530
Schanker LS, Shore PA, Brodie BB, Hogben CAM (1957) Absorption of drugs from the stomach. I. The rat. J Pharmacol Exp Therap 120:528–539
Schanker LS, Tocco DJ, Brodie BB, Hogben CAM (1958) Absorption of drugs from the rat small intestine. J Pharmacol Exp Therap 123:81–88
Schnaitman CA (1969) Comparison of rat liver mitochondrial and microsomal membrane proteins. Proc Natl Acad Sci USA 63:412–419
Sha'afi RI, Rich GT, Sidel VW, Bossert W, Solomon AK (1967) The effect of the unstirred layer on human red cell water permeability. J Gen Physiol 50:1377–1399
Sherrill BC (1978) Kinetic characteristics of the hepatic transport of chylomicron remnants. In: Dietschy JM, Gotto AM, Ontko JA (eds) Disturbances in lipid and lipoprotein metabolism. Am Physiol Soc, Bethesda, pp 99–109
Sherrill BC, Dietschy JM (1975) Permeability characteristics of the adipocyte cell membrane and partitioning characteristics of the adipocyte triglyceride core. J Membr Biol 23:367–383
Sherrill BC, Albright JG, Dietschy JM (1973) Diffusion studies of bile acids, fatty acids and sucrose-NaCl-water systems at 37 °C by a modified capillary cell apparatus and then application to membrane transport studies. Biochim Biophys Acta 311–261–271
Shore PA, Brodie BB, Hogben CAM (1957) The gastric secretion of drugs: a pH partition hypothesis. J Pharmacol Exp Therap 119:361–369
Simmonds WJ (1972) The role of micellar solutilization in lipid absorption. Aust J Exp Biol Med Sci 50:403–421
Simmonds WJ, Redgrave TG, Willix RLS (1968) Absorption of oleic and palmitic acids from emulsions and micellar solutions. J Clin Invest 47:1015–1025
Siperstein MD, Chaikoff IL, Reinhardt WO (1952) C^{14}-cholesterol. V. Obligatory function of bile in intestinal absorption of cholesterol. J Biol Chem 198:111–114
Smulders AP, Wright EM (1971) The magnitude of nonelectrolyte selectivity in the gall bladder epithelium. J Membr Biol 5:297–318
Smulders AP, Tormey JM, Wright EM (1972) The effect of osmotically induced water flows on the permeability and ultrastructure of the rabbit gallbladder. J Membr Biol 7:164–197
Solomon AK (1960) Measurement of the equivalent pore radius in cell membranes. In: Kleinzeller A, Kotyk A (eds) Membrane transport and metabolism. Academic, New York, p 94

Solomon AK (1968) Characterization of biological membranes by equivalent pores. J Gen Physiol 51:335s
Staverman AJ (1951) The theory of measurement of osmotic pressure. Red Trav Chim Pays-Bas 70:344
Stirling CE (1967) High-resolution radioautography of phlorizin-^{3}H in rings of hamster intestine. J Cell Biol 35:605–618
Stirling CE, Kinter WB (1967) High-resolution radioautography of galactose-3H accumulation in rings of hamster intestine. J Cell Biol 35:585–604
Stirling CE, Schneider AJ, Wong MD, Kinter WB (1972) Quantitative radioautography of sugar transport in intestinal biopsies from normal humans and a patient with glucose-galactose malabsorption. J Clin Invest 51:438–451
Stoeckenius W, Engelman DM (1969) Current models for the structure of biological membranes. J Cell Biol 42:613–646
Suzuki A, Highuchi WI, Ho NFH (1970a) Theoretical model studies of drug absorption and transport in the gastrointestinal tract. J Pharm Sci 59:644–650
Suzuki A, Highuchi WI, Ho NFH (1970b) Theoretical model studies of drug absorption and transport in the gastrointestinal tract. II. J Pharm Sci 59:651–659
Teorell T (1936) A method of studying conditions within diffusion layers. J Biol Chem 113:735–748
Teorell T (1953) Transport processes and electrical phenomena in ionic membranes. Prog Biophys Mol Biol 3:305–369
Teorell T (1956) Transport phenomena in membranes. Eighth Spiers Memorial Lecture. Faraday Soc 21:9–26
Teorell T (1958) Transport processes in membranes in relation to the nerve mechanism. Exp Cell Res [Suppl] 5:83–100
Thau G, Bloch R, Kedem O (1966) Water transport in porous and non-porous membranes. Desalination 1:116–129
Thomson ABR (1978) Intestinal absorption of lipids: influence of the unstirred water layer and bile acid micelle. In: Am Physiol Soc (ed), Disturbances in lipid and lipoprotein metabolism. American Physiological Society, Bethesda, pp 29–55
Thomson ABR (1979a) Unstirred water layer and age-dependent changes in rabbit jejunal D-glucose transport. Am J Physiol 236:E685–E691
Thomson ABR (1979b) Limitations of Michaelis-Menten kinetics in presence of intestinal unstirred layer. Am J Physiol 5:E701–E709
Thomson ABR (1979c) Limitations of the Eadie-Hofstee plot to estimate kinetic parameters of intestinal transport in the presence of an unstirred water layer. J Membr Biol 47:39–57
Thomson ABR (1979d) Kinetic constants for intestinal transport of four monosaccharides determined under conditions of variable effective resistance of the unstirred water layer. J Membr Biol 50:141–163
Thomson ABR (1980a) Influence of site and unstirred layers on the rate of uptake of cholesterol and fatty acids into rabbit intestine. J Lipid Res 21:1097–1107
Thomson ABR (1980b) Effect of age on uptake of homologous series of saturated fatty acids into rabbit jejunum. Am J Physiol 239:6363–6371
Thomson ABR (1980c) Unidirectional flux rate of cholesterol and fatty acids into the intestine of rats with drug-induced diabetes mellitus. J Lipid Res 21:687–698
Thomson ABR (1980d) Limitations in the use of the Lineweaver-Burk plot to estimate kinetic parameters of intestinal transport in the presence of unstirred layers. Dig Ds Sci
Thomson ABR (1980e) Effect of diet on intestinal uptake of fatty acids and cholesterol in drug-induced diabetes mellitus, in two animal species
Thomson ABR, Cleland L (1981) Intestinal cholesterol uptake from phospholipid vesicles, and from single and mixed micelles. Lipids 16:881–887
Thomson ABR, Dietschy JM (1977) Derivation of the equations that describe the effects of unstirred water layers on the kinetic parameters of active transport processes in the intestine. J Theor Biol 64:277–294
Thomson ABR, Dietschy JM, (1980a) Experimental demonstration of the effect of the unstirred water layer on the kinetic constants of the membrane transport of D-glucose in rabbit jejunum. J Membr Biol 54:221–229

Thomson ABR, Dietschy JM (1980b) Intestinal kinetic parameters: effects of unstirred layers and transport preparation. Am J Physiol 239:6372–6377
Thomson ABR, O'Brien BD (1980) Uptake of a homologous series of saturated fatty acids into rabbit intestine using three in vitro techniques. Dig Dis Sci 25:209–215
Thomson ABR, Weinstein WM (1979) Transport kinetics of D-glucose in human small intestinal mucosa. Dig Dis Sci 24:442–448
Thomson ABR, Hotke CA, O'Brien BD, Weinstein WM (1983) Intestinal uptake of fatty acids and cholesterol in four animal species and man: role of unstirred water and bile micelle. Comp Biochem Physiol 75A:221–232
Thornton AG, Vahouny GU, Treadwell CR (1968) Absorption of lipids from mixed micellar bile salt solutions. Proc Soc Exp Biol Med 127:629
Toner PG (1968) Cytology of intestinal epithelial cells. Int Rev Cytol 24:233–343
Treadwell CR, Vahouny GV (1968) Cholesterol absorption. In: Code CF (ed) Handbook of physiology. Sect 6, vol III, Alimentary canal. Am Physiol Soc, Washington, DC, pp 1407–1438
Trier JS (1967) Structure of the mucosa of the small intestine as it relates to intestinal function. Fed Proc 26:1391–1404
Trier JS (1968) Morphology of the epithelium of the small intestine. In: Code CF (ed) Handbook of physiology, sect 6, vol III. Alimentary canal. Intestinal absorption. Am Physiol Soc, Washington, DC, pp 1125–1175
Ugolev AM (1965) Membrane (contact) digestion. Physiol Rev 45:555–595
Ugolev AM (1968) Physiology and pathology of membrane digestion. Stekol JA transl. Plenum, New York
Van Deenen LLM, De Grier J, Houtsmuller VMT, Montfoort A, Mulder E (1963) In: Frazer A (ed) Biochemical problems of lipids, Elsevier, Amsterdam, p 404
Van Os CH, Slegers JFG (1973) Path of osmotic water flow through rabbit gall bladder epithelium. Biochim Biophys Acta 291:197–207
Villegas R, Barton TC, Solomon AK (1958) The entrance of water into beef and dog red cells. J Gen Physiol 42:355–369
Wade JB, Karnovsky MJ (1974) The structure of the zonula occludens. J Cell Biol 60:168–180
Wedner HJ, Diamond JM (1969) Contributions of unstirred-layer effects to apparent electrokinetic phenomena in the gall bladder. J Membr Biol 1:92–108
Westergaard H, Dietschy JM (1974a) Delineation of dimensions and permeability characteristics of the two major diffusion barriers to passive mucosal uptake in rabbit intestine. J Clin Invest 54:718–732
Westergaard H, Dietschy JM (1974b) Normal mechanisms of fat absorption and derangements induced by various gastrointestinal diseases. Med Clin North Am 58:1413–1427
Westergaard H, Dietschy JM (1976) The mechanism whereby bile acid micelles increase the rate of fatty acid and cholesterol uptake into the intestinal mucosal cell. J Clin Invest 58:97–108
Wilbrandt W, Rosenberg T (1961) The concept of carrier transport and its corollaries in pharmacology. Pharmacol Rev 13:109–183
Willix RLS (1970) Solute fluxes in fat absorption. J Pharm Sci 59:1439–1444
Wilson FA, Dietschy JM (1972) Characterization of bile acid absorption across the unstirred water layer and brush border of the rat jejunum. J Clin Invest 51:3015–3025
Wilson FA, Dietschy JM (1974) The intestinal unstirred layer: its surface area and effect on active transport kinetics. Biochim Biophys Acta 363:112–126
Wilson FA, Treanor LL (1975) Characterization of the passive and active transport mechanisms for bile acid uptake into rat isolated intestinal epithelial cells. Biochim Biophys Acta 406:280–293
Winne D (1973) Unstirred layer, source of biased Michaelis constant in membrane transport. Biochim Biophys Acta 298:27–31
Winne D (1975) The influence of villous counter current exchange on intestinal absorption. J Theor Biol 53:145–176
Winne D (1976) Unstirred layer thickness in perfused rat jejunum in vivo. Experientia 1278–1279

Winne D (1977) The influence of unstirred layers on intestinal absorption. In: Kramer M, Lauterbach F (eds) Intestinal permeation, International congress series no 391. Excerpta Medica, Amsterdam, pp 58–64

Winne D (1978) The permeability coefficient of the wall of a villous membrane. J Math Biol 6:95–108

Winne D, Kopf S, Ulmer ML (1979) Role of unstirred layer in intestinal absorption of phenylalanine in vivo. Biochim Biophys Acta 550:120–130

Wright EM (1972) Mechanisms of ion transport across the choroid plexus. J Physiol 226:545–571

Wright EM, Bindslev N (1976) Thermodynamic analysis of nonelectrolyte permeation across the toad urinary bladder. J Membr Biol 29:289–312

Wright EM, Diamond JM (1969a) An electrical method of measuring non-electrolyte permeability. Proc R Soc Lond [Biol] 172:203–225

Wright EM, Diamond JM (1969b) Patterns of non-electrolyte permeability. Proc R Soc Lond [Biol] 172:227–271

Wright EM, Pietras RJ (1974) Routes of nonelectrolyte permeation across epithelial membranes. J Membr Biol 17:293–312

Wright EM, Prather JW (1970) The permeability of the frog choroid plexus to nonelectrolytes. J Membr Biol 2:127–149

Wright EM, Barry PH, Diamond JM (1971) The mechanism of cation permeation in rabbit gallbladder. Conductances, the current voltage relation, the concentration dependence of anion-cation discrimination and the calcium competition effect. J Membr Biol 4:331–357

Wright EM, Smulders AP, Tormey JMcD (1972) The role of the lateral intercellular spaces and solute polarization effects in the passive flow of water across the rabbit gallbladder. J Membr Biol 7:198–219

CHAPTER 22

Intestinal Permeation of Organic Bases and Quaternary Ammonium Compounds

F. LAUTERBACH

A. Introduction

Organic bases taken up orally and thus subject to intestinal absorption may be divided into two classes: (1) regular constituents of food participating in intermediary metabolism like purine and pyrimidine bases and amino acids; and (2) xenobiotic substances amongst which drugs form an important group. Studies on the absorption mechanisms led to the discovery of specific and active transport systems for purine and pyrimidine bases (CSÁKY 1961; SCHANKER and TOCCO 1960, 1962; SCHANKER et al. 1963; KOLASSA et al. 1977; SCHARRER et al. 1981) and for amino acids (for reviews see WISEMAN 1974; SCHULTZ and FRIZZELL 1975) capable of transferring these substances against an electrochemical gradient from the gut lumen into the interstitial space equilibrating with the bloodstream. These transport mechanisms are not the subject of the present chapter.

Basic xenobiotics, on the other hand, have until recently been believed to permeate the intestinal wall simply by passive diffusion across the lipid membrane matrix. This notion dates back to the observations by OVERTON (1899, 1902) and COLLANDER and BÄRLUND (1933) that there exists a positive correlation between lipid solubility and permeation of various organic solutes across cell membranes. In studies with amides and alcohols HÖBER and HÖBER (1937) demonstrated this principle to hold true for intestinal absorption as well.

The situation is more complex in the case of electrolytes which may exist in a lipophilic, uncharged and a hydrophilic, charged form. Augmentation of permeation of organic bases into plant cells by increasing the proportion of the uncharged free base was observed by OVERTON as early as 1896. Four decades later TRAVELL (1940) made the momentous discovery that dogs easily survived lethal strychnine doses when propulsion of the alkaloid from the acidic gastric environment into the more alkaline intestinal fluid was prohibited by a pyloric ligature; she concluded that strychnine absorption is restricted to the uncharged free base. This principle was later generalized and named "nonionic diffusion" (MILNE et al. 1958). According to the principle of nonionic diffusion, a few simple rules should govern intestinal absorption of organic bases.

1. Absorption is dependent on the lipophilicity of the free base and parallels its proportion to total base concentration. Since, according to the HENDERSON–HASSELBALCH equation

$$\log \frac{[B]}{[BH^+]} = pH - pK_a,$$

(where [B] and [BH^+] are the concentrations of free and protonated base), it follows that: (a) absorption is increased by increasing the pH of the solution; and (b) absorption is decreased by increasing the pK_a of the bases.

2. Absorption is proportional to the concentration or, under constant experimental conditions, to the dose, i.e. absorption *rate* is independent of the intestinal concentration.

3. Absorption follows a first-order reaction as long as experimental conditions (intestinal volume, area etc.) are constant. Thus it is virtually complete after sufficiently long periods of time.

4. The transepithelial flux ratio in both directions is unity under symmetric conditions and in the absence of additional driving forces. This is an important though often unproved prerequisite for permeation by diffusion.

The simplicity and intellegibility of this theory as well as the number of confirmatory results (for reviews see BRODIE 1964; SCHANKER 1960, 1962, 1964, 1971; KURZ 1975) led to the widespread opinion that intestinal absorption of xenobiotics is fully understood. On the other hand, it is obvious that incompatible results did not receive the appropriate attention.

In Sect. B, therefore, a critical survey of results compatible and incompatible with the general rules of absorption by nonionic diffusion will be attempted. Here as well as in later sections, considerations on the behaviour of the protonated, cationic form of organic bases will be extended to the quaternary ammonium compounds, the intestinal permeation of which poses especially exciting questions owing to their permanent positive charge. Section C will deal with the phenomenon of intestinal secretion of organic cations by active transport mechanisms against an electrochemical gradient from the blood into the gut lumen. In Sect. D, a unifying concept for the intestinal permeation of organic cations by diffusion and a transport mechanism which (owing to its secretory nature) opposes, but might eventually also mediate absorption will be developed. In Sect. E, some comparative aspects of the intestinal permeation of other classes of xenobiotics and the permeation of organic bases in other organs will be included.

B. Absorption of Organic Bases and Quaternary Ammonium Compounds

I. Dependence on Polarity

The validity of the first rule of nonionic diffusion has been substantiated for numerous organic bases. The absorption rate of basic drugs was increased by increasing the pH of the luminal perfusion fluid both in the small intestine (HOGBEN et al. 1959) and the colon (SCHANKER 1959). Likewise, absorption rate tended to decrease with increasing pK_a values of the drugs under investigation (SCHANKER et al. 1958; SCHANKER 1959). From the stomach, only the extremely weak organic bases are absorbed (SCHANKER et al. 1957; HOGBEN et al. 1957). Also, in accordance with the pH partition hypothesis, organic bases accumulate in the gastric juice after parenteral administration (SHORE et al. 1957; ZAWOISKI et al. 1958).

On the other hand, the early investigations of HOGBEN et al. (1959) indicated that the situation is far more complex than predicted by the partitioning of nonionized species between two compartments separated by a lipid barrier. The lowest pK_a compatible with rapid absorption was about 3 for an acid, but about 7.8 for bases, i.e. under the experimental conditions, the favourable ratio of nonionized to ionized species for acids and bases was 1:4,000 and 1:16, respectively. Moreover, the equilibrium between concentrations in gut lumen and blood plasma did not conform to the theoretical value (JACOBS 1940) which under the assumption of partitioning of the nonionized moiety of a base between two compartments (1 and 2) of different pH is given by

$$\frac{c_1}{c_2} = \frac{1+10^{(pK_a - pH_1)}}{1+10^{(pK_a - pH_2)}}.$$

At equilibrium the concentration ratio lumen: plasma for organic bases was higher, and for organic acids it was lower than predicted. These observations led to the postulate that at the absorbing surface a "virtual" pH lower than that in the bulk luminal solution exists. Though this "acid microclimate" has been confirmed by experimental means (see Chap. 20) its responsibility for the observed deviations from the nonionic diffusion theory has been questioned. D. WINNE (1972, personal communication) has pointed to the obvious fact that a small zone of lower pH, negligible in size, cannot shift an equilibrium calculated on the basis of the amount in the total luminal fluid. JACKSON et al. (1978) found no reason to assume an acid microclimate in influx experiments with organic acids.

Conflicting results were also observed in the rat jejunum in vitro. Even under short-circuit conditions the ratio of the transepithelial fluxes from the mucosal to serosal side J_{ms} and from the serosal to mucosal side J_{sm} deviated from unity for a number of weak organic bases and acids (JACKSON et al. 1974; JACKSON and MORGAN 1975). Generally it was: for a base

$$\frac{J_{ms}}{J_{sm}} < 1$$

and for an acid

$$\frac{J_{ms}}{J_{sm}} > 1.$$

To explain these results JACKSON et al. (1974) and JACKSON and KUTCHER (1977) further developed a three-compartment model originally proposed by HOGBEN et al. (1959). This model consists of two boundaries in series characterized by a finite permeability not only for the nonionized P_{ni}, but also for the ionized moiety P_i. The values of P_i/P_{ni} at the two boundaries are different. Whereas the pH values in the two outer compartments are identical, that of the intermediate compartment is different. In such a model the relationship between the transepithelial fluxes is described by

$$\frac{J_{ms}}{J_{sm}}=\frac{\left[1+\left(\frac{P_i}{P_{ni}}\right)_a 10^{\alpha_m}\right]\left[1+\left(\frac{P_i}{P_{ni}}\right)_b 10^{\alpha_x}\right]}{\left[1+\left(\frac{P_i}{P_{ni}}\right)_a 10^{\alpha_x}\right]\left[1+\left(\frac{P_i}{P_{ni}}\right)_b 10^{\alpha_m}\right]},$$

where $(P_i/P_{ni})_a$ and $(P_i/P_{ni})_b$ are the discrimination coefficients for the weak base in the two barriers, $\alpha_m = pK_a - pH_m$ and $\alpha_x = pK_a - pH_x$ with m and x referring to the bulk solution and the intermediate compartment, respectively (JACKSON et al. 1974; JACKSON 1977).

The situation may be complicated further by the existence of a transepithelial potential difference (JACKSON 1977; JACKSON et al. 1981). So far observations in the rat jejunum are compatible with only one of the possible versions of the model where: (1) discrimination between ionized and nonionized moieties is more pronounced in the boundary proximal to the gut lumen than in that more distally, hence $(P_i/P_{ni})_a < (P_i/P_{ni})_b$; and (2) the pH of the intermediate compartment is higher than that of the outer ones.

Therefore, the authors concluded that boundary a is formed by the mucosal epithelium whereas the basement membrane shows the low but significant discrimination between ionized and nonionized species required for boundary b (TAI and JACKSON 1981). Thus, for the intermediate compartment the interstitial paracellular space would be a morphological correlate where an augmented pH might exist owing to vectorial release of intracellularly generated metabolites and protons (JACKSON and MORGAN 1975; JACKSON and KUTCHER 1977).

According to the strict nonionic diffusion theory, quaternary ammonium compounds should not be absorbed at all, and according to its modifications as described, only to the very limited extent determined by the permeability for the ionized species of organic bases. However, the range of absorption rates reported for these substances varies from practically nil to almost complete. The disappearance rate of several quaternary drugs from the intestinal fluid was only a few percent in the rat (SCHANKER et al. 1958; SCHANKER 1959; KUNZE et al. 1971). Also in the rat, absorption of the quaternary ammonium surfactant cetyltrimethylammonium bromide was poor (ISOMAA 1975). On the other hand, *N*-methylatropine was absorbed to approximately 25% within 3 h (LEVINE 1959; ALBANUS et al. 1969) and *N*-methylhomatropine to 28% even after rectal administration (CRAMER et al. 1978). In humans absorption rates of less than 20% were calculated from intestinal tube investigations or cumulative urinary excretion for bevonium methylsulphate (BEERMANN et al. 1971a,c), *N*-methylscopolamine (BEERMANN et al. 1971b), *N*-methylatropine (BEERMANN et al. 1971c), emepronium (SUNDWALL et al. 1973) and thiazinamium methylsulphate (JONKMAN et al. 1977). Absorption rates varying between less than 10% within 12 h and 36% within 3 h have been reported for *N*-butylscopolamine (WICK 1967; WALDECK 1969; DUCHENE-MARULLAZ et al. 1969; BEERMANN et al. 1971c; PENTIKÄINEN et al. 1973).

Poor absorption was observed for the bisquaternary herbicides paraquat in guinea-pigs and rats (MURRAY and GIBSON 1974) and in humans (VAN DIJK et al.

1975), and diquat in dogs (BENNETT et al. 1976). The most remarkable behaviour was displayed by monoquaternary pyridinium aldoximes, which were absorbed by rats considerably or even completely within 3 h (whereas their bisquaternary analogs reached absorption rates of only 34%–38%) (LEVINE and STEINBERG 1966).

Permeation through aqueous pores has been suggested to explain the high absorption rate of pyridinium aldoximes (CRONE and KEEN 1969) as well as of other quaternary ammonium compounds (BREITER and OHNESORGE 1971; KUNZE et al. 1971). The finding that absorption of the small tetraethylammonium cation is lower than that of the large *N*-methylscopolamine suggests that other factors are involved at least (TURNHEIM and LAUTERBACH 1980).[1] As a second mechanism, formation of lipophilic ion pairs by quaternary ammonium compounds has been suggested (for references see JONKMAN et al. 1977). However, the operation of this mechanism under physiological conditions has been questioned (RUIFROK 1981), since a 10–50-fold excess of the acidic counterion is necessary (IRWIN et al. 1969).

II. Dependence on Concentration

Proportionality between intestinal concentration and absorbed amount has been proved only occasionally and with conflicting results. Constancy of the absorption rate in spite of increasing doses was observed for primary and tertiary amines in rat small intestine (SCHANKER et al. 1958) and colon (SCHANKER 1959). Tissue uptake of the bisquaternary compound paraquat in rat gut proved to be linear between 10^{-5} and 10^{-2} *M* (STEFFEN and KONDER 1979). On the other hand, LEVINE and PELIKAN (1961) described a peculiar absorption behaviour of the quaternary compound benzomethamine. Under all conditions, absorption was a curvilinear function of dose, characterized by a steep rise within a narrow, intermediate dose range (Fig. 1). Linearity between absorbed amount and administered dose was observed only in the lower (I) and upper (III) segments. No significant differences in the slope of the two segments, calculated from the individual values, could be detected; the authors concluded that absorption of benzomethamine is consistent with diffusion within these dose ranges, whereas an additional, possibly carrier-mediated process must be operative in the intermediate range. It is important to note, however, and will be discussed later (see Sect. D) that the absorption curve can also be interpreted as demonstrating an *increase* of the absorption rate from a constant, low value at low doses to another, also constant but higher value at higher doses. Similar absorption curves have been described under certain conditions for the nonquaternary bases quinine and quinidine (RAGOZZINO and MALONE 1963).

In contrast, a *decrease* of the absorption rate with increasing concentrations, consistent with saturation of the absorption process, was demonstrated for several quaternary pyridinium aldoximes and 2-allyloxy-4-chloro-*N*-(2-diethyl-

---

1 According to dipole moment and infrared data, the dissociated, basic form of *N*-methylpyridinium-2-aldoxime can exist as a resonance hybrid of zwitterionic and uncharged form (LARSSON and WALLERBERG 1962). Saturation and inhibition of pyridinium aldoxime absorption (see Sect. B. II) render the possibility unlikely that formation of an uncharged moiety is the sole reason for the high absorption rate

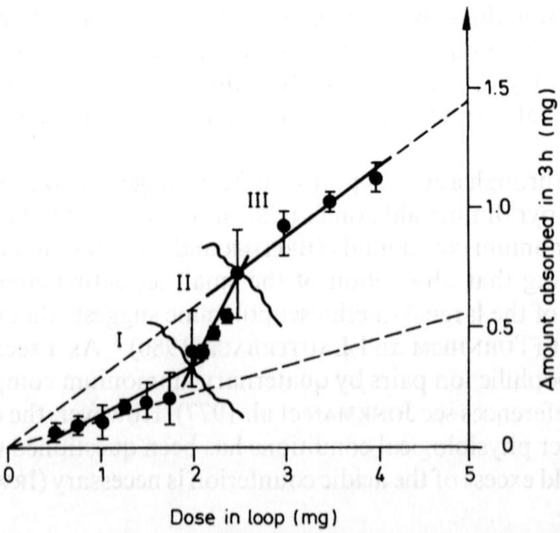

Fig. 1. Dose–absorption curve for benzomethamine. Doses indicated on the abscissa were placed in a 10-cm loop about 26 cm from the pylorus. *Full lines* represent calculated regression lines for the three segments. *Broken lines* drawn by the author. After LEVINE and PELIKAN (1961)

aminoethyl)benzamide, a tertiary amine of pK_a 7.9. Absorption of the pyridinium aldoximes was competitively inhibited by their congeners and the tertiary amine (Fig. 2). It was also suppressed by other basic, nonquaternary drugs (KAKEMI et al. 1969; SUZUKI et al. 1975).[2] The claim that the unusually high absorption rate of bisquaternary paraquat in the dog decreases with increasing doses (BENNETT et al. 1976) has been questioned because of its basis on pharmacokinetic data (STEFFEN and KONDER 1979).

III. Dependence on Time

Substantiation of absorption as a diffusional, first-order reaction by recording its time course has been neglected even more than controlling the concentration dependence. Corresponding investigations by R. LEVINE and her group with several monoquaternary ammonium compounds yielded a peculiar result. After a rapid initial phase, absorption came to a complete halt, although 70%–90% of the administered dose still remained in the intestine (LEVINE et al. 1955; LEVINE and CLARK 1957a, b; LEVINE 1959, 1960, 1961). In contrast, absorption of the bisquaternary hexamethonium proceeded linearly and thus reached a higher absorption rate at 3 h than its monoquaternary derivative whose absorption ceased at 2 h (LEVINE 1960). A comparable progressive decrease of the absorption coeffi-

2 Choline uptake into intestinal tissue has also been demonstrated to proceed by a saturable, mediated process (HERZBERG and LERNER 1973; KUCZLER et al. 1977). Whether this normal body constituent shares the transport systems for xenobiotic cations is not known. In kidney slices, choline inhibited uptake and stimulated efflux of tetraethylammonium (HOLM 1977)

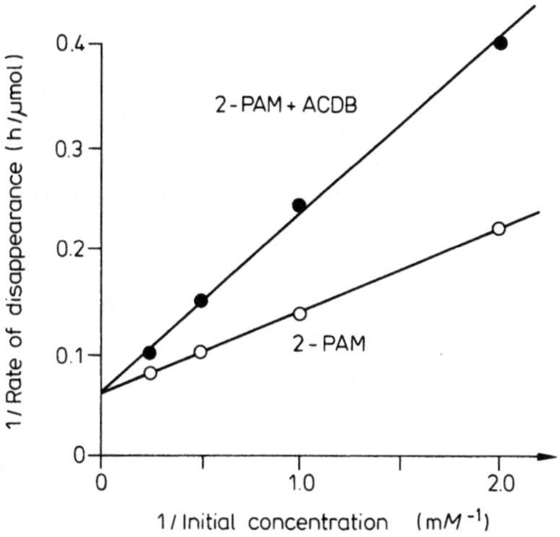

Fig. 2. Lineweaver–Burk plots for pralidoxime iodide (2-PAM) in the absence or presence of 1 m*M* 2-allyloxy-4-chloro-*N*-(2-diethylaminoethyl)benzamide hydrochloride (ACDB). SUZUKI et al. (1975)

cient with increasing absorption time has been reported for atropine (SUND 1971) and recently for several ergot alkaloids, guanfacin and ketotifen (FRANZ et al. 1980).

C. Intestinal Secretion of Organic Cations

I. Secretion by the Isolated Mucosa of Guinea-Pig Small Intestine

Summarizing the knowledge on the absorption of quaternary ammonium compounds reviewed in the preceding section there are three main discrepancies which exclude their absorption by simple diffusion across lipid barriers:

1. Certain quaternary ammonium compounds reveal high absorption rates in spite of their considerable polarity.
2. Absorption rate can be concentration dependent and may either decrease or even increase with rising doses.
3. Time course of absorption does not follow first-order kinetics; absorption may even come to a halt in spite of a large unabsorbed residue.

Therefore, participation of a carrier-mediated process in the overall absorption of these compounds was suggested by several authors. However, neither the increase in absorption rate with rising doses which may be deduced from the results of LEVINE and PELIKAN (1961) nor the standstill of absorption in spite of large amounts of unabsorbed quaternary base can be explained by the existence of a system favouring absorption by facilitated diffusion or active transport. Hence, the hypothesis was put forward, and evidence reported, that the suspected transport system might in fact be an active secretion system for ammonium compounds located in the intestinal mucosa (LAUTERBACH 1970). This hypothesis was based on two reasons. First, active intestinal secretion of cardiac glycosides had just been discovered (LAUTERBACH 1969a, b, 1971). Second, by participation of an active secretory system in intestinal permeation of quaternary bases, all peculiar phenomena observed so far could be unequivocally explained (see Sect. D).

Validation of this hypothesis was greatly facilitated by the method of the isolated mucosa of guinea-pig small intestine (LAUTERBACH 1977a, 1981). As compared with other in vitro methods, studies with the isolated mucosa mounted in a flux chamber are distinguished by a number of advantages. The most important of these might be considered to be the omission of the additional diffusion barriers formed by the connective and muscular tissue layers and, hence, the determination of transepithelial fluxes in both directions under identical conditions and with equal accuracy, the simultaneous determination of drug uptake from the luminal as well as from the blood side of the mucosal tissue, and the suitability for the large series of experiments needed for kinetic studies.

As exemplified by the observations with *N*-methylscopolamine, intestinal permeation of quaternary ammonium compounds across the isolated mucosa re-

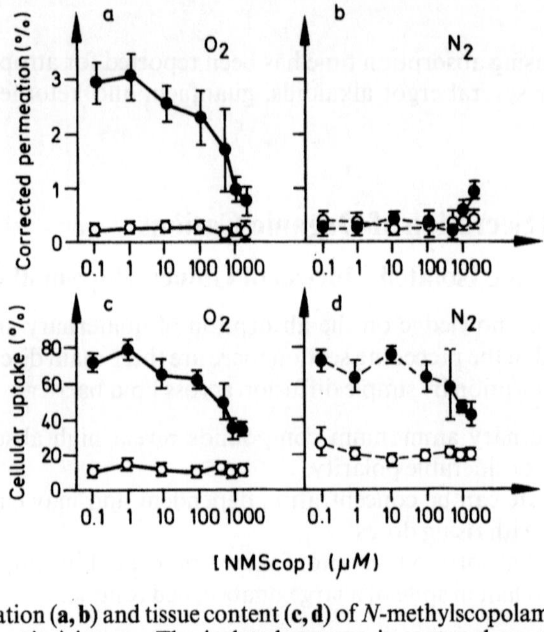

Fig. 3a–d. Permeation (**a, b**) and tissue content (**c, d**) of *N*-methylscopolamine in the isolated mucosa of guinea-pig jejunum. The isolated mucosa is captured on a nylon mesh and placed between two fenestrated polyvinyl chloride sheets, thus forming a separating membrane between two flux chambers. Window diameter 5 mm. The chambers are filled with 0.2 ml incubation solution and continuously gassed through drill holes in the chamber walls. The concentrations indicated on the abscissa (logarithmic scale) were administered under aerobic (O_2) or anaerobic conditions (N_2) either from the luminal (*open circles*) or the blood side (*full circles*). Incubation time 45 min; 37 °C. Permeation has been corrected for fluxes across inulin-permeable shunt pathways. Ordinates: concentration of *N*-methylscopolamine in the tissue, referred to the intracellular space and concentration in the countercompartment, as percentages of the concentration administered. Mean ± standard error. TURNHEIM and LAUTERBACH (1977a)

vealed a number of characteristic features (Fig. 3; TURNHEIM and LAUTERBACH 1977 a).

1. The permeation from the blood side of the isolated mucosa to the luminal side was significantly higher than in the reverse direction with concentrations lower than 500 μ*M*. At 1 μ*M*, a flux ratio of 12:1 was achieved. Since a potential difference of 2–4 mV has been measured in the preparation used in this study (LAUTERBACH 1971, 1977 a), the value far exceeds that to be expected for passive distribution of charged species according to Ussing's flux ratio test (USSING 1949). Secretion against a concentration gradient could be demonstrated by simultaneous administration of 1 μ*M* *N*-methylscopolamine to both sides of the mucosa. Within 3 h, concentration on the blood side dropped to 74% of its initial value, whereas it increased to 122% on the luminal side.

2. The permeation from blood to lumen was dependent on the concentration administered. With increasing concentrations the permeation rate decreased and at 2 m*M* the permeations in both directions across the mucosa were not significantly different from one another. Even at the highest concentration investigated, however, the permeation rate did not approach zero, indicating that the total transcellular flux from blood to lumen consists of a saturable and a nonsaturable term.

3. The permeation from lumen to blood did not exhibit nearly as marked a concentration dependence as was observed with the permeation from blood to lumen.

4. Secretion was dependent on aerobic metabolism. Under anaerobic conditions, a flux ratio of unity was achieved by a slight increase in the permeation from lumen to blood and a drastic decrease in the permeation from blood to lumen.

5. The cellular content exhibited a pattern similar to that of the permeation: it was significantly higher from the blood side than from the luminal side. As with the permeation rate, a dependence on the concentration administered was observed. When increased concentrations were administered from the blood side, the cellular uptake decreased. Although the difference in uptake from the two sides of the mucosa decreased with increasing concentrations administered, it was not abolished completely even with the highest concentration. The uptake from the lumen side did not display as striking a concentration dependence as was observed with the uptake from the blood side.

6. Under anaerobic conditions, uptake of *N*-methylscopolamine from the luminal side was increased, whereas uptake from the blood side remained unchanged.

II. Substrate Specificity

The characteristics of *N*-methylscopolamine permeation and uptake were shared by five other monoquaternary ammonium compounds tested in the isolated mucosa. There were, however, remarkable quantitative differences. Secretory rates comparable to that of *N*-methylscopolamine were observed with two other tropanium derivatives, ipratropium and α-phenylcyclopentane acetic acid-*N*-iso-

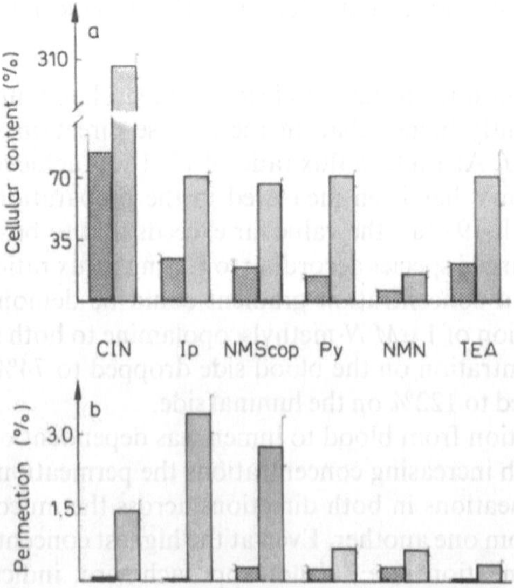

Fig. 4a, b. Cellular content (**a**) and permeation (**b**) of monoquaternary ammonium compounds in the isolated mucosa of guinea-pig jejunum. Administration in 10 μ*M* solution either from the luminal side (*stippled bars*) or from the blood side (*hatched bars*). Incubation time 45 min; 37 °C. *CIN*, α-phenylcyclopentane acetic acid-*N*-isopropylnortropin ester methobromide; *Ip*, ipratropium; *NMScop*, *N*-methylscopolamine; *Py*, pyridostigmine; *NMN*, *N*-methylnicotinamide; *TEA*, tetraethylammonium. Ordinates: concentration in the tissue, referred to the intracellular space, and concentration in the countercompartment, as percentages of the concentration administered. Mean ± standard error. TURNHEIM and LAUTERBACH (1977a), B. PIEPER and F. LAUTERBACH (1979, unpublished work)

propylnortropin ester methobromide. With smaller cations (*N*-methylnicotinamide, pyridostigmine, tetraethylammonium), much smaller secretion rates were observed (TURNHEIM and LAUTERBACH 1977a; PIEPER and LAUTERBACH 1979). Tissue content was always found to be higher after blood side than after luminal administration, though no correlation between tissue content and secretory rate existed (Fig. 4).

Secretion and tissue content after blood side administration of *N*-methylnicotinamide were progressively inhibited by increasing concentrations of *N*-methylscopolamine, suggesting that a common transport system is shared by both quaternary substances (TURNHEIM and LAUTERBACH 1977a). Inhibition of *N*-methylscopolamine secretion by the tertiary amine atropine (pK_a 9.9) suggests, furthermore, that nonquaternary amines in their protonated form might be substrates of the intestinal system for secretion of organic cations (R. B. SUND, F. LAUTERBACH, and K. TURNHEIM 1972, unpublished work). So far, no unequivocal evidence has been obtained for intestinal secretion of bisquaternary ammonium compounds. Experiments with decamethonium (Fig. 5) as well as with the herbicides diquat and paraquat revealed a strict correlation between the simultaneous transmucosal permeation of the bisquaternary compound and polyethylene glycol. The ordinate intercepts of the respective regression lines were not significant-

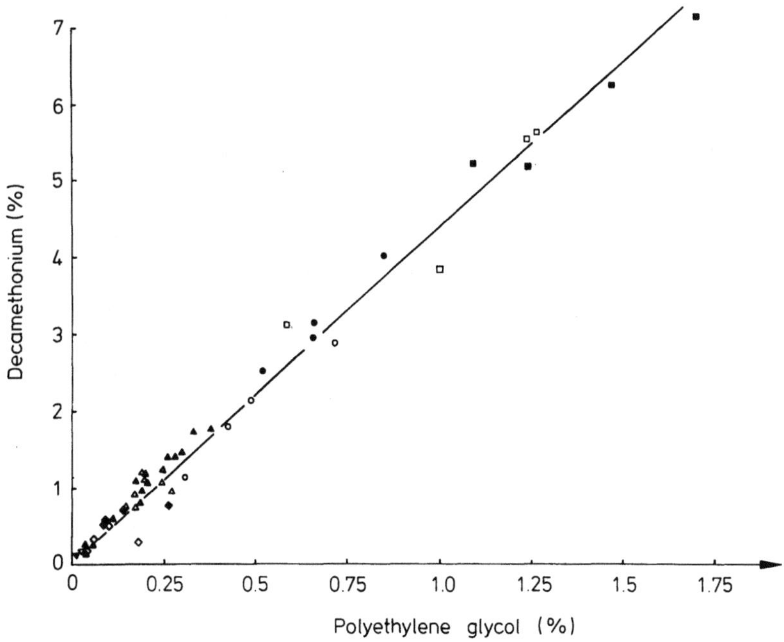

Fig. 5. Correlation between permeation of polyethylene glycol, molecular weight 900, (abscissa) and decamethonium (ordinate). Isolated mucosa of guinea-pig jejunum. Administration of 10 μ*M* decamethonium either to the luminal side (*open symbols*) or to the blood side (*full symbols*). Coordinates indicate concentration in the countercompartment as percentage of the concentration administered after: 10 (*downward triangles*); 20 (*lozenges*); 45 (*upward triangles*); 90 (*circles*); and 180 min (*squares*). Each point represents one single experiment. Regression line calculated from all data: $y=4.32x+0.077$; $R=0.994$. B. PIEPER and F. LAUTERBACH (1980, unpublished work)

ly different from zero. Hence it was concluded that the transepithelial permeation of these compounds is almost completely restricted to polyethylene glycol-permeable paracellular shunt pathways. This conclusion is supported by the extremely low tissue content. After 45 min incubation with 10 μ*M* decamethonium, cellular content after luminal and blood side administration was only 7% and 9%, respectively (compare Fig. 4 for respective values of monoquaternary amines; PIEPER and LAUTERBACH 1979). The higher uptake from the blood side, however, observed under all circumstances and likewise with all other xenobiotics undergoing intestinal secretion suggests further investigations to exclude or substantiate a residual affinity of bisquaternary compounds for the intestinal secretory system.

III. Localization of the Secretory System in the Enterocyte

The demonstration of the intestinal secretion of quaternary ammonium compounds poses the question of where in the enterocyte the secretory system is located. In principle, an active uptake across the basolateral membrane followed by passive release across the brush border or a diffusional entrance across the basolateral followed by active extrusion across the luminal membrane, is conceivable as well as a combination of both possibilities. Several attempts have been made to elucidate the situation.

1. Countertransport

Existence of accelerated exchange diffusion was demonstrated in two experimental setups (TURNHEIM et al. 1977). When isolated mucosae were preloaded with 1 μ*M* labelled *N*-methylscopolamine, 1 m*M* of the unlabelled compound, added to the blood side during a subsequent efflux period, stimulated the release of activity to the blood side accompanied by a compensatory decrease of activity released to the luminal side. An excess of unlabelled *N*-methylscopolamine added to the luminal side had no effect. Vice versa, when isolated mucosae were preloaded with 1 m*M* unlabelled *N*-methylscopolamine, influx of 1 μ*M* labelled *N*-methylscopolamine across the basolateral membrane was stimulated, whereas influx across the luminal membrane remained unchanged. The demonstration of the phenomenon of countertransport was regarded as evidence for the existence of a mediated transport system in the basolateral membrane. No clear indication of the existence of a transport system in the luminal membrane was found in these experiments. However, a decrease in the secretion rate accompanying the stimulated uptake of *N*-methylscopolamine from the blood side was regarded as evidence for an additional luminal system.

2. Influence of Anaerobiosis and Cyanide

Further hints were obtained by interpreting the influence of anaerobiosis on permeation and uptake of several quaternary ammonium compounds. Secretion of *N*-methylscopolamine was depressed under anaerobic conditions. If this were due to a decreased influx across the basolateral membrane, tissue content should have also decreased. On the other hand, if this were due to an inhibition of efflux across the brush border membrane, tissue content should have increased. In fact, tissue content remained unchanged, from which it can be concluded that anaerobiosis inhibited influx across the basolateral as well as efflux across the brush border membrane. Thus, a cell model emerges where transepithelial secretion is brought about by two transport mechanisms in series: the first in the basolateral membrane mediating influx into the cell; and the second in the brush border membrane extruding its substrates into the intestinal lumen. A parallel, diffusional pathway has to be assumed to complete the model since a nonsaturable component (compare Fig. 3) obviously contributes to the secretory flux (Fig. 6; TURNHEIM et al. 1977). In fact, this system is quite similar to that inferred previously for the secretion of cardiac glycosides (LAUTERBACH 1971, 1981).

At present, no definite answer can be given concerning the possible active nature of both transport mechanisms. Owing to the negative cell interior, influx across the basolateral membrane follows an electrochemical gradient and might be decreased by a reduction of the potential difference in anaerobiosis. Such reduction, however, should simultaneously favour efflux across the luminal membrane. Since the latter was decreased in anaerobiosis, and *N*-methylscopolamine was secreted against an electrochmical gradient provided there was no compartmentation within the cell, the luminal extrusion system might well be an active one.

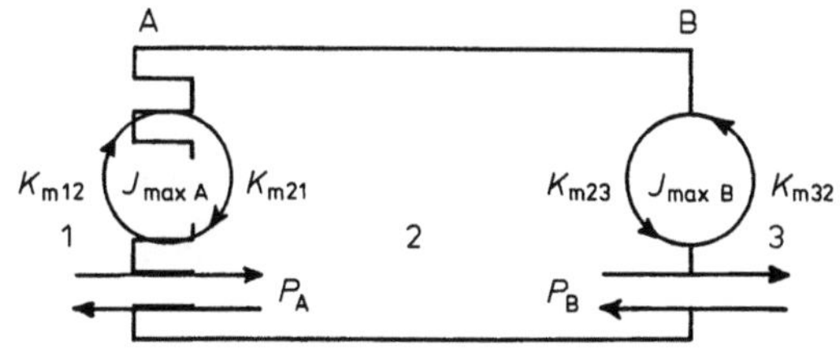

Fig. 6. Kinetic model for the description of the intestinal permeation of quaternary ammonium compounds. The model consists of compartment 1 (intestinal lumen), compartment 2 (enterocyte), and compartment 3 (interstitial space on the blood side). Permeation of the luminal A and basolateral B membranes proceeds by transport mechanisms (*circles*) as well as by passive diffusion (*arrows*). The transport mechanisms are characterized by their maximal velocities J_{max} and different half-saturation constants K_m at the inner and the outer faces of the respective membrane. Diffusion is determined by the passive permeability *P*. LAUTERBACH (1975)

The assumption of two transport systems in series is further supported by the increase in transepithelial permeation and tissue content observed in anaerobiosis after luminal administration of monoquaternary compounds. It can be attributed to a diminished resecretion of quaternary molecules following influx across the luminal membrane. Tissue content after blood side administration either remained unchanged (*N*-methylscopolamine) or decreased (*N*-methylnicotinamide and tetraethylammonium) (TURNHEIM and LAUTERBACH 1977a), which may be explained by changes in the activity of the basolateral system. Theoretically, an increase in tissue content due to a more pronounced inhibition of the luminal system is also conceivable. So far, this has not been observed with quaternary ammonium compounds, but with cardiac glycosides (LAUTERBACH 1971, 1981).

The metabolic dependence of the luminal extrusion system was further substantiated in efflux experiments. After preloading the isolated mucosa, efflux of *N*-methylscopolamine was influenced by cyanide such that only the efflux coefficient across the luminal membrane was significantly reduced (TURNHEIM et al. 1977).

3. Effect of Inhibitors

Characterization of the secretory systems for quaternary ammonium compounds has been further attempted by looking for specific inhibitors. Renal secretion of *N*-methylnicotinamide in vivo was effectively and irreversibly inhibited by phenoxybenzamine (ROSS et al. 1968). In aqueous solutions at pH 7, this *β*-haloalkylamine forms an intermediate cyclic ethylenimonium cation with a half-life of 0.6 min which either acts as an alkylating agent or undergoes hydrolysis to the respective alcohol with a half-life of 19 min (HARVEY and NICKERSON 1953; ADAMS 1974; HENKEL et al. 1976).

In the isolated mucosa of guinea-pig jejunum, pretreatment of the tissue by blood side administration of phenoxybenzamine inhibited secretion and decreased tissue content of *N*-methylscopolamine, the size of the effect being dependent on the total amount of phenoxybenzamine and its contact time. After 30 min

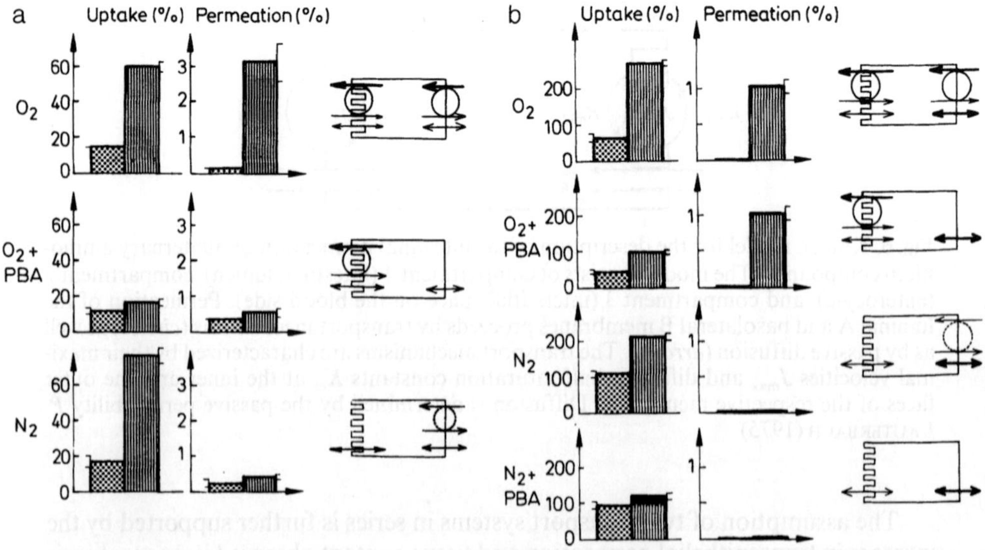

Fig. 7 a, b. Influence of phenoxybenzamine (PBA) and anaerobiosis (N_2) on cellular content and permeation of *N*-methylscopolamine (**a**) and α-phenylcyclopentane acetic acid *N*-isopropyl-nortropin ester methobromide (**b**). 10 μ*M* quaternary ammonium compounds were administered from the luminal side (*stippled bars*) or blood side (*hatched bars*) under aerobic conditions (O_2; control), after a 30-min superfusion period with 100 μ*M* phenoxybenzamine on the blood side (O_2+PBA), under anaerobic conditions (N_2) or under anaerobic conditions after pretreatment with PBA (N_2+PBA). Incubation time 45 min; 37 °C. Ordinates: left, concentration of quaternary compound in the tissue, referred to the intracellular space, and right, concentration in the countercompartment, corrected for flux across shunt pathways, as a percentage of the concentration administered. Schematic cell diagrams depict possible explanation for the observed changes; for further discussion see text. B. PIEPER and F. LAUTERBACH (1980, unpublished work)

superfusion with a 100 μ*M* solution of phenoxybenzamine, tissue content of *N*-methylscopolamine administered in a 10 μ*M* solution was reduced by 72% and permeation from blood to lumen by 82%, which corresponded to a flux ratio of nearly unity (Fig. 7: PIEPER and LAUTERBACH 1979; PIEPER 1979). The inhibitory effect of phenoxybenzamine on *N*-methylscopolamine secretion appeared to be irreversible. Even after a subsequent continuous superfusion with phenoxybenzamine-free solution for 60 min, no restoration of secretion and only a slight rise of tissue uptake above the inhibited level was observed. In contrast, so far all attempts have failed to demonstrate an unequivocal effect of phenoxybenzamine from the luminal side. Likewise, addition of phenoxybenzamine to the blood side did not influence uptake and permeation of *N*-methylscopolamine from the luminal side (PIEPER and LAUTERBACH 1979). Hence it was concluded that only the basolateral entrance mechanism is inhibited by phenoxybenzamine, whereas the luminal mechanism is either insensitive or inaccessible to this inhibitor.

Concerning the existence of the luminal extrusion mechanism, particularly interesting results were obtained by comparing the effects of phenoxybenzamine and anaerobiosis on uptake and secretion of *N*-methylscopolamine and α-phenyl-

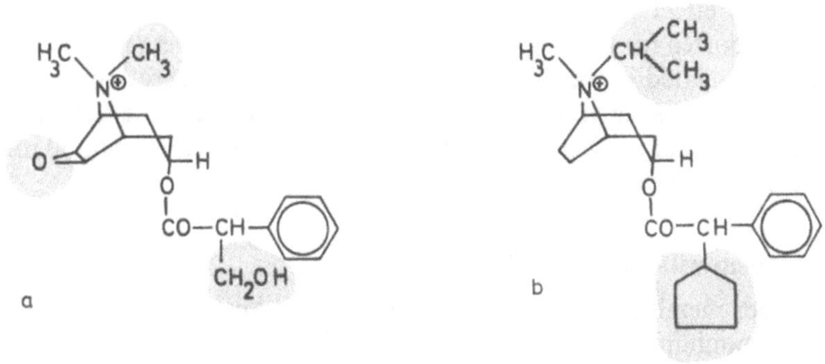

Fig. 8a, b. Structural formula of *N*-methylscopolamine (**a**) and α-phenylcyclopentane acetic acid-*N*-isopropylnortropin ester methobromide (**b**). *Shaded areas* depict changes which increase the chloroform/water partition coefficient from 0.013 to 0.065

cyclopentane acetic acid-*N*-isopropylnortropin ester methobromide (CIN). The latter differs from *N*-methylscopolamine by omission of the epoxide bridge, quaternization by an isopropyl instead of a methyl group and substitution of the primary alcohol group by a cyclopentyl group (Fig. 8). All these changes contribute to an increase in lipophilicity, resulting in chloroform/water partition coefficients of 0.013 and 0.065, respectively. As observed with *N*-methylscopolamine, preincubation with phenoxybenzamine reduced tissue content of CIN. However, in contrast to *N*-methylscopolamine, secretion of CIN was not inhibited at all (see Fig. 7b). As depicted in the schematic cell diagrams of Fig. 7, this has been regarded as evidence that the more lipophilic CIN crosses the basolateral membranes by diffusion in sufficient quantities to sustain secretion, in spite of a reduction in tissue content which possibly does not involve the transport pool. Anaerobiosis, however, abolishes the secretion completely as observed for *N*-methylscopolamine, but causes only a slight decrease of tissue content by one-fifth. Referring to the proposed model, this has been interpreted as evidence that the luminal extrusion mechanism came to a halt owing to the lack of oxidative energy, whereas the basolateral mechanism might mediate uptake of the quaternary base, even under anaerobic conditions, though at a reduced rate, perhaps functioning as a facilitated diffusion system (PIEPER 1979).

Comparable results have been obtained with another β-haloalkylamine, dibenamine. Addition of the inhibitor to the blood side resulted in reduction of *N*-methylscopolamine content and complete suppression of secretion. Dibenamine added to the luminal side was ineffective (B. PIEPER and F. LAUTERBACH 1979, unpublished work). Another inhibitor of intestinal secretion of quaternary ammonium compounds is cyanine dye # 863 (1′-ethyl-3,6-dimethyl-2-phenyl-4-pyrimido-2′-cyanine chloride) whose inhibitory effect on the renal secretion of *N*-methylnicotinamide and tetraethylammonium had been reported previously (PETERS et al. 1955; RENNICK et al. 1956). As compared with the β-haloalkylamines, the 60-min preincubation with 1 m*M* cyanine dye # 863 necessary to suppress the secretion of 10 μ*M* *N*-methylscopolamine indicated a lower inhibitory potency. Though formation of covalent bonds is not to be expected in that case, the inhibitory effect was resistent to subsequent washout. Similar observations have been reported for the dog kidney, where several days were needed to excrete the dye accumulated in the tissue and to restore fully the secretion of *N*-methylnicotinamide (PETERS et al. 1955; RENNICK et al. 1956). In contrast, in the chicken kidney the inhibitory effect disappeared almost completely within 50 min after stopping the cyanine dye infusion (VOLLE et al. 1960).

4. Experiments with Membrane Vesicles

Brush border membrane vesicles from rat intestine were used to study five quaternary ammonium compounds (RUIFROK 1981). Uptake could be observed of only the two most lipophilic molecules and appeared to be a passive process stimulated by a transmembrane electrical potential difference. For equilibration, 10 min was needed by methyldeptropine, but 90 min by *d*-tubocurarine. No saturation of methyldeptropine uptake was measured up to a concentration of 9 m*M*. More interesting contributions to an understanding of the intestinal permeation of quaternary ammonium compounds might be expected by using this promising method for efflux with brush border vesicles and studies with basolateral membranes.

IV. In Vivo Secretion

Secretion of quaternary ammonium compounds inferred from in vitro experiments with isolated mucosae was substantiated by in vivo studies (LAUTERBACH 1970; TURNHEIM and LAUTERBACH 1972, 1977b). After intravenous administration, concentration of *N*-methylnicotinamide and *N*-methylscopolamine in the intestinal fluid exceeded the plasma level 6.5- and 4.3-fold within 75 min. As in the isolated mucosa, tetraethylammonium revealed the smallest secretory rate, a gradient of only 2 was established within 3 h. The concentration gradient for *N*-methylscopolamine decreased with increasing doses, indicating saturation of the secretory mechanisms and was diminished by simultaneous intravenous administration of an excess of *N*-methylnicotinamide.

The possibility of intestinal excretion of organic cations seems to have been widely ignored, not least owing to the usually rapid biliary and/or renal excretion. NEEF et al. (1978) suspected intestinal secretion of thiazinamium and thiazinamium sulphoxide. Within 1 h, 36% and 47%, respectively, of the administered radioactivity were excreted with the bile, but additionally 12% and 9%, were found in a homogenate of gut tissue and contents; no attempts were reported to determine concentration gradients between blood and intestinal fluid. Intestinal secretion of a nonquaternary base, erythromycin, by the rabbit was observed by HOLLAND and QUAY (1976).

D. A Concept for the Intestinal Permeation of Organic Cations

The discovery of an active secretion of organic cations by the mucosal epithelium led to the formulation of a uniform concept for the permeation kinetics of organic bases, consistent with or even predicting peculiarities in the absorption behaviour of these substances, e.g. an increase in the absorption rate with rising doses and a standstill of absorption in spite of large unabsorbed residues. This concept is based on the assumption that the intestinal transport mechanisms for quaternary ammonium compounds are as reversible as those for other substrates, i.e. they facilitate membrane permeation in both directions, notwithstanding their preference for one. The cell model developed for the description of secretory processes (compare Fig. 6) thus applies equally well to transcellular absorption. Permeation in both directions has to be described by at least a system of three compartments formed by the luminal solution, the enterocyte, and the interstitial space, and separated by the brush border and basolateral membrane. Permeation of both membranes can proceed by a transport mechanism whose preference for one direction may be described by different K_m values at the *cis* and *trans* side as well as by a parallel diffusion pathway.[3] Hence, the total system is defined by at least eight principally independent parameters.

The system displays some characteristic features most easily visualized by computer simulation. Figure 9 gives two examples. In both, the two transport mechanisms are assumed to favour the secretory direction by setting $K_{m21} < K_{m12}$ and $K_{m32} < K_{m23}$. Irrespective of the parameter settings, there are two concentration ranges where the permeation rate is independent of concentration.

1. At low concentrations, where $c \ll K_m$ and hence all transport processes work in their proportionality range. In spite of the complexity of the system, participation of transport processes would not be detected by mere determination of absorption or secretion rates at different concentrations, even if these are varied over several orders of magnitude. However, comparison of fluxes in both directions, as may be easily performed with the isolated mucosa preparation, would readily reveal the secretory nature of the system.

2. At high concentrations, where $c \gg K_m$, and hence, transport processes do not contribute measurably to total permeation because of saturation. Transepithelial fluxes are restricted to diffusion and, therefore, equal rates in both directions are observed (compare Fig. 3a).

The intermediate dose range is of particular interest. In both examples, the secretory rate decreases, as has been observed in vitro as well as in vivo, with increasing concentrations. In contrast, absorption rate shows a dual pattern. It may fall (Fig. 9a) as observed with pyridinium aldoximes (compare Fig. 2). It may, on the other hand, rise (Fig. 9b) a behaviour described for benzomethamine (compare Fig. 1). Reversion of the absorption characteristic from falling to rising is brought about by variation of only two half-saturation constants, namely reducing K_{m21} and increasing K_{m23}. These changes favour accumulation in the small, intermediate, cellular compartment and, thereby, saturation of the luminal secretory mechanism. In consequence, absorption is increased since resecretion of substrate which had entered the cell during the course of absorption is reduced.

The peculiar time course of quaternary ammonium compound absorption is most easily understood by regarding another computer simulation performed for

3 Clearly, this system is still a simplification. In reality, further parameters would have to be considered, i.e. the permeability of the paracellular shunt pathways (compare Fig. 5) and most likely, multiple cellular compartments

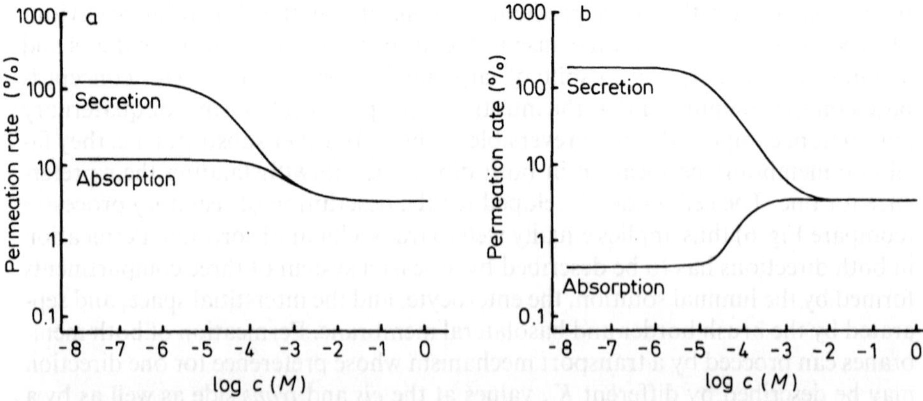

Fif. 9a, b. Computer simulation of the permeation kinetics in the three-compartment system depicted in Fig. 6. Abscissa shows the logarithm of the initial concentration on the side of administration. Ordinate shows permeation rate, i.e. amount disappearing from 1 ml luminal solution after luminal administration (absorption) or amount appearing in 1 ml luminal solution after administration on the blood side (secretion) as percentages of the amount contained initially in 1 ml solution at the side of administration. In approximate accordance with a tied-loop experiment in a small animal, the volumes of compartments 1, 2 and 3 were assumed to be 1, 0.6 and 300 cm^3, respectively and the membrane area A = B = 20 cm^2. The kinetic parameters had the following values:

	a	*b*
$P_A = P_B$(cm min^{-1})	2×10^{-4}	2×10^{-4}
$J_{maxA} = J_{maxB}$(mol min^{-1} cm^{-2})	3.6×10^{-11}	3.6×10^{-11}
$K_{m12}(M)$	8×10^{-5}	8×10^{-5}
$K_{m21}(M)$	1×10^{-5}	1×10^{-6}
$K_{m32}(M)$	2.5×10^{-5}	2.5×10^{-5}
$K_{m23}(M)$	5×10^{-5}	2.5×10^{-3}

LAUTERBACH (1975)

a simplified two-compartment system (TURNHEIM and LAUTERBACH 1980). The outstanding result is cessation of absorption in spite of huge amounts of unabsorbed drug owing to the establishment of an equilibrium between absorption and resecretion (Fig. 10a). However, this interruption is observed only within dose ranges sufficiently low to allow the secretory system to cope with the drug appearing at the transluminal side of the secretory system. If doses are increased and the secretory capacity is surpassed, absorption tends to continue. The higher the dose, the later equilibrium is approached; it may never be reached. Absorption rate thus becomes not only a function of the dose, but also of the absorption time (Fig. 10b). It may even pass through a maximum. Observation of a rising or falling absorption characteristic may depend not only on the properties of the respective substrate (determining affinities and passive permeabilities), but also on the time of observation.

The theoretical curves have been experimentally verified (TURNHEIM and LAUTERBACH 1980). Intrajejunal administration of only 1 nmol/g *N*-methylscopolamine resulted in a rapid initial absorption and complete standstill after 15 min, when only 20% of the dose had been absorbed. Absorption of a 100-fold

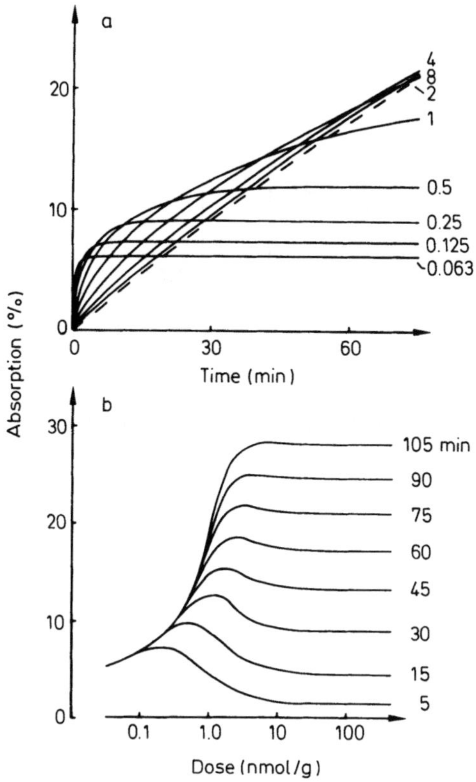

Fig. 10 a, b. Computer simulation of the absorption kinetics as a function of time and concentration in a two-compartment system. The substrate permeates the separating membrane by a secretory transport system and a parallel, diffusional pathway. Absorption is assumed to proceed in an animal of weight 350 g from the intestinal lumen (volume 1 cm^3) across an epithelium (area 30 cm^2) into an apparent distribution volume (800 cm^3). The parameters used for calculation have the following values: $P = 10^{-4}$ cm min^{-1}; $J_{max} = 0.3$ nmol min^{-1} cm^{-2}; $k_{12} = 8 \times 10^{-5}$ *M*; $k_{21} = 1.2 \times 10^{-8}$ *M*. **a** time dependence of absorption at the indicated dose (nmol/g). The *broken line* represents the asymptote of the time course of absorption which is approached at very high intestinal substrate concentration; **b** dose dependence of absorption at the indicated absorption periods. TURNHEIM and LAUTERBACH (1980)

dose, however, started slowly, but proceeded steadily (Fig. 11). Hence, at short absorption intervals, absorption rate dropped with increasing dose. At 75 min there was no longer a difference in the absorption rate of 1 and 100 nmol/g doses. Extending the dose range to still lower levels, however, revealed that, in accordance with the simulated model, an increase of the 75-min absorption rates with rising doses was observed (Fig. 12). A similar standstill of absorption, though at different levels, was observed with *N*-methylnicotinamide and tetraethylammonium.

Interpretation of the interruption of absorption as an equilibrium was substantiated by its perturbation (TURNHEIM and LAUTERBACH 1980). This was achieved first by transfering the intestinal content into an isolated loop of an untreated guinea-pig after absorption had stopped. As expected, absorption

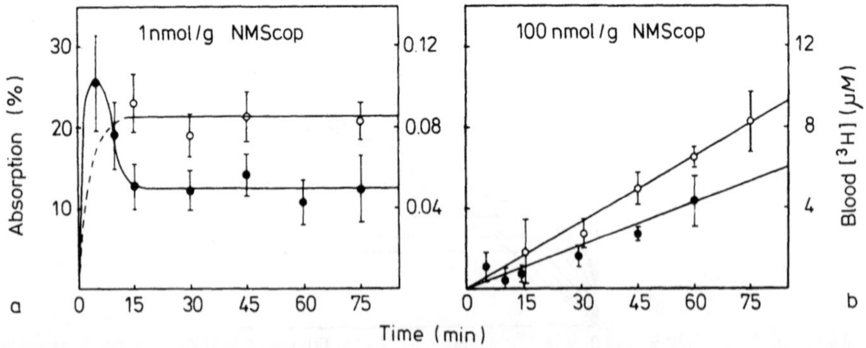

Fig. 11 a, b. Time course of absorption, as a percentage of the dose given (*open circles*) and blood levels of radioactivity (*full circles*) after administration of 1 nmol/g (**a**) or 100 nmol/g (**b**) *N*-methylscopolamine ^{3}H into an isolated jejunal loop. Mean ± standard error of 4–7 experiments. TURNHEIM and LAUTERBACH (1980)

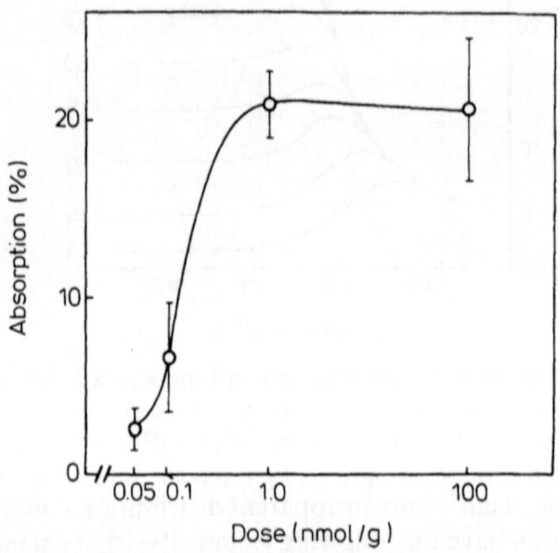

Fig. 12. Relationship between dose of *N*-methylscopolamine ^{3}H administered into an isolated jejunal loop and the percentage absorbed within 75 min. Mean ± standard error of 4–7 experiments. TURNHEIM and LAUTERBACH (1980)

restarted, resulting in the uptake of another aliquot of the dose. Hence, formation of unabsorbable complexes as proposed earlier (LEVINE et al. 1955) cannot be the sole reason for cessation of absorption. Second, absorption of labelled *N*-methylscopolamine or *N*-methylnicotinamide could be enhanced by simultaneous intravenous administration of an excess of unlabelled *N*-methylnicotinamide.

In summary, all phenomena predicted by the hypothesis that absorption of quaternary ammonium compounds is the result of simultaneous working of diffusion and transport (where the secretory transport system might oppose or, under suitable conditions, favour the absorption) are verified by at least one example. Although intestinal secretion of further quaternary bases remains to be investigated it seems reasonable to assume that the peculiar absorption behaviour of numerous organic cations so often reported in the earlier literature can be ascribed to the same principles.

E. Comparative Aspects of Organic Cation Secretion

I. Intestinal Secretion of Other Xenobiotics

The ability of the intestinal mucosa to excrete foreign compounds is not restricted to organic cations. Intestinal secretion has been demonstrated previously for cardiac glycosides (LAUTERBACH 1969a, b, 1971). As compared with quaternary ammonium compounds, very similar observations have been made. In the isolated jejunal mucosa, cardiac glycosides are also taken up preferentially from the blood side, in contrast to the favoured uptake from the luminal side of nutrients like sugars and amino acids. Anaerobiosis caused the same effects on tissue content, absorption and secretion, as mentioned for quaternary ammonium compounds. An identical system of two transport mechanisms in series has thus been deduced to be responsible for secretion of cardiac glycosides (for reviews see LAUTERBACH 1977b, 1981). Insensitivity of secretion of cardiotonic steroids to phenoxybenzamine (PIEPER and LAUTERBACH 1979) as well as other results demonstrate that these drugs do not share the transport system for quaternary ammonium compounds. In vivo, secretion interferes with absorption in the same way as elucidated for quaternary ammonium compounds (SEIDENSTÜCKER and LAUTERBACH 1976; SEIDENSTÜCKER 1978; LAUTERBACH 1981). Intestinal secretion of organic acids has likewise been demonstrated for some sulphonic acids (SUND and LAUTERBACH 1978; LAUTERBACH 1979) and salicylic acid (LAUTERBACH and STEINKE 1981). As with the other xenobiotics, secretion seems to be favoured by an enlargement of the lipophilic part of the molecule (LAUTERBACH 1979). Some evidence has accumulated that more than one transport system for organic acids with different substrate specificities might exist in the intestine (LAUTERBACH and STEINKE 1981; LAUTERBACH et al. 1982).[4]

In the guinea-pig, at least, considerable differences between these groups of xenobiotics exist with respect to the distribution of secretory activity along the gastrointestinal tract. Secretion of quaternary ammonium compounds in the isolated colonic mucosa proceeds at rates comparable to or even less than those observed in the jejunum (B. PIEPER and F. LAUTERBACH 1980, unpublished work). In contrast, much higher secretory rates for cardiac glycosides (KILIAN et al. 1978; KILIAN and LAUTERBACH 1979) and the sulphonic acid β-naphthol orange (U. KILLIAN and F. LAUTERBACH 1980, unpublished) were observed in the colon than in the jejunum, but no secretion of salicylic acid could be detected (LAUTERBACH et al. 1982). Furthermore, secretory processes in the colon were inhibited only slightly by anaerobiosis (KILIAN et al. 1978; KILIAN and LAUTERBACH 1979).

II. Secretion of Organic Cations by Other Organs

1. Substrate Specificity

Transport of xenobiotic organic cations has been observed in a number of tissues; the system in the choroid plexus (TOCHINO and SCHANKER 1965; ASGHAR and

---

4 Intestinal secretion of normal body constituents has been demonstrated with hypoxanthine and xanthine in the golden hamster (BERLIN and HAWKINS 1968a, b) and the guinea-pig (KOLASSA et al. 1980)

ROTH 1971) has been shown to be sensitive to Dibenamine (MILLER and ROSS 1976). Most studies were engaged with the main excretory organs of the body: kidney (for reviews see PETERS 1960; WEINER 1971, 1973; HOLM 1975; GREVEN 1981; RENNICK 1981) and liver (for reviews see SCHANKER 1968; SMITH 1971; MEIJER 1977). In contrast to the intestine where only preliminary data are available, suggesting the secretion of nonquaternary amines in their protonated form by the transport system for quaternary ammonium compounds, ample evidence has accumulated that in the kidney nonquaternary and quaternary cations share the same transport system (TORRETTI et al. 1962; for reviews see preceding citations). Affinity of monoquaternary ammonium compounds to the secretory system seems to be favoured by increasing the lipophilicity of the uncharged part of the molecule in the intestine as well as in kidney (FARAH et al. 1959; GREEN et al. 1959; VOLLE et al. 1959; REYNARD 1968) and liver (SMITH 1971; SCHANKER 1972; HIROM et al. 1974).

Intestinal secretion of bisquaternary ammonium compounds has not been unequivocally detected so far. Likewise, these substances are secreted in the kidney only slowly or not at all (VOLLE et al. 1960; HOLM 1975) and only in the case of very pronounced lipophilicity in the liver (MEIJER 1977). In contrast to the observations made in the intestine, considerable accumulation of bisquaternary ammonium compounds in kidney slices has been observed (MCISAAC 1965, 1969) though with marked species differences. It remains to be investigated whether these might also account for the deviations between kidney and intestine.

2. Cellular Localization of Transport Mechanisms

As in the intestine, secretion by two transport mechanisms in series has been inferred both for the liver (for review see MEIJER 1977) and the kidney (for reviews see FOULKES 1981; RENNICK 1981). Experiments with renal membrane vesicles revealed different mechanisms for the function of the transporters in the luminal and antiluminal membrane consistent with a "carrier" and "gated pore" model, respectively (KINSELLA et al. 1979; HOLOHAN and ROSS 1980). Energy for the transport across the luminal membrane was supplied by two functionally linked $Na^+:H^+$ and H^+ : *N*-methylnicotinamide antiport systems (HOLOHAN and ROSS 1981).

F. Conclusions

Intestinal permeation of organic bases cannot be explained consistently by simple nonionic diffusion. Several models have been developed to explain deviations from flux ratios calculated on the basis of this theory. Moreover, intestinal secretion of monoquaternary ammonium compounds has been unequivocally demonstrated; secretion of organic bases as cations by this route is very likely. Hence, two main consequences emerge.

First, absorption of organic cations has to proceed against a secretory mechanism. Well-known peculiarities in the absorption behaviour of organic bases and quaternary ammonium compounds can now be explained by a concept of the interaction of diffusion and a secretory transport system which either opposes or, eventually, mediates the absorptive flux. It is a consequence of this concept – and substantiated by experimental evidence – that absorption becomes dependent on intestinal concentration and absorption time in a complex manner. Hence, no extrapolation of absorption rates determined at a given dose and given time is allowed as long as participation of a secretory transport process has not been excluded.

Second, the intestine joins the liver and the kidney as a third potent organ for the excretion of xenobiotic substances. Further investigations are needed to establish the quantitative contribution of intestinal secretion to the overall elimination of drugs and other foreign compounds. The fact that 15 cm of guinea-pig jejunum excreted 2% of a dose of intravenous quaternary ammonium compound within 75 min (TURNHEIM and LAUTERBACH 1977 b) suggests that the role of intestinal secretion might be substantial, not least in cases of hepatic and/or renal insufficiency.

References

Adams WP (1974) Kinetics and reaction mechanism of phenoxybenzamine decomposition in aqueous and aqueous ethanolic solutions. Dissertation, University of Kentucky

Albanus L, Sundwall A, Vangbo B (1969) On the metabolic disposition of methylatropine in animals and man. Acta Pharmacol Toxicol (Copenh) 27:97–111

Asghar K, Roth LJ (1971) Entry and distribution of hexamethonium in the central nervous system. Biochem Pharmacol 20:2787–2795

Beermann B, Hellström K, Rosen A (1971 a) Uptake in the human small intestine of a quaternary anticholinergic compound (Acabel). Eur J Clin Pharmacol 3:93–96

Beermann B, Hellström K, Rosen A (1971 b) Absorption of ^{14}C-methylscopolamine from the digestive tract. Eur J Clin Pharmacol 4:46–51

Beermann B, Hellström K, Rosen A (1971 c) The gastrointestinal absorption of anticholinergic drugs: Comparison between individuals. Acta Pharmacol Toxicol (Copenh) 29, [Suppl] 3:98–102

Bennett PN, Davies DS, Hawkesworth GM (1976) In vivo absorption studies with paraquat and diquat in the dog. Br J Pharmacol 58:284P

Berlin RD, Hawkins RA (1968 a) Secretion of purines by the small intestine: general characteristics. Am J Physiol 215:932–941

Berlin RD, Hawkins RA (1968 b) Secretion of purines by the small intestine: transport mechanism. Am J Physiol 215:942–950

Breiter K, Ohnesorge FK (1971) On the enteral absorption of tertiary and quaternary amines from the isolated guinea pig jejunum. Acta Pharmacol Toxicol (Copenh) 29 [Suppl] 4:42

Brodie BB (1964) Physico-chemical factors in drug absorption. In: Binns TB (ed) Absorption and distribution of drugs. Livingstone, Edinburgh, London, pp 16

Collander R, Bärlund H (1933) Permeabilitätsstudien an Chara ceratophylla. II. Die Permeabilität für Nichtelektrolyte. Acta Bot Fenn 11:1–114

Cramer MB, Cates LA, Clarke DE (1978) Rectal absorption of homatropine (^{14}C)methylbromide in the rat. J Pharm Pharmacol 30:284–286

Crone HD, Keen TEB (1969) An in vitro study of the intestinal absorption of pyridinium aldoximes. Br J Pharmacol 35:304–312

Csáky TZ (1961) Significance of sodium ions in active intestinal transport of nonelectrolytes. Am J Physiol 201:999–1001

Duchene-Marullaz P, Constantin M, Talvard J, Beau G (1969) A propos de l'absorption intestinale du N-butyl hyoscine. Therapie 24:621–625

Farah A, Frazer M, Porter E (1959) Studies on the uptake of N′-methylnicotinamide by renal slices of the dog. J Pharmacol Exp Ther 126:202–211

Foulkes EC (1981) Asymmetry of membrane functions in transporting cells. In: Greger R, Lang F, Silbernagl S (eds) Renal transport of organic substances. Springer, Berlin Heidelberg New York, pp 45–54

Franz JM, Vonderscher JP, Voges R (1980) Contribution to the intestinal absorption of ergot peptide alkaloids. Int J Pharm 7:19–28

Green RE, Ricker WE, Attwood WL, Koh YS, Peters L (1959) Studies of the renal tubular transport characteristics of N^1-methylnicotinamide and tetraalkylammonium compounds in the avian kidney. J Pharmacol Exp Ther 126:195–201

Greven J (1981) Renal transport of drugs. In: Greger R, Lang F, Silbernagl S (eds) Renal transport of organic substances. Springer, Berlin Heidelberg New York, pp 262–277

Harvey SC, Nickerson M (1953) The chemical transformation of dibenamine and dibenzyline and biological activity. J Pharmacol Exp Ther 109:328–339

Henkel JG, Portoghese PS, Miller JW, Lewis P (1976) Synthesis and adrenoreceptor blocking action of aziridinium ions derived from phenoxybenzamine and dibenamine. J Med Chem 19:6–10

Herzberg GR, Lerner J (1973) Intestinal absorption of choline in the chick. Biochim Biophys Acta 307:234–242

Hirom PC, Hughes RD, Millburn P (1974) The physicochemical factor required for the biliary excretion of organic cations and anions. Biochem Soc Trans 2:327–330

Höber R, Höber J (1937) Experiments on the absorption of organic solutes in the small intestine of rats. J Cell Physiol 10:401–422

Hogben CAM, Schanker LS, Tocco DJ, Brodie BB (1957) Absorption of drugs from the stomach. II. The human. J Pharmacol Exp Ther 120:540–545

Hogben CAM, Tocco DJ, Brodie BB, Schanker LS (1959) On the mechanism of intestinal absorption of drugs. J Pharmacol Exp Ther 125:275–282

Holland DR, Quay JF (1976) Intestinal secretion of erythromycin base. J Pharm Sci 65:417–419

Holm J (1975) Uptake of monoquaternary and polymethylene-bisquaternary amines by kidney slices. Thesis, University of Copenhagen

Holm J (1977) Effect of choline on tetraaethylammonium transport in mouse kidney cortex slices. Biochem Pharmacol 26:1935–1939

Holohan PD, Ross CR (1980) Mechanisms of organic cation transport in kidney plasma membrane vesicles: 1. Countertransport studies. J Pharmacol Exp Ther 215:191–197

Holohan PD, Ross CR (1981) Mechanisms of organic cation transport in kidney plasma membrane vesicles: 2. ΔpH studies. J Pharmacol Exp Ther 216:294–298

Irwin GM, Kostenbauder HB, Dittert LW, Staples R, Misher A, Swintosky JV (1969) Enhancement of gastrointestinal absorption of a quaternary ammonium compound by trichloroacetate. J Pharm Sci 58:313–315

Isomaa B (1975) Absorption, distribution and excretion of (^{14}C)CTAB, a quaternary ammonium surfactant, in the rat. Food Cosmet Toxicol 13:231–237

Jackson MJ (1977) Epithelial transport of weak electrolytes. Properties of a model of the three-compartment system. J Theor Biol 64:771–788

Jackson MJ, Morgan BN (1975) Relations of weak-electrolyte transport and acid-base metabolism in rat small intestine in vitro. Am J Physiol 228:482–487

Jackson MJ, Kutcher LM (1977) The three-compartment system for transport of weak electrolytes in the small intestine. In: Kramer M, Lauterbach F (eds) Intestinal permeation. Excerpta Medica, Amsterdam, pp 65–73

Jackson MJ, Shiau YF, Bane S, Fox M (1974) Intestinal transport of weak electrolytes. Evidence in favor of a three-compartment system. J Gen Physiol 63:187–213

Jackson MJ, Williamson AM, Dombrowski WA, Garner DE (1978) Intestinal transport of weak electrolytes. Determinants of influx at the luminal surface. J Gen Physiol 71:301–327

Jackson MJ, Tai CY, Steane JE (1981) Weak electrolyte permeation in alimentary epithelia. Am J Physiol 240:G191–G198

Jacobs MH (1940) Some aspects of cell permeability to weak electrolytes. Cold Spring Harbor Symp Quant Biol 8:30–39

Jonkman JHG, van Bork LE, Wijsbeek J, DeZeeuw RA, Orie NGM (1977) Variations in the bioavailability of thiazinamium methylsulfate. Clin Pharmacol Ther 21:457–463

Kakemi K, Sezaki H, Kondo T (1969) Absorption and excretion of drugs. XLI. Studies on the gastrointestinal absorption of 2-pyridine aldoxime methiodide and its derivatives. Chem Pharm Bull (Tokyo) 17:1864–1870

Kilian U, Lauterbach F (1979) Intestinal secretion of drugs by isolated mucosae of the small and large intestine in guinea-pig and man. Gastroenterol Clin Biol 3:178

Kilian U, Lauterbach F, Pieper B (1978) Investigations on the intestinal secretion of drugs by the isolated mucosa of guinea-pig colon. Naunyn-Schmiedebergs Arch Pharmacol 302:R2

Kinsella JL, Holohan PD, Pessah NI, Ross CR (1979) Transport of organic ions in renal cortical luminal and antiluminal membrane vesicles. J Pharmacol Exp Ther 209:443–450

Kolassa N, Stengg R, Turnheim K (1977) Adenosine uptake by the isolated epithelium of guinea pig jejunum. Can J Physiol Pharmacol 55:1033–1038

Kolassa N, Schützenberger WG, Wiener H, Turnheim K (1980) Active secretion of hypoxanthine and xanthine by guinea pig jejunum in vitro. Am J Physiol 238 (Gastrointest Liver Physiol 1):G141–149

Kuczler FJ, Nahrwold DL, Rose RC (1977) Choline influx across the brush border of guinea pig jejunum. Biochim Biophys Acta 465:131–137

Kunze H, Blinne K, Vogt W (1971) Intestinal absorption of a mono-quaternary drug, ^{14}C-neostigmine. Naunyn-Schmiedebergs Arch Pharmacol 270:161–168

Kurz H (1975) Principles of drug absorption. In: Forth W, Rummel W (eds) Pharmacology of intestinal absorption: gastrointestinal absorption of drugs, vol 1. Pergamon, Oxford, pp 245–296 (International encyclopedia of pharmacology and therapeutics, sect 39B)

Larsson L, Wallerberg G (1962) The structure of N-methylpyridinium-2-aldoxime. Acta Chem Scand [B] 16:788–789

Lauterbach F (1969a) Metabolismus und enterale Resorption herzwirksamer Glykoside. Naunyn-Schmiedebergs Arch Pharmacol 263:26–39

Lauterbach F (1969b) Die enterale Sekretion kardiotoner Steroide – Untersuchungen zum Mechanismus des Resorptionsvorganges. Naunyn-Schmiedebergs Arch Pharmacol 264:267–268

Lauterbach F (1970) Werden quaternäre Ammoniumverbindungen über einen enteralen Sekretionsmechanismus resorbiert? Naunyn-Schmiedebergs Arch Pharmacol 266:388

Lauterbach F (1971) Untersuchungen über den Mechanismus der Permeation cardiotoner Steroide durch die Mucosa des Dünndarmes – ein Beitrag zur Theorie der Resorption von Pharmaka. Habilitationsschrift, University of Bochum

Lauterbach F (1975) Resorption und Sekretion von Arzneistoffen durch die Mukosaepithelien des Gastrointestinaltraktes. Arzneimittelforsch 25:479–488

Lauterbach F (1977a) Passive permeabilities of luminal and basolateral membranes in the isolated mucosal epithelium of guinea pig small intestine. Naunyn-Schmiedebergs Arch Pharmacol 297:201–212

Lauterbach F (1977b) Intestinal secretion of organic ions and drugs. In: Kramer M, Lauterbach F (eds) Intestinal permeation. Excerpta Medica, Amsterdam, pp 173–194

Lauterbach F (1979) Enterale Resorptions- und Sekretionsmechanismen. In: Rietbrock N, Schnieders B (eds) Bioverfügbarkeit von Arzneimitteln. Fischer, Stuttgart, pp 109–126

Lauterbach F (1981) Intestinal absorption and secretion of cardiac glycosides. In: Greeff K (ed) Cardiac glycosides. Springer, Berlin Heidelberg New York, pp 105–139 (Handbook of experimental pharmacology, vol 56/II)

Lauterbach F, Steinke W (1981) Comparative aspects of the intestinal secretion of organic acids and its inhibition by probenecid and phenoxybenzamine. Naunyn-Schmiedebergs Arch Pharmacol 316 [Suppl]:R50

Lauterbach F, Giese M, Kilian U, Steinke W (1982) Comparative aspects of diffusion and transport of drugs across the mucosa of small intestine and colon. Naunyn-Schmiedebergs Arch Pharmacol 321:R55

Levine RM (1959) The intestinal absorption of the quaternary derivatives of atropine and scopolamine. Arch Int Pharmacodyn Ther 121:146–149

Levine RM, Clark BB (1957a) The physiological disposition of oxyphenonium bromide (antrenyl) and related compounds. J Pharmacol Exp Ther 121:63–70

Levine RM, Clark BB (1957b) A note on the intestinal absorption of penthienate (monodral). Arch Int Pharmacodyn Ther 112:458–462

Levine RM, Blair MR, Clark BB (1955) Factors influencing the intestinal absorption of certain monoquaternary anticholinergic compounds with special reference to benzomethamine [N-diethylaminoethyl-N′-methyl-benzilamide methobromide (MC-3199)]. J Pharmacol Exp Ther 114:78–86

Levine RR (1960) The physiological disposition of hexamethonium and related compounds. J Pharmacol Exp Ther 129:296–304

Levine RR (1961) The influence of the intraluminal intestinal milieu on absorption of an organic cation and an anionic agent. J Pharmacol Exp Ther 131:328–333

Levine RR, Pelikan EW (1961) The influence of experimental procedures and dose on the intestinal absorption of an onium compound, benzomethamine. J Pharmacol Exp Ther 131:319–327

Levine RR, Steinberg GM (1966) Intestinal absorption of pralidoxime and other aldoximes. Nature 15:269–271

McIsaac RJ (1965) The uptake of hexamethonium-C^{14} by kidney slices. J Pharmacol Exp Ther 150:92–98

McIsaac RJ (1969) The binding of organic bases to kidney cortex slices. J Pharmacol Exp Ther 168:6–12

Meijer DKF (1977) The mechanisms for hepatic uptake and biliary excretion of organic cations. In: Kramer M, Lauterbach F (eds) Intestinal permeation. Excerpta Medica, Amsterdam, pp 196–207

Miller TB, Ross CR (1976) Transport of organic cations and anions by choroid plexus. J Pharmacol Exp Ther 196:771–777

Milne MD, Scribner BH, Crawford MA (1958) Non-ionic diffusion and the excretion of weak acids and bases. Am J Med 24:709–729

Murray RE, Gibson JE (1974) Paraquat disposition in rats, guinea pigs and monkeys. Toxicol Appl Pharmacol 27:283–291

Neef K, Jonkman JHG, Meijer DKF (1978) Hepatic disposition and biliary excretion of the organic cations thiazinamium and thiazinamium sulfoxide in rats. J Pharm Sci 67:1147–1150

Overton E (1896) Über die osmotischen Eigenschaften der Zelle in ihrer Bedeutung für die Toxikologie und Pharmakologie (mit besonderer Berücksichtigung der Ammoniake und Alkaloide). Vierteljahresschr Naturforsch Ges Zuerich 41:383–406

Overton E (1899) Über die allgemeinen osmotischen Eigenschaften der Zelle, ihre vermutlichen Ursachen und ihre Bedeutung für die Physiologie. Vierteljahresschr Naturforsch Ges Zuerich 44:88–135

Overton E (1902) Beiträge zur allgemeinen Muskel- und Nervenphysiologie. Pfluegers Arch 92:115–280

Pentikäinen P, Penttilä A, Vapaatalo H, Hackman R (1973) Intestinal absorption, intestinal distribution, and excretion of (^{14}C)labelled hyoscine N-butylbromide (butylscopolamine) in the rat. J Pharm Pharmacol 25:371–375

Peters L (1960) Renal tubular excretion of organic bases. Pharmacol Rev 12:1–35

Peters L, Fenton KJ, Wolf ML, Kandel A (1955) Inhibition of the renal tubular excretion of N′-methylnicotinamide (NMN) by small doses of a basic cyanine dye. J Pharmacol Exp Ther 113:148–159

Pieper B (1979) Influence of phenoxybenzamine on the intestinal secretion of various quaternary ammonium compounds by two transport mechanisms in series. Naunyn-Schmiedebergs Arch Pharmacol 307:R5

Pieper B, Lauterbach F (1979) Specificity, localization and inhibition of intestinal transport systems for quaternary ammonium compounds. Gastroenterol Clin Biol 3:167–168

Ragozzino PW, Malone MH (1963) Biodynamics of thiourea-alkaloid combinations. J Pharmacol Exp Ther 141:363–368

Rennick BR (1981) Renal tubular transport of organic cations. In: Greger R, Lang F, Silbernagl S (eds) Renal transport of organic substances. Springer, Berlin Heidelberg New York, pp 178–188

Rennick BR, Kandel A, Peters L (1956) Inhibition of the renal tubular excretion of tetraethylammonium and N′-methylnicotinamide by basic cyanine dyes. J Pharmacol Exp Ther 118:204–219

Reynard AM (1968) The reversible and irreversible inhibition of N^1-methylnicotinamide uptake into rat kidney cortex slices. J Pharmacol Exp Ther 163:461–467

Ross CR, Pessah NI, Farah A (1968) Inhibitory effects of β-haloalkylamines on the renal transport of N-methylnicotinamide. J Pharmacol Exp Ther 160:375–380

Ruifrok PG (1981) Uptake of quaternary ammonium compounds into rat intestinal brush border membrane vesicles. Biochem Pharmacol 30:2637–2641

Schanker LS (1959) Absorption of drugs from the rat colon. J Pharmacol Exp Ther 126:283–290

Schanker LS (1960) On the mechanism of absorption of drugs from the gastrointestinal tract. J Med Pharmaceut Chem 2:343–359

Schanker LS (1962) Passage of drugs across body membranes. Pharmacol Rev 14:501–530

Schanker LS (1964) Physiological transport of drugs. Adv Drug Res 1:71–106

Schanker LS (1968) Secretion of organic compounds in bile. In: Code CF (ed) Bile, digestion, ruminal physiology. American Physiological Society, Washington, DC, pp 2433–2449 (Handbook of physiology, sect 6, Alimentary Canal, vol V)

Schanker LS (1971) Absorption of drugs from the gastrointestinal tract. In: Brodie BB, Gillette JR (eds) Concepts in biochemical pharmacology, P 1. Springer, Berlin Heidelberg New York, pp 9–24 (Handbook of experimental pharmacology, vol 28/1)

Schanker LS (1972) Transport of drugs. In: Hokin LE (ed) Metabolic pathways, metabolic transport, Vol IV. Academic, London, pp 543–579

Schanker LS, Tocco DJ (1960) Active transport of some pyrimidines across the rat intestinal epithelium. J Pharmacol Exp Ther 128:115–121

Schanker LS, Tocco DJ (1962) Some characteristics of the pyrimidine transport process of the small intestine. Biochim Biophys Acta 56:469–473

Schanker LS, Shore PA, Brodie BB, Hogben CAM (1957) Absorption of drugs from the stomach. I. The rat. J Pharmacol Exp Ther 120:528–539

Schanker LS, Tocco DJ, Brodie BB, Hogben CAM (1958) Absorption of drugs from the rat small intestine. J Pharmacol Exp Ther 123:81–88

Schanker LS, Jeffrey JJ, Tocco DJ (1963) Interaction of purines with the pyrimidine transport process of the small intestine. Biochem Pharmacol 12:1047–1053

Scharrer E, Raab W, Tiemeyer W, Amann B (1981) Active absorption of hypoxanthine by lamb jejunum in vitro. Pfluegers Arch 391:41–43

Schultz SG, Frizzell RA (1975) Amino acid transport by the small intestine. In: Csáky TZ (ed) Intestinal absorption and malabsorption. Raven, Newlett, p 77

Seidenstücker R (1978) Beziehungen zwischen enteraler Sekretion und Resorption herzwirksamer Glycoside. Ph. D. Thesis, Bochum

Seidenstücker R, Lauterbach F (1976) Mediation of intestinal absorption of cardiotonic steroids by a secretory transfer mechanism. Naunyn-Schmiedebergs Arch Pharmacol 293:R45

Shore PA, Brodie BB, Hogben CAM (1957) The gastric secretion of drugs: A pH partition hypothesis. J Pharmacol Exp Ther 119:361–369

Smith RL (1971) Excretion of drugs in bile. In: Brodie BB, Gillette JR (eds) Concepts in biochemical pharmacology, pt 1. Springer, Berlin Heidelberg New York, pp 354–389 (Handbook of experimental pharmacology, vol 28/1)

Steffen C, Konder H (1979) Absorption of paraquat by rat gut in vitro. Arch Toxicol 43:99–103

Sund RB (1971) The absorption of atropine from the small intestine of anaesthetized rats. Medd Nor Farm Selskap 33:154–162

Sund RB, Lauterbach F (1978) Intestinal secretion of sulphanilic acid by the isolated mucosa of guinea pig jejunum. Acta Pharmacol Toxicol (Copenh) 43:331–338

Sundwall A, Vessman J, Strindberg B (1973) Fate of emepronium in man in relation to its pharmacological effects. Eur J Clin Pharmacol 6:191–195

Suzuki E, Doi K, Kondo T, Matsui H, Sezaki H (1975) Effect of some cationic drugs on the intestinal absorption of pralidoxime iodide. Chem Pharm Bull (Tokyo) 23:899–908

Tai CY, Jackson MJ (1981) Weak-acid transport in the small intestine: Discrimination in the lamina propria. J Membr Biol 59:35–43

Tochino Y, Schanker LS (1965) Active transport of quaternary ammonium compounds by the choroid plexus in vitro. Am J Physiol 208:666–673

Torretti J, Weiner IM, Mudge GH (1962) Renal tubular secretion and reabsorption of organic bases in the dog. J Clin Invest 41:793–804

Travell J (1940) The influence of the hydrogen ion concentration on the absorption of alkaloids from the stomach. J Pharmacol Exp Ther 69:21–33

Turnheim K, Lauterbach F (1972) Intestinal transport of quaternary ammonium compounds in vivo. Naunyn-Schmiedebergs Arch Pharmacol 274:R118

Turnheim K, Lauterbach F (1977 a) Absorption and secretion of monoquaternary ammonium compounds by the isolated intestinal mucosa. Biochem Pharmacol 26:99–108

Turnheim K, Lauterbach F (1977 b) Secretion of monoquaternary ammonium compounds by guinea pig small intestine in vivo. Naunyn-Schmiedebergs Arch Pharmacol 299:201–205

Turnheim K, Lauterbach F (1980) Interaction between intestinal absorption and secretion of monoquaternary ammonium compounds in guinea pigs – a concept for the absorption kinetics of organic cations. J Pharmacol Exp Ther 212:418–424

Turnheim K, Lauterbach F, Kolassa N (1977) Intestinal transfer of the quaternary ammonium compound N-methyl-scopolamine by two transport mechanisms in series. Biochem Pharmacol 26:763–767

Ussing HH (1949) The distinction by means of tracers between active transport and diffusion. Acta Physiol Scand 19:43–56

Van Dijk A, Maes RAA, Drost RH, Douze JMC, van Heyst ANP (1975) Paraquat poisoning in man. Arch Toxicol 34:129–136

Volle RL, Huggins CG, Rodriguez GA, Peters L (1959) Inhibition of the renal tubular transport of N^1-methylnicotinamide (NMN) by 1,1-dialkylpiperidinium compounds in the avian kidney. J Pharmacol Exp Ther 126:190–194

Volle RL, Peters L, Green RE (1960) Inhibition of the renal tubular excretion of N^1-methylnicotinamide (NMN) in the avian kidney by a cyanine dye and by bisquaternary compounds. J Pharmacol Exp Ther 129:377–387

Waldeck F (1969) The intestinal absorption of scopolamine-N-butylbromide (Buscopan®) from isolated loops in conscious rats. Eur J Pharmacol 8:108–113

Weiner JM (1971) Excretion of drugs by the kidney. In: Brodie BB, Gillette JR (eds) Concepts in biochemical pharmacology, P 1. Springer, Berlin Heidelberg New York, pp 328–353 (Handbook of experimental pharmacology, vol 28/1)

Weiner JM (1973) Transport of węak acids and bases. In: Orloff I, Berliner RW, Geiger SR (eds) Renal physiology. American Physiological Society, Washington, DC, pp 521–554 (Handbook of physiology, sect 8)

Wick H (1967) Enteral absorption of hyoscine N-butylbromide. J Pharm Pharmacol 19:779

Wiseman G (1974) Absorption of protein digestion products. In: Smyth DH (ed) Biomembranes 4A, intestinal absorption, Plenum, London, chap 8, pp 363

Zawoiski EJ, Baer JE, Braunschweig LW, Paulson SF, Shermer A, Beyer KH (1958) Gastrointestinal secretion and absorption of 3-methylaminoisocamphane hydrochloride (Mecamylamine). J Pharmacol Exp Ther 122:442–448

CHAPTER 23

Role of Blood Flow in Intestinal Permeation*

D. WINNE

A. Introduction

The net transfer of a substance from the intestinal lumen into the intestinal venous blood can be defined as intestinal absorption. The substances, drugs and nutrients, permeate from the bulk phase of the luminal fluid through the unstirred fluid layer adjacent to the mucosal surface to the intestinal cells (Fig. 1). The intestinal epithelium is passed on cellular and/or paracellular pathways by passive and active transport mechanisms, respectively. After having traversed the subepithelial interstitial space and the capillary walls, the molecules are picked up by the blood in the subepithelial capillaries. Finally the drugs and nutrients appear in the intestinal venous blood, eventually together with their metabolites. In rodents the intestinal wall is thin, so that a small fraction of the substances is not drained by the blood, but reaches the serosal side. Usually this fraction penetrates into neighbouring intestinal segments or into the peritoneum, appearing finally in the systemic blood. Under experimental conditions, if the intestinal segment is placed outside the abdominal cavity, this fraction enters the tissue covering the intestine or the solution bathing the segment (OCHSENFAHRT 1971, 1979). Permeation from the intestinal lumen into the serosal fluid is the pathway when the in-

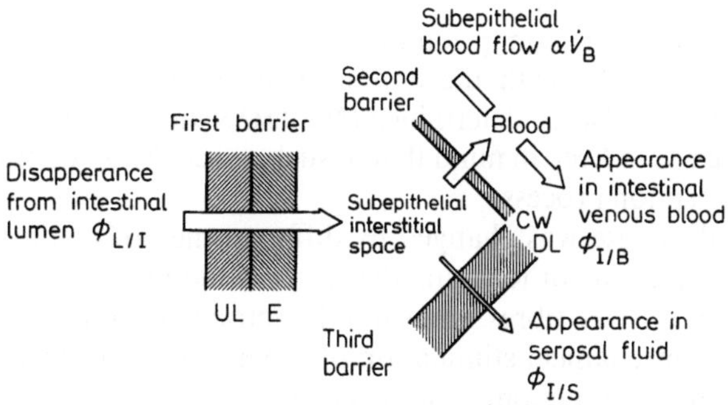

Fig. 1. Schematic view of intestinal permeation and drainage by blood. *UL*, unstirred fluid layer adjacent to mucosal surface; *E*, epithelium; *CW*, capillary wall; *DL*, deeper layers of intestinal wall; $\Phi_{L/I}$, disappearance rate from intestinal lumen; $\Phi_{I/B}$, appearance rate in intestinal venous blood; $\Phi_{I/S}$, appearance rate in serosal fluid; α, fraction of subepithelial blood flow rate or absorption site blood flow rate; $\dot{V}_B$, total blood flow rate of intestinal segment

* This chapter submitted in April 1980 covers the literature up to 1979

testinal segment is excised and investigated in vitro. According to the quantity measured we distinguish: the disappearance rate from the intestinal lumen, the appearance rate in the intestinal venous blood and the appearance rate in the serosal fluid (Fig. 1). If necessary, we have to consider storage and metabolism in the intestinal cells. In this chapter "absorption rate" is used as the preferred term.

In general, the absorption rate depends on the luminal concentration, the resistances of the mucosal unstirred layer and the intestinal epithelium and on the efficiency of the drainage system. In this chapter, the influence of the drainage system, i.e. the influence of blood flow, on the intestinal permeation process will be described. The role of the lymphatic system in intestinal absorption has been reviewed by BARROWMAN (1978). More general aspects of the intestinal circulation have been discussed by LUNDGREN and JODAL (1975) and SVANVIK and LUNDGREN (1977).

B. Methods

If the relationship between blood flow and intestinal absorption is to be studied, it is necessary to measure simultaneously the blood flow rate and the absorption rate in the intestinal segment under study. Moreover, the blood flow rate has to be varied. Table 1 lists the methods which were applied in the investigations discussed in the rest of this chapter. The experiments were performed in the small intestine of dogs, cats, rats, guinea-pigs, rabbits, frogs or toads.

When the blood flow rate was measured by collecting the intestinal venous outflow, the blood loss was compensated by reinfusion of the blood or by infusion of blood obtained from donor animals. The circulation was closed when an electromagnetic or bubble flow meter was used. The blood flow rate was determined also by measurement of the cardiac output and the fractional blood flow rate in the intestine or by means of microspheres. From the luminal clearance of tritiated water and its arteriovenous concentration difference the total blood flow rate can be calculated. Under the assumption that the venous blood at the site of absorption is equilibrated fully with the luminal concentration the "absorption site blood flow rate" can also be determined (MAILMAN and JORDAN 1975; MAILMAN 1978 b), but one has to keep in mind that in such a case the blood flow rate is measured by an absorption process.

The blood flow rate was changed by different methods: constriction of the mesenteric artery, raising or lowering the systemic blood pressure, stimulation of the vasoconstrictor nerve fibres, transmural electric field stimulation, raising the venous pressure, mechanical stimulation of the intestinal mucosa, distension of the intestinal lumen, reduction of body temperature, upward tilting of the head or administration of drugs. In some investigations only the natural variability of the blood flow rate was recorded. Absorption was measured by determination of the disappearance rate from the intestinal lumen and/or the appearance rate in the intestinal venous blood or was derived from the concentration curves in the systemic blood after luminal and intravenous administration of the substance under investigation. In addition, the intestinal lymph flow was measured when the fluid absorption was studied in more detail. When the substance was offered

Table 1. Methods used to investigate the relationship between intestinal absorption and blood flow

	Dog	Cat	Rat	Guinea-pig	Rabbit	Frog or toad
Blood circulation						
Closed	[11–13, 23, 26–31, 37, 45]	[19]	[7, 18, 54]	[20]	[14]	
Open						
with reinfusion	[36, 39, 42–44]	[5, 6, 9, 10, 15, 21, 40, 41]				
Single-pass perfusion	[17, 36, 38, 42–44]		[2–4, 16, 22, 24, 25, 32–34, 46–53, 55]		[1]	[8, 35]
Measurement of blood flow rate						
Venous outflow						
Weight or volume	[17, 23, 36, 39, 42–44]		[2–4, 22, 24, 25, 32, 33, 34, 46–53, 55]		[1]	
Drop recorder	[38]	[5, 6, 9, 10, 15, 21, 40, 41]				
Portal bubble flow meter				[20]		
Electromagnetic flow meter around mesenteric artery	[11–13, 26–28, 31, 37	[19]				
Cardiac output + fractional blood flow rate			[7, 54]			
Microspheres			[7]		[14]	
Luminal clearance of tritiated water	[29, 30]					
Given by arterial inflow rate of vascularly perfused intestinal segment	[45]		[16, 18, 22, 32]			[8, 35]
Variation of blood flow rate						
Constriction of mesenteric artery	[11–13, 26–28, 31, 37, 42, 43]	[21, 40, 41]				
Changing systemic blood pressure			[24, 25, 34, 46–53]			
Stimulation of vasoconstrictor nerve fibres		[9, 40, 41]				
Transmural electric field stimulation		[5]				
Raising venous pressure		[40, 41]	[22]			
Drugs	[23, 29, 30, 36–38, 44]	[5, 6, 9, 10, 15, 19, 21, 40]	[2, 4, 7, 46]		[14]	

Table 1 (continued)

	Dog	Cat	Rat	Guinea-pig	Rabbit	Frog or toad
Mechanical stimulation of intestinal mucosa			[3]			
Distension of intestine	[17]					
Reduction of body temperature			[54]			
Upward tilting of head	[39]					
Natural variability			[55]	[20]	[1]	
Changing arterial inflow rate of vascularly perfused intestinal segment	[45]		[16, 18, 22, 32, 33]			[8, 35]
Measurement of absorption rate						
Disappearance rate from intestinal lumen	[11–13, 29, 30, 38, 39, 42–45]	[9, 10, 15, 19, 21]	[7, 24, 25, 32, 33, 47, 48, 50–53]		[1, 14]	[8]
Appearance rate in intestinal venous blood	[17, 36, 37, 42]	[5, 6, 40, 41]	[2–4, 16, 18, 22, 24, 25, 32–34, 46, 48, 50–53, 55]	[20]	[1]	[8, 35]
Appearance rate in intestinal lymph			[22]			
Appearance rate in intestinal lumen, when substance offered from blood side	[23]		[2, 3, 49, 54]			
Deconvolution of systemic blood concentration curves after luminal and intravenous administration	[26–28, 31]					

[1] BARR and RIEGELMAN (1970); [2, 3] BEUBLER and JUAN (1977, 1978); [4] BEUBLER and LEMBECK (1976); [5] BIBER (1974); [6] BIBER et al. (1973b); [7] BOLTON et al. (1975); [8] BOYD and PARSONS (1978); [9] BRUNSSONS et al. (1979); [10] CEDGÅRD et al. (1978); [11, 12] CROUTHAMEL et al. (1970, 1975); [13] DIAMOND et al. (1970); [14] DONOWITZ et al. (1979); [15] EKLUND et al. (1979); [16] FORTH (1967); [17] GATCH and CULBERTSON (1935); [18] GITS and GERBER (1973); [19] GANGER et al. (1979a); [20] HAASS et al. (1972); [21] JODAL et al. (1977); [22] LEE and DUNCAN (1968); [23] LEE and SILVERBERG (1976); [24, 25] LICHTENSTEIN and WINNE (1973, 1974); [26] LOVE (1976); [27] LOVE and MATTHEWS (1972); [28] LOVE et al. (1972); [29] MACFERRAN and MAILMAN (1977); [30] MAILMAN (1978a); [31] MATHEWS and LOVE (1974); [32, 33] OCHSENFAHRT (1973, 1979); [34] OCHSENFAHRT and WINNE (1969); [35] PARSONS and PRICHARD (1968); [36] PYTKOWSKI and LEWARTOWSKI (1972); [37] PYTKOWSKI and MICHALOWSKI (1977); [38] REES (1920); [39] SAN MARTIN and MAILMAN (1972); [40, 41] SVANVIK (1973a, b); [42] VARRÓ and CSERNAY (1967); [43, 44] VARRÓ et al. (1965, 1967); [45] WILLIAMS et al. (1964); [46–50] WINNE (1966, 1970a, 1972a, b, 1973); [51–53] WINNE and REMISCHOVSKY (1970, 1971a, b); [54] CSÁKY and VARGA (1975); [55] LASKER and RICKERT (1978)

from the blood side the blood–lumen flux could be studied by measuring the appearance rate in the intestinal lumen.

The artificial vascular perfusion of an intestinal segment represents a more difficult method (for further references see Chap. 5; WINNE 1979a). It has been used successfully to study the exit mechanism at the basolateral border of the intestinal cells (BOYD et al. 1975; BOYD 1977, 1978; BOYD and PARSONS 1976, 1978, 1979; CHEESEMAN 1979). The blood flow rate can easily be varied by changing the vascular inflow rate. If the segment is suspended in a bath (OCHSENFAHRT 1973, 1979), the disappearance rate from the intestinal lumen and the appearance rates in the intestinal venous blood as well as in the serosal bath solution can be measured simultaneously. The vascularly perfused intestinal segment is especially suitable for study of the blood–lumen flux of a substance, since a constant arterial inflow concentration can easily be maintained, if the vascular perfusate is not recirculated (OCHSENFAHRT 1976).

C. Theoretical Considerations

In order to facilitate the understanding and discussion of the experimental results simple equations are derived which describe the relationship between intestinal absorption and blood flow rate. In the analysis of experimental data the special conditions of the experiments have to be taken into account. Appropriate equations have been derived previously (WINNE and OCHSENFAHRT 1967; WINNE 1971). In these papers the theoretical aspects are treated in more detail. In order to describe the dependence of intestinal absorption on blood flow rate a set of models has been used or proposed (WINNE 1978a). Often several models are compatible with experimental results. We have to remember that a model simplifies reality, accentuates certain aspects and neglects others. In this chapter the model depicted in Fig. 1 is used to elucidate the theoretical background.

The net transfer $\Phi_{L/I}$ of a substance through the first barrier, from the intestinal lumen through the mucosal unstirred layer and the intestinal epithelium into the subepithelial interstitial space (Fig. 1), is assumed to be the difference of the unidirectional fluxes. The flux from the intestinal lumen into the interstitial space is proportional to the concentration C_L in the luminal bulk phase, the unidirectional permeability coefficient k_1 and the area A_1. The flux in the reverse direction is proportional to the concentration C_I in the interstitial space, the corresponding permeability coefficient k_2, and the area A_1

$$\Phi_{L/I} = k_1 A_1 C_L - k_2 A_1 C_I \,. \tag{1}$$

The unidirectional permeability coefficients k_1 and k_2 are descriptive in character. They are constant and equal in the case of a passive transport, provided modifying influences (e.g. solvent drag, electrical potential) are not effective. In the other cases, including carrier transport, the coefficients k_1 and k_2 are different and depend on the concentration and additional parameters. Because of the villous structure of the intestinal mucosa the area A_1 can be defined in different ways: area of the unstirred layer, area perpendicular to the permeation direction, area of the epithelial surface, area of the tips of the villi. The permeability coefficients have to be defined correspondingly. The determination of the permeability of the wall of a villous membrane has been described elsewhere (WINNE 1978b). If only the products k_1A_1 and k_2A_1 are examined, they can be regarded as permeability parameters of the layer between the luminal bulk phase and interstitial space. In the following, they are used in this sense.

The interstitial space is drained by the blood flowing through the subepithelial capillaries, the "effective mucosal blood flow" (SOERGEL et al. 1968) or "absorption site blood flow rate" (MAILMAN and JORDAN 1975). The amount of substance absorbed $\Phi_{I/B}$ appearing in the intestinal venous blood per unit time is the arteriovenous concentration difference multiplied by the blood flow rate

$$\Phi_{I/B} = \dot{V}_B(C_{BV} - C_{BA}) = \alpha \dot{V}_B(C^*_{BV} - C_{BA})$$
$$= \alpha a_1 \dot{V}_B(C^*_{PWV} - C_{PWA}) = \alpha a_1 E_1 \dot{V}_B(C_I - C_{PWA}) \,, \tag{2}$$

where C_{BV} is the concentration in the venous blood leaving the intestinal segment, C_{BA} the arterial concentration, and $\dot{V}_B$ the total blood flow rate of the segment; α is the fraction of the total flow rate passing the capillaries involved in the drainage process and C^*_{BV} is the concentration in the venous blood of these vessels. The right-hand side of Eq. (2) is obtained by introduction of $a_1 = C_{BV}/C^*_{PWV} = C_{BA}/C_{PWA}$, the concentration in the blood divided by the concentration in the plasma water, and the quantity E_1 (WINNE and OCHSENFAHRT 1967; WINNE 1979a)

$$E_1 = \frac{C^*_{PWV} - C_{PWA}}{C_I - C_{PWA}} = 1 - \exp(-k_{CW}A_{CW}/\alpha a_1 \dot{V}_B) \,. \tag{3}$$

E_1 characterizes the deviation from the concentration equilibrium at the venous end of the capillary and becomes unity when equilibrium is reached at this point ($C^*_{PWV} = C_I$). E_1 depends on the permeability of the capillary wall, the second barrier (k_{CW} = capillary permeability coefficient, A_{CW} = area of the capillary wall), and the blood flow rate. The factor a_1 accounts for protein binding and storage in the red cells.

The permeation rate of the substance through the deeper layers of the intestinal wall, the third barrier, into the serosal fluid is assumed to be proportional to the concentration difference $C_I - C_S$, the permeability coefficient k_S and the area A_S of the third barrier

$$\Phi_{I/S} = k_S A_S (C_I - C_S) \,. \tag{4}$$

C_S is the concentration in the serosal fluid.

In the steady state the disappearance rate from the intestinal lumen $\Phi_{L/I}$ is equal to the sum of the appearance rates in the intestinal venous blood $\Phi_{I/B}$ and in the serosal fluid $\Phi_{I/S}$, provided metabolism and storage in the intestinal wall can be neglected

$$\Phi_{L/I} = \Phi_{I/B} + \Phi_{I/S} \,. \tag{5}$$

After introducing Eq. (1), the right-hand side of Eq. (2), and Eq. (4) into Eq. (5) this equation can be solved for C_I

$$C_I = \frac{k_1A_1C_L + \alpha a_1 E_1 \dot{V}_B C_{PWA} + k_S A_S C_S}{k_2 A_1 + \alpha a_1 E_1 \dot{V}_B + k_S A_S} \,. \tag{6}$$

Inserting Eq. (6) into Eqs. (1), (2) and (4) yields the disappearance rate from the intestinal lumen,

$$\Phi_{L/I} = \frac{C_L - R(\alpha a_1 E_1 \dot{V}_B C_{PWA} + k_S A_S C_S)/(\alpha a_1 E_1 \dot{V}_B + k_S A_S)}{1/k_1 A_1 + R/(\alpha a_1 E_1 \dot{V}_B + k_S A_S)} \quad (7)$$

the appearance rate in the intestinal venous blood,

$$\Phi_{I/B} = \frac{C_L - (R + k_S A_S/k_1 A_1) C_{PWA} + k_S A_S C_S/k_1 A_1}{1/k_1 A_1 + (R + k_S A_S/k_1 A_1)/\alpha a_1 E_1 \dot{V}_B} \quad (8)$$

and the appearance rate in the serosal fluid

$$\Phi_{I/S} = \frac{C_L + \alpha a_1 E_1 \dot{V}_B C_{PWA}/k_S A_S - (R + \alpha a_1 E_1 \dot{V}_B/k_1 A_1) C_S}{1/k_1 A_1 + (R + \alpha a_1 E_1 \dot{V}_B/k_1 A_1)/k_S A_S}. \quad (9)$$

$R = k_2/k_1$ represents the ratio of the unidirectional permeability coefficients of the first barrier.

The units of the quantities are, for example: $\Phi_{L/I}$, $\Phi_{I/B}$, $\Phi_{I/S}$ mol/min or mol min^{-1} g^{-1}, if the rates are related to wet tissue weight of the segment; C_L, C_{PWA}, C_S mol/l; k_1, k_2, k_S ml min^{-1} cm^{-2}; $\dot{V}_B$ ml/min or ml min^{-1} g^{-1}, if related to wet tissue weight; A_1, A_S cm^2 or cm^2/g, if the absorption and blood flow rates are related to wet tissue weight; α, a_1, E_1 and R are dimensionless. Equations (7)–(9) will be simplified further for the discussion of special aspects and special cases.

D. Experimental Data

I. Dependence of Intestinal Absorption on Total Intestinal Blood Flow Rate

The measurement of the total blood flow rate of an intestinal segment is much easier than the determination of the flow rate in the subepithelial capillaries involved in the drainage process. Therefore, in most investigations of the relationship between intestinal absorption and blood flow the total blood flow rate of an intestinal segment is recorded.

1. Influence of Blood Flow on the Appearance Rate in the Intestinal Venous Blood

The dependence of intestinal absorption of drugs and nutrients has been studied intensively in the rat jejunum (WINNE 1966, 1970a, 1972a, b, 1973; OCHSENFAHRT and WINNE 1969; WINNE and REMISCHOVSKY 1970, 1971a, b; LICHTENSTEIN and WINNE 1973, 1974). Jejunal segments, 5–9 cm in length, were perfused without recirculation (single-pass perfusion), so that the luminal inflow concentration was constant in time and successive periods could be compared. The jejunal vein draining the segment was punctured, the blood collected and weighed (to give the blood flow rate). The concentration of the absorbed substances in the blood was determined yielding, with the flow rate, the appearance rate in the intestinal venous blood. Heparinized blood from donor rats was infused into the jugular vein to compensate the blood loss. The intestinal blood flow rate was varied by raising or lowering the systemic blood pressure (increase and reduction of blood infusion rate). In separate experiments the blood flow was changed in three steps from high to low or from low to high rates. In Fig. 2a some results are given. The appearance rate in the intestinal venous blood was divided by the mean luminal concentration to facilitate the comparison of the curves for different substances. The dimensions of this standardized absorption rate are volume per unit time per unit weight and it can be regarded as the clearance rate. The arrows indicate the direction of blood flow change. The appearance rate of tritiated water decreased and increased almost linearly with decreasing and increasing blood flow. On the other hand, the appearance rate of ribitol was independent of the blood flow rate in the range measured. Compared with the absorption rate of tritiated water the rate of ribitol was small. Erythritol and urea were absorbed at a higher rate than ribitol. Their absorption rates increased or decreased slightly when the outflow was varied between low and intermediate rates. When the blood flow rate was raised above 1 ml min^{-1} g^{-1} the absorption rate of erythritol and urea did not increase further. Ethanol, antipyrine and aniline were absorbed to a higher extent. Their absorption rates showed a marked dependence on blood flow rate. Their curves first increase and then become less steep at higher blood flow rates, so that concave curves are obtained. The curves of amidopyrine (OCHSENFAHRT and WINNE 1969) and methanol (WINNE and REMISCHOVSKY 1970, 1971a) are not depicted.

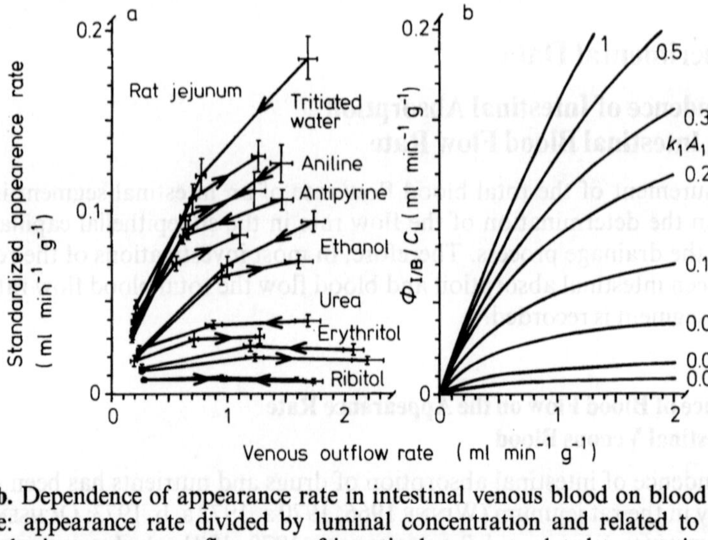

Fig. 2a, b. Dependence of appearance rate in intestinal venous blood on blood flow rate. Ordinate: appearance rate divided by luminal concentration and related to wet tissue weight; abscissa: venous outflow rate of intestinal segment related to wet tissue weight. **a** experimental data obtained in rat jejunum (OCHSENFAHRT and WINNE 1969; WINNE and REMISCHOVSKY 1970, 1971a, b; WINNE 1972a), blood flow varied from high to low or from low to high rates (*arrows*), *bars* indicate ± standard error of the mean; **b** theoretical curves calculated by Eq. (10) with $\Phi_{I/B}/C_L$ as ordinate, $\dot{V}_B$ as abscissa, $\alpha a_1 E_1 = 0.2$, $k_S A_S = 0.07$ ml min^{-1} g^{-1}, $k_1 A_1$ varied

They correspond to the curve of ethanol. The absorption rates of mannitol (WINNE and REMISCHOVSKY 1971 b), sorbose (WINNE 1979 a), diethylstilbestrol and its glucuronide (LASKER and RICKERT 1978) were lower than the rate of ribitol and were independent of the venous outflow rate. The curves in Fig. 2 b seem to converge towards the origin.

In other species similar results have been obtained. When salicylamide was perfused through rabbit small intestine, the appearance of this substance in the mesenteric blood changed in parallel to the blood flow rate. The appearance rate of the glucuronide, which was synthesized during the transfer through the epithelial cells, was independent of the blood flow rate (BARR and RIEGELMAN 1970). Constriction of the mesenteric artery of the dog reduced the venous outflow rate from a jejunal segment and the appearance rate of glucose (VARRÓ and CSERNAY 1967) resulting in a linear relationship between flow rate and absorption. In the vascularly perfused frog small intestine a linear relationship between the appearance rate of glucose (PARSONS and PRICHARD 1968) and 3-*O*-methylglucose (BOYD and PARSONS 1978) in the intestinal venous blood and the vascular perfusion rate was also observed. Inhibition of the active transport component by phlorhizin diminished the absorption rate of 3-*O*-methylglucose and this rate was independent of the vascular perfusion rate. After loading the mucosa with 3-*O*-methylglucose from the lumen and after abruptly washing out the lumen the rate of appearance in the vascular effluent decreased with time according to a double exponential function (BOYD and PARSONS 1978). The rate constant of the fast component increased linearly with the vascular flow rate, while the rate constant of the slow component was independent of flow rate. L-Leucine showed a similar behaviour (CHEESEMAN 1979). The washout rate constant of α-methyl-D-glucoside was relatively independent of vascular flow over a wide range (BOYD and PARSONS 1979). When cardiac glycosides were infused into the duodenum of guinea-pigs (HAASS et al. 1972), the appearance rate of ouabain in the portal blood was nearly independent of the portal flow rate (Fig. 3 a). The natural variation of the portal flow rate was measured by means of a bubble flow meter. The appearance rate of digitoxin and digoxin were linearly correlated to the portal flow rate, but contrary to the results obtained in the rat jejunum (Fig. 2 a) the extrapolated regression lines intersect the abscissa at positive values. The same type of relationship between blood flow and the appearance rate in the intestinal venous blood was observed for phenylalanine and serine in the dog ileum (PYTKOWSKI and LEWARTOWSKI 1972; PYTKOWSKI and MICHALOWSKI 1977). When the vascular perfusion rate in the vascularly perfused rat jejunum was raised, the appearance rate of ^{22}Na increased (GITS and GERBER 1973), while the rate of iron decreased (FORTH 1967). Distension of canine small intestine by raising the intraluminal pressure up to the level of the diastolic blood pressure reduced the blood flow of the segment, but the absorption rates of sodium bromide and ethanol remained relatively constant (GATCH and CULBERTSON 1935). The results obtained with krypton in the cat small intestine will be discussed in Sect. D.II.

Now, we have a look at the predictions based on the model depicted in Fig. 1. The curves in Fig. 2 b were drawn for the special case of a passively transported xenobiotic, for which the unidirectional permeability coefficients are equal ($k_2 = k_1$, $R = 1$). The concentrations in the arterial blood and the serosal fluid were set

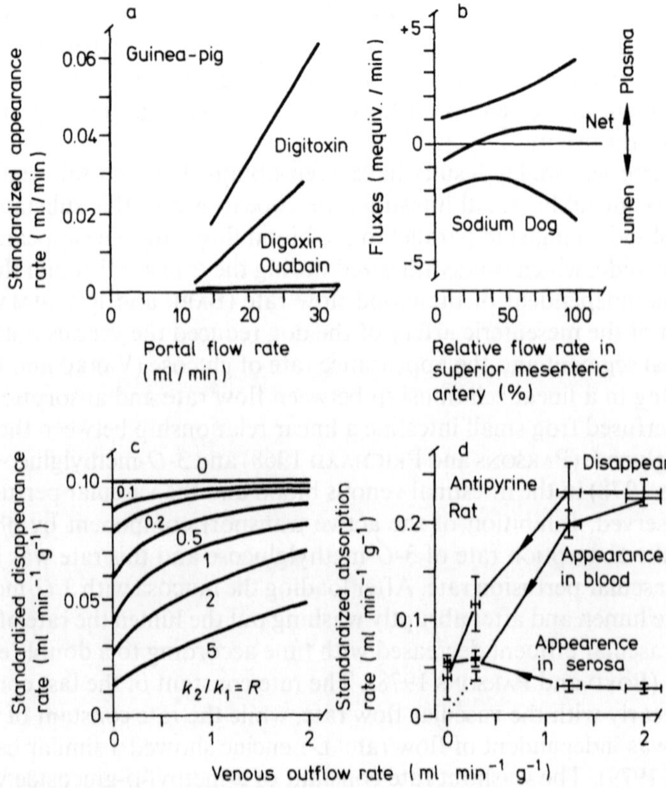

Fig. 3. a Relationship between appearance rate of cardiac glycosides in portal blood and portal flow rate in guinea-pigs. Appearance rate divided by luminal concentration, portal flow rate varied by natural variability. After HAASS et al. (1972). **b** Relationship between net and unidirectional fluxes of sodium in dog jejunum and blood flow rate. Flow rate in superior mesenteric artery related to initial value before constriction of the artery, unidirectional sodium fluxes calculated from systemic plasma concentration after intravenous and luminal administration of labelled sodium (double labels). After LOVE (1976). **c** Dependence of disappearance rate from intestinal lumen on blood flow rate in the case of an actively transported substance ($k_2/k_1=R<1$). Theoretical curves calculated by Eq. (12) with $\Phi_{L/l}/C_L$ as ordinate, $\dot{V}_B$ as abscissa, $\alpha a_1 E_1=0.2$, $k_1 A_1=0.1$ ml min^{-1} g^{-1}, $k_S A_S=0.07$ ml min^{-1} g^{-1}, R varied. **d** Influence of blood flow on intestinal absorption of antipyrine. Vascularly perfused rat jejunal segment suspended in a bath; blood flow reduced in four steps from high flow rate to zero (OCHSENFAHRT 1973). Ordinate: disappearance rate from intestinal lumen, appearance rates in the intestinal venous blood and serosal fluid divided by luminal concentration and related to wet tissue weight; *bars* indicate $\pm$ standard error of the mean

to zero ($C_{PWA}=C_S=0$). We get from Eq. (8)

$$\Phi_{I/B}=\frac{C_L}{1/k_1A_1+(1+k_SA_S/k_1A_1)/\alpha a_1 E_1 \dot{V}_B}. \tag{10}$$

The permeability × area product k_1A_1 of the first barrier and the blood flow rate $\dot{V}_B$ of the intestinal segment were varied, $\alpha a_1 E_1$ and $k_S A_S$ were held constant. The ordinate represents the standardized appearance rate $\Phi_{I/B}/C_L$. The curves start at the origin, rise and level off in the horizontal direction (concave curvature). When k_1A_1 is low, e.g. 0.01 ml min^{-1} g^{-1}, the curve lies near the abscissa and the horizontal section is reached even at low blood flow rates: "blood flow-independent absorption". With increasing k_1A_1, i.e. with increasing permeability (or decreasing resistance) of the first barrier, the horizontal section of the curves shifts to the right and to higher ordinate values. The ascending nonlinear section of the curves dominates. At very high values of k_1A_1 the curves approach an ascending straight line. This line represents the case of "blood flow-limited absorption". The theoretical curves demonstrate that the dependence of the intestinal absorption on the blood flow rate increases with increasing permeability of the unstirred fluid layer and the intestinal epithelium, more generally with increasing absorbability. The curves intersect the origin; at zero blood flow rate the appearance rate is obviously zero. This does not mean that the substances having traversed the first barrier do not enter the capillaries. They enter the capillaries (BOYD and PARSONS 1978), but they cannot appear in the veins, since blood drainage is absent. The special aspects of an actively transported substance will be discussed in Sect. D.I.2.

Comparison of the theoretical curves with the experimental ones obtained in the rat jejunum (Fig. 2) shows that the model of Fig. 1 describes the experimental data sufficiently, but similar models are also compatible with the experimental results (WINNE 1978a; see also DOBSON 1978). Among the experimental findings in other species, the results obtained with digitoxin and digoxin (HAASS et al. 1972) as well as with phenylalanine and serine (PYTKOWSKI and LEWARTOWSKI 1972; PYTKOWSKI and MICHALOWSKI 1977) deviate from the theoretical predictions. The extrapolated regression lines do not intersect the origin, but cross the abscissa at positive values (Fig. 3a). This deviation will be discussed in Sect. D.II. For the deviant behaviour of iron (FORTH 1967) – decreasing appearance rate with rising vascular perfusion rate – no explanation can be given.

Further insight into the theoretical background permits the analysis of Eq. (10). According to this equation the appearance rate in the intestinal venous blood is proportional to the luminal concentration C_L in the case of a passively transported substance with zero concentration in the blood and serosal fluid. By analogy with Ohm's law the denominator can be regarded as resistance. The total resistance is subdivided into two partial resistances. The first term of the denominator $1/k_1A_1$, the reciprocal of the permeability × area product of the first barrier, represents the resistance of the layers between the luminal bulk phase and the subepithelial interstitial space. If necessary, this partial resistance can be subdivided further into the resistance of the mucosal unstirred fluid layer and the resistance of the epithelium. The second term represents the resistance of the drainage system with $\alpha\dot{V}_B$, the subepithelial blood flow rate, as the main factor. The resistance of the capillary wall is included in the factor E_1, see Eq. (3). If the first barrier is highly permeable, k_1A_1 is large and its reciprocal small. Thus, the first term of the denominator can be neglected compared with the second term. Therefore, the blood flow rate determines the appearance rate (blood flow-limited absorption). Since lipophilic substances and tritiated water are highly permeable, the absorption rates of these substances show a marked dependence on blood flow rate. Therefore, their absorption rates can be used to determine the "absorption site blood flow rate" (COBURN 1968; FORSTER 1967; HAMILTON et al. 1967; DOBSON et al. 1971; BIBER et al. 1973a; BOND et al. 1974; MAILMAN and JORDAN 1975; MICFLIKIER et al. 1976; LOVE et al. 1977; MACFERRAN and MAILMAN 1977; MAILMAN 1978b). A low permeability of the first barrier means a high resistance and the first term of the denominator is large compared with the second term, so that the blood flow rate plays little or no role (blood flow-independent absorption). In the case of an intermediate permeability the influence of the blood flow rate on the appearance rate decreases as the flow rate increases since the second term of the denominator becomes smaller with increasing $\dot{V}_B$. When the blood flow rate approaches zero, the second term of the denominator increases infinitely resulting in a zero appearance rate.

2. Influence of Blood Flow on the Disappearance Rate from the Intestinal Lumen

In absorption experiments using the rat jejunum (Fig. 2) the disappearance rate from the intestinal lumen was also measured. The data are depicted in Fig. 4a. The disappearance rate was divided by the mean luminal concentration. The differences in the curves obtained in the experiments with decreasing and increasing blood flow rate will be discussed in Sect. D.I.6. For the present, this deviation will be ignored. The curves for ethanol were omitted, they correspond to the curves of aniline. The relationship between the disappearance rate and the intestinal blood flow differs in one point from the analogous relationship of the appearance rate described in the preceding section. The curves do not converge towards the

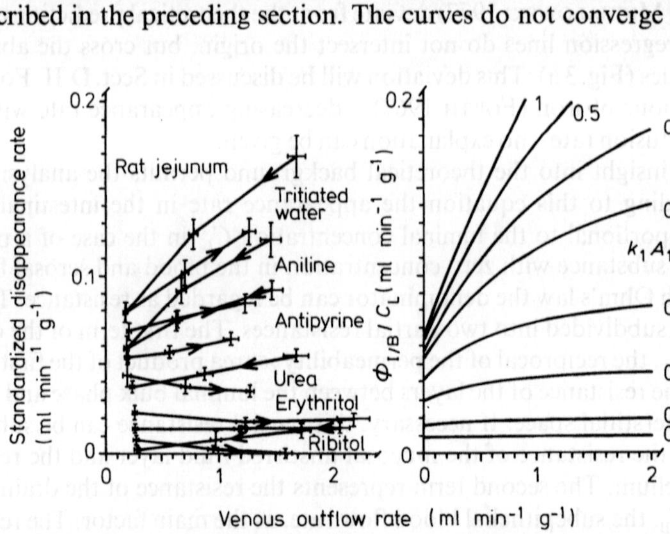

Fig. 4a, b. Dependence of disappearance rate from intestinal lumen on blood flow rate. Ordinate: disappearance rate divided by luminal concentration and related to wet tissue weight; abscissa: venous outflow rate of intestinal segment related to wet tissue weight. **a** experimental data obtained in rat jejunum (H. OCHSENFAHRT and D. WINNE 1969, unpublished work; WINNE and REMISCHOVSKY 1970, 1971a, b; WINNE 1972a); blood flow varied from high to low or from low to high rates (*arrows*), *bars* indicate ± standard error of the mean; **b** theoretical curves calculated by Eq. (11) with $\Phi_{L/l}C_L$ as ordinate, $\dot{V}_B$ as abscissa, $\alpha a_1 E_1 = 0.2$, $k_S A_S = 0.07$ ml min^{-1} g^{-1}, $k_1 A_1$ varied origin, but they seem to intersect the ordinate at positive values. In consequence, the curves are less steep. The dependence of the disappearance rate on the total blood flow rate increases as the absorbability of the substances increases.

In the dog analogous results have been observed. Constriction of the mesenteric artery reduced the disappearance rates of glycine and glucose from the jejunal lumen, resulting in a straight line for glycine and a concave curve for glucose (VARRÓ et al. 1965); on the contrary, the disappearance rate of sorbose was independent of the blood flow rate. Concave curves were also obtained for sulphaethidole (CROUTHAMEL et al. 1970, 1975; DIAMOND et al. 1970), glucose and xylose (WILLIAMS et al. 1964). In investigations with no measurement of blood flow rate (MCIVER et al. 1926; LLUCH TRULL 1954; NELSON and BEARGIE 1965; PALS and STEGGERDA 1966) the same general tendency was observed: reduced disappearance rate when the blood circulation was restricted. The unidirectional sodium fluxes in canine small intestine were diminished when the mesenteric artery was gradually constricted (LOVE and MATTHEWS 1972; LOVE et al. 1972; MATTHEWS and LOVE 1974; LOVE 1976), but convex curves were obtained (Fig. 3 b). The net sodium flux from lumen to blood decreased at low flow rates until its direction changed. In the dog, upward tilting of the head decreased the blood flow in the ileum and increased the sodium absorption from a saline solution (SAN MARTIN and MAILMAN 1972). In analogous experiments with a NaCl–$MgSO_4$ solution in the intestinal lumen the net sodium flux was directed into the lumen and was reversed by upward tilting of the head.

Equation (7) yields for a xenobiotic ($R=1$, $C_{PWA}=C_S=0$)

$$\Phi_{L/I}=\frac{C_L}{1/k_1A_1+1/(\alpha a_1E_1\dot{V}_B+k_SA_S)}. \tag{11}$$

The theoretical curves calculated by this equation are depicted in Fig. 4 b. They simulate satisfactorily the experimental curves. At zero blood flow rate the disappearance rate has positive values and is equal to the appearance rate in the serosal fluid. In that case a substance having entered the subepithelial space from the intestinal lumen is not drained by the blood, but leaves this space through the deeper layers of the intestinal wall and appears in the serosal fluid. With increasing blood flow rate the drainage of the subepithelial tissue becomes more efficient. The concentration of the permeating substance in the interstitial space decreases so that the concentration gradient through the first barrier becomes steeper. Hence, the disappearance rate increases. A comparison with Fig. 2 b shows that the dependence of the disappearance rate on blood flow is less pronounced than the dependence of the appearance rate. From Eq. (11) the same conclusions can be drawn directly. The first term in the denominator is the resistance of the first barrier and the second term is the resistance of the second (drainage system) and third barrier (deeper layers) together. The second and third barrier are parallel resistances. In the case of zero blood flow rate the second term does not increase infinitely, but approaches the resistance $1/k_SA_S$ of the deeper layers of the intestinal wall in series to the resistance of the first barrier. If the permeability of the first barrier is low (high resistance), the first term of the denominator is large and the second term with the blood flow rate plays a minor role (blood flow-independent absorption). If the permeability of the first barrier is high (low resistance), the first term is small and the second term, i.e. the blood flow rate, dominates. The disappearance rate depends more or less on the blood flow rate. Finally, blood flow-limited absorption is obtained. If the luminal perfusion rate of an intestinal segment is reduced, the thickness of the intraluminal unstirred layer, i.e. the resistance of the first barrier, increases and the dependence of absorption on blood flow decreases as shown in absorption experiments with krypton in cat small intestine (JODAL et al. 1977).

A reduction of protein binding should have the same effect as a reduction of blood flow rate, i.e. a diminution of the absorption rate, since a reduction of the factor a_1 in Eqs. (7), (8), (10), and (11) has the same effect as a reduction of $\dot{V}_B$. This prediction was confirmed in rabbits (IMAMURA and ICHIBAGASE 1977). The intravenous administration of salicylic acid and phenylbutazone diminished the disappearance rate of sulphadimethoxine by reducing the binding capacity of the plasma proteins. On the other hand, the disappearance rate of sulphanilamide was not affected, since this substance shows little binding to plasma proteins.

In order to discuss the influence of blood flow on the intestinal absorption of an actively transported substance Eq. (7) was simplified to the case of zero concentration in blood and serosal fluid ($C_{PWA} = C_S = 0$)

$$\Phi_{L/I} = \frac{C_L}{1/k_1 A_1 + R/(\alpha a_1 E_1 \dot{V}_B + k_S A_S)}. \tag{12}$$

Active transport from the lumen to the interstitial space means that $R(=k_2/k_1)$ is smaller than unity. When R decreases the second term in the denominator of Eq. (12) becomes smaller, indicating a smaller influence of blood flow on the absorption in the case $k_2 < k_1$, see Fig. 3c. The curves shift to higher ordinate values and become less steep. From Eq. (12) it follows also that a condition for the influence of blood flow on the absorption is the existence of a unidirectional flux from the interstitial space into the lumen ($k_2 > 0$) which increases with increasing concentration in the interstitial space, i.e. a concentration-dependent leakage into the lumen is necessary, since in the case $k_2 = R = 0$ the second term in the denominator of Eq. (12) vanishes, excluding a dependence of absorption on blood flow. It should be mentioned that Eq. (12) describes only the drainage effect of the blood flow on the absorption rate. If at low blood flow rates the oxygen supply becomes insufficient, the active transport mechanism may be impaired, thus reducing the absorption rate by increasing the resistance of the first barrier (decreasing k_1).

The dependence of the glucose disappearance rate on blood flow observed in the dog (WILLIAMS et al. 1964; VARRÓ et al. 1965) corresponds to the predictions of Eq. (12) while the sodium fluxes in dog small intestine (SAN MARTIN and MAILMAN 1972; LOVE 1976, see also Fig. 3b, do not. This deviation may be attributed to the complicated absorption mechanism of sodium and its interrelationship with nonelectrolyte and water transport which have not been taken into account in the underlying model. Moreover, a variation in the proportion of subepithelial blood flow and the influence of countercurrent exchange may also play a significant role (see Sects. D.II and D.III).

3. Influence of Blood Flow on the Appearance Rate in the Serosal Fluid

In the usual in vitro experiments intestinal absorption is investigated by measuring the transfer of a substance from the lumen into the fluid bathing the serosal side of an excised intestinal segment. Using an isolated jejunal segment of the rat suspended in a serosal bath OCHSENFAHRT (1973, 1979) measured simultaneously the disappearance rate from the intestinal lumen and the appearance rates in the venous outflow and the serosal fluid. The blood vessels of the segment were perfused artificially via a silicone rubber tube from a donor rat.

The blood flow rate was varied from zero to high values or vice versa by clamping the arterial inflow cannula or raising or lowering the systemic blood pressure of the donor rat. By this method the absorption could be investigated under in vitro (zero blood flow rate) and in vivo (nonzero blood flow rate) conditions in one and the same intestinal segment. As an example the results for antipyrine are given in Fig. 3d. The disappearance rate and the appearance rate in the venous blood decreased nonlinearly (concave curves), the latter rate was always smaller than the former. At zero flow rate the disappearance rate was equal to the appearance rate in the serosal fluid. This rate became smaller at nonzero blood flow rates, but did not approach zero even at high blood flow rates. In spite of the drainage by blood, about 10% of the amount leaving the intestinal lumen reached the serosal side of the intestinal wall. This was due to the small thickness of the rat intestinal wall. Also in the vascularly perfused rat jejunum more or less different curves were observed for the blood flow dependence of the absorption, when the blood flow was varied from high to low and from low to high rates (OCHSENFAHRT 1973).

Theoretical curves for the appearance rate in the serosal fluid are not given, they correspond to the experimental results (WINNE 1979a). In Eq. (9) the first term of the denominator represents the resistance of the first barrier as in Eqs. (7) and (8). At zero blood flow rate the second term reduces to $R/k_S A_S$, the resistance of the third barrier, and Eqs. (9) and (7) become equal. In that case the disappearance rate from the lumen is equal to the appearance rate in the serosal fluid; this is the typical situation of in vitro experiments. With increasing blood flow rate the second term in the denominator of Eq. (9) increases so that the appearance rate in the serosal fluid decreases as demonstrated by the experimental data.

4. Influence of Blood Flow on the Appearance Rate in the Intestinal Lumen

If a substance is offered from the blood side its appearance in the intestinal lumen can be measured. Only for tritiated water in rat jejunum has the blood flow dependence of the luminal appearance rate been investigated systematically (OCHSENFAHRT et al. 1966; WINNE 1972b). The appearance rate of tritiated water in the intestinal lumen increased or decreased as the blood flow rate was raised or lowered. The resulting curves are concave and correspond to the curves in Fig. 2a, but with a more pronounced divergence. The luminal clearance of intravenously administered barbital in the ileum of rats was linearly related to the total blood flow rate of the segment when the blood flow rate was reduced by lowering the body temperature (CSÁKY and VARGA 1975). The straight line crossed the origin.

Table 2. Influence of vasoactive drugs on intestinal blood flow and absorption

Drug	Total blood flow rate	Preparation	Absorption of		Reference
Isoprenaline 2–10 μg/min i.a.	Increased	Cat jejunum	Krypton	(A) increased (D) increased	BIBER et al. (1973b); JODAL et al. (1977)
Secretin 2.5–10.5 U kg^{-1} h^{-1} i.a.	Increased	Cat jejunum	Krypton	(A) increased	BIBER (1974)
Cholecystokinin 2.5–10.5 U kg^{-1} h^{-1} i.a.	Increased	Cat jejunum	Krypton	(A) increased	
Caffeine 0.5 mg intraluminal	Increased	Rat jejunum	Salicylic acid	(A) increased	BEUBLER and LEMBECK (1976)
Theophylline 0.5 mg intraluminal	Increased	Rat jejunum	Antipyrine Urea Salicylic acid	(A) increased (A) increased (A) increased	
Pilocarpine 20–50 μg i.a.	Decreased	Dog jejunum	DL-Serine DL-Phenylalanine	(A) decreased (A) decreased	PYTKOWSKI and LEWARTOWSKI (1972)
Pilocarpine 2.5–70 μg/min i.a.	Decreased	Dog jejunum	L-Serine L-Phenylalanine	(A) decreased (A) decreased	PYTKOWSKI and MICHALOWSKI (1977)
Vasoacitive intestinal polypeptide 175 ng/min i.a.	Decreased	Dog ileum	Sodium	(D) decreased	MAILMAN (1978a)

Glucagon 0.05 μg kg^{-1} min^{-1} indirectly i.a.	Decreased	Dog ileum	Sodium	(D) decreased	MacFerran and Mailman (1977)
0.5 μg kg^{-1} min^{-1} indirectly i.a.	Unchanged	Dog ileum	Sodium	(D) decreased	
0.05 μg kg^{-1} min^{-1} directly i.a.	Unchanged	Dog ileum	Sodium	(D) unchanged	
0.5 μg kg^{-1} min^{-1} directly i.a.	Increased	Dog ileum	Sodium	(D) unchanged	
Pentagastrin 10 μg/min i.a.	Unchanged	Dog ileum	Sodium	(D) decreased	Mailman (1979)
Acetylcholine 2.33–266.6 μg/min i.a.	Increased	Dog jejunum	Glucose	(A) decreased	Varró et al. (1967)
Histamine 3.33–13.3 μg/min i.a.	Increased Unchanged	Dog jejunum	Glucose	(A) decreased (A) unchanged	
Epinephrine 0.66–6.60 μg/min i.a.	Increased Decreased	Dog jejunum	Glucose	(A) decreased	

Abbreviations: i.a. = intraarterial; directly = into the artery of the segment; indirectly = into the artery of the neighbouring segment; (A) = appearance rate in intestinal venous blood; (D) = disappearance rate from intestinal lumen

The barbital clearance represented 45%–53% of the total flow rate. Equations for the relationship between luminal appearance rate and blood flow can be derived analogously to Eqs. (1)–(9) and have been published previously (WINNE 1971, 1972b).

5. Influence of Vasoactive Drugs on Intestinal Absorption

Vasoactive drugs can influence the intestinal absorption of drugs and nutrients by changing the intestinal blood flow and/or by affecting the transfer mechanism through the epithelium. In the case of an altered blood flow rate it is difficult to discriminate between a direct effect on the transport mechanism and an influence on the absorption rate via the changed blood flow rate. Blood flow and absorption may be altered independently. Moreover, total blood flow rate and absorption site blood flow rate may vary in parallel or not (see Sect. D.II).

The data collected in Table 2 show that, in general, the absorption varied in parallel to the blood flow. Investigations of net and unidirectional water fluxes will be discussed in Sect. D.I.7. Isoprenaline, secretin and cholecystokinin increased the blood flow rate and the absorption rate of krypton in cat jejunum. These experiments will be discussed further in Sect. D.II. Caffeine and theophylline administered intraluminally increased the blood flow and the absorption of antipyrine, salicylic acid, and urea in rat jejunum. On the other hand, pilocarpine reduced the blood flow rate and the absorption of serine and phenylalanine by increasing the motility. This effect was observed mainly during tonic contractions. The sodium absorption did not always change in parallel to the blood flow variation induced by vasoactive intestinal polypeptide, glucagon, and pentagastrin, indicating that a direct effect on the transfer mechanism of sodium may contribute to the overall effect.

Acetylcholine and histamine increased, epinephrine both increased and decreased total intestinal blood flow rate. The absorption of glucose was reduced or remained unchanged. The adverse effects of these drugs on blood flow and absorption lead one to suppose that the transfer of glucose through the epithelium may be the site of drug action, but complementary experiments (intraarterial filling with Indian ink, benzidine dyeing of intestinal villi) indicated that during the infusion of acetylcholine the blood flow in the villi was reduced. Since the total blood flow rate was increased, the blood flow pattern in the intestinal wall was changed to the detriment of the villi. This observation represents a further explanation for the adverse effect on total blood flow rate and glucose absorption.

6. Influence of Direction of Blood Flow Change on Intestinal Absorption

In the rat jejunum intestinal absorption apparently depends on the direction of blood flow change (Figs. 2a and 4a). When the blood flow rate was reduced from high to low rates steeper curves were obtained than in the opposite case. It should be mentioned that the variation of blood flow was started 10 min after the begin-

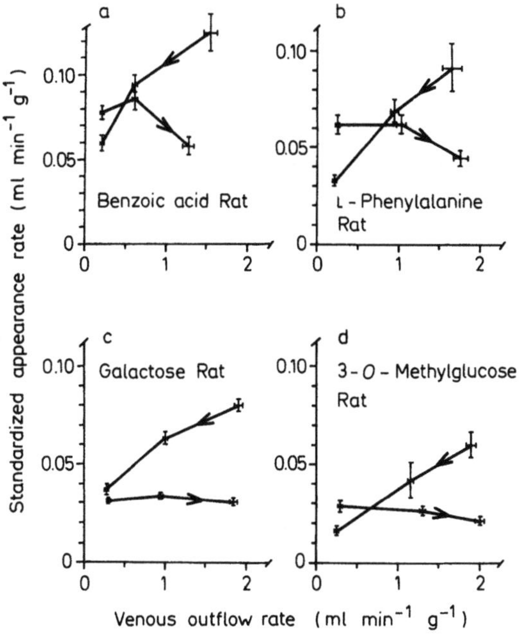

Fig. 5. Influence of blood flow on intestinal absorption of benzoic acid, L-phenylalanine, galactose and 3-*O*-methylglucose. Ordinate: appearance rate in intestinal venous blood divided by luminal concentration and related to wet tissue weight; abscissa: venous outflow rate of intestinal segment related to wet tissue weight. Experimental data obtained in rat jejunum (Ochsenfahrt and Winne 1969; Winne 1973; Lichtenstein and Winne 1973, 1974); blood flow varied from high to low or from low to high rates (*arrows*); *bars* indicate ± standard error of the mean

ning of the luminal perfusion with a period of high *or* low rate in separate experiments. The examples depicted in Fig. 5 show that the divergence may become extreme. The appearance rate of benzoic acid increased when the blood flow was raised from low to intermediate rates, but decreased when the flow rate was raised further to higher values. Thus, crossing curves were obtained. Salicylic acid showed the same behaviour (Ochsenfahrt and Winne 1969). The appearance rate of L-phenylalanine and 3-*O*-methylglucose decreased when the blood flow rate was raised from low to high values, while the appearance rate of galactose remained constant. Phlorhizin reduced the galactose absorption and curves similar to the curves of urea in Fig. 2a were obtained for the blood flow dependence (Lichtenstein and Winne 1974).

The investigations undertaken to clarify the reason for the diverging curves are not yet finished, so that only preliminary results and suggestions can be given. In control experiments with luminal single-pass perfusion and *constant* intermediate blood flow rate the appearance rate in the intestinal venous blood decreased more or less with time in the range measured (10–60 min after starting the luminal perfusion). The decrease of the appearance rate was more pronounced for the substances which showed a marked divergence of the curves for the blood flow

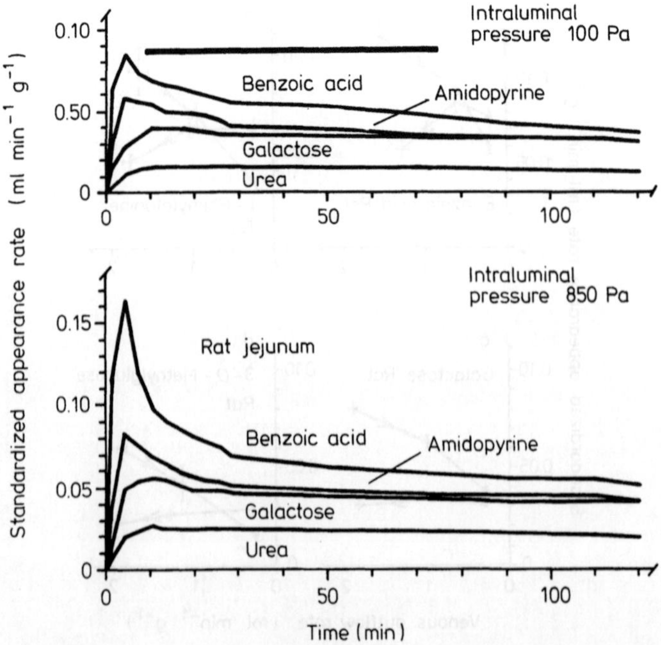

Fig. 6 a, b. Time dependence of intestinal absorption during single-pass perfusion of rat jejunal segment. Ordinate: appearance rate in intestinal venous blood divided by luminal concentration and related to wet tissue weight; abscissa: time after starting luminal perfusion (initial perfusion rate 10 ml/min until solution appeared in outflow cannula, subsequently perfusion continued at a rate of 0.1 ml/min). Experimental data of D. WINNE and H. SUCCO-MEISTER (1977, unpublished work). **a** intraluminal hydrostatic pressure 100 Pa, *thick line* represents the range where the experiments depicted in Figs. 2 a, 4 a, and 5 were performed; **b** intraluminal hydrostatic pressure 850 Pa (10 Pa ~ 1 mm H_2O)

dependence. A constant appearance rate is expected at constant intermediate blood flow after achieving the steady state, provided secondary changes do not occur, since the luminal inflow concentration of the substances is constant. Recently, the time dependence of the absorption rate in the rat jejunum at constant intermediate blood flow rate by luminal single-pass perfusion was investigated in more detail (D. WINNE and H. SUCCU-MEISTER 1977, unpublished work). The appearance rate of substances which are absorbed at a high rate showed, just after starting the luminal perfusion, a peak which declined exponentially to a lower level (Fig. 6 a). Subsequently, the appearance rate decreased at a lower rate. The height of the initial absorption peak decreased as the absorbability of the substances decreased. The thick line in Fig. 6 a indicates the period studied in previous experiments with varying blood flow rate. The initial absorption peak was more pronounced when the intraluminal pressure was elevated by fixing the opening of the luminal outflow cannula 8.5 cm above the intestinal segment (Fig. 6 b). It must be stressed that the appearance rate declined from the peak value in spite of a constant blood flow rate and a constant intraluminal pressure. The initial absorption peak is induced presumably by the quick filling of the intestinal lumen at the start of the intraluminal perfusion and by the distension of the intestinal wall – the intraluminal perfusion was started at a rate of 10 ml/min until the perfusion solution appeared in the outflow cannula and was continued at the rate of 0.1 ml/min. The initial distension of the intestinal wall seems to be the main stimulus, since an absorption peak could also be induced during a luminal perfusion by suddenly raising the intraluminal pressure; the blood flow rate remained constant or was reduced slightly for 1 min. The initial absorption peak, but not the subsequent slight decrease of the absorption rate, could be circumvented by a 30-min preperfusion with a buffer solution, omitting the substance under investigation (compare Fig. 7a and b). By the preperfusion the process leading to the absorption peak is brought forward in time.

A computer analysis (WINNE 1979a) has shown that an increase of the resistance of the first barrier (unstirred layer and intestinal epithelium) and/or a decrease of the fraction of the absorption site blood flow rate, thus simulating the declining section of the intestinal absorption peak, result in divergent curves for the dependence of the absorption rate on the total blood flow rate similarly to the curves in Fig. 5. Figure 7d demonstrates schematically that a superposition of a time-dependent decrease of the absorption on its normal blood flow dependence yields crossed curves. When the blood flow is reduced from high to low rates, the time-dependent decrease of the absorption rate is added to the decrease of the absorption rate due to the reduction of the total blood flow rate. A steeper decreasing curve for the absorption rate is obtained. When the blood flow is raised from low to high rates, the increase of the absorption rate due to the increase of the blood flow rate is increasingly reduced by the time-dependent reduction of the absorption with the greatest effect at high flow rates. In this way, the absorption rate can decrease although the total blood flow rate increases.

Since mechanical stimulation of the intestinal mucosa induced an increase of the total blood flow rate in cats (BIBER et al. 1970, 1971, 1974; FAHRENKRUG et al. 1978) and rats (BEUBLER and JUAN 1978), it is supposed that the initial absorption peak in rat jejunum described previously is caused by an initial increase of the absorption site blood flow rate, the total blood flow rate remaining unchanged. Therefore, the blood flow pattern in the intestinal wall is changed in favour of the villous blood flow rate. In cats the vasodilation induced by mechanical stimulation of the intestinal mucosa could be abolished by tetrodotoxin, lidocaine, 2-bromo-LSD (BIBER et al. 1971) and dihydroergotamine (BIBER et al. 1974), suggesting that the vasodilation is evoked via an intramural nervous reflex in some way dependent on the release of 5-hydroxytryptamine. On the other hand, mechanical stimulation of the mucosa released vasoactive intestinal polypeptide in cats (FAHRENKRUG et al. 1978) and prostaglandin E_1 in rats (BEUBLER and JUAN 1978), so that these two substances may be involved in the whole process. The initial absorption peak in rat jejunum could be reduced by an intraarterial infusion of lidocaine and could be abolished by infusion of dihydroergotamine (D. WINNE 1977, unpublished work). The infusion of papaverine had no effect (Fig. 7c). Lidocaine and papaverine augmented the total blood flow rate which remained at a constant high level during the transient absorption peak.

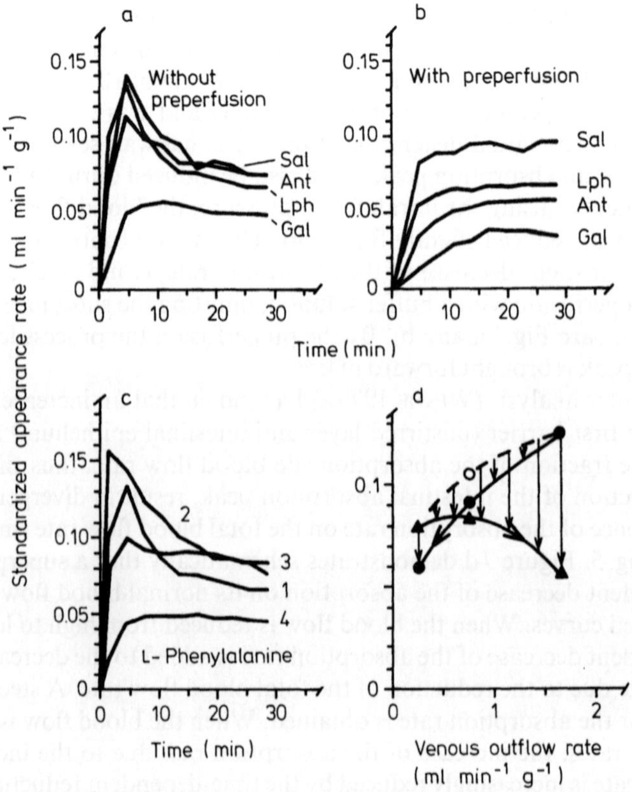

Fig. 7. a, b Influence of preperfusion on time dependence of intestinal absorption during single-pass perfusion of rat jejunal segment. Intraluminal hydrostatic pressure 850 Pa; data of D. WINNE and H. SUCCU-MEISTER (1977, unpublished work); *Sal*, salicylic acid, *LpH*, L-phenylalanine, *Ant*, antipyrine, *Gal*, galactose. **c** Modification of initial absorption peak of L-phenylalanine by intraarterial infusion of 50 µl/min isotonic saline solution (*curve 1*), 100 µg/min papaverine (*Curve 2*), 1 mg/min lidocaine (*curve 3*), and 50 µg/min dihydroergotamine (*curve 4*); data of D. WINNE (1977, unpublished work). Intraluminal hydrostatic pressure 850 Pa. **d** Schematic view of effect of decrease of absorption with time on blood flow dependence of intestinal absorption (LICHTENSTEIN and WINNE 1973). *Broken line:* dependence of absorption on blood flow rate in the absence of decrease of absorption with time; details in text. Ordinate: appearance rate in intestinal venous blood divided by luminal concentration and related to wet tissue weight; abscissa: (**a–c**) time after starting the luminal perfusion with the substances mentioned (preperfusion started 30 min earlier), (**d**) venous outflow rate of intestinal segment related to wet tissue weight

There is a second explanation for the initial absorption peak. Since at the beginning of the perfusion the intestinal lumen was filled quickly (perfusion rate 10 ml/min), the concentration of the permeating substance at the mucosal surface was everywhere the same and equal to the inflow concentration. Subsequently, when the perfusion rate was reduced to 0.1 ml/min, a longitudinal and radial concentration gradient in the intestinal lumen was built up (WINNE 1979 b; WINNE and MARKGRAF 1979) diminishing the concentration at the mucosal surface, so that the absorption rate decreased. In this way, the picture of an initial absorption peak resulted. The radial concentration gradient in a laminar flow is the consequence of the intraluminal diffusion resistance which functions like an unstirred fluid layer. The longitudinal and radial concentration gradient increases with increasing epithelial permeability of the substance and increasing intraluminal radius (distension of intestine). The gradient is influenced by the blood flow rate only indirectly (by variation of the absorption rate), so that the small and variable effect of a blood flow change on the initial absorption peak can be understood. At present, the experimental data to hand are insufficient to clarify the cause of the initial absorption peak.

The slight decrease of the absorption rate after the initial absorption peak contributes to the divergence of the curves describing the blood flow dependence of the absorption rate in the rat jejunum and may be evoked by a slow increase of the resistance of the first barrier, for example by continuous secretion of mucus. Alterations in the epithelium or in the interstitial space inducing the same effect cannot be excluded. For instance, an increase of the water content in the epithelial cells and subepithelial tissue would lengthen the diffusion pathway and would contribute to an increase of the resistance of the first barrier. In the experiments of OCHSENFAHRT and WINNE (1969) luminal perfusion of rat jejunum in vivo increased the water content of the intestinal wall by 3% compared with nonperfused segments (H. OCHSENFAHRT and D. WINNE 1969, unpublished work). This change of water content seems to be too small to explain sufficiently the divergent absorption curves. Since ischaemia increases the secretion of mucus (CHIU et al. 1970; OCHSENFAHRT 1973, 1979), a period of zero or low blood flow rate may increase the unstirred layer thickness by secretion of mucus which is also effective in subsequent periods with normal and high blood flow rates. In this way a different resistance of the first barrier in the experiments with decreasing and increasing blood flow rate can be explained. In the case of actively transported substances an additional factor can be effective. During a period of low blood flow rate the oxygen supply may be insufficient, so that the active transport mechanism is impaired and the reduced absorption rate after such a period can be explained. An ischaemia of 5–10 min seems to be the critical period for the active transport in the intestine (see Sect. D.I.8).

From this discussion the following working hypothesis is deduced for the apparent influence of direction of blood flow change on the intestinal absorption in rat jejunum. There exists an absorption peak at the beginning of the luminal single-pass perfusion. The declining section of the absorption peak is superimposed on the normal dependence of absorption on total blood flow rate, resulting in more or less crossing curves. The absorption peak is attributed to an increase of the absorption site blood flow rate (the total blood flow rate remaining unchanged) or results from the building up of the intraluminal longitudinal and radial concentration gradient, thus reducing the concentration at the mucosal surface. In addition, the resistance of the first barrier increases slowly with time by secretion and/or swelling of mucus. This secretion of mucus may be more pronounced in the experiments with increasing blood flow rate owing to the initial period of low blood flow rate. In the case of actively transported substances the impairment of the transport mechanism in the initial period of low blood flow rate may play an additional role.

Table 3. Influence of blood flow on intestinal fluid absorption and secretion

After/during	Total blood flow rate	Preparation	Luminal solution	Net water flux	Reference
Vasoactive intestinal polypeptide up to 24 ng/min i.a.	Increased	Cat jejunum	Isotonic Krebs–glucose	Fluid absorption reduced and changed to secretion	EKLUND et al. (1979)
175 ng/min i.v.	Decreased	Dog ileum	Isotonic saline		MAILMAN (1978 a)
Crude cholera toxin 50–200 mg/10 cm intestine intraluminal	Increased	Cat jejunum	Isotonic Krebs–Henseleit without glucose		CEDGÅRD et al. (1978)
Purified cholera toxin 50 μg intraluminal for 2 h before absorption measurement	Unchanged	Rabbit ileum	Ringer–bicarbonate		DONOWITZ et al. (1979)
Prostaglandin E_1 0.1–10 μg/min i.a.	Increased	Cat ileum	Isotonic Tyrode		GRANGER et al. (1979 a)
Histamine 2 mg/h i.a.	Increased	Dog jejunum		Induction of secretion	LEE and SILVERBERG (1976)
Raising venous pressure	Decreased	Rat jejunum	Isotonic Ringer–bicarbonate	Fluid absorption reduced	LEE and DUNCAN (1968)
Pituitary extract 0.5–1.0 ml s.c.	Decreased	Dog small intestine	Tap water		REES (1920)
Reduction of systemic blood pressure	Decreased	Rat jejunum	Hypotonic Ringer		WINNE (1970 a)
Glucagon 0.05 μg kg^{-1} min^{-1} i.a. indirectly	Decreased	Dog ileum	Isotonic saline		MACFERRAN and MAILMAN (1977)

Pentagastrin 10 μg/min i.v.	Unchanged	Dog ileum	Isotonic saline		MAILMAN (1979)
Angiotensin 590 ng kg^{-1} min^{-1} i.v.	Unchanged	Rat jejunum	Isotonic Krebs–bicarbonate		BOLTON et al. (1975)
Reduction of systemic blood pressure	Decreased	Rat jejunum	Hypertonic Ringer	Secretion reduced	WINNE (1970a)
Upward tilting of head	Decreased	Dog ileum	Isotonic $NaCl–MgSO_4$		SAN MARTIN and MAILMAN (1972)
Reduction of systemic blood pressure	Decreased	Rat jejunum	Isotonic Ringer	Fluid absorption unchanged	WINNE (1970a)
Isoprenaline graded i.a. infusion	Increased	Cat jejunum	Isotonic Krebs–Henseleit		BRUNSSON et al. (1979)
Glucagon 0.5 μg kg^{-1} min^{-1} i.a. directly	Increased	Dog ileum	Isotonic saline		MACFERRAN and MAILMAN (1977)
Methylprednisolone acetate 3 mg/100 g s.c. per day for 3 days	Increased	Rabbit ileum	Ringer–bicarbonate	Fluid absorption increased	DONOWITZ et al. (1979)
Angiotensin 0.59 ng kg^{-1} min^{-1} i.v.	Unchanged	Rat jejunum	Isotonic Krebs–bicarbonate		BOLTON et al. (1975)
Upward tilting of head	Decreased	Dog ileum	Isotonic saline		SAN MARTIN and MAILMAN (1972)
Electrical stimulation of regional sympathetic nerve fibres	Decreased	Cat jejunum	Isotonic Krebs–Henseleit		BRUNSSON et al. (1979)

Abbreviations: i.a. = intraarterial; i.v. = intravenous; s.c. = subcutaneous; directly = into the artery of the segment; indirectly = into the artery of neighbouring segment

7. Influence of Blood Flow on Intestinal Fluid Absorption and Secretion

It is very difficult to analyse the influence of blood flow on intestinal net water flux since too many interacting factors are involved in this process: arterial and venous pressure (WELLS 1940; SHIELDS and CODE 1961; LEE and DUNCAN 1968; LEE 1973; YABLONSKI and LIFSON 1976), luminal hydrostatic pressure (WELLS 1931; LEE 1965), osmotic pressure (RABINOVITCH 1927; LEE 1973, 1974; DUFFY et al. 1978), motility (LEE 1965), contractility of lymph vessels (LEE 1963, 1965), motility of the villi (LEE 1971), salt and nonelectrolyte absorption (SMYTH 1965; SCHULTZ and CURRAN 1968; TURNBERG 1973; BINDER 1977; HENDRIX and PAULK 1977; BRESLER 1978), intestinal countercurrent exchange (HALJAMÄE et al. 1973; JODAL et al. 1978a; HALLBÄCK 1979), lymph drainage (RUSZNYÁK et al. 1957, p 724; BARROWMAN 1978), and pressure (LEE 1979). Variations of the blood flow rate depend on changes of arterial and venous blood pressure and/or vascular resistance. The intravasal pressure gradient influences directly the net water flux. Therefore, the effect of the drainage process cannot be discriminated from the effect of factors varied simultaneously. If drugs are used, the effects on blood flow rate and net water flux may be independent or related. Since the problems of intestinal fluid absorption cannot be discussed in detail, only those investigations are referred to in which the blood flow rate was varied.

The investigations listed in Table 3 demonstrate that a change of intestinal fluid absorption and secretion induced by drugs or other methods is accompanied by different changes of blood flow rate. The administration of vasoactive intestinal polypeptide, cholera toxin, prostaglandin E_1, and histamine reduced the fluid absorption and changed it finally to secretion into the lumen. The blood flow rate was increased, unchanged or decreased. In these experiments changes of capillary permeability, capillary pressure and/or effects on the epithelial fluid transport mechanism determined the direction of net water flux. The drainage effect of the blood apparently played only a minor role. The data of LEE and DUNCAN (1968) obtained in the vascularly perfused rat jejunum in vitro demonstrate the role of lymph drainage. On raising the venous pressure, the arterial pressure being kept constant, the blood flow rate and the disappearance of fluid from the intestinal lumen decreased in general, while the lymph flow rate increased. The appearance rate of fluid in the venous outflow decreased and reached negative values at high venous pressure (15–25 mmHg), i.e. in that case the lymphatic fluid originated from the luminal solution and the blood. These experiments and others (BARROWMAN 1978; GRANGER and TAYLOR 1978; BRUNSSON et al. 1979) show that absorbed fluid is partially drained by the lymphatic system. In vitro, without blood drainage, the main fraction of the absorbed fluid appeared in the lymph (LEE 1961, 1963, 1969).

The reduction of absorption of hypotonic Ringer solution and the reduction of secretion into hypertonic Ringer or NaCl–$MgSO_4$ solution by reduction of the systemic blood pressure or upward tilting of the head can be explained by the smaller washout effect, since the blood flow rate was decreased in these experiments. Theoretical considerations suggest a greater influence of blood drainage on the net water flux induced by nonisotonic solutions than on the net water flux observed when using isotonic solutions (WINNE 1970b). In this way, the unchanged fluid absorption, in spite of increased blood flow rate induced by isoprenaline or glucagon infusion or in spite of reduced blood flow rate by reduction of systemic blood pressure, can be understood. The increased fluid absorption during decreased blood flow rate induced by upward tilting of the head or electrical stimulation of regional sympathetic nerve fibres and the reduced fluid absorption with no effect on the blood flow rate induced by pentagastrin and angiotensin indicate an action in the epithelium. The parallel reaction of fluid absorption and blood flow rate during indirect administration of glucagon (reduction), after subcutaneous injection of pituitary extract (reduction) and after methylprednisolone administration (enhancement) may be accidental.

The unidirectional water fluxes are determined by measuring the absorption and secretion rate of labelled water or by measuring the net water flux and the absorption rate of labelled water. In the latter case the secretory unidirectional water flux follows from the difference. On the one hand, labelled water, e.g. tritiated water, can be regarded as a hydrophilic xenobiotic, on the other, labelled water molecules have about the same behaviour as the unlabelled molecules. In rat jejunum the absorption and secretion of tritiated water increased and decreased almost linearly with increasing and decreasing total blood flow rate (Figs. 2 and 4, Table 4). Moreover, the direction of net water flux modified the absorption and secretion rate (WINNE 1972a, b). A net water flux directed from the lumen into the blood augmented the absorption, reduced the secretion of tritiated water, and vice versa. The influence of net water flux consists of two components: first, the solvent drag effect during the transfer through the first barrier (unstirred layer and epithelium), second, the change of the volume flow through the subepithelial capillaries, thus varying the drainage efficiency (OCHSENFAHRT and WINNE 1972a, 1973; see also KOJIMA et al. 1972; OCHSENFAHRT and WINNE 1972b, 1974a, b; KOJIMA and MIYAKE 1975).

The influence of drugs on unidirectional water fluxes can be attributed to changes of the drainage effect of the blood, of the net water flux (solvent drag effect), and of the epithelial permeability to water. The other data of Table 4 show in most cases the absorption and secretion of tritiated water in the small intestine varied in parallel to the change of the total blood flow rate induced by administration of drugs. Thus, histamine, theophylline, and caffeine increased the blood flow rate and the absorption rate of tritiated water in rat jejunum. The effect of atropine was similar, but short-lived and small. Norepinephrine, vasopressin, and serotonin had the opposite effect. Mechanical stimulation of the jejunal mucosa in the rat increased the absorption and secretion of tritiated water and the blood flow rate. Simultaneously, prostaglandin E_1 was released into the lumen and venous blood. The effect was reduced by indomethacin. A low dose of prostaglandin E_1 did not affect the blood flow rate, increased the secretion and reduced the absorption rate of tritiated water, presumably by inducing a net water secretion into the lumen (the net water flux was not measured in these experiments). Higher doses increased the blood flow rate, resulting in an increase of the absorption rate of tritiated water at the highest dose. In that case, the effect of blood flow surmounted the effect of net water flux on tritiated water transfer. The effects of glucagon, pentagastrin, indomethacin, and vasoactive intestinal polypeptide are further examples of the complicated relationship between the different effects of

Table 4. Influence of blood flow on unidirectional water fluxes in the intestine as determined by the absorption and/or secretion of tritiated water

After/during	Total blood flow rate	Preparation	Net water absorption	Unidirectional water flux		Reference
				Absorptive	Secretory	
Raising systemic blood pressure	Increased	Rat jejunum		Increased	Increased	WINNE (1972a, b)
Histamine 50 μg/min i.v.	Increased	Rat jejunum		Increased		WINNE (1966)
Atropine 150 μg i.v.	Increased	Rat jejunum		Increased		
Theophylline 0.5 mg intraluminal	Increased	Rat jejunum		Increased		BEUBLER and LEMBECK (1976)
Caffeine 0.5 mg intraluminal	Increased	Rat jejunum		Increased		
Mechanical stimulation of intestinal mucosa	Increased	Rat jejunum		Increased	Increased	BEUBLER and JUAN (1978)
Prostaglandin E_1 intraluminal						
6.5 μg/ml	Increased	Rat jejunum		Increased	Increased	BEUBLER and JUAN (1977)
0.5 μg/ml	Increased			Unchanged	Increased	
0.1 μg/ml	Unchanged			Decreased	Increased	
Glucagon directly i.a.						
0.5 $\mu g\,kg^{-1}\,min^{-1}$	Increased	Dog ileum	Unchanged	Increased	Increased	MACFERRAN and MAILMAN (1977)
0.05 $\mu g\,kg^{-1}\,min^{-1}$	Unchanged		Unchanged	Increased	Increased	

Pentagastrin 10 µg/min i.v.						
Fed	Unchanged	Dog ileum	Unchanged	Decreased		MAILMAN (1979)
Fasted	Unchanged		Decreased	Decreased		
Neostigmine 15 µg i.v.	Unchanged	Rat jejunum		Unchanged		WINNE (1966)
Lowering systemic blood pressure	Decreased	Rat jejunum		Decreased	Decreased	WINNE (1972a, b)
Norepinephrine 6 µg/min i.v.	Decreased	Rat jejunum		Decreased		WINNE (1966)
Vasopressin 0.02 U/min i.v.	Decreased	Rat jejunum		Decreased		
Serotonin 8 µg/min i.v.	Decreased	Rat jejunum		Decreased		
Indomethacin 1 µg/ml intraluminal	Decreased	Rat jejunum		Increased	Decreased	BEUBLER and JUAN (1977)
Vasoactive intestinal polypeptide 175 ng/min i.a.	Decreased	Dog ileum	Decreased	Decreased	Unchanged	MAILMAN (1978a)
Glucagon indirectly i.a.						
$0.05\ \mu g\ kg^{-1}\ min^{-1}$	Decreased	Dog ileum	Decreased	Decreased	Decreased	MACFERRAN and MAILMAN (1977)
$0.5\ \mu g\ kg^{-1}\ min^{-1}$	Unchanged		Decreased	Decreased	Unchanged	

Abbreviations: i.a. = intraarterial; i.v. = intravenous; directly = into the artery of the segment; indirectly = into the artery of neighbouring segment

Table 5. Influence of ischaemia on intestinal absorption

During ischaemia of 5 min duration or less			
In vivo			
Rat Jejunum	Uptake of cholesterol, sitosterol, monoolein, octadecane, oleic acid	Unchanged	SYLVÉN (1970)
After ischaemia of 5 min duration or less			
In vitro			
Rat jejunum	Uptake of L-isoleucine	Unchanged	ROBINSON et al. (1964, 1965)
Dog jejunum	Uptake of L-phenylalanine	Unchanged	ROBINSON et al. (1965)
In vivo			
Rat small intestine	Disappearance of glucose	Unchanged	LLUCH TRULL (1954)
During ischaemia of 10 min duration or more			
In vivo			
Rat jejunum	Uptake of cholesterol, sitosterol, monoolein, oleic acid, octadecane	Decreased	SYLVÉN (1970)
	Disappearance of antipyrine, salicylic acid, L-phenylalanine, 3-*O*-methylglucose	Decreased	OCHSENFAHRT (1973, 1979)
	Disappearance of urea	Unchanged	
Rat small intestine	Uptake of cholesterol	Decreased	SYLVÉN (1971)
	Disappearance of iodide	Decreased	NYLANDER and WIKSTRÖM (1968)
Dog small intestine	Disappearance of fluid, sodium, chloride, glucose	Decreased	HUECKEL et al. (1973); MIRKOVITCH et al. (1975)
	Appearance of triolein in thoracic duct lymph	Decreased	AHONEN et al. (1972)

blood flow rate, net water flux and epithelial permeability on the absorption and secretion of tritiated water.

The author doubts that the unidirectional water fluxes determined in the intestine in vivo by means of the absorption and secretion of labelled water give reliable information about water exchange through the epithelium – the topic of investigation in most cases – since the absorption and secretion rate of labelled water depends heavily on the blood flow rate which may or not influence the water exchange through the epithelium.

8. Influence of Ischaemia on Intestinal Absorption

When the intestinal blood flow is stopped (ischaemia) the drainage of substances ceases. But the disappearance rate from the intestinal lumen does not fall to zero since the substances permeate through the deeper layers of the intestine wall and appear on the serosal side. The disappearance rate is markedly reduced and equal to the appearance rate in the serosal fluid (OCHSENFAHRT 1973, 1979), see also Sect. D.I.3. Since in an ischaemic period the oxygen supply is also stopped, active transport mechanisms are progressively damaged. For example, during an isch-

Table 5. (continued)

After ischaemia of 10 min duration or more			
In vitro			
Rat small intestine	Uptake of L-phenylalanine, L-isoleucine	Decreased	ROBINSON (1966); ROBINSON et al. (1964, 1965, 1966); ROBINSON and MIRKOVITCH (1977)
	Transfer of iodide	Increased	NYLANDER and WIKSTRÖM (1968); WIKSTRÖM (1968)
Guinea-pig small intestine	Transfer of glucose Transfer of sorbose	Decreased Unchanged	GUTHRIE and QUASTEL (1956)
Dog jejunum	Uptake of L-phenylalanine	Decreased	ROBINSON et al. (1965)
Dog small intestine	Uptake of L-phenylalanine, β-methylglucoside	Decreased	MIRKOWITCH et al. (1975); ROBINSON et al. (1973, 1976); ROBINSON and MIRKOVITCH (1972)
Dog colon	Uptake of L-phenylalanine, β-methylglucoside	Decreased	ROBINSON et al. (1975)
	Net transfer of sodium	Decreased	RAUSIS et al. (1972); ROBINSON et al. (1972, 1975)
In vivo			
Rat small intestine	Uptake of iron	Decreased	PRASAD and OSBORNE (1963)
	Disappearance of glucose	Decreased	LLUCH TRULL (1954)
	Disappearance of olive oil	Decreased	HOVING et al. (1977)
Rat colon	Disappearance of olive oil	Decreased	HOVING et al. (1977)
Rabbit small intestine	Luminal appearance of intravenously administered polyvinylpyrrolidone, inulin, vitamin B_{12}, creatinine	Increased	KINGHAM et al. (1976)
	Urea	Unchanged	
Dog small intestine	Disappearance of glucose	Decreased	MIRKOVITCH et al. (1975); ROBINSON et al. (1976)
	Net flux of fluid, sodium, chloride	Absorption reversed to secretion	HUECKEL et al. (1973); MIRKOVITCH et al. (1975); ROBINSON et al. (1976)

aemia of 90 min duration the disappearance rate of L-phenylalanine and 3-*O*-methylglucose from rat jejunum decreased continuously to 20% of the initial level (OCHSENFAHRT 1973). In contrast, the disappearance rate of salicylic acid and antipyrine was reduced because of the stopped blood drainage, but did not change with time. This demonstrates that the lack of oxygen supply does not impair the transfer of passively transported substances. Table 5 shows that the critical duration of an intestinal ischaemia seems to be 5–10 min. During and after an ischaemia of 5 min or less the absorption is not impaired. An ischaemia of more than 5 min reduces the absorption capacity of the intestine for actively transported substances. This was demonstrated in absorption studies in vitro as well as in vivo. After ischaemia the permeability of the epithelium for passively transported substances can be increased, since the appearance rate of intravenously administered substances in the intestinal lumen was increased (KINGHAM et al. 1976).

The deleterious effect of ischaemia can be alleviated by rinsing the intestinal lumen with buffer solutions with and without glucose, oxygenated or not, either before or during the ischaemic period (ROBINSON et al. 1966; CHIU et al. 1970; MCARDLE et al. 1972; ROBINSON and MIRKOVITCH 1972, 1977; ÅHRÉN and HAGLUND 1973; MIRKOVITCH et al. 1975) or by breathing pure oxygen (AHONEN et al. 1972).

The intestinal functions are partially recovered as early as 24 h after the ischaemia (ROBINSON et al. 1975). Full recovery is reached after 2 or 7 days (ROBINSON et al. 1965, 1966, 1974, 1976; ROBINSON 1966). If the segment has been filled with glucose-containing buffer during the period of ischaemia, the structural and functional recovery is complete after 1 day (ROBINSON and MIRKOVITCH 1972; ROBINSON et al. 1973). The response of the ileal mucosa to ischaemia above and below a mechanical obstruction and the recovery follow the same pattern as when there is no superimposed occlusion (MIRKOVITCH et al. 1976).

II. Dependence of Intestinal Absorption on Intramural Blood Flow Pattern

When a substance is absorbed in the intestinal tract, it permeates first through the mucosal unstirred layer, then it is transported through the epithelium by active or passive mechanisms and is finally drained by the blood in the subepithelial capillaries. Therefore, the blood flow rate in these capillaries, "absorption site blood flow rate" (MAILMAN and JORDAN 1975), determines the absorption rate. Since usually the total blood flow rate of the intestinal segment is measured, the fraction α of the flow rate at the absorption site represents an additional variable. Therefore, the intramural blood flow pattern influences the intestinal absorption.

The absorption site blood flow rate is smaller than the mucosal blood flow rate. On the assumption that α is constant, values about 10%–40% were calculated for the fraction of absorption site blood flow rate from the absorption data obtained in rat jejunum (OCHSENFAHRT and WINNE 1969; WINNE and REMISCHOVSKY 1971 a, b; WINNE 1972 a). The fraction of mucosal flow rate determined by other methods in rat small intestine amounted to 60%–70% (CSERNAY et al. 1965; CSÁKY and VARGA 1975; GORE and BOHLEN 1977; BOHLEN et al. 1978). In dog small intestine the absorption site blood flow rate represents about 3%–8% of the total flow rate (MAILMAN and JORDAN 1975; MACFERRAN and MAILMAN 1977; MAILMAN 1978 a, b) and was calculated from the absorption rate of tritiated water. According to measurements with other methods the fraction of mucosal blood flow in dog small intestine amounted to 65%–70% (GRIM and LINDSETH 1958; YU et al. 1975) and the fraction of villous flow rate varied between 30% and 50% (BOND and LEVITT 1979). In cat small intestine about 10%–15% of the total blood flow rate was fully equilibrated with krypton in the lumen (BIBER et al. 1973 b; BIBER 1974; SVANVIK 1973 b). In studies with other methods the fraction of mucosal flow rate was measured as 10%–60% (ROSS 1971; GREENWAY and MURTHY 1972; FARA and MADDEN 1975) and of mucosal–submucosal flow rate it was about 80% (HULTEN et al. 1976). The fraction of villous flow rate amounted to 10%–20% (SVANVIK 1973 a).

The intramural blood flow pattern varies under different experimental conditions. According to measurements with microspheres the fraction of mucosal or mucosal–submucosal blood flow rate in the small intestine of the cat was decreased by an intraarterial infusion of secretin (FARA and MADDEN 1975) and adenosine (GRANGER et al. 1978), by raising the venous pressure (GRANGER et al. 1979b) or during the reactive hyperaemic response after arterial occlusion for 120 s (PARKER and GRANGER 1979) and was increased by an infusion of cholecystokinin (FARA and MADDEN 1975; FARA and CAMPBELL 1976), glucagon (FARA and CAMPBELL 1976) or isoprenaline (FARA and MADDEN 1975). Krypton washout curves indicated an increased fraction of mucosal–submucosal blood flow rate during an isoprenaline infusion (LUNDGREN 1967; KAMPP and LUNDGREN 1968), during preganglionic sympathetic vasoconstrictor fibre stimulation (HULTÉN et al. 1977) and after exposure to cholera toxin (CEDGÅRD et al. 1978). The fraction of villous plasma flow rate measured by means of ^{198}Au-labelled plasma particles (SVANVIK 1973a) was increased during the steady state phase of regional vasoconstrictor fibre stimulation (SVANVIK 1973c), during an intraarterial infusion of isoprenaline (BIBER et al. 1973c), after constriction of the mesenteric artery (LUNDGREN and SVANVIK 1973) and after raising the venous outflow pressure (LUNDGREN and SVANVIK 1973). In human small intestine the fraction of regional blood flow to mucosal–submucosal flow becomes augmented as total intestinal flow is increased (HULTEN et al. 1976).

The different intramural blood flow pattern is clearly demonstrated by the dependence of krypton absorption on total blood flow rate in cat small intestine (Fig. 8a). Constriction of the mesenteric artery (SVANVIK 1973a, b) reduced the venous outflow rate and in parallel the krypton appearance rate in the intestinal venous blood (curve 1). A similar effect was observed when the venous blood pressure was raised (SVANVIK 1973a, b). Stimulation of the regional vasoconstrictor fibres (SVANVIK 1973a, b) reduced the venous outflow rate, but the krypton appearance rate fell to a lesser extent (curve 4) than in the experiments with constriction of the artery. A graded infusion of isoprenaline into the mesenteric artery increased the venous outflow rate (curve 2) and the krypton appearance rate (SVANVIK 1973a; BIBER et al. 1973b). Curves 1 and 2 can be regarded as concave similar to the curves in Fig. 2. The intraarterial infusion of secretin increased the venous outflow rate (curve 3) and the krypton appearance rate (BIBER 1974). However, curve 3 is steeper than curve 2, indicating that secretin increased the absorption site blood flow rate more intensively than isoprenaline. A similar effect was observed during the intraarterial infusion of cholecystokinin and transmural electric field stimulation (BIBER 1974). The different absorption rates of krypton at the same venous outflow rate under different experimental conditions (arterial constriction, regional sympathetic stimulation, isoprenaline, secretion, cholecystokinin, intramural electric field stimulation) points strictly to different blood flow rates at the site of absorption, i.e. to a different intramural blood flow pattern.

In some investigations discussed earlier in this chapter a change of the blood flow pattern probably contributed to the observed effect. Thus, in rat jejunum the intraluminal application of theophylline and caffeine increased the venous outflow rate and appearance rate of tritiated water, urea, antipyrine, and salicylic acid in the

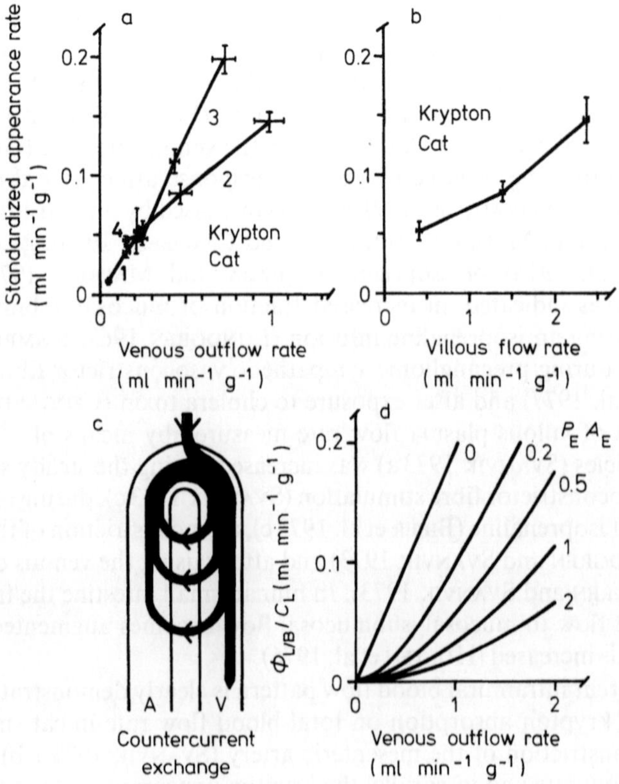

Fig. 8. a Influence of blood flow on the absorption of krypton in cat small intestine. Ordinate: appearance rate in intestinal venous blood divided by luminal concentration and related to wet tissue weight; abscissa: venous outflow rate of intestinal segment related to wet tissue weight. Blood flow reduced by constriction of mesenteric artery (*curve 1*) or stimulation of regional vasoconstrictor fibres (*curve 4*) and raised by intraarterial infusion of isoprenaline (*curve 2*) or secretin (*curve 3*), *bars* indicate ± standard error of the mean. After SVANVIK (1973b), BIBER et al. (1973b), BIBER (1974). **b** Curve 2 of **a** plotted versus the villous blood flow rate related to 1 g villous tissue. **c** Schematic view of villous countercurrent exchange; *A*, arterial limb, *V*, venous limb. **d** Dependence of the appearance rate in intestinal venous blood on blood flow rate in the presence of countercurrent exchange. Curves calculated by Eq. (13) with $\Phi_{L/B}/C_L$ as ordinate, $\dot{V}_B$ as abscissa, $\alpha a_1 E_1 = 0.2$, $k_1 A_1 = 10$ ml min^{-1} g^{-1}, $P_E A_E$ varied

intestinal venous blood (BEUBLER and LEMBECK 1976). Immediately after the administration of the drugs the increase of venous outflow and absorption ran in parallel. But after 5 min the absorption of the substances did not increase further, while the blood flow rate continued to increase except in the experiment with caffeine and tritiated water. On the contrary, a declining tendency of the absorption rate was seen. The authors explained this observation in the following way. The drugs augmented the blood flow rate first in the subepithelial vessels, so that the absorption rate was increased in parallel. Subsequently, the dilation of the vessels in the deeper layers of the intestinal wall further increased the venous outflow without increasing the absorption rate. The different curves obtained for the blood flow dependence of the absorption of some substances in rat jejunum were explained by a change of the blood flow pattern with time, as discussed in detail in Sect. D.I.6.

In Sect. D.I.1 it was mentioned that the influence of blood flow on the appearance rate of cardiac glycosides (HAASS et al. 1972) as well as of phenylalanine and serine (PYTKOWSKI and LEWARTOWSKI 1972; PYTKOWSKI and MICHALOWSKI 1977) did not agree with the predictions of Eq. (10) when assuming a constant α. The linear extrapolation of the regression lines results in a positive intercept on the abscissa (Fig. 3 a) and the nonlinear extrapolation to the origin results in convex curves. As shown by computer simulation (WINNE 1979 a) convex curves can be expected if the fraction α of the absorption site flow rate decreases with decreasing total blood flow rate. Therefore, the deviation from the prediction can be attributed to a variation of the intramural blood flow pattern. The convex curves for the blood flow dependence of the sodium fluxes (Fig. 3 b) can be explained similarly.

III. Role of Villous Countercurrent Exchange in Intestinal Absorption

The relationship between blood flow and intestinal absorption is complicated by villous countercurrent exchange. In the cat, highly permeable substances are shunted extravascularly between the venous and arterial limbs in the intestinal villi (Fig. 8 c) so that a countercurrent exchange is built up (LUNDGREN and KAMPP 1966; KAMPP and LUNDGREN 1966 a, b, 1968; LUNDGREN 1967, 1970, 1974; KAMPP et al. 1968 a–c; HAGLUND et al. 1972, 1973 a; HAGLUND and LUNDGREN 1974; see also the controversial discussion by KOKKO 1978; HALLBÄCK and JODAL 1978; LEVITT 1978; JODAL et al. 1978 b). In dogs, similar results have been obtained (BOND et al. 1977). The relationship between absorption of tritiated water and mucosal blood flow (measured by microspheres) in sheep rumen can be explained best by the assumption of a countercurrent exchange (DOBSON 1979). Investigations in rabbits and rats yielded no signs of an intestinal countercurrent exchange (LEVITT and LEVITT 1973; BOND et al. 1974; LEVITT et al. 1974). This species difference can be explained by the different morphology of the villi: finger-like villi in the cat and dog with a small distance between the arterial and venous limbs; leaf-like, tongue-like, trapezoidal or triangular villi in rodents (KULENKAMPFF 1975; WINNE 1977). Since a hypertonic region (see the following paragraph) was also observed in the villous tips of rabbit small intestine (JODAL et al. 1977), the presence of a countercurrent exchanger in the villi of rodents cannot be excluded completely.

The countercurrent exchange in the villi reduces the efficiency of the blood drainage. The absorbed substances are concentrated near the tips and steeper apical–basal concentration gradients are built up (KAMPP et al. 1968 a; HALJAMÄE et al. 1971, 1973; JODAL 1973; JODAL and LUNDGREN 1973 a, b). The accumulation of sodium chloride in the apical part of the villi increases the local osmotic pressure and may play a relevant role in the absorption of water (HALJAMÄE et al. 1971, 1973; JODAL 1974, 1977; NORRIS and SUMNER 1974; JODAL and LUNDGREN

1975; JODAL et al. 1978a; HALLBÄCK et al. 1978; LUNDGREN and HAGLUND 1978; HALLBÄCK 1979). A marked osmolar gradient from tip to base was found in the large filiform papillae of the feline tongue (HALLBÄCK et al. 1979).

Intestinal absorption or secretion rate of a substance is reduced by countercurrent exchange in the steady state and absorption or secretion is retarded in the nonsteady state, since the molecules are partly trapped in the countercurrent exchanger (HAGLUND et al. 1972; SVANVIK 1973a, b; BIBER et al. 1973b; LUNDGREN and SVANVIK 1968). Thus, the countercurrent exchanger represents an additional resistance as shown by the third term in the following equation (HALLBÄCK 1979; DOBSON 1979)

$$\Phi_{L/B} = \frac{C_L}{1/k_1 A_1 + 1/\alpha a_1 E_1 \dot{V}_B + P_E A_E/(\alpha a_1 \dot{V}_B)^2}. \tag{13}$$

Equation (13) follows from Eqs. (10) and (11) be neglecting the transfer into the serosal fluid ($k_S = 0$) and introducing countercurrent exchange. For a detailed derivation of the equation see WINNE (1975). A shorter theoretical treatment of intestinal countercurrent exchange was given by BOND et al. (1977). $P_E A_E$ characterizes the exchange capacity between the arterial and venous limbs of the villi. The third term in the denominator of Eq. (13) increases with decreasing $(\alpha a_1 \dot{V}_B)^2$ – notice the square – which means that the countercurrent exchanger becomes more effective when the villous flow rate (the linear velocity of the blood in the villous vessels) decreases. The absorption rate is more reduced at low blood flow rates than at high rates, yielding convex curves for the relationship between blood flow and absorption (Fig. 8d). The curvature becomes more pronounced with increasing $P_E A_E$, i.e. with increasing permeability of the layers between the arterial and venous blood in the villi.

When the krypton appearance rate during isoprenaline infusion (curve 2 in Fig. 8a) is plotted versus the villous flow rate (Fig. 8b) a convex curve is obtained (BIBER et al. 1973b) corresponding to the theoretical prediction. The villous blood flow rate has been calculated from the correlation between venous outflow rate and villous plasma flow observed in separate experiments (BIBER et al. 1973a). If the villous blood flow rate is changed by the number of open capillaries, the effect of the countercurrent exchange does not vary (WINNE 1975). Under experimental conditions the villous flow rate is varied by the number of open capillaries as well as by the linear velocity of blood flow. Therefore, the relationship between intestinal absorption and blood flow rate is more complicated in the presence of countercurrent exchange. This may be the reason why the curve in Fig. 8b apparently does not cross the origin as do the theoretical curves in Fig. 8d. Countercurrent exchange may also contribute to the deviation from the theoretical prediction of blood flow dependence of sodium flux (Fig. 3b) and phenylalanine and serin absorption in dog small intestine (PYTKOWSKI and LEWARTOWSKI 1972; PYTKOWSKI and MICHALOWSKI 1977). Distension of the gut reduces the efficiency of the countercurrent exchanger (JODAL et al. 1977). In that case, a substance is absorbed not only through the tips of the villi, but also through the lateral walls, shortening the effective length of the countercurrent exchanger. The extravascular shunting of oxygen in the villi diminishes the oxygen tension in the tips of the villi and this may be the cause of the lesions observed first in the tips of the villi in hypotension (LUNDGREN 1967; KAMPP et al. 1967, 1968b; HAGLUND 1973; HAGLUND et al. 1973b, 1975; LUNDGREN and HAGLUND 1978).

E. Concluding Remarks

The experimental data described and discussed in Sect. D demonstrate the role of blood flow in intestinal permeation. With increasing permeability the dependence on blood flow shifts from blood flow-independent to blood flow-limited absorption, since the influence of the drainage process increases when the resistance of the epithelium and the mucosal unstirred layer decreases. Since it is mainly the subepithelial capillaries which are involved in the drainage process, the intramural blood flow pattern and the effect of villous countercurrent exchange have to be taken into account in the analysis of absorption data. It is possible that in future the blood flow pattern in the intestinal villi will also have to be considered. The investigations of LEVITT et al. (1979) and LIFSON et al. (1979) represent an interesting and promising starting point for this problem.

Details about the relationship between blood flow and intestinal absorption have been obtained from investigations in animals. There is no reason why the results should not generally be transferred to the human. Thus, based on the experimental data in animals the reduction of intestinal absorption in the elderly is attributed partly to the diminution of the splanchnic blood flow (BENDER 1965, 1968; RICHEY and BENDER 1975, 1977). In the ileum of rats the luminal clearance of barbital and the blood flow rate measured by means of microspheres decreases with increasing age of the animals (CSÁKY and VARGA 1975). Further comparative investigations with simultaneous measurements of blood flow and intestinal absorption are not known to the author.

The equations derived in Sect. C for the relationship between blood flow and intestinal absorption cover only the drainage effect of the blood flow. The blood flow is not only important for the transport of the absorbed substances to the liver. This can be recognized by comparing experiments in vitro and in vivo. In vitro the lack of blood drainage causes an accumulation of the absorbed substances (DAVIDSON and LEESE 1977) and fluid in the intestinal wall, so that their concentration at the basal side of the epithelial cells rises above the usual arterial level (PARSONS 1975). This may influence the metabolism of the cells, e.g. the metabolic rate of glucose and lactate production is higher in vitro than in vivo (PARSONS 1975; HANSON and PARSONS 1976). Under in vitro conditions the subepithelial tissue functions as a thick unstirred layer and the concentration on the basal side of the epithelial cells does not coincide with the concentration in the solution bathing the serosal surface of the intestine. For highly lipid-soluble substances the transfer through the subepithelial tissue represents the rate-limiting step (GIBALDI and GRUNDHOFER 1972). The supply of oxygen and nutrients is another function of the blood circulation. In experiments without blood drainage oxygen and nutrients have to diffuse from the mucosal bulk phase or the serosal bath through the mucosal unstirred layer of through the subepithelial tissue to the epithelial cells. It seems that in vitro the oxygen supply is often not optimal (OCHSENFAHRT 1973; FISHER and GARDNER 1974a; DUGAS and CRANE 1975; HANSON and PARsons 1976). In vivo the oxygen is supplied directly to the basal side of the epithelial cells.

An undisturbed blood circulation provides not only for the drainage of the absorbed substances, but also maintains a positive hydrostatic pressure in the capillaries and the tissue. In this way the net absorption of fluid is influenced (see Sect. D.I.7). The different effect of laxatives in vivo and in vitro is attributed to the lack of tissue pressure under in vitro conditions. Oxyphenisatin and other substances abolish the sodium and fluid absorption in the colon in vitro and in vivo. However, only in vivo can a net flux into the lumen be observed at higher concentrations of the laxatives (FORTH et al. 1966; NELL et al. 1973; EWE and HÖLKER 1974; RUMMEL et al. 1975; WANITSCHKE et al. 1977 b). If in vitro the physiological hydrostatic pressure on the contraluminal side of isolated rat colonic mucosa is simulated by a pressure of 5 cm H_2O, a net transfer of fluid and sodium chloride into the mucosal bath is also observed in vitro (WANITSCHKE et al. 1977 a), for further details see also Chap. 29 and RUMMEL et al. (1975).

References

Ahonen J, Inberg MV, Jääskeläinen AJ, Havia T, Aho AJ, Scheinin TM (1972) Effect of oxygen ventilation in mesenteric arterial occlusion in the dog. Scand J Gastroenterol 7:9–16

Åhrén C, Haglund U (1973) Mucosal lesions in the small intestine of the cat. Acta Physiol Scand 88:541–550

Barr WH, Riegelman S (1970) Intestinal drug absorption and metabolism. I. Comparison of methods and models to study physiological factors of in vitro and in vivo intestinal absorption. J Pharm Sci 59:154–163

Barrowman JA (1978) Physiology of the gastro-intestinal lymphatic system. Cambridge University Press, Cambridge

Bender AD (1965) The effect of increasing age on the distribution of peripheral blood flow in man. J Am Geriatr Soc 13:192–198

Bender AD (1968) Effect of age on intestinal absorption: Implications for drug absorption in the elderly. J Am Geriatr Soc 16:1331–1339

Beubler E, Juan H (1977) The function of prostaglandins in transmucosal water movement and blood flow in the rat jejunum. Naunyn Schmiedebergs Arch Pharmacol 299:89–94

Beubler E, Juan H (1978) PGE-release, blood flow and transmucosal water movement after mechanical stimulation of the rat jejunal mucosa. Naunyn Schmiedebergs Arch Pharmacol 305:91–95

Beubler E, Lembeck F (1976) Methylxanthines and intestinal drug absorption. Naunyn Schmiedebergs Arch Pharmacol 292:73–77

Biber B (1974) The effects of intestinal vasodilator mechanisms on the rate of ^{85}Kr absorption in the cat. Acta Physiol Scand 90:578–582

Biber B, Jodal M, Lundgren O, Svanvik J (1970) Intestinal vasodilatation after mechanical stimulation of the jejunal mucosa. Experientia 26:263–264

Biber B, Lundgren O, Svanvik J (1971) Studies on the intestinal vasodilatation observed after mechanical stimulation of the mucosa of the gut. Acta Physiol Scand 82:177–190

Biber B, Lundgren O, Stage L, Svanvik J (1973 a) An indicator-dilution method for studying intestinal hemodynamics in the cat. Acta physiol Scand 87:433–447

Biber B, Lundgren O, Svanvik J (1973 b) The influence of blood flow on the rate of absorption of ^{85}Kr from the small intestine of the cat. Acta Physiol Scand 89:227–238

Biber B, Lundgren O, Svanvik J (1973 c) Intramural blood flow and blood volume in the small intestine of the cat as analyzed by an indicator-dilution technique. Acta Physiol Scand 87:391–404

Biber B, Fara J, Lundgren O (1974) A pharmacological study of intestinal vasodilator mechanisms in the cat. Acta Physiol Scand 90:673–683

Binder HJ (1977) Mechanisms underlying the absorption of water and ions. Int Rev Physiol 12:285–304
Bohlen HG, Henrich H, Gore RW, Johnson PC (1978) Intestinal muscle and mucosal blood flow during direct sympathetic stimulation. Am J Physiol 235:H40–H45
Bolton JE, Munday KA, Parsons BJ, York BG (1975) Effects of angiotensin II on fluid transport, transmural potential difference and blood flow by rat jejunum in vivo. J Physiol (Lond) 253:411–428
Bond JH, Levitt MD (1979) Use of microspheres to measure small intestinal villous blood flow in the dog. Am J Physiol 236:E577–E583
Bond JH, Levitt DG, Levitt MD (1974) Use of inert gases and carbon monoxide to study the possible influence of counter current exchange on passive absorption from the small bowel. J Clin Invest 54:1259–1265
Bond JH, Levitt DG, Levitt MD (1977) Quantitation of countercurrent exchange during passive absorption from dog small intestine – evidence for marked species differences in efficiency of exchange. J Clin Invest 59:308–318
Boyd CAR (1977) Amino acid inhibition of the exit of monosaccharide from the intestinal epithelium. J Physiol (Lond) 271:48P–49P
Boyd CAR (1978) A classification of systems available for amino acid exit from small intestine into the blood. J Physiol (Lond) 276:52P–53P
Boyd CAR, Parsons DS (1976) Movement of sugars between compartments of vascularly perfused intestine. J Physiol (Lond) 258:12P–13P
Boyd CAR, Parsons DS (1978) Effects of vascular perfusion on the accumulation, distribution and transfer of 3-*O*-methyl-D-glucose within and across the samll intestine. J Physiol (Lond) 274:17–36
Boyd CAR, Parsons DS (1979) Movement of monosaccharides between blood and tissues of vascularly perfused small intestine. J Physiol (Lond) 287:371–391
Boyd CAR, Cheeseman CI, Parsons DS (1975) Amino acid movements across the wall of anuran small intestine perfused through the vascular bed. J Physiol (Lond) 250:409–429
Bresler EH (1978) A model for transepithelial fluid transport. Am J Physiol 235:F626–F637
Brunsson I, Eklund S, Jodal M, Lundgren O, Sjövall H (1979) The effect of vasodilatation and sympathetic nerve activation on net water absorption in the cat's small intestine. Acta Physiol Scand 106:61–68
Cedgård S, Hallbäck DA, Jodal M, Lundgren O (1978) The effects of cholera toxin on intramural blood flow distribution and capillary hydraulic conductivity in the cat small intestine. Acta Physiol Scand 102:148–158
Cheeseman CI (1979) Factors affecting the movement of amino acids and small peptides across the vascularly perfused *anuran* small intestine. J Physiol (Lond) 293:457–468
Chiu CJ, Scott HJ, Gurd FN (1970) Intestinal mucosal lesion in low-flow states. II. The protective effect of intraluminal glucose as energy substrate. Arch Surg 101:484–488
Coburn RF (1968) Carbon monoxide uptake in the gut. Ann NY Acad Sci 150:13–21
Crouthamel W, Doluisio JT, Johnson RE, Diamond L (1970) Effect of mesenteric blood flow on intestinal drug absorption. J Pharm Sci 59:878–879
Crouthamel W, Diamond L, Dittert LW, Doluisio JT (1975) Drug absorption VII: influence of mesenteric blood flow on intestinal drug absorption in dogs. J Pharm Sci 64:664–671
Csáky TZ, Varga F (1975) Subepithelial capillary blood flow estimated from blood-to-lumen flux of barbital in ileum of rats. Am J Physiol 229:549–552
Csernay L, Wolf F, Varró V (1965) Der Kreislaufgradient im Dünndarm. Z Gastroenterol 3:261–265
Davidson RE, Leese HJ (1977) Sucrose absorption by the rat small intestine in vivo and in vitro. J Physiol (Lond) 267:237–248
Diamond L, Doluisio JT, Crouthamel WG (1970) Physiological factors affecting intestinal drug absorption. Eur J Pharmacol 11:109–114
Dobson A (1978) Tritiated water clearance and capillary blood flow to the epithelium of the rumen. J Physiol (Lond) 277:74P

Dobson A (1979) The choice of models relating tritiated water absorption to subepithelial blood flow in the rumen of sheep. J Physiol (Lond) 297:111–121
Dobson A, Sellers AF, Thorlacius SO (1971) Limitation of diffusion by blood flow through bovine ruminal epithelium. Am J Physiol 220:1337–1343
Donowitz M, Wicklein D, Reynolds DG, Hynes RA, Charney AN, Zinner MJ (1979) Effect of altered intestinal water transport on rabbit ileal blood flow. Am J Physiol 236:E482–E487
Duffy PA, Granger DN, Taylor AE (1978) Intestinal secretion induced by volume expansion in the dog. Gastroenterology 75:413–418
Dugas MC, Crane RK (1975) Response of transmural electrical parameters across in vitro everted sacs of hamster jejunum to variations in oxygenation rate. Biochim Biophys Acta 401:486–501
Eklund S, Jodal M, Lundgren O, Sjöqvist A (1979) Effects of vasoactive intestinal polypeptide on blood flow, motility and fluid transport in the gastrointestinal tract of the cat. Acta Physiol Scand 105:461–468
Ewe K, Hölker B (1974) Einfluß eines diphenolischen Laxans (Bisacodyl) auf den Wasser- und Elektrolyttransport im menschlichen Colon. Klin Wochenschr 52:827–833
Fahrenkrug J, Haglund U, Jodal M, Lundgren O, Olbe L, Schaffalitzky de Muckadell OB (1978) Nervous release of vasoactive intestinal polypeptide in the gastrointestinal tract of cats: possible physiological implications. J Physiol (Lond) 284:291–305
Fara JW, Campbell R (1976) Intestinal vascular and secretory responses to gastrointestinal hormones. Fed Proc 35:449
Fara JW, Madden KS (1975) Effect of secretin and cholecystokinin on small intestinal blood flow distribution. Am J Physiol 229:1365–1370
Fisher RB, Gardner MLG (1974) A kinetic approach to the study of absorption of solutes by isolated perfused small intestine. J Physiol (Lond) 241:211–234
Forster RE (1967) Measurement of gastrointestinal blood flow by means of gas absorption. Gastroenterology 52:381–386
Forth W (1967) Eisen- und Kobalt-Resorption am perfundierten Dünndarmsegment. 3. Konferenz der Gesellschaft für Biologische Chemie, Oestrich/Rheingau, 27.–29. April 1967: Springer, Berlin Heidelberg New York, pp 242–250
Forth W, Rummel W, Baldauf J (1966) Wasser- und Elektrolytbewegung am Dünn- und Dickdarm unter dem Einfluß von Laxantien, ein Beitrag zur Klärung ihres Wirkungsmechanismus. Naunyn Schmiedebergs Arch Pharmacol 254:18–32
Gatch WD, Culbertson CG (1935) Circulatory disturbances caused by intestinal obstruction. Ann Surg 102:619–635
Gibaldi M, Grundhofer B (1972) Rate-limiting barriers in intestinal absorption. Proc Soc Exp Biol Med 141:564–568
Gits J, Gerber GB (1973) Absorption of sodium ions from rat intestine in vivo and from a perfused isolated preparation. Biophysik 10:39–43
Gore RW, Bohlen HG (1977) Microvascular pressures in rat intestinal muscle and mucosal villi. Am J Physiol 233:H685–H693
Granger DN, Taylor AE (1978) Effect of solute-coupled transport on lymph flow and oncotic pressures in cat ileum. Am J Physiol 235:E429–E436
Granger DN, Valleau JD, Parker RE, Lane RS, Taylor AE (1978) Effects of adenosine on intestinal hemodynamics, oxygen delivery, and capillary fluid exchange. Am J Physiol 235:H707–H719
Granger DN, Shackleford JS, Taylor AE (1979a) PGE_1-induced intestinal secretion: mechanism of enhanced transmucosal protein efflux. Am J Physiol 236:E788–E796
Granger DN, Richardson PDI, Taylor AE (1979b) Volumetric assessment of the capillary filtration coefficient in the cat small intestine. Pfluegers Arch 381:25–33
Greenway CV, Murthy VS (1972) Effects of vasopressin and isoprenaline infusions on the distribution of blood flow in the intestine; criteria for the validity of microsphere studies. Br J Pharmacol Chemother 46:177–188
Grim E, Lindseth EO (1958) Distribution of blood flow to the tissues of the small intestine of the dog. Univ Minn Med Bull 30:138–145

Guthrie JE, Quastel JH (1956) Absorption of sugars and amino acids from isolated surviving intestine after experimental shock. Arch Biochem Biophys 62:485–496

Haass A, Lüllmann H, Peters T (1972) Absorption rates of some cardiac glycosides and portal blood flow. Eur J Pharmacol 19:366–370

Haglund U (1973) Vascular reactions in the small intestine of the cat during hemorrhage. Acta Physiol Scand 89:129–141

Haglund U, Lundgren O (1974) The small intestine in hemorrhagic shock. Gastroenterology 66:625–627

Haglund U, Jodal M, Lundgren O (1972) The importance of the intestinal countercurrent exchanger for the absorption of fatty acids. Acta Physiol Scand 84:27A

Haglund U, Jodal M, Lundgren O (1973a) An autoradiography study of the intestinal absorption of palmitic and oleic acid. Acta Physiol Scand 89:306–317

Haglund U, Lundgren O, Svanvik J (1973b) On the pathogenesis of the intestinal mucosal lesions in shock. Acta Physiol Scand 87:49A–50A

Haglund U, Hultén L, Åhrén C, Lundgren O (1975) Mucosal lesions in the human small intestine in shock. Gut 16:979–984

Haljamäe H, Jodal M, Lundgren O, Svanvik J (1971) The distribution of Na in intestinal villi during absorption of sodium chloride. Acta Physiol Scand 83:283–285

Haljamäe H, Jodal M, Lundgren O (1973) Countercurrent multiplication of sodium in intestinal villi during absorption of sodium chloride. Acta Physiol Scand 89:580–593

Hallbäck DA (1979) Fluid and electrolyte transport in the small intestine as related to the countercurrent exchanger. Physiological and pathophysiological aspects. University of Göteborg

Hallbäck DA, Jodal M (1978) Intestinal countercurrent. Gastroenterology 75:553–554

Hallbäck DA, Hultén L, Jodal M, Lindhagen J, Lundgren O (1978) Evidence for the existence of a countercurrent exchanger in the small intestine in man. Gastroenterology 74:683–690

Hallbäck DA, Jodal M, Lundgren O (1979) Vascular anatomy and tissue osmolality in the filiform and fungiform papillae of the cat's tongue. Acta Physiol Scand 105:469–480

Hamilton JD, Dawson AM, Webb J (1967) Limitation of the use of inert gases in the measurement of small gut mucosal blood flow. Gut 8:509–521

Hanson PJ, Parsons DS (1976) The utilization of glucose and production of lactate by in vitro preparations of rat small intestine: effects of vascular perfusion. J Physiol (Lond) 255:775–795

Hendrix TR, Paulk HT (1977) Intestinal secretion. Int Rev Physiol 12:257–284

Hoving J, Wilson JHP, Valkema AJ, Woldring MG (1977) Estimation of fat absorption from single fecal specimens using ^{131}I-triolein and ^{75}Se-triether. Gastroenterology 72:406–412

Hueckel HJ, Chiu CJ, Hinchey EJ (1973) The effect of intraluminally administered glucose in reducing fluid and electrolyte loss from the ischemic intestine. Surg Gynecol Obstet 136:780–784

Hultén L, Jodal M, Lindhagen J, Lundgren O (1976) Blood flow in the small intestine of cat and man as analyzed by inert gas washout technique. Gastroenterology 70:45–51

Hultén L, Lindhagen J, Lundgren O (1977) Sympathetic nervous control of intramural blood flow in the feline and human intestines. Gastroenterology 72:41–48

Imamura Y, Ichibagase H (1977) Effect of simultaneous administration of drugs on absorption and excretion. VIII. Effect of plasmaprotein binding displacement on the intestinal absorption of sulfonamides in rabbits. Chem Pharm Bull (Tokyo) 25:3400–3405

Jodal M (1973) The significance of the intestinal countercurrent exchanger for the absorption of sodium and fatty acids. Akademisk Avhandling, Göteborg

Jodal M (1974) An autoradiographic study of the intestinal absorption of ^{22}Na. Acta Physiol Scand 90:79–85

Jodal M (1977) The intestinal countercurrent exchanger and its influence on intestinal absorption. In: Kramer M, Lauterbach F (eds) Intestinal Permeation. Workshop Conference Hoechst, vol 4. Excerpta Medica, Amsterdam, pp 48–55

Jodal M, Lundgren O (1973 a) The distribution of absorbed ^{3}H-palmitic acid in the intestinal villi of the cat during various circulatory conditions. Acta Physiol Scand 89:318–326
Jodal M, Lundgren O (1973 b) Studies on the in vivo absorption of butyric acid in the small intestine of the cat. Acta Physiol Scand 89:327–333
Jodal M, Lundgren O (1975) Demonstration of tissue hyperosmolarity in the tips of intestinal villi during sodium chloride absorption. Acta Physiol Scand 95:7A–8A
Jodal M, Svanvik J, Lundgren O (1977) The importance of the intestinal countercurrent exchanger for ^{85}Kr absorption from the feline gut. Acta Physiol Scand 100:412–423
Jodal M, Hallbäck DA, Lundgren O (1978 a) Tissue osmolality in intestinal villi during luminal perfusion with isotonic electrolyte solutions. Acta Physiol Scand 102:94–107
Jodal M, Lundgren O, Sjöquist A, Haglund U (1978 b) Countercurrent controversy. Gastroenterology 75:767–769
Kampp M, Lundgren O (1966 a) Blood flow and flow distribution within the small intestine of the cat. Acta Physiol Scand 68 [Suppl 277]:102
Kampp M, Lundgren O (1966 b) Evidence for countercurrent exchange in intestinal villi. Acta Physiol Scand 68 [Suppl 277]:103
Kampp M, Lundgren O (1968) Blood flow and flow distribution in the small intestine of cat as analysed by the Kr^{85} wash-out technique. Acta Physiol Scand 72:282–297
Kampp M, Lundgren O, Nilsson NJ (1967) Extravascular short-circuiting of oxygen indicating countercurrent exchange in the intestinal villi of the cat. Experientia 23:197
Kampp M, Lundgren O, Sjöstrand J (1968 a) The distribution of intravascularly administered lipid soluble and lipid insoluble substances in the mucosa and the submucosa of the small intestine of the cat. Acta Physiol Scand 72:469–480
Kampp M, Lundgren O, Nilsson NJ (1968 b) Extravascular shunting of oxygen in the small intestine of the cat. Acta Physiol Scand 72:396–403
Kampp M, Lundgren O, Sjöstrand J (1968 c) On the components of the Kr^{85} wash-out curves from the small intestine of the cat. Acta Physiol Scand 72:257–281
Kingham JGC, Whorwell PJ, Loehry CA (1976) Small intestinal permeability. 1. Effects of ischaemia and exposure to acetyl salicylate. Gut 17:354–361
Kojima S, Miyake J (1975) Factors influencing absorption and excretion of drugs. IV. Effect of hypertonic and hypotonic solutions on in situ rat intestinal absorption of several drugs. Chem Pharm Bull (Tokyo) 23:1247–1255
Kojima S, Smith RB, Crouthamel WG, Doluisio JT (1972) Drug absorption VI: water flux and drug absorption in an *in situ* rat gut preparation. J Pharm Sci 61:1061–1064
Kokko JP (1978) Countercurrent exchanger in the small intestine of man: is there evidence for its existence? Gastroenterology 74:791–792
Kulenkampff H (1975) The structural basis of intestinal absorption. In: Forth W, Rummel W (eds) Pharmacology of intestinal absorption: gastrointestinal absorption of drugs, vol I. Pergamon, Oxford, pp 1–69 (International encyclopedia of pharmacology and therapeutics, section 39B)
Lasker J, Rickert DE (1978) Absorption and glucuronylation of diethylstilbestrol by the rat small intestine. Xenobiotica 8:665–672
Lee JS (1961) Flows and pressures in lymphatic and blood vessels of intestine in water absorption. Am J Physiol 200:979–983
Lee JS (1963) Role of mesenteric lymphatic system in water absorption from rat intestine in vitro. Am J Physiol 204:92–96
Lee JS (1965) Motility, lymphatic contractility, and distention pressure in intestinal absorption. Am J Physiol 208:621–627
Lee JS (1969) Role of lymphatic system in water and solute transport from rat intestine in vitro. Q J Exp Physiol 54:311–321
Lee JS (1971) Contraction of villi and fluid transport in dog jejunal mucosa in vitro. Am J Physiol 221:488–495
Lee JS (1973) Effects of pressures on water absorption and secretin in rat jejunum. Am J Physiol 224:1338–1344
Lee JS (1974) Glucose concentration and hydrostatic pressure in dog jejunal villus lymph. Am J Physiol 226:675–681

Lee JS (1979) Lymph capillary pressure of rat intestinal villi during fluid absorption. Am J Physiol 237:E301–E307

Lee JS, Duncan KM (1968) Lymphatic and venous transport of water from rat jejunum: a vascular perfusion study. Gastroenterology 54:559–567

Lee JS, Silverberg JW (1976) Effect of histamine on intestinal fluid secretion in the dog. Am J Physiol 231:793–798

Levitt MD (1978) Countercurrent controversy. Gastroenterology 75:767

Levitt MD, Levitt DG (1973) Use of inert gases to study the interaction of blood flow and diffusion during passive absorption from the gastrointestinal tract of the rat. J Clin Invest 52:1852–1862

Levitt MD, Bond JH, Levitt DG (1974) Does contercurrent exchange influence small-bowell function? Am J Dig Dis 19:771–774

Levitt DG, Sircar B, Lifson N, Lender EJ (1979) Model for mucosal circulation of rabbit small intestine. Am J Physiol 237:E373–E382

Lichtenstein B, Winne D (1973) The influence of blood flow on the absorption of 3-*O*-methylglucose from the jejunum of the rat. Naunyn Schmiedebergs Arch Pharmacol 279:153–172

Lichtenstein B, Winne D (1974) The influence of blood flow on the phlorizine-insensitive and sensitive galactose absorption in rat jejunum. Naunyn Schmiedebergs Arch Pharmacol 282:195–212

Lifson N, Sircar B, Levitt DG, Lender EJ (1979) Heterogeneity of macroscopic and single villus blood flow in rabbit small intestine. Microvasc Res 17:158–180

Lluch Trull M (1954) Influencia del aporte de oxígeno en la absorción intestinal de glucosa. Rev Esp Fisiol 10:275–314

Love AHG (1976) Intestinal blood flow and sodium exchange. In: Robinson JWL (ed) Intestinal ion transport. The proceedings of the international symposium on intestinal ion transport, Titisee, may 1975. MTP Press, Lancaster, pp 261–265

Love AHG, Matthews J (1972) Intestinal absorption and blood flow. Eur J Clin Invest 2:294

Love AHG, Matthews JGW, Veall N (1972) Intestinal blood flow and sodium transport. Gut 13:853–854

Love AHG, Chen LC, Reeve J, Veall N (1977) The relative transfer rates for sodium and xenon from gut lumen to plasma in man. Clin Sci Mol Med 52:249–254

Lundgren O (1967) Studies on blood flow distribution and countercurrent exchange in the small intestine. Acta Physiol Scand [Suppl] 303:1–42

Lundgren O (1970) Counter current exchange in the small intestine. Am Heart J 79:285–288

Lundgren O (1974) The circulation of the small bowel mucosa. Gut 15:1005–1013

Lundgren O, Haglund U (1978) The pathophysiology of the intestinal countercurrent exchanger. Life Sci 23:1411–1422

Lundgren O, Jodal M (1975) Regional blood flow. Annu Rev Physiol 37:395–414

Lundgren O, Kampp M (1966) The wash-out of intraarterially injected krypton^{85} from the intestine of the cat. Experientia 22:268–270

Lundgren O, Svanvik J (1968) Uptake of Kr^{85} from the lumen of the small intestine to the intestinal blood in the cat. Acta Physiol Scand 74:20A–21A

Lundgren O, Svanvik J (1973) Mucosal hemodynamics in the small intestine of the cat during reduced perfusion pressure. Acta Physiol Scand 88:551–563

MacFerran SN, Mailman D (1967) Effects of glucagon on canine intestinal sodium and water fluxes and regional blood flow. J Physiol (Lond) 266:1–12

Mailman D (1978a) Effects of vasoactive intestinal polypeptide on intestinal absorption and blood flow. J Physiol (Lond) 279:121–132

Mailman DS (1978b) Absorptive site (ASBF) and total (TBF) intestinal blood flow measured by ^3H_2O clearances. Physiologist 21:75

Mailman D (1979) Effects of pentagastrin (G5) on canine intestinal absorption and blood flow. Fed Proc 38:1315

Mailman D, Jordan K (1975) The effect of saline and hyperoncotic dextran infusion on canine ileal salt and water absorption and regional blood flow. J Physiol (Lond) 252:97–113

Matthews JGW, Love AHG (1974) Interrelationship of mesenteric ischemia and diarrhoea. Proc R Soc Med 67:12

McArdle AH, Chiu CJ, Gurd FN (1972) Intraluminal glucose. Substrate for ischemic intestine. Arch Surg 105:441–445

McIver MA, Redfield AC, Benedict EB (1926) Gaseous exchange between the blood and the lumen of the stomach and intestines. Am J Physiol 76:92–111

Micflikier AB, Bond JH, Sircar B, Levitt MD (1976) Intestinal villus blood flow measured with carbon monoxide and microspheres. Am J Physiol 230:916–919

Mirkovitch V, Menge H, Robinson JWL (1975) Protection of the intestinal mucosa during ischaemia by intraluminal perfusion. Res Exp Med (Berl) 166:183–191

Mirkovitch V, Robinson JWL, Menge H, Cobo F (1976) The consequences of ischaemia after mechanical obstruction of the dog ileum. Res Exp Med (Berl) 168:45–55

Nell G, Overhoff H, Forth W, Rummel W (1973) The influence of water gradients and oxyphenisatin on the net transfer of sodium and water in the rat colon. Naunyn Schmiedebergs Arch Pharmacol 277:363–372

Nelson RA, Beargie RJ (1965) Relationship between sodium and glucose transport in canine jejunum. Am J Physiol 208:375–379

Norris HT, Sumner DS (1974) Distribution of blood flow to the layers of the small bowel in experimental cholera. Gastroenterology 66:973–981

Nylander G, Wikström S (1968) Propulsive gastrointestinal motility in regional and graded ischemia of the small bowel. An experimental study in the rat. I. Immediate results. Acta Chir Scand [Suppl] 385:1–67

Ochsenfahrt H (1971) The mucosal-serosal transfer of drugs in the rat jejunum with and without blood flow. Naunyn Schmiedebergs Arch Pharmacol 270:Suppl R 102

Ochsenfahrt H (1973) Untersuchungen zur Resorption von Arzneimitteln aus der isolierten, vaskular perfundierten Jejunumschlinge der Ratte mit und ohne Durchblutung am Beispiel einiger organischer Substanzen. Habilitationsschrift, Fachbereich Theoretische Medizin, Eberhard-Karls-Universität, Tübingen

Ochsenfahrt H (1976) The blood-to-lumen flux of drugs in the vascularly perfused jejunum of the rat. Naunyn Schmiedebergs Arch Pharmacol 293:Suppl R 45

Ochsenfahrt H (1979) The relevance of blood flow for the absorption of drugs in the vascularly perfused, isolated intestine of the rat. Naunyn Schmiedebergs Arch Pharmacol 306:105–112

Ochsenfahrt H, Winne D (1969) Der Einfluß der Durchblutung auf die Resorption von Arzneimitteln aus dem Jejunum der Ratte. Naunyn Schmiedebergs Arch Pharmacol 264:55–75

Ochsenfahrt H, Winne D (1972a) The contribution of blood flow changes to solvent drag phenomenon. Life Sci 11:1105–1113

Ochsenfahrt H, Winne D (1972b) Solvent drug influence on the intestinal absorption of basic drugs. Life Sci 11:1115–1122

Ochsenfahrt H, Winne D (1973) The contribution of solvent drag to the intestinal absorption of tritiated water and urea from the jejunum of the rat. Naunyn Schmiedebergs Arch Pharmacol 279:133–152

Ochsenfahrt H, Winne D (1974a) The contribution of solvent drag to the intestinal absorption of the basic drugs amidopyrine and antipyrine from the jejunum of the rat. Naunyn Schmiedebergs Arch Pharmacol 281:175–196

Ochsenfahrt H, Winne D (1974b) The contribution of solvent drag to the intestinal absorption of the acidic drugs benzoic acid and salicylic acid from the jejunum of the rat. Naunyn Schmiedebergs Arch Pharmacol 281:197–217

Ochsenfahrt H, Winne D, Sewing KF, Lembeck F (1966) Die Ausscheidung von Tritium-Wasser in das Jejunum der Ratte unter dem Einfluß von 5-Hydroxytryptamin und Noradrenalin. Naunyn Schmiedebergs Arch Pharmacol 254:461–469

Pals DT, Steggerda FR (1966) Relation of intraintestinal carbon dioxide to intestinal blood flow. Am J Physiol 210:893–896

Parker RE, Granger DN (1979) Effect of graded arterial occlusion on ileal blood flow distribution. Proc Soc Exp Biol Med 162:146–149
Parsons DS (1975) Energetics of intestinal transport. In: Csáky TZ (ed) Intestinal absorption and malabsorption. Raven, New York, pp 9–36
Parsons DS, Prichard JS (1968) A preparation of perfused small intestine for the study of absorption in amphibia. J Physiol (Lond) 198:405–434
Prasad KN, Osborne JW (1963) Influence of β-mercaptoethylamine, mesenteric vessel clamping and pH on intestinal absorption of Fe^{59} in rats. Proc Soc Exp Biol Med 114:523–527
Pytkowski B, Lewartowski B (1972) Motility dependent absorption of amino acids in canine small intestine segment hemoperfused in vitro. Pfluegers Arch Ges Physiol 335:125–138
Pytkowski B, Michalowski Y (1977) Motility- and blood flow-dependent absorption of amino acids in canine small intestine. Eur J Clin Invest 7:79–86
Rabinovitch J (1927) Factors influencing the absorption of water and chlorides from the intestine. Am J Physiol 82:279–289
Rausis C, Robinson JWL, Mirkovitch V, Saegesser F (1972) Ischémie colique nécrosante et gangreneuse: faits cliniques et recherche expérimentale. Helv Chir Acta 39:251–258
Rees MH (1920) The influence of pituitary extracts on the absorption of water from the small intestine. Am J Physiol 53:43–48
Richey DP, Bender AD (1975) Effects of human aging on drug absorption and metabolism. In: Goldman R, Rockstein M, Sussman ML (eds) The physiology and pathology of human aging. Academic, New York, pp 59–93
Richey DP, Bender AD (1977) Pharmacokinetic consequences of aging. Annu Rev Pharmacol Toxicol 17:49–65
Robinson JWL (1966) Certain aspects of intestinal amino-acid absorption. Thèse de Doctorat, Faculté des Sciences, Université de Lausanne
Robinson JWL, Mirkovitch V (1972) The recovery of function and microcirculation in small intestinal loops following ischaemia. Gut 13:784–789
Robinson JWL, Mirkovitch V (1977) The roles of intraluminal oxygen and glucose in the protection of the rat intestinal mucosa from the effects of ischaemia. Biomedicine 27:60–62
Robinson JWL, Jéquier JC, Taminelli F (1964) The measurement of amino-acid absorption in vitro. Gastroenterologia 102:292–299
Robinson JWL, Jéquier JC, Felber JP, Mirkovitch V (1965) Amino acid absorption by the intestinal mucosa. Its dependence on the blood supply and its recovery after ischemia. J Surg Res 5:150–152
Robinson JWL, Antonioli JA, Mirkovitch V (1966) The intestinal response to ischaemia. Naunyn Schmiedebergs Arch Pharmacol 255:178–191
Robinson JWL, Rausis C, Basset P, Mirkovitch V (1972) Functional and morphological response of the dog colon to ischaemia. Gut 13:775–783
Robinson JWL, Mirkovitch V, Rausis C (1973) Récupération fonctionelle et morphologique de l'intestin grêle de chien après ischémie aiguë. Helv Chir Acta 39:287–290
Robinson JWL, Haroud M, Winistörfer B, Mirkovitch V (1974) Recovery of function and structure of dog ileum and colon following two hour's acute ischaemia. Eur J Clin Invest 4:443–452
Robinson JWL, Menge H, Mirkovitch V (1975) The response of the dog colon mucosa one hour's ischaemia. Res Exp Med (Berl) 165:127–134
Robinson JWL, Menge H, Sepúlveda FV, Cobo F, Mirkovitch V (1976) The functional response of the dog ileum to one hour's ischaemia. Clin Sci Mol Med 50:115–122
Ross G (1971) Effects of norepinephrine infusions on mesenteric arterial blood flow and its tissue distribution. Proc Soc Exp Biol Med 137:921–924
Rummel W, Nell G, Wanitschke R (1975) Action mechanisms of antiabsorptive and hydragogue drugs. In: Csáky TZ (ed) Intestinal absorption and malabsorption. Raven, New York, pp 209–227
Rusznyák I, Földi M, Szabó G (1957) Physiologie und Pathologie des Lymphkreislaufes. Fischer, Jena

San Martin R, Mailman D (1972) Effect of head upward tilting on unidirectional Na and H_2O fluxes across the canine ileum. Proc Soc Exp Biol Med 140:694–699

Schultz SG, Curran PF (1968) Intestinal absorption of sodium chloride and water. In: Code CF (ed) Intestinal absorption. American Physiological Society, Washington, DC, pp 1245–1275 (Handbook of physiology, vol 3/6)

Shields R, Code CF (1961) Effect of increased portal pressure on sorption of water and sodium from the ileum of dogs. Am J Physiol 200:775–780

Smyth DH (1965) Water movement across the mammalian gut. Symp Soc Exp Biol 19:307–328

Soergel KH, Whalen GE, Harris JA, Geenen JE (1968) Effect of antidiuretic hormone on human small intestinal water and solute transport. J Clin Invest 47:1071–1082

Svanvik J (1973 a) Mucosal blood circulation and its influence on passive absorption in the small intestine. Acta Physiol Scand [Suppl] 385:1–44

Svanvik J (1973 b) The effect of reduced perfusion pressure and regional sympathetic vasoconstrictor activation on the rate of absorption of ^{85}Kr from the small intestine of the cat. Acta Physiol Scand 89:239–248

Svanvik J (1973 c) Mucosal hemodynamics in the small intestine of the cat during regional sympathetic vasoconstrictor activation. Acta Physiol Scand 89:19–29

Svanvik J, Lundgren O (1977) Gastrointestinal circulation. In: Crane RK (ed) Gastrointestinal physiology. University Park Press, Baltimore, pp 1–34 (International review of physiology II, vol 12)

Sylvén C (1970) Influence of blood supply on lipid uptake from micellar solutions by the rat small intestine. Biochim Biophys Acta 203:365–375

Sylvén C (1971) Uptake of micellar lipids by small intestinal segments (under different experimental conditions). Acta Physiol Scand 83:289–299

Turnberg LA (1973) Absorption and secretion of salt and water by the small intestine. Digestion 9:357–381

Varró V, Csernay L (1967) The portal transfer of glucose in the dog. Am J Dig 12:775–784

Varró V, Blahó G, Csernay L, Jung I, Szarvas F (1965) Effect of decreased local circulation on the absorptive capacity of a small intestine loop in the dog. Am J Dig Dis 10:170–177

Varró V, Jung I, Szarvas F, Csernay L, Sávay G, Ökrös J (1967) The effect of vasoactive substances on the circulation and glucose absorption of an isolated jejunal loop in the dog. Am J Dig Dis 12:46–59

Wanitschke R, Nell G, Rummel W (1977 a) Influence of hydrostatic pressure gradients on net transfer of sodium and water across isolated rat colonic mucosa. Naunyn Schmiedebergs Arch Pharmacol 297:191–194

Wanitschke R, Nell G, Rummel W, Specht W (1977 b) Transfer of sodium and water through isolated rat colonic mucosa under the influence of deoxycholate and oxyphenisatin. Naunyn Schmiedebergs Arch Pharmacol 297:185–190

Wells HS (1931) The passage of materials through the intestinal wall. I. The relation between intra-intestinal pressure and the rate of absorption of water. Am J Physiol 99:209–220

Wells HS (1940) The balance of physical forces which determine the rate and direction of flow of fluid through the intestinal mucosa. Am J Physiol 130:410–419

Wikström S (1968) Propulsive gastrointestinal motility in regional and graded ischemia of the small bowel. An experimental study in the rat. II. Late results. Acta Chir Scand [Suppl] 386:1–53

Williams JH Jr, Mager M, Jacobson ED (1964) Relationship of mesenteric blood flow to intestinal absorption of carbohydrates. J Lab Clin Med 63:853–863

Winne D (1966) Der Einfluß einiger Pharmaka auf die Darmdurchblutung und die Resorption tritiummarkierten Wassers aus dem Dünndarm der Ratte. Naunyn Schmiedebergs Arch Pharmacol 254:199–224

Winne D (1970 a) Der Einfluß der Durchblutung auf die Wasser- und Salzresorption im Jejunum der Ratte. Naunyn Schmiedebergs Arch Pharmacol 265:425–441

Winne D (1970 b) Formal kinetics of water and solute absorption with regard to intestinal blood flow. J Theor Biol 27:1–18

Winne D (1971) Die Pharmakokinetik der Resorption bei Perfusion einer Darmschlinge mit variabler Durchblutung. Naunyn Schmiedebergs Arch Pharmacol 268:417–433
Winne D (1972a) The influence of blood flow and water net flux on the absorption of tritiated water from the jejunum of the rat. Naunyn Schmiedebergs Arch Pharmacol 272:417–436
Winne D (1972b) The influence of blood flow and water net flux on the blood-to-lumen flux of tritiated water in the jejunum of the rat. Naunyn Schmiedebergs Arch Pharmacol 274:357–374
Winne D (1973) The influence of blood flow on the absorption of L- and D-phenylalanine from the jejunum of the rat. Naunyn Schmiedebergs Arch Pharmacol 277:113–138
Winne D (1975) The influence of villous counter current exchange on intestinal absorption. J Theor Biol 53:145–176
Winne D (1977) The vasculature of the jejunal villus. In: Kramer M, Lauterbach F (eds) Intestinal permeation. Proceedings of the fourth workshop conference Hoechst, 19–22 October 1975. Excerpta Medica, Amsterdam, pp 56–57
Winne D (1978a) Blood flow in intestinal absorption models. J Pharmacokinet Biopharm 6:55–78
Winne D (1978b) The permeability coefficient of the wall of a villous membrane. J Math Biol 6:95–108
Winne D (1979a) Influence of blood flow on intestinal absorption of drugs and nutrients. Pharmacol Ther [B] 6:333–393
Winne D (1979b) Rat jejunum perfused in situ: effect of perfusion rate and intraluminal radius on absorption rate and effective unstirred layer thickness. Naunyn Schmiedebergs Arch Pharmacol 307:265–274
Winne D, Markgraf I (1979) The longitudinal intraluminal concentration gradient in the perfused rat jejunum and the appropriate mean concentration for calculation of the absorption rate. Naunyn Schmiedebergs Arch Pharmacol 309:271–279
Winne D, Ochsenfahrt H (1967) Die formale Kinetik der Resorption unter Berücksichtigung der Darmdurchblutung. J Theor Biol 14:293–315
Winne D, Remischovsky J (1970) Intestinal blood flow and absorption of non-dissociable substances. J Pharm Pharmacol 22:640–641
Winne D, Remischovsky J (1971a) Der Einfluß der Durchblutung auf die Resorption von Harnstoff, Methanol und Äthanol aus dem Jejunum der Ratte. Naunyn Schmiedebergs Arch Pharmacol 268:392–416
Winne D, Remischovsky J (1971b) Der Einfluß der Durchblutung auf die Resorption von Polyalkoholen aus dem Jejunum der Ratte. Naunyn Schmiedebergs Arch Pharmacol 270:22–40
Yablonski ME, Lifson N (1976) Mechanism of production of intestinal secretion by elevated venous pressure. J Clin Invest 57:904–915
Yu YM, Yu LCC, Chou CC (1975) Distribution of blood flow in the intestine with hypertonic glucose in the lumen. Surgery 78:520–525

CHAPTER 24

Hormonal Effects on Intestinal Permeability

V. VARRÓ

A. Introduction

In addition to various amounts of nutrients, the intestines contain endogenous digestive secretions such as saliva, gastric juice, pancreatic secretion, bile, and intestinal secretion. The total amount of intestinal fluid has been estimated to represent about 7–9 l/day. Fortunately nearly all of the water, electrolytes, and most of the other constituents are reabsorbed in the small and large intestine, because even a small decrease in this efficient reabsorption (e.g., of water) would cause profuse, severe, fatal diarrhea.

The basic mechanisms regulating the absorption of water, electrolytes, carbohydrate, protein, fat, etc., are relatively well known, but the role of endogenous and exogenous factors regulating permeation processes have been less intensively studied. A new field of research is the influence of the digestive polypeptide hormones on secretion and excretion in the gut. The effect of the recently characterized and synthesized gut polypeptides on secretory function of the stomach, pancreas, and biliary tract has been reasonably well analyzed; however, investigation of the intestines, which are the site of origin of most of these hormones, has been overshadowed by other studies. The recognition that the gut hormones possess not only endocrine and neurocrine, but also paracrine functions rendered the intestine even more important as the target organ of various polypeptides.

On the other hand, our knowledge of the nature of the cells through which electrolyte transport occurs is also inadequate. It is not clear whether or not there are separate cells for absorption and secretion. Although it is generally accepted that the crypt cells of the gland of Lieberkühn possess a primary role in intestinal secretion, while absorption occurs through the villi, the possibility that the observed absorptive response in the intestine is the net result of *two* processes linked to *two* types of cells cannot be ruled out (LEWIN 1980).

The primary function of intestine is absorption not secretion, but we know that under physiologic conditions the intestine is capable of active secretion of several substances, first of all of water and salt. Both processes are primarily linked to the activity of Na^+K^+-ATPase that regulates the transepithelial transport of Na^+.

This chapter will discuss only the pancreatic and gastrointestinal hormones with regard to small intestinal and colonic permeation. An attempt is made to give all the information which seems important for the proper evaluation of the data presented. Thus, the method and species (in vitro or in vivo; animal or human studies) and the quality and quantity of the polypeptide hormone used are mentioned whenever possible. Every effort has been made to indicate properly the net movement of fluid and substances across the intestinal mucosa. Net movements from (secretion) or into (absorption) the mucosa represent the difference between the sometimes rapid bidirectional fluxes. Accurate designation is not always possible owing to lack of information in the text cited. Differences between active and passive transport mechanisms are noted by indicating the concentration of the ingredients of the solute in question.

The study of bidirectional fluxes tells us more about the permeability properties of the enterocyte membrane than about transport processes. In the latter, intracellular metabolic processes may contribute a lot to the difference between the lumen : plasma ratio of a given substance which was put into the intestine. In this context the words "transfer" and "transport" have been used according to the authors' designation, otherwise "transfer" refers to movement of fluid and/or substances (e.g., glucose) in vitro between the mucosal and serosal sides, while "transport" means the appearance of a substance in the venous effluent of a gut segment.

Although the effects of some peptide hormones on intestinal absorption are well established by both in vitro and in vivo experiments, we do not as yet know whether these agents have a physiologic role in the control of intestinal transport. The changes observed during animal experiments may represent pharmacologic actions which can be observed during life only under exceptional pathologic conditions (e.g., Verner–Morrison syndrome).

Special attention has been paid therefore, to the effect of the endocrine tumors which produce severe loss of water and electrolyte through the intestinal epithelium. Verner–Morrison syndrome (pancreatic cholera) offers a unique possibility of studying the effect of one or more hormones on the absorptive and/or excretory function of the gut.

B. Gastrin

I. In Vitro Studies

GARDNER et al. (1967), working with everted gut sacs of the distal portion of the hamster small intestine, observed an inhibition of the net transfer of water and ions from the mucosal to the serosal side with crude porcine gastrin. This same effect could not be demonstrated in the proximal and middle portions of the gut; potassium transport was not affected at all. Their incubation medium contained glucose (15.1 m*M*), thus, the mechanism of inhibition might have been influenced by the stimulation of hexose-induced sodium transfer.

As to the mechanism of this in vitro effect; gastrin and pentagastrin failed to stimulate adenylate cyclase activity or alter the stimulation of the same by vasoactive intestinal polypeptide (VIP) or prostaglandin E_1 (PGE_1) in homogenates of human jejunal mucosal biopsies (KLAEVEMAN et al. 1975). These experiments, however, do not exclude the possibility that, in *intact* cells, the hormone might increase adenylate cyclase activity and cellular cAMP. This assumption is weakened by the finding of SCHWARTZ et al. (1974) who reported that pentagastrin did not alter cellular cAMP in rabbit ileal mucosa.

II. In Vivo Studies

In dogs, gastrin inhibited fluid absorption (or increased secretion) from the intact jejunum (WRIGHT et al. 1968). GINGELL et al. (1968) found a marked reduction of water and sodium absorption in isolated segments of the dog ileum during intravenous infusion of pentagastrin in doses of 4 and 8 μg kg^{-1} h^{-1}. The pentapeptide had no effect upon the net transport of these substances in the jejunum or colon. Net secretion of potassium was increased in the lumen of the small intestine with the dose of 4 μg kg^{-1} h^{-1}, but neither with the larger dose, nor with both doses combined in the colon. BYNUM et al. (1971) found that water and electrolyte absorption were inhibited by both endogeneous gastrin and exogenous pentagastrin in jejunal and ileal loops of the dog, but their instillation fluid also contained glucose in a concentration of 0.5%. BARBEZAT (1973) clearly demonstrated a significant stimulation of secretion in both jejunal and ileal Thiry–Vella pouches of dogs with doses of pentagastrin as low as 1 μg kg^{-1} h^{-1}. As dose–response curves indicated that this dose is well within the physiologic range of pentagastrin, he considered that this hormone may well play a part in the normal control of gut secretion. In the rat with in situ prepared small intestinal loops, pentagastrin increased net duodenal and decreased net ileal sodium and water absorption from a test solution containing 138 m*M* NaCl. This effect was largely due to decreased efflux in the duodenum and ileum. No changes were observed in the jejunum. There was no correlation between the doses of pentagastrin administered (1, 2.5, 5, and 20 μg/100 g) and intestinal absorption, the smallest dose generally having maximal effect. The authors conclude that gastrin modulates intestinal transport in rats and this effect is partly specific to the intestinal segment and, we may add, the species under study (PANSU et al. 1980).

Using isolated segments, the artificial nature of these preparations must be borne in mind. To assess the physiologic role of hormones upon intestinal handling of water and electrolytes the same investigations have to be repeated with normal anatomic relationships preserved, so that the intestinal mucosa are in contact with food and digestive secretions. Furthermore, pure porcine gastrin II (4 μg kg^{-1} h^{-1}) weakly stimulated fluid secretion of the Brunner's glands in the dog (STENING and GROSSMAN 1969).

Both exogenous pentagastrin (5 μg kg^{-1} h^{-1}) and endogenously released gastrin inhibited jejunal and ileal active absorption of glucose from 0.5% solution in the presence of sodium (150 mequiv./l) (BYNUM et al. 1971) and the same was observed with 2.5% glucose solution in the distal small intestine by MOSHAT et al. (1970).

In humans, the effect of synthetic human gastrin I was thoroughly studied using segmental perfusion with a proximal occlusive balloon by MODIGLIANI et al. (1976). Infusing different doses of gastrin, they found a significant reduction of net absorption of water and electrolytes from a glucose–saline solution with doses of 0.5–1.0 and 2.0 μg kg^{-1} h^{-1}, but not from a mannitol–saline solution.

Ileal absorption of the same substances was not influenced either from the glucose–saline or from the mannitol–saline solution. Glucose-stimulated sodium absorption was significantly depressed by synthetic human gastrin I (MODIGLIANI and BERNIER 1972). Comparing the effect of pentagastrin, the same authors

(MODIGLIANI et al. 1976) concluded that the pentapeptide of gastrin is about 30% less potent on a molar basis than the synthetic heptadecapeptide in inhibiting water and ion absorption in human jejunum.

Summarizing the results of gastrin and its active COOH terminal analog on jejunal absorption, one may speculate on the probable role of this hormone during normal digestion. It might be hypothesized that the inhibitory effect of gastrin on absorption in dogs and humans occurs only in the initial phase of digestion at a time when food and secretions have not reached the gut. When acid gastric contents reach the duodenum, antral release is turned off and the braking effect of gastrin is lifted. This inhibitory effect on fluid and solutes absorption might also contribute to the watery diarrhea in Zollinger–Ellison syndrome, characterized by excess production of circulating gastrin.

C. Cholecystokinin

The effects of cholecystokinin (CCK) on transintestinal water and ion movement in humans and in most animal species studied are very similar to that of secretin and gastrin. The very similar biologic effect of CCK and gastrin could be attributed to the common COOH terminal tetrapeptide amide constituent of the molecule which is the bioactive part of gastrin.

In vitro studies with CCK (Vitrum 30 U)[1] added to the incubation medium inhibited mucosal–serosal water and ion transfer in the distal portion of the hamster intestine with the everted gut sac technique; net transfer of fluid was also inhibited in the proximal and middle portion. Secretin and gastrin produced the same effect only in the distal segment (GARDNER et al. 1967). As reported later with secretin, the incubation medium contained glucose; thus, a hexose-induced stimulation of sodium transfer could have influenced the results obtained with CCK. In the rat, no effect of CCK was found on fluid and ion absorption in vivo (HUBEL 1972a; NASSET and JU 1970; PANSU et al. 1980). Species differences seem to influence the results obtained as BUSSJAEGER and JOHNSON (1973) reported that pure CCK in doses of 4 U kg^{-1} h^{-1} inhibited the absorption of fluid, sodium, potassium, and chloride in both the jejunal and ileal Thiry–Vella loop of dog from a Krebs–Ringer bicarbonate solution. Instillation of fat into the duodenojejunal portion of the bowel duplicated the effects of exogenous CCK in the ileal loop. In the same experiment, the buffer solution also contained glucose (100 mg%); CCK slightly increased glucose absorption from the jejunum, but not from the ileum. Interestingly, endogenous CCK released by fat instillation evoked a significant decrease of glucose absorption from the ileal loop. On the other hand the spontaneous secretion of fluid and electrolytes was not stimulated by the COOH teminal octapeptide of CCK (CCK-OP) even with supramaximal doses for other actions (BARBEZAT 1973). It was quite unexpected, therefore, that CCK-OP given alone in a dose of 1 µg kg^{-1} h^{-1} produced diarrhea in three of the five dogs tested; when it was given together with glucagon diarrhea appeared in all five animals (BARBEZAT 1973).

1 Pure CCK contains 3,000 Ivy dog units per milligram

In human studies, MATUCHANSKY et al. (1972) studied the effect of intravenous CCK infusion on jejunal fluid and electrolyte movement by intubation. CCK administration resulted in decreased net water, sodium, and chloride absorption (or increased net secretion). Further analysis revealed that a decrease in lumen–plasma movement was induced by CCK without significant change in blood–lumen transfer. As at the same time CCK also significantly reduced the mean transit time, decreased the volume of fluid in the intestinal segment, and perhaps altered the mucosal blood flow, additional studies are required to asses the definite importance of the single factors. MORITZ et al. (1973) reported that CCK infusion in humans resulted in net fluid and electrolyte secretion. In both studies CCK doses of 1–6 Ivy dog units kg^{-1} h^{-1} were used.

In conclusion; although the evidence is somewhat equivocal, CCK, like secretin and gastrin, seems to inhibit net fluid and ion absorption (or increase net secretion) in humans. The results in animals seem to depend on the species and experimental design used.

D. Vasoactive Intestinal Polypeptide

Vasoactive intestinal polypeptide (VIP) is a highly basic polypeptide which has a structural similarity to secretin, glucagon, and gastric inhibitory polypeptide (GIP). Clinical interest in the effect of VIP on fluid and electrolyte movement relates to the problem of identifying the hormonal agent responsible for the excessive fluid and electrolyte losses in Verner–Morrison syndrome.

I. In Vitro Studies

VIP has been reported to stimulate cAMP accumulation in isolated enterocytes in concentrations as low a 10^{-10} M (LABURTHE et al. 1979). Specific binding of ^{125}I-labeled VIP has been demonstrated in various intestinal cell preparations in both rats and humans (LABURTHE et al. 1979; PRIETO et al. 1979).

Several authors have reported that, in muscle-stripped everted sacs of rat colon, VIP decreased net absorption of sodium and water or increased the secretion of water (RACUSEN and BINDNER 1977; WALDMAN et al. 1977b). Both groups found that VIP stimulated adenylate cyclase activity in homogenates of colonic mucosa, while SCHWARTZ et al. (1974) demonstrated the same effect in homogenates of rabbit and/or dog small intestinal mucosa. KLAEVEMAN et al. (1975) tested VIP for its ability to alter adenylate cyclase activity in vitro in homogenates of human jejunal biopsies: VIP activated adenylate cyclase activity. This effect was detectable at concentrations of 10^{-7} M and maximal stimulation occurred at 10^{-4} M. In homogenates of human ileal mucosa at a concentration of 2 μg/ml, VIP caused a fivefold increase in the cAMP level. Glucagon, GIP, and pentagastrin (the latter also in combination with glucagon) failed to alter cAMP levels after 1, 5, and 10 min incubation (SCHWARTZ et al. 1974). In the rat colon, secretin had the same effect as VIP, but their respective affinities were in the ratio 1:100 and the combined effect of both peptides was not additive (WALDMAN et al. 1977a). It seems, therefore, that the effect of secretin on the enterocyte is mediated through the VIP receptors (LABURTHE et al. 1979).

These experiments strongly suggest that there are specific VIP receptors in the intestine and their occupancy is thought to initiate the production of cAMP as intracellular "second messenger". Definite proof, however, of the physiologic implication of VIP in electrolyte transport through the enterocytes awaits further evidence as little if anything is known about either its concentration at the effector cell or the factors regulating its release. Presently employed methods demonstrate the presence, but not the function of this peptide in the intestine.

II. In Vivo Studies

In the rat, COUPAR (1976) infused VIP ($\sim$97.5 μg kg^{-1} h^{-1}) via the arterial route and noted net jejunal secretion, while intravenous infusion of VIP (14.3 μg kg^{-1} h^{-1}) inhibited net absorption of water and electrolytes in the ileum and reversed net absorption to net secretion in the colon (WU et al. 1979). VIP induces a marked secretion of fluid in Thiry–Vella loops of dogs when infused over a 15-min period; a marked increase was noted in the jejunum, while a small response was observed in the ileum (BARBEZAT 1973). VIP seems to be a more potent secretory agent than glucagon and potentiates the effect of the latter when the two are given in combination (SCHEBALIN et al. 1974). KREJS et al. (1978) studied intestinal transport in the dog jejunum by intraarterial infusion of VIP (4.8 μg kg^{-1} h^{-1}) and found net jejunal secretion. VIP at a dose of 175 ng/min caused reduced gut absorption (net secretion) of sodium and water, due mainly to significant decreases in the unidirectional absorptive fluxes in anesthetized dogs and also in dogs given guanethidine to block sympathetic reflexes. Associated with the reduced absorption were a decrease in absorptive site blood flow and a decrease in arterial pressure. Atropine blocked most of the effects of VIP (MAILMAN 1978). VIP is one of the few gastrointestinal hormones which has been shown to increase adenylate cyclase activity in vitro, but even the hormones which do not activate this enzyme may reduce net absorption, primarily by reducing mucosal–serosal flux (SCHWARTZ et al. 1974). The influence of VIP on cAMP metabolism, Na, and Cl fluxes in rabbit are similar to those seen with cholera enterotoxin and certain prostaglandins.

III. VIP-Secreting Tumors

Several hormones have been suggested as the agent responsible for the watery diarrhea, hypokalemia, and achlorhydria seen in Verner–Morrison syndrome mostly caused by an islet cell tumor. Many of these studies were initiated to evaluate the role of these hormones as potential mediators of the excessive fluid loss associated with these tumors. Although these studies verified that several peptide hormones may influence water and electrolyte transport, the problem arises whether the observed effects were not pharmacologic phenomena. Among them the most prominent role is attributed to VIP, although current opinion favors the concept that more than one hormone is involved in the diarrhea in these patients. Substantial amounts of VIP have been extracted from these tumors (consequently called vipomas), originating not only in the pancreas, but in also other organs, e.g., lungs. The following lines of evidence favor the role of VIP as a causative agent in Verner–Morrison syndrome.

Plasma levels of VIP were elevated in most, but not all patients with Verner–Morrison syndrome (SAID and FALOONA 1975). No other gastrointestinal peptide hormone level was elevated in the cases reported by RAMBAUD et al. (1975). As some of the first radioimmunoassays of VIP were not quite reliable, these findings were greatly fortified by the same results achieved by EBEID et al. (1978) and FAHRENKRUG et al. (1979) using specific immunoassays for VIP. The elevated plasma levels returned to normal after successful removal of the tumor (EBEID et al. 1978; FAHRENKRUG et al. 1979). VIP has been demonstrated in high concentration in the tumor tissue (RAMBAUD et al. 1975; FAHRENKRUG et al. 1979).

KREJS and FORDTRAN (1980) examined whether elevation of plasma VIP concentration to the levels noted in patients with Verner–Morrison syndrome, would reduce absorption or cause secretion in the small bowel of normal subjects. They found that changes in plasma VIP concentration even slightly above the normal range have little if any effect on ion transport rates by the human jejunum. At higher infusion rates (200 and 400 pmol kg^{-1} h^{-1}), VIP concentrations rose to levels commonly seen in patients with Verner–Morrison syndrome. At these levels, VIP caused a dose-dependent decrease of water and sodium absorption. Chloride absorption changed to secretion while bicarbonate movement remained unaffected. The electrogenic anion-secretory process stimulated by VIP appeared to be specific for chloride. It is important to note that all changes induced by VIP were reversible.

The small intestine was found to be the site of the water and electrolyte losses in fasting patients with Verner–Morrison syndrome. The absorption rate of glucose was unchanged in the jejunum with a perfusion solution of 30 m*M*, but decreased at a concentration of 100 m*M*, whereas ileal glucose absorption was diminished, even with 30 m*M* glucose solution. The most striking finding was that the stimulatory effect of glucose and leucine on sodium transport could not be elicited with 30 m*M* solution; there was even a *stimulation* of sodium secretion (RAMBAUD et al. 1975). The water and ion loss seemed to be the most abnormal in the ileum: here fluid losses of 9 l/day could be registered (BERNIER et al. 1979). Colonic mucosa in the studies of RAMBAUD et al. (1975) seemed to reduce water and ion losses, except for potassium, which was excreted mainly by the colonic mucosa.

Pure natural porcine VIP infused continuously at 5–10 pmol kg^{-1} min^{-1} for 12 h to conscious pigs provoked copious watery diarrhea indistinguishable from that of Verner–Morrison syndrome. This diarrhea developed at VIP blood levels of (90–120 pmol/l) which were similar to those found in patients (MODLIN et al. 1977).

Although most of the evidence speaks in favor of the decisive role of VIP in the pathophysiology of Verner–Morrison syndrome, the coincident effect of other gastrointestinal peptides cannot be excluded. Thus SCHMITT et al. (1975) demonstrated the presence of five hormones (secretin, glucagon, serotonin, enteroglucagon, and VIP) in the pancreatic tumor which caused watery diarrhea. VIP was shown to potentiate the effect of glucagon in inducing intestinal secretion (BARBEZAT 1973; SCHEBALIN et al. 1974). In a clinical picture presenting the same symptoms as those seen in Verner–Morrison syndrome, but with no demonstrable tumor (pancreatic or extrapancreatic), normal plasma values of VIP were measured both by BLOOM (1978) and EBEID et al. (1978). Similar findings were also reported by KAHN et al. (1975) and LARSSON et al. (1976).

Further investigations are needed to clarify the relation of other biologically active substance besides those mentioned (e.g., prostaglandins, calcitonin) to VIP in producing the water and ion derangement observed in this pathologic state. Thus, RAMBAUD et al. (1975) found in their patients, besides elevated levels of VIP, high plasma concentrations of PGE, PGF, and calcitonin.

E. Secretin

Certain endocrine tumors cause profuse watery diarrhea and at the same time produce some of the gastrointestinal hormones in excess. The suspected link between diarrhea and the overproduction of these peptides prompted several research groups to investigate the effect of gastrointestinal hormones on the absorption of water and electrolytes in the small intestine. *The majority of studies in animals did not show any effect of secretin on intestinal absorption of water and ions.* Thus, negative results were reported by BYNUM et al. (1971) in dog jejunum and ileum using a potent secretin extract prepared by JORPES ($1\ U\ kg^{-1}\ h^{-1}$).[2] BARBEZAT (1973) did not detect any effect with pure synthetic secretin in Thiry–Vella loops prepared either from the upper jejunum or the lower ileum of dogs. In the rat, HUBEL (1967) and NASSET and JU (1970) could not influence the net flux of water, bicarbonate, chloride, sodium, or potassium when perfusing the lumen of the ileum with a solution containing a single dose of secretin, which caused maximal pancreatic secretion. PANSU et al. (1980), however, reported that secretin (GIH) in various doses (0.17, 0.85, 3.5 CU/100 g) diminished net ileal absorption of sodium and water. No effect was observed in the jejunum. However, all these studies were performed in loops separated from the digestive system.

Similarly, HUBEL (1972a) reported a reduction of water and ion absorption in the rat small intestine, when secretin was administered intravenously in very high doses (100 Boots units/kg). Employing an everted sac preparation of the hamster, GARDNER et al. (1967) reported that secretin (Vitrum 30 units) inhibited the net transfer of sodium, chloride, and fluid. The diminution of net transfer of sodium resulted from a decrease in the mucosal–serosal component; serosal uptake was not altered. It should be mentioned that the incubation medium in these experiments always contained glucose (15.1 m*M*), thus, a hexose-induced stimulation of sodium transfer could have complicated the results. Fluid secretion of the duodenal Brunner's glands was stimulated in cats and dogs by both natural and synthetic secretin (STENING and GROSSMAN 1969).

The first studies in humans were performed by MODIGLIANI et al. (1971) with the intestinal perfusion technique using a tube with a proximal occlusive balloon. They could not observe any effect of Boots secretin infused at a rate sufficient to cause maximal bicarbonate response ($3\ U\ kg^{-1}\ h^{-1}$). Subsequently, all other studies using the triple lumen nonocclusive tube and injecting GIH secretin reported reduced net absorption (or induced net secretion) of water, sodium, and

2 Both pure natural porcine and pure synthetic secretin have between 3,000 and 4,000 clinical units (CU) per milligram (JORPES 1968)

chloride in the proximal jejunum (MEKHJIAN et al. 1972; MORITZ et al. 1973; HICKS and TURNBERG 1973) with doses of 1.2 or 4 U kg^{-1} h^{-1}. Bicarbonate secretion was uninfluenced. No effect of secretin was detected in the lower segments (HICKS and TURNBERG 1973).

HICKS and TURNBERG (1973) postulated that the physiologic role of secretin might consist in preventing too rapid dehydration of the upper jejunal contents which might interfere with adequate mixing and digestion. To clarify the discrepancy between the two techniques, MODIGLIANI et al. (1977) repeated their experiment using the triple lumen tube and GIH secretin and obtained the same reduction in absorption as the other authors. They postulate that: (a) Boots secretin is contaminated with a substance possessing an opposite effect on intestinal absorption, possibly VIP; and (b) the occlusive balloon reduced the inhibition of absorption caused by secretin.

The mechanism whereby secretin reduces water absorption, or induces secretion, is open to speculation. Changes of blood supply and/or motor activity in the small intestine are most probably not involved, because secretin and CCK have similar effects on transintestinal fluxes in spite of their divergent action on motility and mucosal blood supply in the human jejunum (FARA and MADDEN 1975). Based on studies with cholera toxin, it is currently accepted that cAMP stimulates secretion and/or inhibits absorption in the intestine. Secretin, however, does not seem to stimulate the adenylate cyclase–cAMP system in the human jejunum (KLAEVEMAN et al. 1975). Another possibility might be the stimulation of the secretion of bile acids which per se could cause inhibition of water absorption or perhaps net water secretion, depending upon their actual concentration in the perfusion fluid (TEEM and PHILLIPS 1972). The possibility that one of the components of secretin-stimulated pancreatic, biliary, or duodenal intraluminal secretion is responsible for the secretin-induced changes, therefore, cannot be excluded by the findings with the triple lumen tube.

It might be of importance to recall the data of MEYER et al. (1970) that about 0.5 U kg^{-1} h^{-1} secretin is likely to be released in the dog after a meal. At the same time, intestinal absorption in humans was shown to be influenced by 1 U kg^{-1} h^{-1}; lower doses were not tried. Thus, the smallest dose of secretin which influences intestinal absorption may be within the physiologic range, although specific information in humans is still lacking (MODIGLIANI et al. 1977).

F. Insulin

The effect of insulin on intestinal absorption is complex since its effects have to be considered not only in vitro and in vivo, but also in normal and diabetic states. Moreover, the importance of the blood level of glucose has been implicated as a factor in the rate of glucose absorption in vivo following the injection of insulin.

I. Influence of Exogenous Insulin on Intestinal Permeability

1. In Vitro Studies

Addition of insulin in vitro neither stimulated nor inhibited the active glucose uptake of the intestinal tissues (LEESE and MANSFORD 1971). The same authors reported that insulin did not modify the increased absorptive capacity of diabetic rats treated either with streptozotocin or with anti-insulin serum. Similarly, CRANE (1961) was unable to detect any effect of insulin, added in vitro, on the accumulation of galactose in rings of everted hamster intestine. Insulin in a concentration of 1 mU/ml increased both the absorption (mucosal glucose transfer) and the serosal transfer of glucose from a solution containing 200 mg-% glucose in everted sacs of rat jejunum. With 3-*O*-methylglucose at the same concentration the mucosal transfer was almost identical, serosal transfer, however, was much less than with D-glucose in the presence of insulin. According to the authors, the results achieved suggest that the insulin effect with physiologic concentrations of the hormone is dependent on activation of the cellular metabolic process (LOVE and CANAVAN 1968). These results are contradictory not only to the in vitro experiments cited, but also to the effects of larger doses of insulin both in an isolated jejunal loop and in humans (see Sect. F.I.2).

Increased net mucosal–serosal active transfer of D-glucose was demonstrated by AULSEBROOK (1967) in the rat after insulin injection, 18 and 1 h prior to killing; simultaneously, sodium transport was decreased. The same increase was found in preparations originating from alloxan-induced diabetic rats, but in this system both sodium and water transport were augmented; insulin treatment failed to increase glucose transfer further, while that of sodium was moderately decreased. The interpretation of intestinal absorption in alloxan-induced diabetic rats is complicated, however, by the toxic side effects and metabolic disturbances associated with the use of this compound (LUKENS 1948). It should be noted, however, that high blood glucose per se in the rat is sufficient to increase glucose absorption (CSÁKY and FISCHER 1981), even when the intestine is removed for incubation in vitro 30 min after glucose load (CASEY et al. 1968). Glycine transport was markedly stimulated in vitro in rat small intestine when insulin (0.4 U/kg) was given for 6 days prior to the determination on the following day. On the contrary, glycine transport in everted sacs from alloxan-induced diabetic rats was reduced (MAHMOOD and VARMA 1971).

2. In Vivo Studies

Earlier studies on the effect of insulin on intestinal absorption of hexoses have been thoroughly reviewed by CASPARY (1973). He emphasized that experiments performed in intact animals did not differentiate between the effect of insulin on the absorption process and other factors that may influence absorption. Some of these factors, e.g., gastric emptying may be critical determinants. Insulin increases gastric emptying and results in increased glucose absorption. Intestinal perfusion techniques help to eliminate the effect of insulin on intestinal motility; the use of isolated intestinal segments assures even more independence from systemic disturbing factors.

The complexity of the problem is illustrated by the experiments of MEHNERT et al. (1967). They were able to prove that accelerated glucose and fructose absorption after insulin application was due to faster emptying of the stomach. If glucose and fructose were perfused through the rat intestine bypassing the stomach, no differences between insulin-treated and control animals were found. Pretreatment with insulin for 1 week also failed to produce accelerated glucose resorption.

Lack of insulin effect was confirmed in isolated jejunal segments with an intact circulation for 3-*O*-methylglucose in the rat (DUBOIS and ROY 1969) and for D-glucose in the dog (VARRÓ and CSERNAY 1966). The latter experiments were repeated by VÁRKONYI (1978) under the same experimental conditions injecting 0.002, 0.02, and 0.2 U insulin directly into the artery of the jejunal segments, confirming fully the findings of VARRÓ and CSERNAY (1966) (Table 1). MANOME and KURIAKI (1961) perfusing the rat intestine with a 2.3 m*M* glucose solution observed no changes in sugar absorption with small doses of insulin (<0.5 U/kg intravenously); administration of substantially larger doses (5 U/kg) resulted in a moderately increased absorption.

Conflicting results have been reported as to the relation of insulin-induced hypoglycemia and glucose absorption. HORVÁTH and WIX (1951) stated that sugar absorption was increased, depending on the degree of the hypoglycemia and this effect could be inhibited by simultaneous glucose administration. MEHNERT et al. (1967) on the contrary observed an inhibition of glucose absorption which they attributed to the hypoglycemic condition created by intravenous insulin injection. BEYREISS et al. (1964), using continuous perfusion, found diminished active D-galactose absorption after insulin administration in rabbit small intestine. Eventual hypoglycemia as the factor responsible for the inhibitory effect was excluded by simultaneous glucose infusion. In their view the inhibitory effect of insulin on active galactose absorption is mediated by a change in the carrier or ion transport system coupled with galactose transfer. This was confirmed by the lack of insulin effect on L-arabinose which is absorbed by passive diffusion (BEYREISS et al. 1965).

In humans, CUMMINS (1952) and VINNIK et al. (1965), perfusing the small intestine with a nearly isotonic glucose solution (278 and 230 m*M*, respectively), did not observe any effect of insulin on glucose absorption. GOTTESBÜREN et al. (1973 a) showed that glucose absorption was decreased in normal subjects after insulin and insulin plus intravenous glucose infusion; they perfused the intestine, however, with a 21 m*M* glucose solution which is in the range of the Na^+-dependent (active) hexose transport process. The same effect was achieved by endogenous insulin as well, liberated by intravenous injection of 1 g tolbutamide (GOTTESBÜREN et al. 1973 b). In insulin-dependent diabetics, there was no decrease in absorption after injection of tolbutamide, which they thought due to the inability to secrete insulin. On the other hand, a decrease in absorption occurred if insulin was applied in insulin-dependent diabetics.

3. Concluding Remarks

Insulin added in vitro to the small intestine did not influence sugar transfer in experimental animals. It is possible that, under the experimental conditions reported, insulin could not enter the intestinal tissues. FROMM (1969) stripped the serosa and the muscularis from rabbit small intestine and were able to demonstrate an effect of insulin on transmucosal transfer of 3-*O*-methylglucose in the ileum. This approach, although interesting from a theoretical point of view, cannot be considered a physiologic one.

Table 1. Effect of various doses of insulin given intraarterially on absorption and portal transport of isotonic glucose solution and on blood flow in an isolated canine jejunal segment ± standard deviation (VÁRKONYI et al. 1980). For details of the method see VARRÓ et al. (1964). I, III control (physiologic saline) period; II experimental (insulin) period

Insulin	0.002 U		$N=7$	0.02 U		$N=7$	0.2 U		$N=7$
Periods (15 min)	I	II	III	I	II	III	I	II	III
Absorption (mg)	126.83 ± 49.53	132.84 ± 39.81 $P>0.05$	146.33 ± 53.12	140.99 ± 25.81	131.33 ± 13.10 $P>0.05$	139.66 ± 21.92	139.16 ± 84.31	138.49 ± 46.94 $P>0.05$	138.99 ± 41.86
Transport (mg)	80.63 ± 35.98	76.76 ± 31.38 $P>0.05$	76.31 ± 17.63	72.61 ± 27.33	76.25 ± 18.28 $P>0.05$	78.23 ± 22.62	62.68 ± 57.52	70.14 ± 51.74 $P>0.05$	67.49 ± 41.66
Blood flow (ml)	202.83 ± 61.75	220.26 ± 69.43 $P>0.05$	227.16 ± 30.74	116.33 ± 54.04	135.66 ± 74.17 $P>0.05$	148.83 ± 99.37	115.31 ± 42.82	123.99 ± 52.60 $P>0.05$	122.83 ± 44.86

Insulin pretreatment seems to increase the sugar and amino acid uptake of the small intestinal preparation. This increase occurs with concentrations in the active transport range. In the case of glucose, sodium transfer is not simultaneously augmented; thus, insulin does not seem to act through the sodium carrier system.

Exogenous insulin administration in rats and dogs does not influence glucose absorption in isolated segments with intact circulation. In perfusion studies, the results are conflicting, but in these investigations the possibility that the changes observed were the result of more general alterations in the absorptive or metabolic capacities of the small intestine cannot be excluded. When evaluating the experimental results reported, note should taken of differences between doses of insulin administered and concentrations of hexose solutions used. Obviously, different mechanisms are at work during active sugar and amino acid absorption than with concentrations necessitating facilitated or passive transfer through the intestinal mucosa.

One of the main mechanisms suggested for insulin action is that it facilitates the entry of glucose into the cells. In the intestine, the process of hexose absorption involves transfer of the sugar from the mucosal to the serosal side of the intestine. Although conflicting results have been presented, analyzing both in vitro and in vivo experiments, the bulk of evidence speaks in favor of the assumption that, under physiologic conditions, the small intestine should be considered as an "insulin-insensitive" structure until indisputable evidence proves the contrary. The ineffectiveness of insulin in facilitating permeation of glucose (or other sugars having a similar configuration) into other tissues has also been reported. Glycogen synthesis by the brain cells of guinea pigs is not affected by insulin. It seems from these observations that the mechanism of insulin action differs from tissue to tissue. The absorptive processes regulating the uptake of glucose by the enterocytes seem to be independent of the direct action of insulin.

G. Glucagon

Numerous claims are to be found in the literature of the action of glucagon directly on intestinal permeability, yet not a single one is completely free from the objection that the change observed may have been secondary to the alteration of another function of the intestine (e.g., blood flow, motility, or metabolism). In some cases, the mediation by other hormonal responses has to be considered. Interpretation of experimental results has to differentiate between the methods (in vitro or in vivo, acute or chronic administration), substances (hexoses or electrolytes), or species (humans or animals) used. Comments will be ordered, therefore, with consideration of these criteria.

I. Effect on Intestinal Water and Electrolyte Movements

Recent interest in evaluating the role of several gastrointestinal biologically active peptides as potential mediators of the diarrhea associated with some hormone-secreting tumors (e.g., Verner–Morrison syndrome), has provided the impetus for renewed investigation of intestinal water and electrolyte permeation. Although in Verner–Morrison syndrome the peptide most frequently identified in the tumor tissue and the blood of these patients is VIP, in some cases the role of other peptides, including that of glucagon, cannot be ruled out (BARBEZAT and GROSSMAN 1971a). BARBEZAT and GROSSMAN (1971a), perfusing electrolyte solutions through Thiry–Vella loops of jejunum and ileum of dog, found that glucagon given by intravenous infusion for 1 h in a dose of 0.5 μg kg^{-1} min^{-1} suppressed absorption and promoted secretion of electrolytes and water by the small intestinal mucosa.

On the other hand, MOORE and LONGACHER (1974) and MOORE and TAVANO (1974) reported paradoxical effects of acute glucagon infusion in rabbit and dog small intestine. A dose of 30 μg kg^{-1} h^{-1}, did not induce secretion, but inhibited sodium and water absorption in the rabbit ileum, while in the dog it induced a significant increase of net water absorption. In sharp contrast jejunal response to glucagon was opposite in direction in the results in the dog and resulted in a highly significant (29-fold) increase in net water secretion, while in the rabbit jejunum water absorption was not influenced by glucagon. Thus, not only may species differences account for the controversial effect of glucagon on water and sodium movements across the intestinal epithelial cells, but also simultaneous ileal and jejunal responses to glucagon may differ greatly in the same animal. HUBEL (1972a) reported that glucagon enhanced absorption of ions and water from the small intestine of the rat when administered intravenously in high doses (4–257 μg/kg). CASPARY and LÜCKE (1976) observed increased absorption of water, sodium, and potassium after chronic administration of glucagon (100 μg twice daily) in rat small intestine using an in vivo perfusion technique. MACFERRAN and MAILMAN (1977) infused glucagon at doses of 0.05–0.5 μg/kg into a mesenteric artery of a canine ileal segment. They found increased absorptive and secretory fluxes of sodium and water without changes in net fluxes. Absorptive blood flow was increased and the unidirectional secretory and absorptive fluxes of both water and sodium were linearly related to the calculated capillary; pressure during glucagon infusion. They conclude that the effects of glucagon on gut transport of both substances are due to local vasodilation.

In humans, the results depend on whether physiologic or pharmacologic doses of glucagon were employed. Thus, GANESHAPPA et al. (1972), using a slow marker perfusion technique in normal subjects, reported that 2.4 μg/min glucagon administered intravenously for 6–8 h induced a decrease in net sodium and water absorption which was not due to increased intestinal secretion; rather they suggest that glucagon interferes with absorptive mechanisms directly. Essentially the same was stated by MEKHJIAN et al. (1972) who investigated the effect of intravenous administration of various doses of glucagon on the jejunal transport of water and electrolytes in healthy humans by the triple lumen perfusion technique; 2 μg/kg glucagon produced 50% reduction in absorption, 5 μg/kg, however, resulted in secretion of water and electrolytes; with 20 μg/kg the changes were not significant. They are of the opinion that glucagon alters jejunal fluid transport and thus may play a role in diarrheal syndromes associated with some pancreatic tumors. Similarly, HICKS and TURNBERG (1974) reported that pancreatic glucagon given by intravenous infusion reduced absorption of sodium, chloride, and water in the human jejunum. A dose–response curve for glucagon indicated almost no effect at the dose of 0.3 μg kg^{-1} h^{-1}, but ion transport was maximal to

0.6 μg kg^{-1} h^{-1}; this dose can be calculated to have probably achieved steady state levels within the plasma some 2–3 times the levels normally found under physiologic conditions. These observations suggest that, in the physiologic range, glucagon exerts little or no influence on ion transport, but in cases when the levels of plasma concentrations calculated to have been achieved by the effective glucagon doses were within the range which could conceivably be found in pathologic conditions, these observations may have some practical relevance. All investigations were done in the jejunum; ileum and colon were not studied.

Summarizing the results obtained in humans and various mammals, one may conclude that the effect of glucagon on small intestinal water and electrolyte permeation is first of all dose dependent. Besides, there seem to exist significant differences between various species and whether jejunal or ileal absorptive surfaces are concerned. There is no evidence that in the physiologic range glucagon significantly influences ion transport. Somewhat higher glucagon doses – which were, however, within the range to be found in some pathologic conditions – may reduce the absorption of sodium, chloride, and water from the human jejunum. With even higher doses (>0.3 μg kg^{-1} h^{-1}), a sharp attack of watery diarrhea developed after the infusion was stopped. Interpretation of the results necessitates careful analysis of the experimental conditions used. Thus, glucagon may initiate watery diarrhea in humans only if fluid is simultaneously infused into the intestine. Lack of simultaneous fluid infusion may explain the observation of BARBEZAT and GROSSMAN (1971 b) that glucagon alone did not induce diarrhea in dogs and human subjects, while its combination with pentagastrin did. Besides, it is important to verify whether glucose was also added to the perfusion medium containing the electrolytes and some inert marker. Thus, the inhibitory effect of glucagon on sodium and water absorption in the rabbit ileum (as mentioned by MOORE and LONGACHER 1974) could be completely reversed by addition of D-glucose to the perfusate, whereas in the dog ileum the increase of net water was further increased by D-glucose (MOORE and TAVANO 1974). More recently, GRANGER et al. (1980) produced evidence that, in the cat ileum, glucagon-induced intestinal secretion after local intraarterial infusion resulted from an alteration in capillary fluid balance, i.e., an increased capillary pressure and permeability.

II. Endogenous Hyperglucagonemia

In humans, elevated plasma glucagon levels can regularly be observed in chronic renal failure, in diabetes mellitus, and in starvation. In uremia, hyperglucagonemia is a consequence of decreased hormonal catabolism; the metabolic clearance rate of glucagon as determined by infusions of pancreatic hormone is decreased by 60% as compared with healthy controls (SHERWIN et al. 1976). In prolonged starvation, the rise in plasma glucagon observed after 3 days is primarily the result of 20% reduction in the metabolic clearance rate of glucagon; no consistent change in glucagon delivery is demonstrable at this time (FISCHER et al. 1976). These studies underline the fact that hyperglucagonemia does not necessarily reflect altered secretion; metabolic processes must also be taken into account when interpreting elevated glucagon levels. Experimentally, arginine infusion stimulates endogeneous glucagon release in humans. It was demonstrated by

WHALEN et al. (1973) that hyperglucagonemia induced by arginine infusion decreases intestinal motor function without altering net water and electrolyte absorption in humans.

In animals, hyperglucagonemia is mainly produced by semistarvation or experimental diabetes mellitus. Thus, RUDO et al. (1973) reported that in rats semistarvation-induced hyperglucagonemia was associated with increased amino acid uptake in an everted ring assay system. Administration of high titered antiglucagon antisera nearly normalized the increased absorption. In contrast to semistarvation, LEVIN (1974) showed that starvation is associated with a decrease of hexose absorption. Interrelations between hyperglucagonemia, insulin deficiency, and glucose absorptive changes are discussed in Section F and G.

III. Effect on Sugar and Amino Acid Absorption In Vivo

Intestinal absorption in experimental animals in response to glucagon have been investigated in a few instances after acute exposure. PONZ et al. (1957) reported no change after subcutaneous glucagon administration while the same doses (0.2–1.0 mg) given intravenously produced a moderate decrease of glucose absorption in the rat. VARRÓ and CSERNAY (1966) observed that big doses of glucagon (50–100 µg) injected directly into the nutrient artery of an isolated jejunal loop from the dog did not alter the absorption of isotonic glucose solution from the lumen, but caused a significant increase of portal glucose transport and of local blood flow. These experiments were repeated by VÁRKONYI (1978) under identical conditions, confirming the earlier results (Table 2). In the rat, however, VÁRKONYI and CSÁKY (1979) succeeded in demonstrating a significant increase of glucose absorption with various concentrations of glucose (2.8–150 m*M*) perfusing a proximal small intestinal segment 15 cm in length. This effect could be evoked in the 15–90-min postinjection periods by a dose of 100 µg/100 g glucagon given intravenously (Table 3); 10 µg glucagon had no effect, while big doses (500 µg) significantly decreased the in vivo glucose absorption. It is interesting to note that 100 µg glucagon did not influence the absorption of fructose, galactose, or 3-*O*-methylglucose neither in the range of active transport (2.8 m*M*) nor above such concentrations (150 m*M*) (Table 4). The divergence of the results obtained in the dog and the rat should not be explained by species differences alone. In the dog, the jejunal segment perfused was completely isolated from other parts of the body, thus, glucagon exerted its effect only locally without the possibility of contraregulatory events. In the rat, the glucagon was injected into the systemic circulation, thus, hormonal or other adaptive processes may have been acting. The opposite effect of moderate to big doses of glucagon speaks in favor of such an assumption.

Chronic administration of glucagon (10 and 100 µg twice daily for 5 days) resulted in increased absorption of 3-*O*-methylglucose as well as in an increase of D-glucose-induced (56 m*M*) transmural potential difference, as examined by an in vivo perfusion technique in the rat (CASPARY and LÜCKE 1976). Bolus injection of glucagon had no such effect. Since potential difference increments induced by D-glucose were achieved before steady state sodium absorption, one may assume

Table 2. Effect of various doses of glucagon given intraarterially on absorption and portal transport of isotonic glucose solution and on blood flow in an isolated canine jejunal segment ± standard deviation (VÁRKONYI et al. 1980). For details of the method see VARRÓ et al. (1964). I, III control (physiologic saline) periods; II experimental (glucagon) period

Glucagon	25 μg		$N=8$	50 μg		$N=8$	100 μg		$N=8$
Periods (15 min)	I	II	III	I	II	III	I	II	III
Absorption (mg)	207.79 ± 66.73	200.19 ± 64.38 $P>0.05$	203.59 ± 98.86	176.99 ± 94.05	187.16 ±119.06 $P>0.05$	177.16 ± 90.16	103.24 ± 59.12	96.99 ± 69.18 $P>0.05$	105.85 ± 90.74
Transport (mg)	64.16 ± 51.32	71.54 ± 54.76 $P>0.05$	65.40 ± 47.12	62.45 ± 36.19	87.74 ± 20.27 $P>0.02$	65.05 ± 39.36	46.64 ± 33.88	84.70 ± 36.42 $P>0.02$	52.88 ± 38.99
Blood flow (ml)	138.59 ± 80.17	238.79 ± 53.63 $P<0.01$	138.39 ± 76.46	112.83 ± 22.37	219.66 ± 63.83 $P<0.01$	113.49 ± 13.04	111.50 ± 31.95	208.43 ± 86.09 $P<0.01$	124.11 ± 29.37

Table 3. Glucose absorption from various concentrations of ^{14}C-labeled glucose solutions (2.8–150 m*M*) perfusing a proximal jejunal segment of 15 cm length in the rat pretreated with glucagon (100 μg/kg intravenously). Isotonicity was assured by sodium sulfate Ringer solution. Values were expressed as m*M* glucose per gram dry intestinal weight ± standard deviation (VÁRKONYI and CSÁKY 1979)

Initial glucose concentration of the perfusate (m*M*)		*N*	15 min	30 min	60 min	90 min
2.8	Control	16	73.21 ± 19.29	108.57 ± 16.79	170.27 ± 31.35	221.01 ± 32.9
	Glucagon	19	126.28 ± 92.12	207.08 ± 113.58	323.33 ± 220.54	390.17 ± 235.0
			P < 0.01	*P* < 0.01	*P* < 0.01	*P* < 0.01
5.6	Control	8	64.78 ± 17.63	93.06 ± 27.29	119.21 ± 22.73	159.89 ± 46.8
	Glucagon	12	85.68 ± 22.31	135.96 ± 38.31	203.35 ± 60.71	266.58 ± 95.6
			P < 0.01	*P* < 0.01	*P* < 0.01	*P* < 0.01
56	Control	7	292.22 ± 116.17	526.15 ± 224.18	923.76 ± 438.93	1,210.18 ± 723.0
	Glucagon	7	406.77 ± 144.47	666.21 ± 140.43	1,170.93 ± 368.83	1,595.27 ± 783.6
			P < 0.01	*P* < 0.01	*P* < 0.01	*P* < 0.01
150	Control	8	554.79 ± 239.15	741.19 ± 397.16	1,156.56 ± 516.34	1,501.95 ± 739.7
	Glucagon	8	918.06 ± 749.04	1,603.54 ± 707.80	2,103.47 ± 943.65	2,652.83 ± 993.0
			P < 0.01	*P* < 0.01	*P* < 0.01	*P* < 0.01

that an increase of sodium influx occurred in the presence of glucose in the glucagon-treated animals. As to the different results for 3-*O*-methylglucose absorption after glucagon administration, one may speculate that different mechanisms are at work in acute and chronic treatment.

With pharmacologic doses of glucagon (0.1 mg/h), EWE et al. (1973) could not evoke any changes in jejunal absorption of glucose in humans. Using the triple lumen perfusion technique, GOTTESBÜREN et al. (1974) investigated the jejunal absorption of glucose solution (380 mg-%) in the presence of electrolytes (Na, K, Cl) in three groups of human subjects: metabolically healthy adults, patients with adult onset diabetes (reduced insulin secretion after glucagon administration) and patients with juvenile onset diabetes (no insulin secretion after glucagon administration). They found an initial short increase of glucose absorption after glucagon administration (1.0 mg intravenously) which was more pronounced in diabetics. In the second phase (30–45 min after glucagon injection) a significant decrease of glucose absorption was seen. Unfortunately, these interesting findings do not provide any evidence as to how much and which of the responses are due to a direct glucagon effect; a series of secondary changes (hormonal, circulatory, or motility) might, alone or in combination, produce the results observed.

In conclusion, in vitro experiments or investigations using totally isolated jejunal segments in vivo do not provide evidence that glucagon directly influences hexose absorption. Systemic administration of or chronic pretreatment with glucagon induce changes in glucose absorption both in animals and in humans; the nature of these changes (increase) seems to be dose dependent. All evidence speaks in favor of the role of secondary, hormonal or other, mechanisms.

Table 4. Absorption of various sugars from a solution of 2.8 or 150 m*M* in the rat pretreated with glucagon (100 µg/kg intravenous). For all other details see Table 3. The differences between pretreated and control animals are not significant ($P > 0.05$) (VÁRKONYI and CSÁKY 1979)

Initial sugar concentration of the perfusate			N	15 min	30 min	60 min	90 min
2.8 m*M*	Fructose	Control		13.48 ± 9.57	28.92 ± 10.99	44.99 ± 16.23	61.90 ± 19.55
150 m*M*				1,071.09 ± 566.30	1,340.80 ± 552.24	2,066.11 ± 562.30	2,180.86 ± 442.98
2.8 m*M*	Fructose	Glucagon		15.20 ± 6.48	26.87 ± 8.98	36.75 ± 7.29	51.08 ± 9.68
150 m*M*				797.95 ± 481.76	1,284.50 ± 958.72	1,533.40 ± 926.18	1,971.17 ± 914.16
2.8 m*M*	Galactose	Control		49.95 ± 8.90	73.14 ± 16.39	94.14 ± 24.12	110.20 ± 36.11
150 m*M*				991.03 ± 339.52	1,136.94 ± 360.20	1,554.26 ± 255.44	2,198.79 ± 853.34
2.8 m*M*	Galactose	Glucagon		38.02 ± 13.38	67.61 ± 13.57	71.60 ± 20.90	89.42 ± 34.66
150 m*M*				1,021.94 ± 370.36	1,521.59 ± 675.19	1,770.25 ± 648.42	2,160.20 ± 719.38
2.8 m*M*	3-*O*-Methyl-glucose	Control		24.55 ± 8.81	38.55 ± 11.03	47.37 ± 15.47	59.41 ± 17.23
150 m*M*				1,152.03 ± 419.84	1,252.51 ± 480.61	1,522.08 ± 827.39	1,760.22 ± 881.11
2.8 m*M*	3-*O*-Methyl-glucose			30.39 ± 21.55	46.81 ± 19.78	56.16 ± 20.51	70.93 ± 20.26
150 m*M*		Glucagon		987.12 ± 560.28	1,348.02 ± 760.72	1,486.90 ± 898.67	1,794.10 ± 519.28

IV. Effect on Sugar and Amino Acid Transfer In Vitro

There are only a few data concerning the effect of glucagon on hexose (glucose) transport by means of the rat everted intestinal loop preparation. Neither NAGLER et al. (1960) nor AULSEBROOK (1965) observed any effect of glucagon added to the incubation medium on intestinal absorption of glucose with this technique. The same was found by RUDO and ROSENBERG (1973) with 0.5 and 5.0 μg/ml glucagon in the incubation medium. If they experimentally induced hyperglucagonemia in rats, however, by 6-hourly injections of glucagon, this treatment resulted in an increased intestinal transport of the hexose, 3-*O*-methylglucose and of the amino acid, 1-aminocyclopentane-1-carboxylic acid (ACPC). These substances were chosen because both are actively transported by the intestinal epithelium, but neither is metabolized nor incorporated into macromolecules by the enterocytes. The effect was observed after a lag of 2 days and increased thereafter with the length of treatment. The doses of glucagon used in this study were large (50 μg every 6 h); it is possible, therefore, that the observed effects were pharmacologic rather than physiologic. Besides, it cannot be excluded that the changes were mediated by other hormonal or metabolic responses. The time lag necessary to increase sugar transport after glucagon administration was not observed by CSÁKY and VÁRKONYI (1979); their experimental design, however, differed significantly from that of RUDO and ROSENBERG (1973). Injecting 100 μg/100 g glucagon intravenously to rats, the D-glucose transport capacity of the in vitro jejunal preparation of the animals was significantly increased after 15–30 min and remained elevated, even after 60 min. They used glucose concentrations of 2.8–300 m*M* at the mucosal side and claimed that the preparation always regained its initial transport capacity after 180 min. The active transport of galactose, 3-*O*-methylglucose, and fructose was not influenced by the same treatment (CSÁKY and VÁRKONYI 1979).

V. Effect on Portal Glucose Transport

In contrast to numerous studies of the in vivo absorption (disappearance rate) of glucose from the intestinal lumen after glucagon administration, only a few studies are known of changes of transfer through the basal membrane of the epithelial cells induced by glucagon. Intracellular metabolic processes which might mediate this altered portal transfer have not been investigated either.

VARRÓ and CSERNAY (1966) were the first to report that the direct intraarterial application of big doses of glucagon (150–100 μg) caused an increased loss of glucose from isotonic solution from the epithelial cells towards the serosa in dogs. They drew attention to the peculiar finding that, in some instances, more glucose was transported than absorbed, i.e., more glucose was detected in the venous effluent of the isolated jejunal segment than the amount which disappeared from the glucose solution put into the lumen during a given experimental period. Because glucagon in the same doses significantly increased the blood flow of the jejunal loop independently whether glucose or physiologic saline were put into the lumen, it had to be excluded that the increased blood supply could have been the

Table 5. Absorption and portal transport of glucose from isotonic solution from an isolated canine jejunal segment during glucagon infusion (100 μg/30 min). For details of the method see VARRÓ et al. (1964). In all instances glucose transport exceeded the quantity of hexose absorbed (VÁRKONYI 1978)

Dog	Absorption (mg/30 min)	Transport (mg/30 min)	Transport (% absorption)	Blood flow (ml/30 min)
1	178.00	278.30	156.34	253.00
2	133.00	199.35	149.88	443.00
3	150.00	244.80	163.20	435.00
4	88.00	118.14	134.25	226.00
5	207.00	225.32	128.17	260.00
6	223.00	346.80	155.55	491.00
Average	163.16 ± 49.90	236.45 ± 76.79	147.89 ± 13.73	351.33 ± 117.15

cause of the intracellular glucose mobilization. This assumption was, however, not compatible with the observation that sometimes increased portal glucose transport was detected, even in connection with unchanged or slightly elevated blood flow. They suggested, therefore, that in the dog jejunal mucosa a "labile glucose pool" may exist from which glucose can be mobilized, e.g., by glucagon. In their view glucose was stored in the form of glycogen in the intestinal mucosa; this would represent another source of mobile glycogen in the body besides that of the liver. These experiments were repeated by VÁRKONYI (1978) under identical conditions. He was able to verify the previous findings not only in the case of physiologic glucose solution (300 m*M*), but also in the range of active glucose transport (2.8 m*M*). Besides lengthening the period of glucagon administration (from 15 to 30 min) the "plus transport" of glucose became so to say a regular phenomenon (Table 5).

To test the hypothesis whether parallel changes of the intracellular glycogen content could be observed after glucagon injection, morphological and functional experiments were carried out. Using histochemical methods it was found that, in the isolated intestinal loop of the dog, glucagon applied intraarterially changed the mucosal localization of glycogen and caused glycogen mobilization from the enterocytes (VÁRKONYI et al. 1977). With the aid of a sensitive method for the determination of tissue glycogen, the glycogen content of the intestinal mucosa of the dog and the rat was investigated. In both species significant glucagon-induced reduction of mucosal glycogen contents was revealed (VÁRKONYI et al. 1979). These experiments raise the possibility that, under special conditions (possibly hepatic insufficiency), the small intestine might be considered as another important organ for the regulation of carbohydrate metabolism and homeostasis.

In this context it should be mentioned that DENCKER et al. (1973) reported, on the basis of their human in vivo studies using umbilical vein catheterization, that the amplitudes of the portal–arterial glucose differences are not directly proportional to the rate of glucose absorption, but rather represent the actual net glucose release to the portal circulation.

VI. Changes of Mucosal cAMP and cGMP Levels After Glucagon Treatment in the Rat Small Intestine

There are few data on the role of the cAMP–adenylate cyclase system in the intestinal mucosa. These investigations were carried out mainly to analyze the mechanism of action of cholera toxin or of aminophylline and epinephrine on intestinal cAMP concentration (FIELD and MCCOLL 1968; FIELD 1971; SHARP and HYNIE 1971; FIELD et al. 1976). To our knowledge, cGMP levels have been studied in rat intestinal mucosa only by ISHIKAWA et al. (1969) after aminophylline administration. Localization of these nucleotides in the intestinal mucosa was achieved by SHU-HOI-ONG et al. (1975) with the aid of immunohistochemistry. According to their findings, while cGMP was localized mainly at the brush border region, cAMP was concentrated at the basal membrane of the epithelial cells. As glucagon was also supposed to influence glucose movement out of the cell at this site, it seemed to be worthwhile to study cAMP and cGMP levels in the intestinal mucosa after glucagon administration. Injecting 100 μg/100 g glucagon intravenously to rats, a highly significant increase in mucosal cAMP concentrations could be observed with the aid of a specific assay technique (Amersham Searle Kit TRK 432). The elevation of the cAMP level showed two peaks: the first 15 min and a second 90 min after the glucagon injection (Table 6). On the contrary, no changes at all could be observed after administration of the same dose of glucagon in the cGMP levels of the mucosa in the same periods. Adding dibutyryl-cAMP in various concentrations to the incubation medium produced no change in the active transport of glucose (2.8 m*M*) when the nucleotide was put on the mucosal side of the in vitro preparation. On the serosal side, cAMP enhanced active glucose absorption in a concentration of 10^{-8} *M*, while a significant inhibition of glucose uptake was demonstrated with concentrations of 10^{-6} and 10^{-4} M (VÁRKONYI and CSÁKY 1981). The results of these investigations suggest that mobilization of glucose from glycogen and the increased portal transport of glucose after glucagon administration could, at least partially, be mediated by the activation of the cAMP–adenylate cyclase system.

Table 6. Changes of cAMP concentrations (pmol per gram dry jejunal mucosa ± standard deviation) after pretreatment with glucagon and insulin (VÁRKONYI and CSÁKY 1983)

Periods	0 min	15 min	30 min	60 min	90 min	180 min
Control (intravenous 0.9% NaCl)	$N=16$ 801.40 ±247.10	$N=6$ 881.47 ± 293.98	$N=6$ 643.67 ± 114.59	$N=6$ 828.11 ± 201.51	$N=6$ 817.30 ± 124.87	$N=6$ 665.69 ± 173.05
Glucagon (1 mg/kg)	$N=16$ 801.40 ±247.10	$N=8$ 3,986.47 ± 268.42 $P<0.001$	$N=14$ 1,432.39 ± 333.07 $P<0.001$	$N=14$ 1,858.81 ± 825.90 $P<0.001$	$N=8$ 3,915.87 ± 946.88 $P<0.01$	$N=14$ 1,379.08 ± 268.37 $P<0.05$
Insulin (10 *U*/kg)	$N=16$ 801.40 ±247.10	$N=8$ 2,003.16 ± 760.02 $P<0.001$	$N=8$ 2,355.42 ± 955.08 $P<0.001$	$N=8$ 1,943.08 ± 496.48 $P<0.001$	$N=8$ 1,552,65 ± 755.15 $P<0.01$	$N=8$ 1,104.32 ± 328.94 $P<0.05$

In homogenates of human jejunal biopsies, KLAEVEMAN et al. (1975) could not demonstrate in vitro stimulation of adenylate cyclase activity with glucagon concentrations of 3×10^{-6} *M*. Species differences and the fact that the effect of glucagon was not tested in intact tissue may explain the contradictory data.

VII. Intestinal Mucosal Adaptation to Glucagon

Experimental diabetes in the rat is associated with changes in intestinal transport capacity, in digestive brush border activity, and with morphological alterations of the mucosal architecture. Both clinical and experimental, diabetes are followed by elevated endogenous glucagon levels; thus glucagon may be considered as one of the causative factors responsible for the adaptive changes observed. Some clinical data support this assumption. GLEESON et al. (1971) and BLOOM (1972) found significantly increased villous height in a patient with a hormone-secreting tumor, and were of the opinion that the morphological changes were caused by the enteroglucagon which was extracted from the tumor.

Experimental results do not lend support to this hypothesis. Short-term glucagon treatment (100 μg twice daily for 5 days) did not affect the disaccharidase (maltase, sucrase, trehalase, lactase) and alkaline phosphatase activities in intestinal mucosa of glucagon-treated rats (CASPARY and LÜCKE 1976). The same dose of a long-acting glucagon preparation given for 26 days resulted in a decrease of villous height and consequently in a diminished absorptive surface similar to the picture seen in nontropical sprue. The activities of intestinal disaccharidases were likewise diminished (LORENZ-MEYER et al. 1977). In conclusion, the hyperplastic intestinal mucosal changes in diabetes mellitus are not caused by elevated levels of glucagon.

H. Other Gastrointestinal Polypeptides

I. Gastric Inhibitory Polypeptide

Gastric inhibitory polypeptide (GIP) given by constant intravenous infusion in varying doses (3.75–120 μg in 15 min) produced a marked jejunal volume response which appeared to be dose related in one dog with a Thiry–Vella loop. The response in another dog with an ileal Thiry–Vella loop was less marked and without clear-cut dose relation (BARBEZAT 1973). In humans, a dose of 1 μg/min reduced water absorption and induced chloride secretion in the jejunum (HELMAN and BARBEZAT 1976). It is known that GIP is a contaminant of most of the commercially available CCK preparations, thus some of the effects ascribed to CCK might have been caused by GIP. GIP was found by immunofluorescence in the tumor of a patient with Verner–Morrison syndrome and might thus contribute to the watery diarrhea and electrolyte loss (ELIAS et al. 1972).

II. Pancreatic Polypeptide

On the basis of a patient with watery diarrhea syndrome, a pancreatic polypeptide (PP) cell tumor, and thousandfold elevated PP, but normal VIP level in the plasma, PP was suggested as an additional causative agent in Verner–Morrison syndrome (LARSSON et al. 1976). PP is patented as a veterinary laxative in the United States (CHANCE and JONES 1974) and it may be assumed that PP could cause the two main symptoms of the syndrome, i.e., watery diarrhea and low gastric acid secretion. It should be emphasized, however, that the question whether PP is, wholly or partially, responsible for the syndrome is irrelevant to the function of PP as a marker for pancreatic tumors (SCHWARTZ 1979).

III. Somatostatin

In vitro, somatostatin has been shown to increase sodium and chloride absorption in rabbit ileum, but not in the jejunum (DHARMSATHAPHORNE et al. 1979). Utilizing an in vivo perfusion technique in the rat, the same research group (DHARMSATHAPHORNE et al. 1980a, b) reported that somatostatin infused intravenously had no effect on basal absorption of water, sodium, or urea, while it increased both sodium and chloride absorption across rabbit ileal mucosa. As this latter effect does not involve adrenergic or cholinergic agonists, DHARMSATHAPHORNE et al. (1980a, b) suggest that somatostatin may have a direct effect on the enterocytes. Steady state perfusion experiments were carried out in the jejunum of healthy subjects with either glucose- and amino acid-containing test solutions or a plasma-like electrolyte solution (KREJS et al. 1980). Somatostatin infusion (8 μg kg^{-1} h^{-1}) significantly reduced both glucose and amino acid absorption (L-glycine and L-lysine). Kinetic analysis revealed that this effect was mainly due to a reduction of V_{max} of glucose transport. There was a significant reduction in both lumen–plasma and plasma–lumen water flux, but net water and electrolyte absorption was not affected. As to the mechanism of the observed changes induced by somatostatin, KREJS et al. (1980) suggest a selective reduction in mucosal surface area. In rats (in contrast to humans), recent results of MÄRKI (1981) seem to indicate that somatostatin does not decrease intestinal absorption of glucose, while it inhibits triacylglycerol absorption. Glucose absorption in vitro by jejunum from rats treated with high doses of somatostatin in vivo was no different from that of untreated rats (MÄRKI 1981).

In a case of vipoma, administration of somatostatin (500 μg/h intravenously) normalized the output of water and electrolytes in the terminal ileum. At the same time, a diminution of the plasma VIP values could be observed which declined in parallel with the quantity of the intraluminal secretion of water and electrolytes. It was concluded that the effect of somatostatin was exerted through an inhibition of the water and electrolyte flux by VIP (RUSKONE et al. 1980).

IV. Sorbin

A peptide substance inducing increase of water and sodium absorption has been partially purified from porcine small intestine. The specificity of the biologic effect was checked by testing under the same conditions hormones and analogs that are known to increase intestinal absorption and those that are present in the porcine duodenal material (e.g., CCK and somatostatin). The name "sorbin" has been proposed for this active principle (PANSU et al. 1981).

J. General Remarks on the Effects of Gastrointestinal Hormones on Intestinal Permeation

Reviewing the data published in the literature, the following impressions were gained regarding the effect of the gut polypeptides on intestinal absorption and/or secretion:

a. Insulin, whether added in vitro or administered in vivo, does not influence the sugar transfer in experimental animals. The bulk of evidence speaks in favor of the assumption that, under physiologic conditions, the small intestine could be considered as an "insulin-insensitive" structure.

b. Glucagon influences water and electrolyte movement differently in various animals and whether jejunal or ileal surfaces are concerned. In humans, it reduces water, sodium, and chloride absorption in doses which are within the range to be found in some pathologic conditions. There is no convincing evidence that in physiologic ranges glucagon significantly reduces water and ion transport. In vitro experiments do not provide evidence that glucagon directly influences hexose absorption. Systemic administration or chronic pretreatment with glucagon induce changes in glucose absorption both in animals or in humans; the nature of these changes (increases) seems to be dose dependent. All the evidence speaks in favor of the role of secondary mechanisms. Experiments in animals demonstrate that glucagon in pharmacologic doses may mobilize glucose from intestinal mucosal "glycogen pools". These experiments raise the possibility that the small intestine might be considered as another important organ for the regulation of carbohydrate metabolism and homeostasis. According to the data presented, it might be supposed that glucose mobilization is mediated by the activation of the cAMP–adenylate cyclase system.

c. Secretin in the majority of studies in animals does not show any effect on intestinal absorption of water and ions. When infused intravenously in humans, secretin was shown by intubation studies to reduce absorption (or induce secretion) of water and ions. It seems that the smallest dose of secretin which influences intestinal permeation may be in the physiologic range.

d. Gastrin (and pentagastrin) and cholecystokinin (and cholecystokinin octapeptide) seem to inhibit net fluid and ion absorption (or increase secretion). In the case of gastrin, this effect has been demonstrated both in dogs and humans. Thus, it cannot be excluded that this inhibitory effect of fluid and solutes might not contribute to the watery diarrhea observed in Zollinger–Ellison syndrome, characterized by excess production of circulating gastrin. The results achieved with CCK are more controversial and seem to depend on the species and experimental design used. In humans, although decreased absorption could be demonstrated, the definite assessment of the changes of other factors (motility, blood flow, etc.) requires additional studies.

e. Vasoactive intestinal polypeptide, studied mostly in animals, evoked copious secretion of water and sodium in dogs. This effect seems to be due to its ability to activate the adenylate cyclase system through special receptor sites. Most of the evidence favors the role of VIP as the most important factor in inducing the watery diarrhea and subsequent fluid and electrolyte loss in patients with Verner–Morrison syndrome.

References

Aulsebrook KA (1965) Intestinal absorption of glucose and sodium: effects of epinephrine and norepinephrine. Biochem Biophys Res Commun 18:165–169

Aulsebrook KD (1967) Intestinal transport of glucose and sodium. Changes in alloxan diabetes and effects of insulin. Experientia 21:346–347

Barbezat GO (1973) Stimulation of gastrointestinal secretion by polypeptide hormones. Scand J Gastroenterol 8 [Suppl 22]:1–21

Barbezat GO, Grossman MI (1971a) Effect of glucagon on water and electrolyte movement in jejunum, and ileum of dog. Gastroenterology 60:762 (abstract)

Barbezat GO, Grossman MI (1971b) Cholera like diarrhoea induced by glucagon plus gastrin. Lancet 1:1025–1026

Bernier JJ, Rambaud JC, Modigliani R, Matuchansky C (1979) Physiopathologie des diarrhées hydro-électrolytiques IIe partie. Gastroenterol Clin Biol 3:433–438

Beyreiss K, Müller F, Strack E (1964) Über die Resorption von Monosacchariden. I. Der Einfluß von Insulin auf die Resorption von Galactose. Z Ges Exp Med 138:227–288

Beyreiss K, Müller F, Strack E (1965) Über die Resorption von Monosacchariden. III. Der aktive Transport von D/+/-Xylose gegenüber L/+/-Arabinose. Z Ges Exp Med 138:546–560

Bloom SR (1972) An enteroglucagon tumour. Gut 13:520–523

Bloom SR (1978) Vasoactive intestinal peptide, the major mediator of the WDHA (pancreatic cholera) syndrome: value of measurement in diagnosis and treatment. Am J Dig Dis 23:373–376

Bussjaeger LJ, Johnson LR (1973) Evidence for hormonal regulation of intestinal absorption by cholecystokinin. Am J Physiol 224:1276–1279

Bynum TE, Jacobson ED, Johnson LR (1971) Gastrin inhibition of intestinal absorption in dog. Gastroenterology 61:858–862

Casey MG, Felber JP, Vannotti A (1968) Biochemical study of the mechanism of intestinal absorption. Effect of blood glucose levels on glucose absorption by the intestine in vitro. Digestion 1:233–237

Caspary WF (1973) Effect of insulin and experimental diabetes mellitus on the digestive-absorptive function of the small intestine. Digestion 9:248–263

Caspary WF, Lücke H (1976) Effect of chronic glucagon administration on the digestive and absorptive function of rat small intestine in vivo. Res Exp Med (Berl) 167:1–13

Chance RE, Jones WE (1974) US Patent Office 3-842-063

Coupar IM (1976) Stimulation of sodium and water secretion without inhibition of glucose absorption in the rat jejunum by vasoactive intestinal polypeptide (VIP). Clin Exp Pharmacol Physiol 3:615–618

Crane RK (1961) An effect of alloxan-diabetes on the active transport of sugars by rat small intestine in vitro. Biochem Biophys Res Commun 4:436–440

Csáky TZ, Fischer E (1981) Intestinal sugar transport in experimental diabetes. Diabetes 30:568–574

Csáky TZ, Várkonyi T (1979) Interrelation between pancreatic glucagon and intestinal absorption. I. The effect of glucagon on sugar transport in vitro (in Hungarian). Kisérl Orvostud 31:310–314

Cummins AL (1952) Absorption of glucose and methionine from the human intestine; the influence of glucose concentration in the blood and in the intestinal lumen. J Clin Invest 31:928–937

Dencker M, Meeuwisse C, Olin T, Tranberg KG (1973) Intestinal transport of carbohydrate as measured by portal catheterisation in man. Digestion 9:514–524

Dharmsathaphorne K, Racusen L, Binder H, Dobbins JW (1979) Somatostatin (SRIF) stimulates Na and Cl absorption in the rabbit ileum. Clin Res 27:265A

Dharmsathaphorne K, Sherwin RS, Dobbins JW (1980a) Somatostatin inhibits fluid secretion in the rat jejunum. Gastroenterology 78:1554–1558

Dharmsathaphorne K, Binder HJ, Dobbins JW (1980b) Somatostatin stimulates sodium and chloride absorption in the rabbit ileum. Gastroenterology 78:1559–1565

Dubois RS, Roy CC (1969) Insulin stimulated transport of 3-*O*-methyl-glucose across the rat jejunum. Proc Soc Exp Biol Med 130:931–934

Ebeid AM, Murray PD, Fischer JE (1978) Vasoactive intestinal peptide and the watery diarrhea syndrome. Ann Surg 187:411–416

Elias E, Bloom SR, Welbourn RB, Kuzio MJM, Pearse AGE, Booth CC, Brown JC (1972) Pancreatic cholera due to production of gastric inhibitory polypeptide. Lancet 2:791–793

Ewe K, Laubenthal G, Hoditz U (1973) Die Wirkung von Pentagastrin und Glucagon auf die Wasser-, Elektrolyt- und Glucoseresorption im menschlichen Jejunum. Report at the 79th Tagung der Dtsch Ges Inn Med, Wiesbaden

Fahrenkrug J, Schaffalitzky de Muckadell OB (1979) Verner-Morrison syndrome and vasoactive intestinal polypeptide (VIP). Scand J Gastroenterol 14 [Suppl 53]:57–60

Fara JW, Madden KS (1975) Effect of secretin and cholecystokinin on small intestinal blood flow distribution. Am J Physiol 229:1365–1370

Field M (1971) Intestinal secretion: effect of cyclic AMP and its role in cholera. N Engl J Med 284:1137–1144

Field M, McColl I (1968) Contrasting effect of epinephrine and cyclic AMP on ion transport across intestine. Fed Proc Fed Am Soc Exp Biol 27:603

Field M, Brasitus TA, Sheerin HE, Kimberg DV (1976) Role of cyclic nucleotides in the regulation of intestinal ion transport. In: Robinson JWL (ed) Intestinal ion transport. MTP Press, Lancaster, pp 233–245

Fischer M, Sherwin RS, Hendler R, Felig P (1976) Kinetics of glucagon in man: effects of starvation. Proc Natl Acad Sci USA 73:1735–1739

Fromm D (1969) Insulin and intestinal sugar absorption. Am J Clin Nutr 22:311–314

Ganeshappa KP, Whalen GE, Soergel KH (1972) The effect of glucagon on small intestinal absorption in man. Gastroenterology 62:750 (abstract)

Gardner JD, Peskin GW, Gerda JJ, Brooks FP (1967) Alterations on in vitro fluid and electrolyte absorption by gastrointestinal hormones. Am J Surg 113:57–64

Gingell JC, Davies MW, Shields R (1968) Effect of a synthetic gastrin-like pentapeptide upon the intestinal transport of sodium, potassium, and water. Gut 9:11–116

Gleeson MH, Bloom SR, Polak JM, Henry K, Dowling RH (1971) Endocrine tumour in the kidney affecting small bowel structure, motility and absorptive function. Gut 12:773–782

Goldman RB, Kim YS, Jones RS (1971) The effect of glucagon on enterokinase secretion from Brunner's gland pouches in dogs. Proc Soc Exp Biol Med 138:562–565

Gottesbüren H, Leising H, Menge H, Lorenz-Meyer H, Riecken EO (1974) Einfluß von Glucagon auf die Glucose-, Wasser- und Elektrolytresorption des menschlichen Jejunums. Klin Wochenschr 52:926–929

Gottesbüren H, Menge H, Schmitt E, Bloch R, Lorenz-Meyer H, Riecken OE (1973 a) Untersuchungen zum Einfluß des Insulins auf die intestinale Resorption beim Menschen. I. Vergleich der Glucose-, Wasser- und Elektrolytresorption bei Diabetikern und bei stoffwechselgesunden Probanden. Res Exp Med (Berl) 160:326–330

Gottesbüren H, Schmitt E, Menge R, Bloch H, Lorenz-Meyer H, Riecken EO (1973 b) Untersuchungen zum Einfluß des Insulins auf die intestinale Resorption beim Menschen. II. Der Einfluß endogenen und intravenös injizierten Insulins auf die Resorption. Res Exp Med (Berl) 161:262–271

Granger DN, Kvietys PR, Wilborn WH, Mortillaro NA, Taylor AE (1980) Mechanism of glucagon-induced intestinal secretion. Am J Physiol 239:G30–G38

Helman CA, Barbezat CO (1976) Effect of gastric inhibitory polypeptide on jejunal water and electrolyte transport in man. Lancet 2:1129

Hicks T, Turnberg LA (1973) The influence of secretion on ion transport in the human jejunum. Gut 14:485–490

Hicks T, Turnberg LA (1974) Influence of glucagon on the human jejunum. Gastroenterology 67:1114–1118

Horváth J, Wix G (1951) Hormonal influences on glucose resorption from the intestine. Acta Physiol Acad Sci Hung 2:445–450

Hubel KA (1967) Effect of secretin on bicarbonate secretion in fluid perfusing the rat ileum. Experientia 23:337–338
Hubel KA (1972a) Effects of secretin and glucagon on intestinal transport of ions and water in the rat. Proc Soc Exp Biol Med 139:656–658
Hubel KA (1972b) Effects of pentagastrin and cholecystokinin on intestinal transport of ions and water in the rat. Proc Soc Exp Biol Med 140:670–672
Isaacs PET, Turnberg LA (1977) Failure of glucagon to influence ion transport across human jejunal and ileal mucosa in vitro. Gut 18:1059–1061
Ishikawa E, Ishikawa S, Davis JW, Sutherland EW (1969) Determination of guanosine 3′,5′-monophosphate in tissues and of guanyl-cyclase in rat intestine. J Biol Chem 244:6371–6376
Jorpes JE (1968) Memorial lecture: the isolation and chemistry of secretin and cholecystokinin. Gastroenterology 55:157–164
Kahn CR, Levy AG, Gardner JD, Miller JV, Gorden P, Schein PS (1975) Pancreatic cholera: beneficial effect of treatment with streptozotocin. N Engl J Med 292:491–945
Klaeveman HL, Conlon TP, Levy AG, Gardner JD (1975) Effects of gastrointestinal hormones on adenylate cyclase activity in human jejunal mucosa. Gastroenterology 68:667–675
Krejs GJ, Fordtran JS (1980) Effect of VIP infusion on water and ion transport in the human jejunum. Gastroenterology 78:722–727
Krejs GJ, Barkley RM, Read NW, Fordtran JS (1978) Intestinal secretion induced by vasoactive intestinal polypeptide. A comparison with cholera toxin in the canine jejunum in vivo. J Clin Invest 61:1337–1345
Krejs GJ, Browne R, Raskin P (1980) Effect of intravenous somatostatin on jejunal absorption of glucose, amino acids and electrolytes. Gastroenterology 78:26–31
Laburthe M, Prieto JC, Amiranoff B, Dupont C, Hui Bon Hoa D, Rosselin G (1979) Interaction of vasoactive intestinal peptide with isolated intestinal epithelial cells from rat. II. Characterisation and structural requirements of the stimulatory effect VIP on adenosine 3′-5′-monophosphate production. Eur J Biochem 96:239–248
Larsson LI, Schwartz TW, Lundquist G, Cance RE, Sundler F, Rehfeld JF, Grimelius L, Fahrenkrug J, Schaffalitzky de Muckadell OB, Moon N (1976) Occurrence of human pancreatic polypeptide in pancreatic endocrin tumours. Am J Pathol 85:675–684
Leese HJ, Mansford KRL (1971) The effect of insulin and insulin deficiency on the transport and metabolism of glucose by rat small intestine. J Physiol (Lond) 212:819–838
Levin RJ (1974) A unified theory for the action of partial or complete reduction of food intake on jejunal hexose absorption in vivo. In: Dowling RH, Riecken EO (eds) Intestinal adaptation. Schattauer, Stuttgart, pp 125–135
Lewin MJM (1980) Hormone receptor control of electrolyte secretion in the gastrointestinal tract. In: Jerzy Glass GB (ed) Gastrointestinal hormones. Raven, New York, pp 477–497
Lorenz-Meyer H, Menge H, Riecken EO (1977) Untersuchungen zur Funktion und Morphologie der Dünndarmschleimhaut der Ratte unter chronischem Glucagoneinfluß. Res Exp Med 170:181–192
Love AHG, Canavan DA (1968) Effects of insulin on intestinal absorption. Lancet 2:1325–1326
Lukens FDW (1948) Alloxan diabetes. Physiol Rev 28:304–329
MacFerran SN, Mailman D (1977) Effects of glucagon on canine intestinal sodium and water fluxes and on regional blood flow. J Physiol (Lond) 266:1–12
Mahmood A, Varma SD (1971) Über die Wirkung des Alloxan-Diabetes, von Insulin und diabetogenen Hormonen (Thyroxin, Hydrocortison, Oxytocin) auf den intestinalen Transport von Glycin. Z Gastroenterol 9:425–428
Mailman D (1978) Effects of vasoactive intestinal polypeptide on intestinal absorption and blood flow. J Physiol (Lond) 279:121–132
Manome SH, Kuriaki K (1961) Effect of insulin, phlorizin and some metabolic inhibitors on the glucose absorption from the intestine. Arch Int Pharmacodyn 130:187–191

Matuchansky C, Huet PM, Mary JY, Rambaud JC, Bernier JJ (1972) Effect of cholecystokinin and metoclopramide on jejunal movements of water and electrolytes and on transit time of luminal fluid in man. Eur J Clin Invest 2:169–175
Märki F (1981) Effect of somatostatin on intestinal absorption of nutrients in the rat. Regul Peptides 2:371–381
Mehnert H, Förster H, Haslbeck G (1967) Zur Frage der Wirkung von Insulin auf die intestinale Resorption von Glucose und Fructose. Diabetologia 3:23–29
Mekhjian H, King D, Sanzenbacher L, Zollinger R (1972) Glucagon and secretin inhibit water and electrolyte transport in the human jejunum. Gastroenterology 62:782 (abstract)
Meyer JH, Way LH, Grossman MI (1970) Pancreatic response to acidification of various length of proximal intestine in the dog. Am J Physiol 219:971–977
Modigliani R, Bernier JJ (1972) Effets du glucose sur les mouvements nets et unidirectionnels de l'eau et des électrolytes dans l'intestin grele de l'homme. Biol Gastroenterol (Paris) 5:165–174
Modigliani R, Mary JY, Bernier JJ (1973) Effect of pentagastrin upon movements of water, electrolytes and glucose across the human jejunum and ileum. Digestion 8:208–219
Modigliani R, Mary JY, Bernier JJ (1976) Effects of synthetic human gastrin I upon movements of water, electrolytes and glucose across the human small intestine. Gastroenterology 71:978–984
Modigliani R, Huet PM, Rambaud JC, Bernier JJ (1971) Effect of secretin upon movements of water and electrolytes across the small intestine in man. Rev Eur Etud Clin Biol 16:361–364
Modigliani R, Bernier JJ, Matuchansky C, Rambaud JC (1977) Intestinal water and electrolyte transport in man under the effect of exogenous hormones of the gut and prostaglandins and in patients with endocrine tumors of the pancreas. In: Glass GBJ (ed) Progress in gastroenterology, vol 3. Grune and Stratton, New York, p 288
Modlin IM, Bloom SR, Mitchell SJ (1977) Role of VIP in diarrhoea. Gut 18:418–419A
Moore EW, Longacher JW (1974) The effect of peptide hormones on simultaneous jejunal and ileal H_2O and electrolyte transport in the rabbit. I. Glucagon: the nature of the effect. Gastroenterology 66:748 (abstract)
Moore EW, Tavano PHJ (1974) The effect of peptide hormones on simultaneous jejunal and ileal H_2O and electrolyte transport in the dog. II. Glucagon: some paradoxical effects. Gastroenterology 66:749 (abstract)
Moritz M, Finkelstein G, Meshkinpour H (1973) Effect of secretin and cholecystokinin on the transport of electrolyte and water in human jejunum. Gastroenterology 64:76–80
Moshat MG, Broitman SA, Zamchek N (1970) Gastrin and absorption. Am J Clin Nutr 23:336–342
Nagler R, Forrest WJ, Shapiro HN (1960) Effect of glucagon on transfer of glucose utilizing everted sac of small intestine. Am J Physiol 198:1323–1325
Nasset ES, Ju JS (1970) Effect of secretin and cholecystokin-pancreozymin (CCK-PZ) on intestinal secretion in the rats. Physiologist 13:268
Pansu D, Bosshard A, Dechelette MA, Vagne M (1980) Effect of pentagastrin, secretin and cholecystokinin on intestinal water, sodium absorption in the rat. Digestion 20:201–206
Pansu D, Vagne M, Bosshard A, Mutt V (1981) Sorbin, a peptide contained in porcine upper small intestine which induces the absorption of water and sodium in the rat duodenum. Scand J Gastroenterol 16:193–199
Ponz F, Llunch M, Planas J (1957) Effectos del glucagon sobre la absorcion intestinal de glucosa. Rev Esp Fisiol 13:25–33
Prieto K, Laburthe M, Rosselin G (1979) Interaction of vasoactive intestinal peptide with isolated intestinal epithelial cells from rat. I. Characterization, quantitative aspects and structural requirements of binding sites. Eur J Biochem 96:229–237
Racusen LC, Binder HJ (1977) Alteration of large intestinal electrolyte transport by vasoactive intestinal peptide. Gastroenterology 73:790–793
Rambaud JP, Modigliani R, Matuchansky C, Bloom S, Said SI, Pessyre D, Bernier JJ (1975) Pancreatic cholera. Studies on tumoral secretions and pathophysiology of diarrhea. Gastroenterology 69:110–122

Rudo ND, Rosenberg IH (1973) Chronic glucagon administration enhances intestinal transport in the rat. Proc Soc Exp Biol Med 142:521–525

Rudo ND, Lawrence AM, Rosenberg IH (1973) Increased intestinal transport in the rat due to hyperglucagonemia in starvation: studies with glucagon antisera. Clin Res 21:522

Ruskone A, René E, Chayvialle JA, Bonfils S, Rambaud JC (1980) Vipomes, somatostatine et absorption intestinale. Gastroenterologie Biol Clin (Paris) 4:938–939

Said SI, Faloona GR (1975) Elevated plasma and tissue levels of VIP in the watery diarrhea syndrome due to pancreatic, bronchogenic and other tumors. N Engl J Med 293:155–160

Schebalin R, Said SI, Makhlouf GM (1974) Interplay of glucagon, vasoactive intestinal peptide (VIP) and synthetic fragments of VIP in intestinal secretion. Clin Res 22:368A

Schmitt MG, Soergel KH, Hensley GT, Chey WY (1975) Watery diarrhea associated with pancreatic islet cell carcinoma. Gastroenterology 69:206–216

Schwartz TW (1979) Pancreatic polypeptide (PP) and endocrine tumours of the pancreas. Scand J Gastroenterol 53 [Suppl 14]:93–100

Schwartz CJ, Kimberg DV, Sheerin HE, Field M, Said SI (1974) Vasoactive intestinal peptide stimulation of adenylate cyclase and active electrolyte secretion in intestinal mucosa. J Clin Invest 54:536–544

Sharp GWG, Hynie S (1971) Stimulation of intestinal adenyl cyclase by cholera toxin. Nature 229:266–269

Sherwin RS, Bastl C, Finkelstein FO, Fischer M, Black H, Hendler R, Felig P (1976) Influence of uremia and hemodialysis in the turnover and metabolic effect of glucagon. J Clin Invest 57:722–731

Shu-Hoi-Ong, Whitley TH, Stowe NW, Steiner AL (1975) Immunohistochemical localisation of 3′,5′-cyclic AMP and 3′,5′-cyclic GMP in rat liver, intestine and testis. Proc Natl Acad Sci USA 72:2022–2026

Stening GF, Grossman MI (1969) Hormonal control of Brunner's gland. Gastroenterology 56:1047–1052

Teem MV, Phillips SF (1972) Perfusion of the hamster jejunum with conjugated and unconjugated bile acids: inhibition of water absorption and effects on morphology. Gastroenterology 62:261–267

Várkonyi T (1978) Sugar absorption from the small intestine. The regulatory role of glucagon (in Hungarian). PhD dissertation, University of Szeged

Várkonyi T, Csáky TZ (1979) Interrelation between pancreatic glucagon and intestinal absorption. II. The effect of glucagon on sugar transport in vivo (in Hungarian). Kisérl Orvostud 31:315–318

Várkonyi T, Csáky T (1983) The effect of insulin, glucagon and endogenous hyperglucagonemia on cAMP and cGMP content of the rat small intestinal mucosa (in Hungarian). Kisérl Orvostud 35:37–42

Várkonyi T, Wittmann T, Varró V (1980) Effect of pancreatic glucagon and insulin on canine intestinal blood flow. Acad Sci Hung 37:395–399

Várkonyi T, Wittmann T, Karácsony G, Varró V (1977) Die Veränderung der strukturellen Lokalisation des Glycogens während der Glucoseresorption. Z Gastroenterol 9:565–571

Várkonyi, T, Kiss ZF, Wittmann T, Varró V (1979) Effect of glucagon on glycogen content of the dog and rat small intestinal mucosa. Acta Hepatogastroenterol (Stuttg) 26:129–132

Varró V, Csernay L (1966) The effect of intra-arterial insulin and glucagon on the glucose metabolism of the small intestine in the dog. Scand J Gastroenterol 1:232–237

Varró V, Csernay L, Blaho G, Szarvas SF (1964) A simple method for the simultaneous recording of blood flow and absorption in isolated segments of dog intestine. Am J Dig Dis 9:138–144

Vinnik IE, Kern PJR, Sussman KE (1965) The effect of diabetes mellitus and insulin on glucose absorption by the small intestine in man. J Lab Clin Med 66:131–136

Waldman DB, Garber JD, Makhlouf GM (1977a) Effect of vasoactive intestinal peptide (VIP), secretin and structurally related peptides on colonic transport and adenylate cyclase activity. In: Bonfils S, Fromageot P, Rosselin G (eds) Hormonal receptors in digestive tract physiology. North-Holland, Amsterdam, pp 507–508
Waldman DB, Gardner JD, Zfass AM, Makhlouf GM (1977b) Effects of vasoactive intestinal peptide, secretin and related peptides on rat colonic transport and adenylcyclase activity. Gastroenterology 73:518–523
Whalen GE, Wu ZC, Ganeshappa KP, Wall MJ, Kalkhoff RK, Soergel KH (1973) The effect of endogenous glucagon on human small bowell function. Gastroenterology 64:822 (abstract)
Wright HK, Kabemba J, Herskovic T (1968) Effect of gastrin on jejunal water absorption. Surg Forum 19:282–283
Wu ZC, O'Dorisio TM, Cataland S, Mekhjian HS, Gaginella TS (1979) Effects of pancreatic polypeptide and vasoactive intestinal polypeptide on rat ileal and colonic water and electrolyte transport in vivo. Dig Dis Sci 24:625–630

CHAPTER 25

The Influence of Opiates on Intestinal Transport

J. S. McKay, S. Hughes, and L. A. Turnberg

A. Introduction

The antidiarrhoeal activity of opiates is usually ascribed to increased smooth muscle tone and inhibition of the propulsive activity of the intestine (Vaughan-Williams and Streeten 1950; Daniel et al. 1959; Dajani et al. 1975; Stewart et al. 1977). Recent work on the pathogenesis of diarrhoea suggests that abnormalities of water and electrolyte transport play a primary role (Binder 1979; Turnberg 1979) and attention has turned to the possibility that opiates may exert their antidiarrhoeal effects by an action on mucosal transport. Of interest too, is the demonstration that the gut has high concentrations of endogenous opiates, the enkephalins, found predominantly in the myenteric plexuses. Leu^5-enkephalin and Met^5-enkephalin, the types found here, almost certainly have a role in the normal control of intestinal motility. The possibility that they also exert some physiological control of mucosal transport is intriguing.

B. In Vivo Studies

An antisecretory role for opiates is not a new concept. Magnus (1906) reported that morphine inhibited "milk diarrhoea" in cats, an effect not influenced by resecting the sympathetic supply to the gut. Morphine and opium also decreased the fluid exudation induced by colocynth in the small and large intestine (Padtberg 1911). More recently, diphenoxylate and morphine were shown to inhibit the secretion induced by cholera toxin in rat and guinea-pig ileal loops (Valiulis and Long 1973), and loperamide and morphine inhibited prostaglandin E_2-(PGE_2)-induced secretion in the rat (Karim and Adaikan 1977). This effect was inhibited by naloxone, suggesting that opiate receptors were involved (Coupar 1978).

Beubler and Lembeck (1979) demonstrated that morphine and levorphanol, but not the inactive isomer dextrorphan, inhibited the intestinal fluid accumulation induced by vasoactive intestinal polypeptide (VIP), PGE_1, bisacodyl and carbachol. Secretion induced by magnesium sulphate, mannitol or bethanechol was unaffected. In addition, naloxone enhanced the activity of PGE_1 and VIP, effects held to be due to inhibition of endogenous enkephalin activity. Furthermore, these authors effectively excluded a central nervous system action by demonstrating that loperamide, which does not cross the blood–brain barrier, had similar antisecretory activity to morphine and that even in pithed rats a synthetic enkephalin analogue inhibited PGE_1-induced secretion (Beubler and Lembeck 1979;

Lembeck and Beubler 1979). However, since these results may be attributable to changes in intestinal motility, blood supply or biliary and pancreatic secretion, each of which may be influenced by opiates, they cannot give a precise indication of the mechanism of action of opiates on intestinal mucosa.

C. In Vitro Studies

These difficulties were eliminated with the in vitro short-circuit current technique and several groups have now reported results of experiments performed on either rabbit ileal mucosa, stripped of muscle layers, or guinea-pig ileum. The addition of a variety of opiates (morphine, codeine, levorphanol, dextromoramide, enkephalins, and loperamide) to the serosal bathing medium has been shown to decrease the potential difference and short-circuit current across the mucosa (Fig. 1).

I. Opiate Receptors

Naloxone has been found to inhibit competitively the response to opiates (Fig. 2) and the stereospecificity of this effect has been further confirmed using laevo- and dextrorotatory isomers (Dobbins et al. 1980; McKay et al. 1981). These two features (a stereospecific response and competitive inhibition by a specific antagonist) provide strong evidence for the presence of specific opiate receptors in these mucosal preparations.

The dose–response curve obtained for morphine ranged from 10^{-6} to 10^{-4} *M* (McKay et al. 1981) which seems high for a "physiological" effect and is much greater than, for example, that required to produce 50% inhibition of electrically evoked contraction of guinea-pig ileal muscle (Kosterlitz and Watt 1968). However, it is clear that Met- and Leu-enkephalins and certain other enkephalin

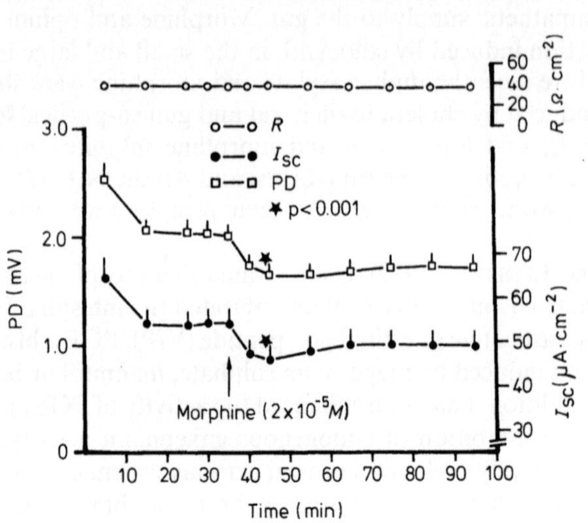

Fig. 1. The effect of morphine on potential difference (*PD*), short-circuit current (I_{sc}) and tissue resistance (*R*) in isolated rabbit ileal mucosa

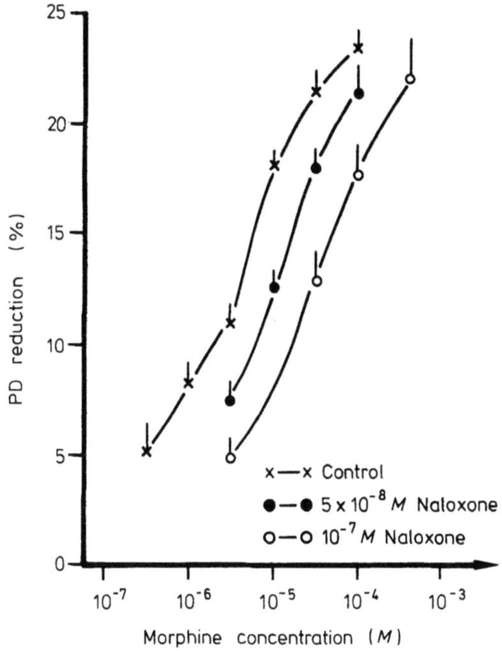

Fig. 2. Effect of varying doses of agonist (morphine) and antagonist (naloxone) on PD responses in isolated rabbit ileal mucosa indicating competitive inhibition

analogues are effective in this mucosal preparation at concentrations as low as 10^{-8} *M* and this order of potency (i.e. enkephalins more potent than morphine) is the reverse of that found in guinea-pig ileal muscle where morphine was more potent than an enkephalin (HUTCHINSON et al. 1975). This observation suggests the possibility that different types of opiate receptor may be involved in these two types of activity. At present there is considerable debate about the existence of multiple opiate receptors. In the guinea-pig ileal muscle, it has been suggested that opiate effects are modulated by μ receptors and here morphine is considerably more potent than Leu-enkephalins. In tissues where morphine is less potent than enkephalins, as in mouse vas deferens (and possibly ileal mucosa) a δ receptor is thought to mediate opiate effects.

II. Possible Neural Mediation

It is uncertain whether these receptors are situated directly on enterocyte membranes or whether opiates exert their effects through some intermediary mechanism. They could, for example, stimulate or inhibit release of another mediator from nerves or paracrine cells. Enkephalin-like immunoreactivity has been reported in considerable concentrations in the nerves of the myenteric plexus (ELDE et al. 1976; POLAK et al. 1977; SCHULTZBERG et al. 1980) while only occasional immunoreactive cells have been identified in the mucosa and submucosa (SCHULTZBERG et al. 1980). However, this distribution may be species dependent since ALU-

METS et al. (1978) reported enkephalin-like reactivity in gut endocrine cells of chicken, mouse, rat, pig, and monkey, but not in those of guinea-pig, cat, and human.

There is also evidence from another source that opiates may act through the mediation of local neurological mechanisms. Tetrodotoxin, a specific neurotoxin, prevents the responses to enkephalin, suggesting that enkephalins are preganglionic neurotransmitters in the stripped mucosal preparation (DOBBINS et al. 1980; TURNBERG et al. 1982). These studies are not absolutely conclusive because it is possible that tetrodotoxin can block a direct effect of enkephalin on the enterocyte as tetrodotoxin itself has been shown to influence intestinal ion transport in high concentrations (HUBEL 1978).

Opiates are, of course, well known to influence the release of neurotransmitters in a variety of systems and this possibility has been investigated in rabbit ileal mucosa with a variety of neurotransmitter antagonists. Cholinergic, adrenergic, and dopaminergic blockade failed to influence opiate responses, suggesting that these divisions of the autonomic system are not involved (DOBBINS et al. 1980; MCKAY et al. 1981). It remains unclear however whether other neural, possibly peptidergic, pathways are involved in the intestinal response to opiates and this possibility requires further investigation.

D. Ion Flux Responses

Three groups of workers have demonstrated that opiates enhance net chloride (Cl^-) absorption in rabbit and guinea-pig ileal mucosa in vitro (KACHUR et al. 1980; DOBBINS et al. 1980; MCKAY et al. 1981). KACHUR et al. (1980) found that etorphine caused both a decreased serosa–mucosa Cl^- flux and a simultaneous enhanced mucosa–serosa flux in the guinea-pig while DOBBINS et al. (1980) found that the enhanced net Cl^- absorption was due predominantly to an increased mucosa–serosa flux. In addition, the latter group demonstrated enhanced net sodium (Na^+) absorption induced by enkephalin which was entirely due to an increased Na^+ flux from mucosa to serosa. RACUSEN et al. (1978) had previously reported a similar response to codeine in rabbit ileal mucosa.

On the basis of these data it was proposed that Met-enkephalin might stimulate a neutral coupled Na^+Cl^- influx across the brush border of the enterocyte. Following extrusion of Na^+ and Cl^- at the basolateral membrane some Na^+ may leak back into the mucosal solution through the tight junction which is cation selective, resulting in excess Cl^- absorption compared with that of Na^+. This in turn might account for the observed decrease in short-circuit current. In addition, it was postulated that opiates might reduce Cl^- permeability at the brush border membrane which could lead to a reduced serosa–mucosa Cl^- flux and short-circuit current (Fig. 3).

On the other hand, the results of MCKAY et al. (1981) are compatible with a different model. In stripped rabbit ileal mucosa, we observed that the increased net Cl^- absorption after administration of morphine was largely due to a decrease in serosa–mucosa Cl^- flux, although a small increase in mucosa–serosa Cl^- movement was also noted. A simultaneous increase in the residual ion flux

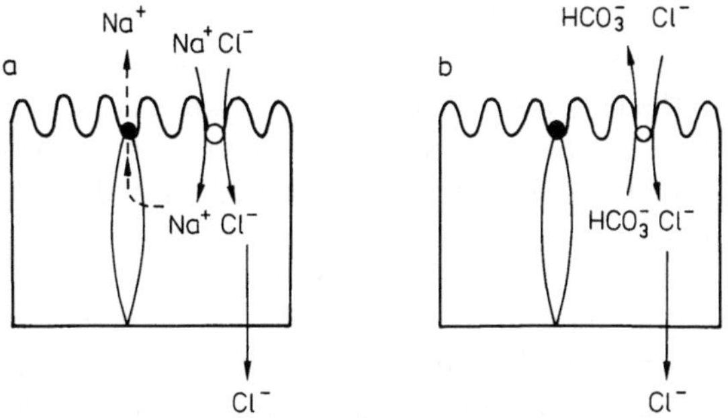

Fig. 3 a, b. Models of ion transport responses to opiates according to (**a**) DOBBINS et al. (1980), (**b**) MCKAY et al. (1981)

was observed while Na^+ transport was unaffected. Since the most likely unmeasured ions making up the residual flux are bicarbonate (HCO_3^-) and hydrogen (H^+), these data are compatible with a morphine-stimulated Cl^-/HCO_3^- exchange, in which HCO_3^- is secreted for Cl^- absorbed, (or possibly a coupled H^+ and Cl^- absorptive process). A similar response was observed after administration of the enkephalin analogue Me-Tyr-D-Met-Gly-Phe-Pro-NH_2. Here, in addition, it was proposed that enhanced electrogenic Cl^- absorption, and/or a change in Cl^- permeability of the paracellular shunt pathway, resulting in a diminished backflux of Cl^- relative to Na^+, might account for the observed decrease in short-circuit current (Fig. 3). It should be noted that DOBBINS et al. (1980) reported that Met-enkephalin induced a 37% increase in tissue conductance whereas KACHUR et al. (1980) found conductivity changes of less than 10% after Leu-enkephalin administration and MCKAY et al. (1981) observed no morphine- or enkephalin-induced changes in tissue conductivity.

The reasons for these discrepancies in conductivity, and in Na^+ and Cl^- fluxes, are not clear but it is possible that, since basal absorption of Na^+ was relatively high in the latter experiments, this may have been maximal prior to the addition of opiate. Differences in experimental technique and rabbit strain may also account for some of the discrepancies. In any event, the currently available evidence does not allow us to distinguish between these models for the ion transport responses to opiates. Both models include a reduction in Cl^- permeability, probably of the paracellular shunt pathway, with, in the former model, an enhanced coupled Na^+Cl^- entry step or, in the latter, an increased Cl^-/HCO_3^- exchange.

E. Antisecretory Activity

In an attempt to elucidate further the mechanisms by which opiates influence intestinal ion transport, we have recently investigated their effects on intestinal secretion induced by a variety of secretagogues (MCKAY et al. 1982). Although these studies showed that the secretory response to acetylcholine (a reduced mucosa–serosa and increased serosa–mucosa Cl^- flux resulting in net Cl^- secretion) was completely inhibited by morphine, further evidence from this study suggested that the antisecretory action of opiates is complex and not simply a direct inhibition of the secretory stimulus. The following pieces of evidence support this conclusion. First, the electrical responses to PGE_2 and acetylcholine were unaffected by morphine, and the response due to cholera toxin was only partially and transiently reduced. Second, PGE_2 caused Cl^- secretion by reducing the mucosa–serosa Cl^- flux, and although morphine prevented this reduction (at least in part) it also reduced the serosa–mucosa Cl^- flux, an effect which occurs in control tissues (Fig. 4). Loperamide has also been shown to inhibit PGE_2-induced secretion by a closely similar mechanism (Hughes et al. 1982). These observations suggest that opiates may simply add their absorption-enhancing action partially to nullify the action of these secretagogues. The secretion induced by the heat-stable and heat-labile toxins of *Escherichia coli* (caused by a reduction in mucosa–serosa and an increase in serosa–mucosa Cl^- flux) were also inhibited by loperamide, largely by decreasing serosa–mucosa Cl^- flux (Hughes et al. 1982). It may thus be inferred that opiates prevent net secretion, first by an absorption-enhancing action and second by inhibiting the action of secretagogues. Even taking into account changes in total tissue conductance, which occur with some secretagogues and

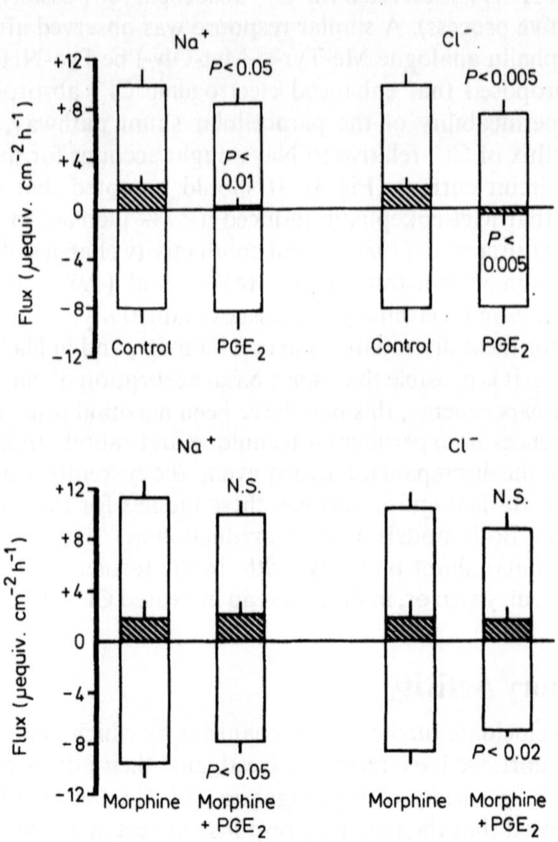

Fig. 4 a, b. Sodium and chloride flux responses to (**a**) PGE_2 (10^{-5} *M*) and (**b**) PGE_2 plus morphine (2×10^{-5} *M*). Positive flux indicates mucosa–serosa; negative flux indicates serosa–mucosa. *Hatched areas* are net fluxes. N.S. = not significant

which clearly influence unidirectional flux determinations, this conclusion is generally supported by the experimental evidence (McKAY et al. 1982).

Na^+ transport was unaffected by morphine in the presence of acetylcholine, which itself did not influence Na^+ transport, but morphine and loperamide prevented the reduction in Na^+ absorption produced by PGE_2. Thus, in some circumstances, it is possible to demonstrate an action on Na^+ transport compatible with an enhanced coupled NaCl uptake mechanism.

Opiates have, therefore, been shown to inhibit the secretion produced by secretagogues which act by at least three different mechanisms. For example, secretion produced by PGE_2, heat-labile *E. coli* toxin and cholera toxin is believed to be mediated by increased production of cAMP in the mucosa (KIMBERG et al. 1971; EVANS et al. 1972). Heat-stable *E. coli* toxin on the other hand, is thought to act via another cyclic nucleotide, cGMP (FIELD et al. 1978) while acetylcholine-induced secretion is mediated by a rise in intracellular calcium (BOLTON and FIELD 1977). In the case of the secretagogues acting through cAMP the data are compatible with the possibility that opiates act either by inhibiting the elaboration of cAMP in the epithelium or by preventing the action of cAMP on the mucosa. The former possibility is supported by the finding that opiates inhibit PGE-stimulated increases in cAMP in a variety of systems, including brain (COLLIER and ROY 1974), neuroblastoma × glioma hybrid cells (SHARMA et al. 1975) and homogenates of full thickness intestinal mucosa (COLLIER and ROY 1974). Recent studies with rat mucosal scrapings have confirmed that morphine prevents PGE-stimulated increases in cAMP content (BEUBLER and LEMBECK 1980). However, our observations suggest that although this mechanism may play a part, it cannot account for its entire antisecretory activity. Since secretion mediated by cGMP or calcium is also inhibited, it seems logical to propose that opiates act at a site in the biochemical pathway common to all three mediators.

Recent studies suggest that intracellular Ca^{2+} concentrations may play a key role in regulating intestinal transport processes (BOLTON and FIELD 1977; FRIZZEL 1977) and there is evidence that cAMP-mediated secretion may involve a calcium-dependent regulator protein, calmodulin (ILUNDAIN and NAFTALIN 1979). The response to morphine is known to be sensitive to changes in Ca^{2+} concentration in brain and guinea-pig ileal longitudinal muscle and this interaction is thought to be competitive in nature (YAMAMOTO et al. 1978; OPMEER and VAN REE 1979). It is also of interest that the morphine-induced electrical response in rabbit ileal mucosa is sensitive to changes in the Ca^{2+} concentration of the bathing medium, being inhibited by increases and enhanced by reductions in serosal Ca^{2+} concentration. It is conceivable therefore that the antisecretory activity of morphine is dependent on this antagonism to calcium. However, a simple direct antagonism to calcium or calmodulin does not provide an adequate explanation for all the experimental observations. Thus opiates, while inhibiting secretagogue-induced flux changes do not prevent the electrical responses to secretagogues. On the other hand agents which inhibit calmodulin activity, such as trifluoperazine, not only inhibit secretion, but also inhibit these electrical responses. Observations by ILUNDAIN and NAFTALIN (1981) indicate that loperamide does not influence the increases in mucosal border conductance to chloride which they have shown to occur with secretagogues. Rather, loperamide apparently prevented net secretion by simultaneously increasing anion permeability of the basolateral border of the epithelial layer (Ilundain and Naftalin 1981).

F. Summary

In conclusion, the studies reviewed here support the hypothesis that opiates do influence intestinal ion transport and that this activity might be responsible for their antidiarrhoeal effects. Indeed, it is possible that enkephalins may have a physiological role in the control of ion transport processes. Although there is good evidence for the presence of specific opiate receptors, it remains unclear whether these are situated on the enterocyte membrane or on nerves or paracrine cells. The ion transport response includes an enhanced net Cl^- absorption and, in some situations, an enhanced Na^+ absorption. The mechanisms underlying this action have not yet been resolved, but might involve activation of either a Cl/HCO_3^- exchange or a coupled NaCl uptake process, either of these being associated with a change in Cl^- permeability of the shunt pathway to account for the decrease in short-circuit current. Finally, the mechanisms by which opiates exert their antisecretory effects are uncertain, but it is conceivable that they are due to a combination of their ability to enhance absorption plus an antisecretagogue action, possibly mediated by an antagonism to intracellular calcium.

References

Alumets J, Hähanson R, Sundler F, Chang KJ (1978) Leu-enkephalin-like material in nerves and enterochromaffin cells in the gut. An immunohistochemical study. Histochemistry 56:187–196

Beubler E, Lembeck F (1979) Inhibition of stimulated fluid secretion in the rat small and large intestine by opiate agonists. Naunyn Schmiedebergs Arch Pharmacol 306:113–118

Beubler E, Lembeck F (1980) Inhibition by morphine of prostaglandin E_1-stimulated secretion and cyclic adenosine 3-5-monophosphate formation in the rat jejunum in vivo. Br J Pharmacol 68:513–518

Binder HJ (1979) Net fluid and electrolyte secretion: the pathophysiologic basis for diarrhoea. In: Binder HJ (ed) Mechanisms of intestinal secretion. Liss, New York, pp 1–15

Bolton JE, Field M (1977) Ca ionophore-stimulated ion secretion in rabbit ileal mucosa: relation to effects of cyclic 3′5′ AMP and carbamylcholine. J Membr Biol 35:159–173

Collier HOJ, Ray AC (1974) Morphine-like drugs inhibit the stimulation by E-prostaglandins of cyclic AMP formation by rat brain homogenate. Nature 248:24–27

Coupar IM (1978) Inhibition by morphine of prostaglandin stimulated fluid secretion in rat jejunum. Br J Pharmacol 63:57–63

Daniel EE, Sutherland WH, Bogoch A (1959) Effects of morphine and other drugs on the motility of the terminal ileum. Gastroenterology 36:510–523

Dajani EZ, Roge EAW, Bertermann RE (1975) Effects of E prostaglandin, diphenoxylate and morphine on intestinal motility in vivo. Eur J Pharmacol 34:105–113

Dobbins J, Racusen L, Binder HJ (1980) Effect of D-alanine methionine enkephalin amide on ion transport in rabbit ileum. J Clin Invest 66:19–28

Elde R, Hölfelt T, Johanson O, Terenius L (1976) Immunohistochemical studies using antibodies to leucine-enkephalin: initial observations on the nervous system of the rat. Neuroscience 1:349–351

Evans DJ, Chen LC, Curlin GT, Evans DG (1972) Stimulation of adenyl cyclase by Escherichia coli enterotoxin. Nature New Biology 236:137–138

Field M, Graf LH, Laird WJ, Smith PL (1978) Heat stable enterotoxin of E. coli in vitro effects on guanylate cyclase activity, cyclic GMP concentrations and ion transport in small intestine. Proc Natl Acad Sci USA 72:2800–2804

Frizzel RA (1977) Active chloride secretion by rabbit colon: calcium-dependent stimulation by ionophore A 23187. J Membr Biol 35:175–187

Hubel KA (1978) The effects of electrical field stimulation and tetrodotoxin on ion transport by the isolated rabbit ileum. J Clin Invest 62:1039–1047

Hughes S, Higgs NB, Turnberg LA (1982) The anti-diarrhoeal activity of loperamide: studies of its influence on ion transport across rabbit ileal mucosa in vitro. Gut 23:974–979

Hutchinson M, Kosterlitz HW, Leslie FM, Waterfield AA (1975) Assessment in the guinea pig ileum and mouse vas deferens of benzomorphans which have strong antinociceptive activity but do not substitute for morphine in the dependent monkey. Br J Pharmacol 55:541–546

Ilundain A, Naftalin RJ (1979) Role of Ca^{2+}-dependent regulator protein in intestinal secretion. Nature 279:446–448

Ilundain A, Naftalin RJ (1981) The effect of loperamide on cellular control of secretion. Europ intest transport group meeting, Berlin, August 1981

Kachur JF, Miller RJ, Field M (1980) Control of guinea pig intestinal electrolyte secretion by a δ-opiate receptor. Proc Natl Acad Sci USA 77:2753–2756

Karim SMM, Adaikan PG (1977) The effect of loperamide on prostaglandin induced diarrhoea in rat and man. Prostaglandins 13:321–331

Kimberg DV, Field M, Johnson J, Henderson A, Gershon E (1971) Stimulation of adenyl cyclase by cholera enterotoxin and prostaglandins. J Clin Invest 50:1218–1230

Kosterlitz HW, Watt AJ (1968) Kinetic parameters of narcotic agonists with particular reference to N-Allynoroxymorphine (naloxone). Br J Pharmacol 33:266–276

Lembeck F, Beubler E (1979) Inhibition of PGE_1-induced intestinal secretion by the synthetic enkephalin analogue FK 33-824. Naunyn Schmiedebergs Arch Pharmacol 308:261–264

Magnus R (1906) Die stopfende Wirkung des Morphins I. Pfluegers Arch Ges Physiol 115:316–333

Magnus R (1908) Die stopfende Wirkung des Morphins II. Pfluegers Arch Ges Physiol 122:210–250

McKay JS, Linaker BD, Turnberg LA (1981) Influence of opiates on ion transport across rabbit ileal mucosa. Gastroenterology 80:279–284

McKay JS, Linaker BD, Higgs NB, Turnberg LA (1982) Studies of the anti-secretory activity of morphine in rabbit ileum in vitro. Gastroenterology 82:243–247

Opmeer FA, Van Ree JM (1979) Competitive antagonist of morphine action in vitro by calcium. Eur J Pharmacol 53:395–397

Padtberg JH (1911) Über die Stopfwirkung von Morphin und Opium bei Koloquinthen-Duralifällen. Pfluegers Arch Ges Physiol 139:318–336

Polak JM, Sullivan SM, Bloom SR, Facer P, Pearse AGE (1977) Enkephalin-like immunoreactivity in the human gastrointestinal tract. Lancet II:972–974

Racusen LC, Binder HJ, Dobbins JW (1978) Effects of exogenous and endogenous opiate compounds on ion transport in rabbit ileum in vitro. Gastroenterology 74:1081

Schultzberg M, Hökfelt T, Nilssen G, Terenius L, Rehfeld JF, Brown M, Elde R, Goldstein M, Said S (1980) Distribution of peptide- and catecholamine-containing neurons in the gastrointestinal tract of rat and guinea-pig. Immunohistochemical studies with antisera to substance P, vasoactive intestinal polypeptide, enkephalins, somatostatin, gastrin/cholecystokinin, neurotension, and dopamine β hydroxylase. Neuroscience 5:689–744

Sharma SK, Niremberg M, Klee WA (1975) Morphine receptors as regulators of adenylate cyclase activity. Proc Natl Acad Sci USA 72:590–594

Stewart JJ, Weisbrodt NW, Burks TF (1977) Centrally mediated intestinal stimulation by morphine. J Pharmacol Exp Ther 202:174–181

Turnberg LA (1979) The pathophysiology of diarrhoea. Clin Gastroenterol 8(3):551–568

Turnberg LA, McKay JS, Higgs N (1982) The role of opiates in the control of small intestinal transport. In: Case M, Garner A, Turnberg LA, Young JA (eds) Electrolyte and water transport across gastrointestinal epithelia. Raven, New York
Valiulis E, Long JF (1973) Effects of drugs on intestinal water secretion following cholera toxin in guinea pigs and rabbits. Physiologist 16:475
Vaughan-Williams EM, Streeten DHP (1950) The action of morphine, pethidine, and amidone upon the intestinal motility of conscious dogs. Br J Pharmacol 5:584–603
Yamamoto H, Harris RA, Loh HH (1978) Effects of acute and chronic morphine treatments on calcium localisation and binding in brain. J Pharmacol Exp Ther 205:255–264

CHAPTER 26

Effect of Cholera Enterotoxin on Intestinal Permeability

T. R. HENDRIX

A. Introduction

An enormous volume of fluid may be lost in the stool during an attack of cholera. If effective fluid replacement is not instituted, hypovolemia, shock, and death occur. In some untreated outbreaks, mortality rates as high as 60% have been recorded (PHILLIPS 1966). The average duration of the illness is 5 days. On the first day of illness, stool losses as great as 16 l (average 8.3 l) have been measured (CARPENTER et al. 1966). The average stool volume measured during hospitalization in one study was 30.8 l (range 5.2–69.1 l) (LINDENBAUM et al. 1965). This devastating illness is caused by the bacterial organism, *Vibrio cholerae*. Although there was compelling evidence to the contrary, the prevailing view of the pathogenesis of cholera was, until recently, that the cholera organism produced severe damage to the epithelium and the fluid loss is exudative, analogous to the fluid losses from severely burned skin surfaces (HENDRIX 1971). It is generally accepted now that *V. cholerae* neither invades nor produces morphologically detectable damage to the intestinal epithelium (ELLIOTT et al. 1970) but, rather, produces an exotoxin, cholera enterotoxin or choleragen, which when instilled into the lumen of the small intestine in the absence of the cholera organism produces all the clinical and physiologic alterations seen in the spontaneously occurring disease (DE 1959; SACK and CARPENTER 1969).

B. Cholera Enterotoxin–Intestinal Interaction

Research in the past 30 years has increased our understanding of the clinical manifestations of cholera and their treatment, led to the isolation and purification of cholera enterotoxin, and clarified the mechanisms of cholera enterotoxin's interaction with the intestinal epithelium. This progress has been made possible by the development of good experimental models for the study of the effects of cholera enterotoxin on the intestinal epithelium (SACK and CARPENTER 1969). Despite these impressive advances, the exact mechanism by which such large volumes of fluid enter the intestinal lumen and are lost in the stool continue ill defined and controversial.

One mechanism, an enterotoxin-induced increase in intestinal permeability is the subject of this chapter. First, however, a brief review of what is known of cholera enterotoxin and its interaction with the intestinal epithelium will be useful in the subsequent consideration of its effect on intestinal permeability.

I. The Enterotoxin

Cholera enterotoxin is a protein with a molecular weight of 82,000–84,000 as determined by ultracentrifugation (LOSPALLUTO and FINKELSTEIN 1972). It contains two types of subunits, A and B (LÖNROTH and HOLMGREN 1973). The A subunit has enterotoxin properties of cholera enterotoxin and a molecular weight of 28,000 (GILL and KING 1975). Whereas there is one A subunit in a molecule of cholera enterotoxin, there are five B subunits each with molecular weight 11,600, arranged in a ring. The B subunit structure is responsible for binding the toxin molecule to the intestinal cell.

II. Enterotoxin–Enterocyte Interaction

The first step in the train of events leading to cholera is the rapid, tight binding of the enterotoxin to the enterocyte. This binding is due to specific reaction between the B subunits of cholera enterotoxin and specific membrane glycolipid, the GM1 ganglioside (HOLMGREN and 1974, 1975). Since all cells have GM1 ganglioside in their plasma membranes, cholera enterotoxin can bind to all cells, but in the course of cholera only the apical plasma membrane of the intestinal cells are exposed for contact with the toxin. The B subunits are essential for delivery of the A subunit to the interior of the cell where it activates adenylate cyclase.

III. Enterotoxin Activation of Adenylate Cyclase

Cholera enterotoxin activation of adenylate cyclase involves a totally different sequence from physiologic hormone activation. Whereas, hormone activation is rapid, reversible, and acts through a mechanism involving a hormone receptor, a catalytic site for conversion of ATP to cAMP, and a guanine nucleotide binding regulatory protein, cholera enterotoxin activation of adenylate cyclase is slow, permanent, and produced by alteration in the guanine nucleotide binding regulatory protein. Before cholera enterotoxin can increase adenylate cyclase activity, the A subunit must be inserted through the plasma membrane. After cleavage of a disulfide bond, it catylyzes the transfer of ADP–ribose to a variety of membrane and cellular proteins. One of these proteins, located on the inner surface of the cell membrane, is cyclase regulatory protein which activates cyclase when GTP is bound and returns cyclase to the inactive form when the bound GTP is hydrolyzed. The cholera enterotoxin-induced ADP ribosylation of the GTP regulatory protein reduces the rate that GTP bound to the protein is hydrolyzed, thus maintaining cyclase in the activated state. At the present time, it is not known whether cholera enterotoxin-induced activation of adenylate cyclase and elevation of intestinal cAMP is responsible for the entire secretory response to cholera toxin.

IV. Cyclic AMP and Intestinal Secretion

Several lines of evidence have suggested that cholera enterotoxin produces intestinal secretion via some mechanism activated by cAMP: (a) cholera enterotoxin elevates intestinal mucosal cAMP in experimental animals (SHAFER et al. 1970). Intestinal mucosal adenylate cyclase activity in acute cholera in humans has been found to be twice the activity found during convalescence (CHEN et al. 1971); (b) exposure of intestinal epithelium in vitro to cAMP or agents that elevate cAMP levels, e.g., the phosphodiesterase inhibitor, theophylline, prostaglandin E, and vasoactive intestinal peptide, decreases Na^+ and Cl^- flux from luminal to serosal surface of the intestinal mucosa and increases Cl^- flux from serosa to lumen in an Ussing chamber when all electrical and chemical gradients are absent (FIELD 1971; KIMBERG et al. 1971; SCHWARTZ et al. 1974); (c) Cholera enterotoxin produces similar changes in ion fluxes in vitro (FIELD et al. 1972). Thus, it is established that cholera enterotoxin causes ileal mucosa in vitro to move chloride ions from the serosal to the mucosal surface in the absence of an electrochemical or hydrostatic gradient (active transport) at the same time that activation of adenylate cyclase is produced. Although in vitro studies have shown that cholera enterotoxin inhibits electrogenic, active, sodium absorption, it does not interfere with the most important jejunal mechanism for the absorption of sodium and water, sodium-coupled glucose absorption (FIELD 1971; SEREBRO et al. 1968; IBER et al. 1969). It is not, however, established that the active secretion of chloride ions and impaired active, electrogenic, sodium absorption observed in vitro are the major factors in the production of the massive fluid movement into the intestine that characterized the disease cholera.

C. Role of Increased Filtration in the Production of Cholera-Induced Intestinal Secretion

When it became obvious that it was necessary to abandon the long-held hypothesis that attributed the voluminous secretion of intestinal fluid seen in cholera to exudation through a grossly damaged intestinal epithelium, attention turned to the possibility that cholera enterotoxin might increase the permeability of the intestinal epithelium. This view would accomodate the observations that: (a) the intestinal epithelium was intact, and (b) the protein content of the intestinal fluid was very low (HENDRIX and BAYLESS 1970). In addition, cholera enterotoxin had been shown to produce striking increases in capillary permeability when injected intracutaneously (CRAIG 1966). The effect on capillary permeability was so reproducible that for many years it provided the most useful assay for cholera enterotoxin potency. In the simplest formulation, fluid movement can be increased through a semipermeable membrane by: (a) increasing the permeability of the membrane; (b) increasing the force driving the fluid through the membrane; or (c) a combination of (a) and (b).

I. Increased Intestinal Permeability

An evaluation of the mechanisms operating to increase the flow of fluid into the intestine is complex because the mucosa is not a simple homogeneous semipermeable membrane. First, the mucosa is topographically complex with tightly arranged villi and simple tubular glands, the crypts of Lieberkühn. Second, the epithelium is composed of a variety of cells. The most numerous are the mature villus cells, transition cells at the base of the villi, immature crypt cells, and goblet cells. Measurement across the mucosa of transmural potential difference, short-circuit current, and solute and water fluxes represent the algebraic sum of these different cell populations. Any formulation of a mechanism based on such determination is flawed to the extent that these different cell types contribute differently to the modality being measured. Third, there are two routes available for the passage of water and small solutes: (a) the transcellular route which requires passage through two cell membranes, the apical brush border and the basolateral plasma membrane; and (b) the paracellular route through the so-called tight junctions that surround each epithelial cell and join it to its neighbors. It has been estimated that 85% of ions move across the intestinal epithelium via this route (FRIZZELL and SCHULTZ 1972). The driving force for absorption via this route is an osmotic gradient generated by the active transport of solute (Na^+) into the lateral intercellular spaces. No analogous model has been developed for the generation of an osmotic gradient to drive bulk fluid flow into the intestinal lumen.

1. Increased Caliber of Epithelial "Channels"

Support for the hypothesis that cholera enterotoxin increased the caliber of the transepithelial "channels" was provided by experiments in which the rate of intraluminal fluid accumulation in response to osmotic gradients produced by uncharged solutes of varying size was compared in control and cholera-infected animals. In these experiments, reflection coefficients for hypertonic (450–500 mosmol/l) mannitol, erythetol, urea, and NaCl were determined within 10–12 h of the infection of intestinal loops. Calculations based on the change in net fluid movement lead to the conclusion that cholera enterotoxin increased the effective radius of the "epithelial pores" from 6 Å found in the control animals to 11–12 Å in cholera-infected animals (LOVE 1969). For such calculations to be applicable, the membrane under study should be homogeneous (not the case in the intestine). Other factors which may have contributed to the finding of increased permeability were the long delay between the inoculation of the intestinal loops and the permeability measurements and the use of toxin-producing organisms in a closed loop rather than the enterotoxin itself.

There are a variety of observations which refute the hypothesis that cholera enterotoxin increases the permeability or enlarges the "pores" in the intestinal epithelium:

1. The clinical observation that the hypersecretion induced by cholera toxin is not associated with any change in the ionic composition of intestinal fluid is not compatible with the notion that cholera enterotoxin increases the caliber of epithelial pores. In normal humans and experimental animals such as the dog, the ionic composition of jejunal and ileal fluid differ. The fluid in both segments has the same sodium and potassium concentrations and is isotonic with plasma.

On the other hand, the bicarbonate concentration in the jejunum is less than in plasma and is higher in the ileum while chloride concentration is higher in the jejunum and lower in the ileum. When these intestinal ion concentrations are measured during cholera at a time when net intestinal fluid flux has changed from absorption to secretion, they are found to be unchanged from concentrations in normal subjects (BANWELL et al. 1970; CARPENTER et al. 1968). If cholera enterotoxin produces any increase in epithelial pore diameter and this is a factor in cholera-induced intestinal secretion, the differences in jejunal and ileal ion concentration should decrease with increasing secretory rates and the concentrations should approach those in plasma.

2. No difference in the clearance of mannitol ^{14}C from plasma to stool was seen in patients studied during and after recovery from cholera, thus indicating that if there is any cholera enterotoxin-induced change in epithelial pore diameter, it is not great enough to allow the passage of mannitol from plasma into the luminal fluid (GORDON et al. 1972).

3. No change in permeability was found when the method of comparing the ratios of two small uncharged water-soluble solutes during their passage from plasma to intestinal lumen was used (SCHERER et al. 1974; RHODE and CHEN 1972). In these studies, labeled water, urea, creatinine, and lactose were given intravenously in pairs, i.e., water–urea, water–creatinine, and the ratios in plasma and luminal fluid were measured in control animals and in animals with intestinal secretion induced by cholera enterotoxin and hypertonic mannitol. Neither the direction nor the rate of net fluid movement influenced the concentration ratios of the solute pairs, thus providing no evidence that the caliber of the epithelial pores was altered by exposure to cholera enterotoxin.

4. When diffusive permeability, expressed as fractional diffusive clearance of a solute, and convective permeability, expressed as the sieving coefficient of a solute (ratio of concentration of solute in convective fluid stream to that in the fluid of origin), were measured before and after cholera enterotoxin exposure, no evidence that cholera enterotoxin produced its effects by altered permeability was found (LIFSON et al. 1972).

5. Similar conclusions, but based on a much less sophisticated model, were reached when the volume and composition of luminal fluid collected from intestinal loops exposed to cholera enterotoxin, a hypertonic solute, or both secretory stimuli in combination were measured (HALSTED et al. 1971). It was found that the secretory response to the combined stimuli was the sum of the individual stimuli whereas, if cholera enterotoxin had increased the caliber of the epithelial pores, the composition of fluid produced in response to the osmotic gradient should have changed.

In summary, no convincing evidence exists that cholera enterotoxin produces its secretory effects by simply increasing the size of intraepithelial pores.

2. Increased Number of Epithelial Channels

It is conceivable that cholera enterotoxin could be some unknown mechanism increase the number of "channels" in the epithelium available for fluid flow. Since the forces driving secretion have not been identified and quantified, it is not possible to assess this possibility.

II. Increased Driving Force

The forces driving transepithelial fluid movement are of 3 types: (a) an osmotic gradient; (b) a hydrostatic gradient; and (c) active transport with the consequent electrochemical gradients generated.

1. Osmotic Gradient

There are many examples of osmotic gradients producing intestinal secretion. In most of these examples, an unabsorbable solute in the lumen, as a consequence of failure of digestion, mucosal transport, or ingestion of certain laxatives, imposes an osmotic gradient between the intestinal lumen and the plasma so that fluid remains in the lumen instead of being absorbed. Cholera enterotoxin-induced secretion is not one of them. The osmolalities of intestinal contents and stool in patients with cholera are unchanged from control values (BANWELL et al. 1970). In fact, hemoconcentration develops in severe cholera so that the osmotic gradient that develops favors absorption rather than secretion. Intestinal secretion continues in spite of the development of an osmotic gradient.

A hypertonic compartment in the lamina propria of the villus tip has been proposed (HALJAMÄE et al. 1973). More recently, direct measurement of the temperature at which thawing of frozen sections of intestinal villi occurs has shown that the absorption of glucose and sodium by the jejunum is associated with osmolalities in the villus tips as high as 1,100–1,200 mosmol/kg H_2O (JODAL et al. 1978). It has been proposed that the vascular arrangement of the villi acts as a countercurrent exchanger and it is this mechanism that produces the high osmolality at the villus tips (LUNDGREN 1967; HALLBÄCK et al. 1978). In a study of the effect of cholera enterotoxin, it was confirmed that cholera enterotoxin produced a *net* secretion of water, sodium, chloride, and potassium. In addition, unidirectional sodium transport from lumen to blood was decreased while the flux in the opposite direction was increased. These changes in water and electrolyte fluxes were associated with a small reduction in villous tip hyperosmolality ($1{,}022 \pm 30 \rightarrow 764 \pm 68$ mosmol/kg H_2O) (HALLBÄCK et al. 1979). While this reduction in tissue osmolality may contribute to the observed reduced absorption, it is insufficient to play any role in cholera enterotoxin-induced secretion. In summary, osmotic driving forces play a role in intestinal absorption. The intestinal secretion produced by cholera enterotoxin, however, is not attributable to increased filtration driven by an identified osmotic gradient.

2. Hydrostatic Gradient

Early in the present era of interest in the pathogenesis of cholera, it was noted that the intracutaneous injection of cholera enterotoxin was followed by local extravasation (CRAIG 1966; FINKELSTEIN et al. 1966). It was reasoned that a similar response occurred in the intestine with increased intestinal tissue pressure and exudation of fluid into the intestine. It is possible in vitro with mounted intestinal mucosa to demonstrate that a small elevation of hydrostatic pressure (4 cm H_2O) on the serosal side reduces fluid absorption to zero and higher pressure results in net secretion. On the basis of these observations, it was suggested that increased hydraulic filtration might explain the net secretion observed in cholera (HAKIN and LIFSON 1969). These studies, however, have no relevance to the intact animal because the hydraulically induced secretion was associated with the appearance of glucose in the mucosal solution, an event that does not occur in vivo even with massive secretion or very high levels of blood glucose. The pressure applied to the stripped mucosa opened unphysiologic pathways. In this context, it is of interest to note that no increase in lumen–serosa fluid flow was induced by mucosal pressures as high as 22 cm H_2O (FINKELSTEIN et al. 1966). The differences in hydraulic conductivity when the pressure is applied first to the mucosal and then to the serosal surfaces may be analogous to the great strength of an arch when a force is applied to its upper surface, but weakness when the force is applied in the opposite direction. On the other hand, increased tissue pressure produced by hypervolemia can lead to intestinal secretion (HUMPHREYS and EARLEY 1971; HIGGINS and BLAIR 1971). This secretory mechanism, unlike cholera enterotoxin-induced secretion, is not associated with any elevation of tissue cAMP (TURJMAN et al. 1977).

Increased hydrostatic pressure leading to filtration through the epithelium has not been believed to play a role in the pathogenesis of cholera-induced secretion because in clinical cholera, diarrhea persists in the face of extreme hypovolemia and hypotension. In addition, superior mesenteric artery pressure has been lowered to below 30% of normal in experimental cholera without producing a decrease in enterotoxin-induced fluid output by the small intestine (CARPENTER et al. 1969). On the other hand, such lowering of arterial flow may not be directly reflected in capillary pressure. In fact, no change in mean capillary hydrostatic pressure was observed when arterial pressures were lowered to 50 mm Hg (HAGLUND and LUNDGREN 1972).

Measurement of intestinal blood flow in experimental cholera has shown an increase of 30% at a time when maximal secretion is occurring (CARPENTER et al. 1969; Cedgord et al. 1978). In addition, the increase in total blood flow was due to a doubling of mucosal–submucosal blood flow (CEDGORD et al. 1978). It seems most likely that this increased blood flow is a response to keep the intestinal secretory mechanism supplied with fluid for secretion rather than the primary cause of cholera-induced secretion.

Histologic studies using large molecular probes (ferritin) have suggested that cholera-induced secretion was associated with an increase in capillary permeability (DALLDORF et al. 1969). In studies using a smaller probe, horseradish peroxidase (molecular weight 40,000), no evidence of heightened permeability of intestinal epithelium could be found. Electron microscopic observation shows no alteration of normal pinocytotic vesicles and fenestrae normally present in intestinal capillaries (YARDLEY and BROWN 1973). Using physiologic rather than histologic criteria, the same conclusion was reached in studies comparing regional blood flow and capillary filtration in control and cholera-infected animals (CEDGORD et al. 1978).

In summary, cholera-induced secretion is associated with increased mucosal blood flow and vasodilation. These hemodynamic changes are not associated with changes in capillary permeability and, as noted, villus hypertonicity is not disturbed; thus, the data at hand are more compatible with the notion that these hemodynamic alterations are the consequence of cholera-induced secretion rather than the cause.

D. Conclusion

A review of studies of the pathogenesis of cholera enterotoxin-induced secretion produce no support for the hypothesis that the primary event is an enterotoxin-mediated increase in epithelial permeability. Nor is there evidence that cholera enterotoxin increases osmotic or hydrostatic gradients so that the increased intestinal fluid characteristic of cholera arises from increased filtration through normal caliber "channels". Physiologic models are available to explain the intestinal absorption phenomenon. These include: (a) active solute transport with the development of a standing gradient in the intercellular spaces which in turn induces osmotic flow through the paracellular route; and (b) development of villus tip hyperosmolality by countercurrent multiplication. With these models, comparisons can be made between the predicted and observed behavior of modalities related to absorption in a variety of physiologic and pathologic states. From the study of the discrepancies, the models and our understanding of intestinal absorption can both be perfected. Unfortunately, the principal model for movement in the opposite direction, secretion, involves passive movement down activity gradients. This model has not proven adequate to explain cholera enterotoxin-induced secretion. Although cholera enterotoxin-induced active transport of chloride ions from serosa to mucosa (active secretion) has been described in vivo, no model has been proposed whereby this active solute secretion might create a hyperosmotic compartment to provide the osmotic gradient to drive intestinal secretion. It is possible that the crypts of Lieberkühn might provide such a model so that the actively secreted ions are contained in a limited space and, thus, the activity gradient generated by active ion secretion is not dissipated before it can induce osmotic flow into the intestine. Whether or not enterotoxin-induced changes in local permeability are necessary or play a role in such a model remains to be determined. Indirect evidence implicating the crypts as the source of cholera enterotoxin-induced secretion has been presented (SEREBRO et al. 1969; ROGGIN et al. 1972; HENDRIX and PAULK 1977).

References

Banwell JG, Pierce NF, Mitra RC, Brigham KL, Caranasos GJ, Keimowitz RI, Fedson DS, Thomas J, Gorbach SL, Sack RB, Mondal A (1970) Intestinal fluid and electrolyte transport in human cholera. J Clin Invest 49:183–195

Carpenter CCJ, Barua D, Wallace CK, Mitra PP, Sack RB, Khanra SR, Wells SA, Dans PE, Chandhuri RN (1966) Clinical studies in asiatic cholera. IV. Antibiotic therapy in cholera. Bull Johns Hopkins Hosp 118:216–229

Carpenter CCJ, Sack RB, Feeley JC, Steenberg RW (1968) Site and characteristics of electrolyte loss and effect of intraluminal glucose in experimental canine cholera. J Clin Invest 47:1210–1220

Carpenter CCJ, Greenough WB, Sack RB (1969) The relationship of superior mesenteric artery blood flow to gut electrolyte loss in experimental cholera. J Infect Dis 119:182–193

Cedgord S, Hallbäck DA, Jodal M, Lundgren O, Redfors S (1978) The effects of cholera toxin on intramural blood flow distribution and capillary hydraulic conductivity in the cat small intestine. Acta Physiol Scand 102:148–158

Chen LC, Rohde JE, Sharp GWG (1971) Intestinal adenyl-cyclase activity in human cholera. Lancet 1:939–941

Craig JP (1966) Preparation of the vascular permeability factor of *Vibrio cholerae*. J Bacteriol 92:793–795

Dalldorf FG, Keusch GT, Livingston HL (1969) Transcellular permeability of capillaries in experimental cholera. Am J Pathol 57:153–160

De SN (1959) Enterotoxicity of bacteria-free culture filtrates of *Vibrio cholerae*. Nature 183:1533–1534

Elliott HL, Carpenter CCJ, Sack RB, Yardley JH (1970) Small bowel morphology in experimental canine cholera. A light and electron microscopic study. Lab Invest 22:112–120

Field M (1971) Ion transport in rabbit ileal mucosa. II. Effects of cyclic 3′,5′-AMP. Am J Physiol 221:992–997

Field M, From D, Al-Awqati Q, Greenough WB (1972) Effect of cholera toxin on ion transport across isolated ileal mucosa. J Clin Invest 51:796–804

Finkelstein RA, Nye SW, Atthasampunna P, Charunmethee P (1966) Pathogenesis of experimental cholera, effect of choleragen on vascular permeability. Lab Invest 15:1601–1609

Frizzell RA, Schultz SG (1972) Ionic conductances of extracellular shunt pathway in rabbit ileum: influence of shunt on transmural sodium transport and electrical potential differences. J Gen Physiol 59:318–346

Gill DM, King CA (1975) The mechanism of action of cholera toxin in pigeon erythrocyte lipates. J Biol Chem 250:424–432

Gordon RS Jr, Gardner JD, Kinzie JL (1972) Low mannitol clearance into cholera stool as evidence against filtration as a source of stool fluid. Gastroenterology 63:407

Haglund U, Lundgren O (1972) Reactions within consecutive vascular sections of the small intestine of the cat during prolonged hypotension. Acta Physiol Scand 84:151–163

Hakin AA, Lifson N (1969) Effects of pressure of water and solute by dog intestinal mucosa in vitro. Am J Physiol 216:276–284

Haljamäe H, Jodal M, Lundgren O (1973) Countercurrent multiplication of sodium in intestinal villi during absorption of sodium chloride. Acta Physiol Scand 89:580–593

Hallbäck DA, Hulten L, Jodal M, Lindhagen J, Lundgren O (1978) Evidence for the existence of a countercurrent exchanger in the small intestine of man. Gastroenterology 74:683–690

Hallbäck DA, Jodal M, Lundgren O (1979) Effects of cholera toxin on villous tissue osmolality and fluid and electrolyte transport in the small intestine of the cat. Acta Physiol Scand 107:239–249

Halsted CH, Bright LS, Leubbers EA, Bayless TM, Hendrix TR (1971) A comparison of jejunal response to cholera exotoxin and to hypertonic mannitol. Johns Hopkins Med J 129:179

Hendrix TR (1971) The pathophysiology of cholera. Proc NY Acad Med 47:1169–1180

Hendrix TR, Bayless TM (1970) Digestion: intestinal secretion. Annu Rev Physiol 32:139–164

Hendrix TR, Paulk HT (1977) Intestinal secretion. Int Rev Physiol 12:257–284

Higgins JT, Blair NP (1971) Intestinal transport of water and electrolytes during extracellular volume expansion in dogs. J Clin Invest 50:2569

Holmgren J, Lindholm L, Lönroth I (1974) Interaction of cholera toxin and toxin derivatives with lymphocytes. J Exp Med 139:801–819

Holmgren J, Lönroth I, Mansson JE, Svennerholm L (1975) Interaction of cholera toxin and membrane G_{M1} ganglioside of the intestine. Proc Natl Acad Sci USA 72:2520–2524

Humphreys MH, Earley LE (1971) The mechanism of decreased intestinal sodium and water absorption after acute volume expansion in the rat. J Clin Invest 50:2355

Iber FL, McGonagle TJ, Serebro HL, Leubbers EL, Bayless TM, Hendrix TR (1969) Unidirectional sodium flux in small intestine in experimental canine cholera. Am J Med Sci 258:340
Jodal M, Hallbäck DA, Lundgren O (1978) Tissue osmolality in intestinal villi during luminal perfusion with isotonic electrolyte solutions. Acta Physiol Scand 102:94–107
Kimberg DV, Field M, Johnson J, Henderson A, Gershaw I (1971) Stimulation of intestinal mucosal adenyl cyclase by cholera enterotoxin and prostaglandins. J Clin Invest 50:1218–1230
Lifson N, Hakim AA, Lender EJ (1972) Effects of cholera toxin on intestinal permeability and transport interactions. Am J Physiol 222:1479–1487
Lindenbaum J, Greenough WB III, Beneson AS, Osedsohn RD, Risvi S, Saad A (1965) Non-vibrio cholera. Lancet 1:1081
Lönroth I, Holmgren J (1973) Subunit structure of cholera toxin. J Gen Microbiol 76:417–427
LoSpalluto JJ, Finkelstein RA (1972) Chemical and physical properties of cholera exo-enterotoxin (choleragen) and its spontaneously formed toxoid (choleragenoid). Biochim Biophys Acta 157:158–1966
Love AHG (1969) Permeability characteristics of the cholera infected small intestine. Gut 10:105–107
Lundgren O (1968) Studies on blood flow distribution and countercurrent exchange in the small intestine. Acta Physiol Scand 72 [Suppl 303]
Phillips RA (1966) Cholera in the perspective of 1966. Ann Intern Med 65:922–930
Rhode JC, Chen LC (1972) Permeability and selectivity of canine and human jejunum during cholera. Gut 13:191–196
Roggin GM, Banwell JG, Yardley JH, Hendrix TR (1972) Unimpaired response of rabbit jejunum to cholera toxin after selective damage to villus epithelium. Gastroenterology 63:981
Sack RB, Carpenter CCJ (1969 a) Experimental canine cholera. II. Production by cell-free filtrates of *Vibrio cholerae*. J Infect Dis 119:150–157
Scherer RW, Harper DT, Banwell JG, Hendrix TR (1974) Absence of concurrent permeability changes of the intestinal mucosa in association with cholera toxin-induced secretion. Johns Hopkins Med J 134:156–167
Schwartz CJ, Kimberg DV, Sheerin HE, Field M, Said SI (1974) Vasoactive intestinal peptide stimulation of adenylate cyclase and active secretion in intestinal mucosa. J Clin Invest 54:536
Serebro HA, Iber FL, Yardley JH, Hendrix TR (1969) Inhibition of cholera toxin action in the rabbit by cycloheximide. Gastroenterology 56:506
Serebro HA, Bayless TM, Hendrix TR, Iber FL, McGonagle T (1968) Absorption of D-glucose by rabbit jejunum during cholera-induced diarrhea. Nature 217:1272
Shafer DE, Lust WD, Sucar B, Goldberg NO (1970) Elevation of adenosine 3′5′ cyclic monophosphate concentration in intestinal mucosa after treatment with cholera toxin. Proc Natl Acad Sci USA 67:851–855
Turjman N, Yardley JH, Hendrix TR, Gotterer GS (1977) Effect of intestinal distention on levels of cyclic AMP and fluid secretion. Johns Hopkins Med J 140:97–99
Yardley JH, Brown GD (1973) Horseradish peroxidase tracer studies in experimental cholera. Lab Invest 28:482–493

CHAPTER 27

Aspects of Bacterial Enterotoxins Other than Cholera on Intestinal Permeability

J. G. BANWELL

A. Introduction

Cholera enterotoxin (CT) (HOLMGREN and LONNROTH 1980) has been the major stimulus for studies of other bacterial enterotoxins. Its features are well described in Chap. 26. Studies of the labile toxin (LT) of *Escherichia coli* (FIELD 1974), demonstrating that its mode of action is very similar to that of CT, and recent studies of the stable toxin (ST) of *E. coli* (FIELD et al. 1978; STAPLES et al. 1980) which have demonstrated that ST specifically activates guanylate cyclase in intestinal mucosal cells, have been the major recent developments in studies of other bacterial enterotoxins. Many enterotoxins have been identified, but have either not been as fully purified as *E. coli* LT and ST or their mode of action on transport processes is less well defined. Information as to their role or significance in bacterial diarrheal disease processes is also limited. Definition of their specific mode of action will, however, be of importance for several reasons. (a) They may help to define normal intestinal physiologic processes in a manner similar to that demonstrated by CT-activated chloride secretion. (b) Other bacterial toxins may cause fluid and electrolyte secretion by activation of secretory processes distinct from those dependent on activation of the cAMP or cGMP systems; for instance, no toxins have yet been identified to cause secretion by mechanisms similar to those accompanying serotonin-induced intestinal secretion and there is no clear knowledge of whether filtrative secretion is a factor in a toxin-mediated process. (c) Finally, purified toxins which have been shown to cause intestinal secretion will need to be integrated with the knowledge of the behavior of the organism as a whole in regard to its adherence factors, mechanism for cytologic damage to the plasma membrane, and active invasion of the mucosal cell in order to provide a full understanding for the action of bacterial organisms in the gastrointestinal tract.

Many advances are to be expected in the forthcoming years with the availability of biochemical techniques to purify and identify small quantities of protein in bacterial culture media and methods for analyzing the interaction of toxins with the intestinal cell membrane. The enterotoxic agents which, so far, have been clearly identified as having effects on intestinal transport will serve as the basis for this chapter.

B. *Escherichia coli*

I. Heat-Labile Toxin

1. Nature and Mode of Action

In early studies, a crude broth culture supernatant obtained from cultures of enterotoxigenic *E. coli* were shown to cause intestinal fluid secretion in a variety of animal models (BANWELL and SHERR 1973) and effects in vitro on the isolated stripped intestinal mucosa in the Ussing chamber (AL-AWQATI et al. 1972). There is now recognized to be an immunologic relationship between the heat-labile enterotoxin (LT) of *E. coli* and enterotoxin (choleragen) of *Vibrio cholerae* (GYLES 1974; CLEMENTS and FINKELSTEIN 1979). The LT and cholera toxin produced diarrhea by the same basic mechanism, namely, activation of adenylate cyclase and increase of intracellular levels of cyclic adenosine monophosphate (HOLMGREN and LONNROTH 1980; CLEMENTS and FINKELSTEIN 1979).

Homogeneous LT has been isolated by CLEMENTS and FINKELSTEIN (1979). The toxin has an isoelectric point of 8.0 and an approximate molecular weight of 91,440 on sedimentation equilibrium measurement. The toxin dissociates into two subunits during gel filtration in the presence of a chaotropic agents, such as 5 *M* guanidine. These subunits, termed A and B, have antigenic determinants common to the isolated subunits of cholera toxin (A and B). They were of similar amino acid composition; within the first 20 amino acids of the two chains, only 5 differed and these could be attributed to single base substitutions (SPICER et al. 1981; DORNER et al. 1979).

LT interacts with GM1 ganglioside which may correspond to its affinity for agarose gels containing lactose and galactose (HOLMGREN 1973). The structure of LT may have 5 or 6 B units and be A_1B_5 or A_1B_6 in total structure which provides another similarity to the structure of CT (CLEMENTS and FINKELSTEIN 1979; GILL 1976).

Cholera toxin, a protein of molecular weight 84,000, is known to consist of three peptides A_1, A_2, and B (molecular weight 1,000, 5,000, and 24,000, respectively). The B chain can be obtained as a single unit; it will not by itself stimulate adenylate cyclase, but binds to the cell membrane with high affinity in a manner similar to the whole toxin molecule. The A subunit is nontoxic for intact cells, but is highly active when added to lysed cells. The toxicity is due to the A_1 fragment which becomes inserted into or through the plasma membrane after binding (GILL 1976).

In the plasma membrane, the A_1 peptide undergoes reorientation which is slow and temperature dependent, resulting in the lag phase before stimulation of adenylate cyclase in the intact cell, although addition of A_1 to a lysate causes measurable activation of cyclase immediately. The A_1 peptide splits NAD in the presence of a macromolecule in the cytosol to adenosine phosphoribose (ADPR) and nicotinamide (GILL 1976; ENOMOTO and GILL 1980). ADPR is covalently bonded to guanosine triphosphatase (GTP). It regulates activity of adenylate cyclase by interconversion to an inactive form which is not bound to GTP. It is likely that *E. coli* LT, on account of its similar structure, will be found to have many features similar to CT in its activation of adenylate cyclase (MOSS and RICHARDSON 1978).

2. Effects on Intestinal Permeation

The addition of broth culture supernatant fluid from enterotoxigenic *E. coli* causes fluid accumulation in isolated intestinal loops as well as causing activation of mucosal adenylate cyclase (GUERRANT et al. 1973). Under normal conditions in humans, the sum of net absorptive processes exceeds that of coexistent secretory processes for fluid and electrolytes. In diarrheal disease, the secretory processes (either those normally present or those stimulated by the intestinal secretagogue) exceed the absorptive processes, thereby causing diarrhea or excessive loss of fecal water and electrolytes. The response to direct instillation of *E. coli* enterotoxin is rapid, but ceases on removal of the toxin from the bowel loop, suggesting that rapid inactivation of toxin occurred.

In vitro studies have demonstrated stimulation of intestinal secretion in rabbit ileal mucosa exposed to broth culture supernatant from *E. coli* cultures in vivo for 1 h and then examined in the flux chamber. (No direct studies demonstrating the effect of pure LT enterotoxin in vitro are presently available.) Short-circuit current (I_{sc} increased from 2.5 ± 0.2 equiv. cm^{-2} h^{-1} in control tissue to 3.0 ± 0.3 equiv. cm^{-2} h^{-1}. Tissue electrical resistance was slightly increased (36–45 mV) (AL-AWQATI et al. 1972). Net Na and Cl fluxes were inhibited such that chloride was secreted and Na not absorbed. Unidirectional flux measurements demonstrated that serosal–mucosal flux for Na and Cl was increased over the mucosal–serosal flux (GUERRANT et al. 1973). These electrical changes are similar to those observed with purified CT or following the addition of cAMP or theophylline (acting to inhibit enzymatic degradation of cAMP) to the bathing medium (FIELD 1979). It is conceived that the brush border membrane of the ileum is equipped with channels or carrier mechanisms to translocate the ion pair Na^+Cl^-. This mechanism is inhibited either by absence of Na^+ or Cl^- reciprocally. The Na^+ that enters the cell is actively extruded across the basolateral membrane by the ouabain-inhibitable Na^+-pump. The low intracellular Na^+ concentration favors accumulation of Cl^- which diffuses out across the basolateral membrane (presumed to be more permeable to chloride than the brush border membrane). Coupled uptake of NaCl at the luminal border of the cell is inhibited by cAMP which, thereby, inhibits "active" Cl^- absorption and a large portion of active Na absorption. The mechanism by which exogenous cAMP or *E. coli* enterotoxin causes net secretion may either depend on unmasking of an underlying secretory process (by inhibition of coupled NaCl absorption); alternatively, they may directly stimulate active secretion by a second mechanism. Since other agents, such as furosemide and acetazolamide, also inhibit coupled NaCl transport, it is likely that cAMP and *E. coli* enterotoxin have a *direct* stimulatory effect on active NaCl secretion to cause fluid secretion. There is some evidence that the crypt cells of the mucosa may be the region susceptible to such active secretory stimuli (FIELD 1974, 1979).

Escherichia coli LT is similar to CT in causing no morphological changes when applied to the intestinal mucosal surface. Fluid secretion in response to exposure of the mucosa to toxin has the composition of an ultrafiltrate of plasma equilibrated to the region of the small intestine from which it is derived. Accumulation of macromolecules, such as albumin, is not a feature of *E. coli* toxin exposure and no change in permeability to large molecules occurs (BANWELL and SHERR 1973).

II. Heat-Stable Toxin

Enterotoxigenic strains of *E. coli* may produce, in addition to LT, or separately, a stable toxin (ST) (BANWELL and SHERR 1973). ST appears to be a very different peptide from LT (ALDERETE and ROBERTSON 1978). ST isolated from a strain of *E. coli* enterotoxigenic for the pig, had a molecular weight of 4,400–5,100. The molecule has a single NH_2 terminal glycine residue, a high proportion of cysteine, and three tyrosine molecules. The toxin is stable to acid, but loses activity at pH 9.0. It does not contain either a lipid or carbohydrate. The molecule is stable to heating and to treatment with pronase, trypsin, proteinase, deoxyribonuclease, and phospholipase. It is poorly antigenic, but serum neutralization of toxicity has been observed. The human ST purified recently by STAPLES et al. (1980) is different from that derived from the animal strains. It is of lower molecular weight.

As a result of the purification of ST by ROBERTSON and GIANELLA and colleagues, in vitro detection of enterotoxigenic strains will be possible to improve assay for ST. Up to the present time the suckling mouse assay model has been used, but it is a cumbersome and expensive biologic assay, although reasonably specific for ST (GIANNELLA 1976).

1. Mode of Action

Several workers have recently demonstrated that intestinal fluid secretion in response to ST exposure may be dependent on the increase in cyclic GMP concentrations which accompanies net fluid secretion (FIELD et al. 1978; STAPLES et al. 1980; GIANNELLA and DRAKE 1979; HUGHES et al. 1978). Under short-circuit conditions in the Ussing chamber, addition of ST to the luminal surface produced a rapid (and within 30 s) an increase in potential difference (PD) which became maximal within 5 min and usually persisted at a similar level indefinitely. The increase in PD could be rapidly reversed by replacing with fresh Ringer solution (FIELD et al. 1978). A further increase followed addition of theophylline (5 µmol/ml), but less than when added alone without enterotoxin. Progressive increase in PD and I_{sc} was observed over a wide range of concentrations without attaining a maximum effect. The secretory process was not dependent on the presence of calcium ions. Under short-circuit conditions, ST abolished net Cl absorption present under basal conditions. Addition of theophylline also caused net secretory changes. Both agents decreased mucosal–serosal chloride flux J_{ms}^{Cl} and increased serosal–mucosal chloride flux J_{sm}^{Cl}, although the effect of theophylline was larger than that of the enterotoxin. Tissue conductance was increased 15% (FIELD et al. 1978).

ST, in contrast to LT, caused a persistent increase in tissue cGMP activity and the increase was constant over the entire range of enterotoxin concentrations tested. The effect was due to an influence on guanylate cyclase and not cGMP phosphodiesterase (FIELD et al. 1978; GIANNELLA and DRAKE 1979; HUGHES et al. 1978).

Guanylate cyclase activity was stimulated by ST when added directly to crude membrane fractions from intestinal cells. It has been suggested that, since guanylate cyclase is present with high specific activity in isolated brush border membranes, cGMP released by activation of guanylate cyclase at this site may, thereby, inhibit net Cl absorption. It has been shown that there is a protein kinase in brush border membranes which phosphorylates the membrane and is more sensitive to cGMP than cAMP. GIANNELLA and HUGHES and co-workers have shown that addition of the 8-Br analog of cGMP and exogenous cGMP both stimulate intestinal secretion (GIANNELLA and DRAKE 1979; HUGHES et al. 1978). The rapidity of onset of secretion on ST exposure and its reversibility make it less likely that NAD or a cytosol component are involved in the reaction as they are for the effects of LT or CT. A similar rapid reversal of the secretory stimulation of ST has been observed in vivo in the perfused rat intestine (EADE and GIANNELLA 1978; HUGHES et al. 1978). No impairment of glucose or glucose-facilitated sodium transport was observed after ST exposure in this model. Although LT and ST were shown to have little effect on net fluid and electrolyte transport in the rat cecum, the highly purified ST was observed to alter fluid transport in the rat colon in a similar manner to the small bowel (EADE and GIANNELLA 1978).

III. Relationship of Surface Adhesion (Colonization Factors) to Fluid Secretion

Some strains of *E. coli* which are enteropathogenic to newborn pigs have surface protein antigens of K88 antigen. The plasmid-mediated K88 antigens allow K88-positive *E. coli* to adhere to porcine intestinal mucosa and proliferate in the intestine (JONES and RUTTER 1972). This antigen is essential for virulence, indicating that enterotoxigenicity, alone, is insufficient to promote pathogenicity. Similar colonization factors are most probably of importance in *E. coli* pathogenic for humans (colonization factor) and other animals (calf K99 antigen) (ISAACSON et al. 1978). Enterotoxigenic K88-negative strains failed to produce illness in piglets (SELLWOOD et al. 1975). However, a mild illness was produced in some animals by K88-positive nontoxigenic *E. coli*, suggesting that colonization, alone, by certain Enterobacteriaceae in the upper small intestine may cause diarrhea. Species specificity is often present; K99 antigen which causes calf scours is antigenically distinct from K88 antigen and is less likely to cause disease in piglets (MOON et al. 1979).

Escherichia coli isolates from infants with gastroenteritis have been serotyped for many years, providing an epidemiologic tool to identify modes of transmission of this significantly lethal and common acute diarrheal disease (GANGAROSA and MERSON 1977). Several "classical serotypes" (EPEC) were subsequently recognized as being associated with these diarrheal outbreaks more frequently than other strains (GANGAROSA and MERSON 1977). Some were later identified as strains which were enterotoxigenic (LT or ST). However, other strains were discovered to be neither enterotoxigenic nor invasive of the mucosa. LEVINE et al. (1978) have shown, in challenge experiments carried out in human subjects, that such strains were still capable of causing diarrhea in adults, suggesting that adherence, alone, without identification of LT or ST also may cause fluid secretion. The mechanism for this secretory process related to colonization is unclear. It may depend on: (a) the interreaction of the mucosal cell with specific adherence proteins; (b) production of toxins in quantities too small to be identified; or (c) toxin of a type, as yet poorly characterized. The mechanisms involved may provide new insights into intestinal secretory physiology in future years.

IV. Surface Mucosal Invasion (Enteroadherence)

Another secretory stimulatory mechanism has been described in which superficial invasion (enteroadherence) of the mucosal surface occurs by *E. coli* organisms. This has been demonstrated in rabbits with the *E. coli* strain 015 RDEC-1 organism (CANTEY and BLAKE 1980) and in a single human patient by ULSHEN and ROLLO (1980) with an *E. coli* strain 0125 (a classical enteropathogenic serotype). The RDEC-1 strain does not produce ST or LT, but when fed to young rabbits adheres to the intestinal epithelium of the terminal ileum and cecum. The organism associates with the mucosa without penetrating it, causing superficial damage to the brush border membrane. There is evidence that RDEC-1 may elaborate a Shiga-like toxin at low concentrations (O'BRIEN et al. 1979). This resembles the findings of KLIPSTEIN et al. (1978) that bacteria from preparation of EPEC caused fluid secretion in the perfused rat ileum. The human enteropathogenic serotype studied by ULSHEN and ROLLO (1980) which was also shown to penetrate the glycocalyx and adhere closely to the mucosal surface, causing disruption of the microvillus border, blunting of the intestinal villi, and crypt hypertrophy might, therefore, also be likely to generate such a toxin (TAKEUCHI et al. 1978).

1. Invasive *E. coli*

Invasive *E. coli* invade the colonic mucosa to produce an illness similar to shigellosis with mucosal ulceration and bleeding into the intestine. The nature of the process is poorly understood, but may be due to the production of cytotoxins analogous to those produced by *Shigella* (TULLOCH et al. 1973).

C. *Shigella*

Diarrhea and dysentery are major problems of infection with *Shigella* organisms. It is generally recognized that pathogenic *Shigella* bacteria cause disease by either invasive or toxigenic mechanisms, although such mechanisms may not be mutually exclusive (LEVIN et al. 1973; KEUSCH et al. 1972). For several years, an enterotoxin has been available in impure form. At first, it was isolated only from *Shigella dysenteriae*, but more recently from *Shigella flexneri* as well (O'BRIEN et al. 1977). Although it was early demonstrated that this toxin could cause fluid accumulation in the ligated rabbit ileal loop preparation, or during perfusion in the rabbit intestine (DONOWITZ et al. 1975), the mechanism of the effect remained obscure. Perfusion at various concentrations caused fluid secretion without evidence of mucosal damage and usually with elevation of activity of adenylate cyclase. However, it has since been shown that the increment in adenylate cyclase occurs several hours after the secretory response and is most probably related to the inflammatory occurrence and not directly involved in the secretory effect (O'BRIEN et al. 1979). The toxin was noted to be lethal when injected into mice and this cytotoxic property to various cell lines were closely related to enterotoxic activity during the purification process. KEUSCH and JACEWICZ (1977) have produced evidence that the toxin exerted its toxicity via binding to a cell membrane receptor identified as oligomeric β-1–4-linked *N*-acetyl-D-glucosamine.

OLSNESS and EIKLID (1980) have recently isolated and characterized Shiga toxin (utilizing the binding features already discussed) by affinity chromatography with acid-treated chitin and elution with 1 *M* sodium chloride. On polyacrylamide gel electrophoresis in the presence of sodium dodecylsulfate, pure Shiga toxin migrated as two bands, corresponding to molecular weights of 30,500 and about 11,000. The intact toxin was thought to consist of one heavy chain and four to five copies of the light chain. The toxin was cytotoxic for only certain cell lines (Vero cells and HeLa cells) in which the *N*-acetylglucosamine surface receptor was identified. The toxin has been shown to induce cytotoxic effects similar to abrin, ricin, and modeccin, but whether this is exerted through similar effects on protein synthesis is at present unclear (BROWN et al. 1980). The *Shigella* organism usually enters the epithelial cells of the colon, thereby, causing an inflammatory response. Thus, an intracellular role for the toxin is, as yet, unclear but may well be, in part, responsible for the cell necrosis observed in *Shigella* dysentery.

In vitro experiments in the Ussing chamber utilizing an impure toxin from *S. dysenteriae* demonstrated that net sodium secretion occurred (-1.0 ± 0.6 μequiv. cm^{-2} h^{-1}) in the absence of change in I_{sc}, although both I_{sc} and PD increased in response to addition of theophylline of dibutyryl-cAMP in both control and treated tissues (DONOWITZ et al. 1975). The responses of these parameters to glucose in the media were slightly less in Shiga toxin-exposed tissues. Mucosal cAMP levels were not augmented in response to Shiga toxin exposure, indicating that although toxin exposure might mediate adenylate cyclase changes, the transport defects were not mediated by the cAMP system.

The fact that exogenous Shiga toxin had no apparent toxic effect when injected into the rat cecum suggests that colonic epithelial cells may be resistant to exogenous toxin. Response of small intestinal mucosa to exogenous toxin may be dependent on the presence of the receptor. Resistant cells in tissue culture, for instance, lack the specific receptor. An intriguing feature of the fluid and electrolyte transport processes accompanying *Shigella* diarrhea is the frequent observation that, at the onset, diarrhea is often watery; bloody diarrhea, such as may follow bacterial tissue invasion, is usually a later phase of the illness. This early phase may be so severe as to mimic cholera-induced diarrhea (O'BRIEN et al. 1979). Whether this is due to a direct toxic effect of an enterotoxin or due to some other indirect mechanism is still unclear. Decreased jejunal absorption of sodium and water have been demonstrated in patients with ulcerative colitis (SCHMID et al. 1969). This suggests that there may be a distant secretory effect owing to inflammation in the colon. This secretory state might be mediated by release of humoral or chemical agents such as prostaglandins from the inflamed bowel wall.

D. Prostaglandin Released from Inflamed Tissue and Fluid and Electrolyte Secretion

Prostaglandins have been shown to have potent effects on intestinal electrolyte and fluid movement in experimental animals (PIERCE et al. 1971) and humans (MATUCHANSKY and BERNER 1973). Net fluid and electrolyte secretion can be induced by PGE or PGF_2 α infused intraluminally or intraarterially. PGE will inhibit ileal sodium absorption. In the colon, PGE_1 and PGA_2 increase I_{sc}, decrease net sodium transport and increase mucosal cAMP levels (RACUSEN and BINDER 1980). Indomethacin, a prostaglandin synthetase inhibitor, inhibited secretion, in part, by inhibition of activation of adenylate cyclase, but also, in part, by a prostaglandin-independent mechanism (SMITH et al. 1981). Prostanglandins have been suggested as a mediators of the diarrhea associated with ulcerative colitis. Increased synthesis and release of prostaglandins has been observed in ulcerative colitis (SHARON et al. 1978). Colonic production of prostaglandins (PGI_2 and PGA_2) is also enhanced in ulcerative colitis (LIGUMSKY et al. 1980). No information is available as to the PG response in other inflammatory bowel disorders, such as shigellosis and salmonellosis, although it has been suggested that acetylsalicylic acid improved diarrhea in radiation-induced diarrheal disease (MENNIE and DALLEY 1973) by such a mechanism. Prostaglandin release could, therefore, be a factor in the local or remote secretory effects of invasive enteric bacterial infections from *Shigella, E. coli, Salmonella, Yersinia, Campylobacter,* and *Bacillus cereus.*

E. *Salmonella*

I. *Salmonella* Enteritis

POWELL et al. (1971) utilized the rat as a model for studying the effect of *Salmonella typhimurium* infection. In the infected animal with diarrhea, net ileal secretion of H_2O, Na, K, and Cl was observed which was accompanied by a 2–3-fold increase in protein content compared with the control animals. Abnormalities of mucosal histology were evident in this secretory inflamed region. GIANNELLA et al. (1973) demonstrated that mucosal invasion and inflammation were necessary prerequisites to the fluid secretory process. (Noninvasive strains produced neither inflammation nor fluid secretion.) Reduction of this mucosal (polymorphonuclear leukocyte) inflammatory response with nitrogen mustard administration ameliorated the fluid secretion in *Salmonella*-exposed animals; whereas, nitrogen mustard treatment did not inhibit cholera toxin-induced secretion nor alter ileal morphology nor mucosal disaccharidase activity (GIANNELLA 1979).

Studies by FROMM et al. (1974) clearly demonstrate that an invasive strain (TML) of *S. typhimurium* caused net chloride secretion and reduction in net sodium transport in the short-circuited state in the Ussing chamber. Glucose-facilitated Na absorption was intact. Addition of theophylline further stimulates Na transport with increased Cl secretion across TML-invaded mucosa. Thus, direct effects on mucosal cell transport are the cause of fluid secretion, albeit the mechanism for the secretory stimulus is poorly defined.

II. Role of Increased Capillary Hydrostatic Pressure and Transmucosal Permeability

The presence of a mucosal inflammatory reaction in association with *Salmonella* enteritis raised the possibility that in association with the ileocolitis of *Salmonella* invasion, altered permeability might occur and favor fluid transudation. KINSEY et al. (1976) examined this problem of increased intestinal permeability by studying the clearance of intravenously injected erythritol ^{14}C and mannitol ^{3}H in normal and *Salmonella*-infected rhesus monkeys. In the normal animals, a gradient of diminished permeability from jejunum to ileum to colon was observed for both erythritol and mannitol. Permeability, as measured by determining permeability coefficients, was not increased by *Salmonella* infection, and, in fact, was significantly reduced for erythritol in the jejunum of infected animals. Perfusion with hypertonic erythritol and mannitol produced similar streaming potentials (ΔPD) in control and infected animals, indicating that no significant differences in transmucosal permeability were evident.

III. Role for a *Salmonella* Enterotoxin

PETERSON and SANDAFEUR (1979) have advanced our understanding of *Salmonella*-induced fluid secretion. Earlier observation by GIANNELLA et al. (1973) concluded that epithelial cell invasion was correlated with the predisposition of *Salmonella* species to cause fluid secretion and diarrhea. Subsequently, MOLINA and PETERSON (1980) demonstrated an enterotoxic principle to be present. This was associated with the cell wall or outer cell membrane fraction and caused fluid loss when administered to infant mice and permeability changes in rabbit skin which could be blocked by both cholera antitoxin and GM1 ganglioside. The toxin was also detectable in the Chinese hamster ovary (CHO) cell assay system. Present evidence would, therefore, suggest that *Salmonella* species do elaborate a cholera-like enterotoxin, but even in the growth conditions employed in broth culture (incorporation of mitomycin C into culture medium), yields are exceedingly low compared with toxins produced by *Vibrio cholerae* and *E. coli* in similar culture media (MOLINA and PETERSON 1980). The pathophysiologic significance of the *Salmonella* toxin, therefore, is uncertain.

F. *Pseudomonas aeruginosa*

Pseudomonas aeroginosa was shown by KOBUTA and LIU (1971) to produce an enterotoxin which was both heat labile and protease sensitive. The role for the toxin in diarrheal disorders remains to be more clearly documented since this organism has not been identified as being a pathogenic species of great importance in the intestinal tract in humans. The main toxic features of *Pseudomonas aeruginosa* infection derives from septicemic spread and widespread release of the toxin which cause effects in reducing cardiac output and causing shock, hypotension, clotting abnormalities, and hepatocellular necrosis.

IGLEWSKI and KABAT (1975) recognized that this exotoxin resembled cholera toxin and *E. coli* LT in being an ADP-ribosyl transferase, causing protein synthesis inhibition in mammalian cells. The toxin has been purified and has been found to be a single-chain polypeptide of molecular weight 71,500 (POLLACK 1980). Its intestinal cellular effects are probably relatively unimportant in contrast to the general influence of this agent, but might be of importance when the organism occurs in the intestinal tract. No detailed study of its effects on intestinal mucosal transport has been made.

G. *Campylobacter fetus*

Campylobacter fetus jejuni and *C. fetus intestinalis* have been identified recently to cause up to 15% of unexplained diarrheal episodes, both sporadic and epidemic (BUTZLER and SKIRROW 1979). The organism has invasive characteristics, producing an enteritis and even a bacteremic spread. A stable toxin has been identified in some strains (BUTZLER and SKIRROW 1979). Its clinical disease pattern, however, closely resembles that of *Shigella* or *Salmonella* and it may well be that, when carefully studied, and enterotoxin may be detected and have a role in pathogenesis. Recently, a heat-labile enterotoxin has been identified which caused changes in the CHO cell assay which was blocked by cholera antitoxin. Antibody response to autologous *C. fetus jejuni* somatic antigen was observed during infections (RUIZ-PALACIOS et al. 1983).

H. *Yersinia enterocolitica*

Yersinia enterocolitica is recognized as an important cause of gastroenteritis in children and sporadically in adults (GUTMAN et al. 1973; BERGSTRAND and WINBLAD 1974). The most usual manifestation of the illness is an acute enterocolitis with acute terminal ileitis associated with fever and diarrhea as the chief symptoms. Animal models of this infection are available (CARTER 1975).

Production of enterotoxin, similar to *E. coli* ST, has been reported for *Y. enterocolitica* organisms (PAI and MORS 1978). Recently, OKAMOTO et al. (1981) purified a toxin from a culture filtrate of *Y. enterocolitica* by ethanol fractionation, protamine sulfate treatment, and gel column chromatography; 408-fold purification was achieved with a yield of 12%. The minimal effective dose of purified ST was about 110 ng in the suckling mouse assay; its molecular weight was 9,900. It retained its stability on heating to 100 °C for 20 min and to exposure to proteolytic enzymes. Two active fractions were identified. Antiserum from guinea pigs immunized with the purified ST neutralized the activity of both *Y. enterocolitica* ST and *E. coli* ST.

RAO et al. (1979) in FIELD's laboratory have obtained and purified an ST by methods similar to those used by them to obtain *E. coli* ST. Such a toxin was found to stimulate particulate guanylate cyclase activity, increase short-circuit current and inhibit active chloride transport in the isolated rabbit ileal mucosa. It is likely, therefore, that there may be a family of ST molecules, including those associated with *Y. enterocolitica, E. coli* ST, *Klebsiella pneumoniae,* and *Enterobacter cloacae* which all cause intestinal fluid secretion. Whether they all exert their effects by similar mechanisms is, at this time, unknown.

J. Noncoliform Enterobacteriaceae

I. *Klebsiella pneumoniae* Toxin

Enterotoxigenic material elaborated by *K. pneumoniae* is heat stable and has a molecular weight less than 10,000. KLIPSTEIN et al. (1975) demonstrated that crude extracts at concentrations of 2 mg/ml produced net secretion of water, sodium, and chloride in both jejunal and ileal segments of the rat: HCO_3 transport was unaffected. The toxin caused a depression of D-xylose absorption in both jejunum and ileum of the rat. It was similar to *E. coli* ST in causing secretion rapidly (within 30 min) and being heat stable. It has not been determined if its effects are mediated by activation of the guanylate cyclase system as has been shown for *E. coli* ST toxin.

II. *Enterobacter cloacae* Toxin

Enterobacter cloacae, an organism identified as causing acute diarrheal disease in children as well as associated with patients with tropical sprue, has been shown by KLIPSTEIN and ENGERT (1976) to produce a stable toxin in broth culture filtrate. It had a molecular weight in the range 1,000–10,000 and was stable to heating (100 °C for 30 min) and pH 1.0 as well as after incubation with pronase or trypsin. The toxin was characterized by causing fluid secretion in the perfused rat intestine model, but has not been fully purified or studied in vitro in the Ussing chamber.

III. *Aeromonas hydrophila* Toxin

Several reports have described *A. hydrophila* as a possible cause for acute diarrheal disease. LJUNGH et al. (1977) have recently studied 11 isolates, all of which were found to produce enterotoxin activity as determined by assay in the rabbit loop, Y_1 adrenal cell, and rabbit skin assay techniques. However, antisera to cholera and *E. coli* were unable to neutralize the *Aeromonas* enterotoxins in these assay systems. Further work, therefore, will be necessary to improve characterization of the toxin.

K. Food Poisoning Organisms

I. *Bacillus cereus* Toxin

Food poisoning by *B. cereus* is characterized by nausea and vomiting 1–5 h after ingestion or by abdominal pain and diarrhea 8–16 h later (TURNBULL 1976). The toxins described as associated with this organism are multiple and include, amongst others, a diarrheagenic toxin, vascular permeability factor, and dermonecrotic factor (TURNBULL 1976). TURNBULL et al. (1979) have produced evidence that all these effects are due to a single relatively unstable protein of molecular weight 50,000. The vascular permeability effect is closely related to the ligated rabbit ileal loop response. The toxin is also capable of causing severe tissue damage and, under some circumstances, activation of the adenylate cyclase system. Some strains possess, in addition, a hemolysin and phospholipase which may also exert deleterious effects on the bowel wall. The concentration of toxin produced by different strains in broth culture filtrate is variable. Further work will be necessary to characterize the mode of action of this toxin on mucosa more clearly.

II. Clostridial Toxin

Several clostridial species are now recognized to be frequent causes of food poisoning, intestinal colic, and diarrhea (BANWELL and SHERR 1973). *Clostridium perfringens* is the most widely distributed of these. Most human diseases are attributable to type A strains. An enterotoxin has been identified as being produced by some of these strains (DUNCAN and STRONG 1969) and studied in detail (MCDONEL 1974, 1979; MCDONEL and ASANO 1975; MCDONEL and MCCLANE 1979). Only recently, however, have studies defined more precisely the pathophysiologic features that result from *C. perfringens* enterotoxin exposure.

Results of intestinal transport studies reveal that there is a threshold of activity (>250 U) above which excess enterotoxin has no augmenting effect upon fluid secretory output. With exposure to toxin, net movement of water, sodium, and chloride are reversed to cause net fluid secretion into the lumen, while potassium and bicarbonate movement are unaffected. Glucose absorption occurs at reduced rates following exposure (MCDONEL 1974). Net secretion of sodium was a result of a significant increase in plasma–lumen unidirectional flux without change in lumen–plasma flux (MCDONEL and ASANO 1975).

The enterotoxin causes metabolic activity to decrease in exposed loops as judged by reduction in oxygen utilization and inhibition of O_2 consumption in rat mitochondria exposed to toxin. Toxin did not apparently change de novo protein synthesis, nor were changes in activity of cAMP detected (MCDONEL 1979). Morphological evidence favored the idea that the enterotoxin had a rapid (within 15–30 min) direct toxic effect on the microvillus membrane of the villus tip epithelial cells. As a result of this action, villus tip cells became damaged and underwent lysis, changes in organelles being secondary to cell wall destruction (MCDONEL and DUNCAN 1975). Lysis of cells was dependent on binding of the toxin, although binding occurred to both sensitive and insensitive Vero cells in culture (MCDONEL and MCCLANE 1979).

This enterotoxin has important differences compared with those of other toxins, such as Shiga, where membrane changes were more likely secondary to damage to intracellular metabolism of the cell itself. For *C. perfringens* toxin, a direct effect on membrane structure and function would appear to be the most likely manner of its initial effect, maximal in the ileum (MCDONEL and DUNCAN 1977). Electron microscopic changes show early deformation of microvilli with bleb formation of the surface cytoplasm (MCDONEL 1979).

L. *Staphylococcus*

Staphylococcal enterotoxins are proteins produced by the *Staphylococcus* in foods and in culture media. Their ingestion by humans causes food-borne illness or staphylococcal food poisoning associated with vomiting and diarrhea, occurring 2–6 h after ingestion (BANWELL and SHERR 1973). Four staphylococcal enterotoxins have been identified (A, B, C, D) (BERGDOLL et al. 1974). The structure of B has been elucidated to be a 239 amino acid polypeptide chain with molecular weight of 28,494 (HUANG andBERGDOLL 1970). The toxins are heat stable and resemble each other in COOH and NH_2 terminal amino acid structure (BERGDOLL et al. 1974). All four have been found to be associated with food poisoning and enteritis.

Pure B toxin has been shown to reverse net fluid secretion in the rat upper intestine (SULLIVAN 1969; SULLIVAN and ASANO 1971). No change occurred in PD in vivo of I_{sc} or resistance in vitro; and rapid reversal of effects occurred after removal of toxin from the infusate or bathing media. It was concluded that the enterotoxin caused a nonelectrogenic secretory stimulus to the small bowel mucosa, leaving the absorptive mechanism intact. Recent studies with the D toxin by O'BRIEN et al. (1978) have demonstrated that, at least with this toxin, inhibition of water transport in the guinea pig ileum accompanied elevation of the cAMP content in tissue. D toxin was unable to cause cAMP changes in Y_1 adrenal cells of CHO cells. In other recent studies D toxin caused an immediate rise in PD and I_{sc} and the extent and direction of the response increased with toxin concentration. In addition, the unidirectional fluxes of sodium and chloride were increased such that net sodium secretion occurred. Evidence, therefore, favored the concept that cAMP elevation was a secondary phenomenon and that secretion most probably reflected the ability of the D toxin to augment intercellular ionic movement.

M. Additional Mechanisms for Toxin-Mediated Permeation Defects

I. Evidence for a Role for Calcium

Increasing the intracellular calcium concentration mimicked the effect of cAMP and caused active electrolyte secretion. BOLTON and FIELD (1977) demonstrated in rabbit ileum and FRIZZELL (1977) in rabbit colon that the calcium ionophore A23187, which acutely increases intracellular calcium, caused chloride secretion and inhibited neutral sodium chloride absorption. Moreover, serosal calcium was essential for the secretory effect of carbamylcholine-induced rabbit ileal secretion. Removal of serosal calcium inhibited the secretory effect of serotonin (5-hydroxytryptamine) on short-circuit current and its stimulation of sodium chloride secretion (DONOWITZ et al. 1977). To date no bacteriologic agents, similar in their effect to carbamylcholine or serotonin, have been identified to have their effect by such a calcium-dependent system. However, the cellular response to messenger substances is an integrated function and the function and metabolism of cAMP, prostaglandins, and calcium are related (CHEUNG 1980). These three systems may function independently or they may modulate or antagonize the effects of each other. Thus, interaction with calcium is a likely feature of toxin activity.

II. Filtration Secretion

The small intestine may secrete large amounts of water and electrolytes by processes that do not depend on active solute excretion, but on passive filtration secretion resulting from excessive accumulation of fluid within the mucosal interstitium (YABLONSKI and LIFSON 1976). Present evidence does not favor the idea that filtration pressure would cause fluid secretion in the absence of changes in hydraulic permeability. Very high hydrostatic pressure gradients (> 380 mm Hg) would be necessary to cause fluid secretion under conditions of normal small intestinal permeability (0.3 ml l $mosmol^{-1}$). However, where mucosal permeability is increased, such mechanisms might have direct relevance to fluid transport in the small intestine in response to enterotoxins. Recent studies of the mechanism for this process suggest that filtration secretion is readily reversible and is mediated by an alteration in plasma oncotic pressure (HAKIM and LIFSON 1969; DUFFY et al. 1978). Disruption of the mucosal membrane is a necessary concomitant to allow extravasation of fluid into the intestinal lumen following transcapillary exchange into the mucosa. Such a mechanism may depend on the loss of actual cells at the villus tip or be associated with widening of intercellular channels. During filtration secretion induced by hydrostatic pressure, the secreted fluid contains amounts of plasma protein up to 50% of the plasma concentration. Secretion caused by volume expansion, however, is relatively devoid of plasma protein, probably in part the result of concurrent dilution of mucosal interstitial proteins.

There is no information available concerning filtration secretion resulting from exposure to bacterial toxins. Histamine infusion, however, has been shown to induce vasodilation, increase capillary permeability, and cause copious intestinal secretion after arterial injection (LEE and SILVERBERG 1976). Evidence favors the idea that the action of histamine is mediated through increase in tissue fluid in the mucosal interstitium. Thus, it is not improbable that toxins which cause tissue damage and inflammation might either cause release from mast cells of histamine or have effects on capillary blood flow and permeability that parallel effects of histamine.

It is clear from this review of toxin action that a variety of enterotoxins may be elaborated by coliform and other enteric organisms. Some toxins, such as CT and *E. coli* LT have very similar modes of action. It is already known, however, that several stable toxins are elaborated which are of different composition and the toxins may have an effect on the surface membrane of the cell and also, perhaps, play a facilitatory role during cell attack by invasive organisms. Future studies and purification of toxins from bacterial organisms will certainly bring about greater understanding of their action at the molecular level on the intestinal mucosal cell.

References

Al-Awqati Q, Wallace CK, Greenough WB (1972) Stimulation of intestinal secretion in vitro by culture filtrates of *Escherichia coli*. J Infect Dis 125:300–303

Alderete JF, Robertson DC (1978) Purification and chemical characterization of the heat stable enterotoxin produced by porcine strains of enterotoxigenic *Escherichia coli*. Infect Immun 19:1021–1030

Banwell JG, Sherr H (1973) Effect of bacterial enterotoxins on the gastrointestinal tract. Gastroenterology 65:467–497

Bergdoll MS, Huang IY, Schantz EJ (1974) Chemistry of the staphylococcal enterotoxins. J Agric Food Chem 22:9–13

Bergstrand CG, Winblad S (1974) Clinical manifestations of infection with *Yersinia enterocolitica* in children. Acta Paediatr Scand 63:875–877

Bolton J, Field M (1977) Ca ionophore-stimulation ion secretion in rabbit ileal mucosa: relation to action of 3′,5′-AMs and carbamylcholine. J Membr Biol 35:159–173

Brown JE, Ussery MA, Leppla SH, Rothman SW (1980) Inhibition of protein synthesis by Shiga toxin. Activation of the toxin and inhibition of peptide elongation. FEBS Let 117:84–88

Butzler JP, Skirrow MB (1979) Campylobacter enteritis. Clin Gastroenterol 8:737–765

Cantey JR, Blake RK (1980) Diarrhea due to *E. coli* in the rabbit: a novel mechanism. J Infect Dis 136:640–648

Carter PB (1975) Animal model of human disease. Yersinia enteritis: animal model: oral *Yersinia enterocolitica* infection of mice. Am J Pathol 81:703–706

Cheung WY (1980) Calmodulin plays a pivotal role in cellular regulation. Science 207:19–27

Clements JD, Finkelstein RA (1979) Isolation and characterization of homogenous heat-labile enterotoxins with high specific activity for *Escherichia coli* culture. Infect Immun 24:760–769

Donowitz M, Keusch GT, Binder HJ (1975) Effect of Shigella enterotoxin on electrolyte transport in rabbit ileum. Gastroenterology 69:1230–1237

Donowitz M, Charney AN, Heffernan JM (1977) Effect of serotonin treatment on intestinal transport in the rabbit. Am J Physiol 232:E85–E94

Dorner F, Hughes C, Nahler G, Hogenauer G (1979) *Escherichia coli* heat labile enterotoxin: DNA-directed in vitro synthesis and structure. Proc Natl Acad Sci USA 76:4832–4836

Duffy DA, Granger DN, Taylor AE (1978) Intestinal secretion induced by volume expansion in the dog. Gastroenterology 75:413–418

Duncan CL, Strong DH (1969) Experimental production of diarrhea in rabbits with *Clostridium perfringens*. Can J Microbiol 15:765–770

Eade MN, Giannella RA (1978) Effect of purified *E. coli* heat-stable enterotoxin (ST) on intestinal transport and possible mechanism of action. Gastroenterology 74:1121

Enomoto K, Gill DM (1980) Cholera toxin activation of adenylate cyclase. Roles of nucleoside triphosphates and a macromolecular factor in the ADP ribosylation of the GTP-dependent regulatory component. J Biol Chem 255:1252–1258

Field M (1974) Intestinal secretion. Gastroenterology 66:1063–1084

Field M (1979) Mechanisms of action of cholera and *Escherichia coli* enterotoxins. Am J Clin Nutr 32:189–196

Field M, Graf LH Jr, Laird WJ, Smith PL (1978) Heat-stable enterotoxin of *Escherichia coli*: in vitro effects on guanylate cyclase activity, cyclic GMP concentration and ion transport in small intestine. Proc Natl Acad Sci USA 75:2800–2804

Frizzell RA (1977) Active chloride secretion by rabbit colon: Calcium dependent stimulation by ionophore A23187. J Membr Biol 35:175–187

Fromm D, Giannella RA, Formal SB, Quijano R, Collins H (1974) Ion transport across isolated ileal mucosa invaded by Salmonella. Gastroenterology 66:215–225

Gangarosa EJ, Merson MH (1977) Epidemiological assessment of the relevance of the so-called enteropathogenic serogroups of *Escherichia coli* in diarrhea. N Engl J Med 296:1210–1218

Giannella RA (1976) Suckling mouse model for detection of heat-stable *Escherichia coli* enterotoxin: characteristics of the model. Infect Immun 14:95–99

Giannella RA (1979) Importance of the intestinal inflammatory reaction in Salmonella-mediated intestinal secretion. Infect Immun 23:140–145

Giannella RA, Drake KW (1979) Effect of purified *Escherichia coli* heat-stable enterotoxin on intestinal cyclic nucleotide metabolism and fluid secretion. Infect Immun 24:19–23

Giannella RA, Formal SB, Dammin GJ, Collins H (1973) Pathogenesis of Salmonellosis. Studies of fluid secretion, mucosal invasion and morphologic reaction in the rabbit ileum. J Clin Invest 52:441–453

Gill DM (1976) The arrangement of subunits in cholera toxin. Biochemistry 15:1242–1248

Guerrant RL, Ganguly U, Casper AGT, Moore EJ, Pierce NF, Carpenter CCJ (1973) Effect of *Escherichia coli* on fluid transport across canine small bowel. Mechanism and time-course with enterotoxin and whole bacterial cells. J Clin Invest 52:1707–1714

Gutman LT, Ottesen EA, Quan TJ, Noce PS, Katz SL (1973) An interfamilial outbreak of *Yersinia enterocolitica* enteritis. N Engl J Med 288:1372–1376

Gyles CL (1974) Relationship among heat-labile enterotoxins of *Escherichia coli* and *Vibrio cholerae*. J Infect Dis 129:277–283

Hakim AA, Lifson N (1969) Effects of pressure on water and solute transport by dog intestinal mucosa in vitro. Am J Physiol 216:276–284

Holmgren J (1973) Comparison of the tissue receptor for *Vibrio cholerae* and *Escherichia coli* enterotoxins by means of ganglioside and natural cholera toxoid. Infect Immun 8:851–859

Holmgren J, Lonnroth I (1980) Structure and function of enterotoxins and their receptors. Cholera and Ralated Diarrheas. 43rd Nobel Symp. Stockholm 1978. Karger, Basel, pp 88–103

Huang IY, Bergdoll MS (1970) The primary structure of staphylococcal enterotoxin B. Isolation, composition and sequence of tryptic peptides from oxidized enterotoxin B. J Biol Chem 245:3493–3510

Hughes JM, Murad F, Chang B, Guerrant RL (1978) Role of cyclic GMP in the action of heat-stable enterotoxin of *Escherichia coli*. Nature 271:755–756

Iglewski BH, Kabat D (1975) NAD dependent inhibition of protein synthesis by *Pseudomonas aeruginosa* toxin. Proc Natl Acad Sci USA 72:2284–2288

Isaacson RE, Fusco PC, Brinton CC, Moon HW (1978) In vitro adhesion of *Escherichia coli* to porcine small intestinal epithelial cells: pili as adhesive factors. Infect Immun 21:392–397

Jones GW, Rutter JM (1972) Role of K88 antigen in the pathogenesis of neonatal diarrhea caused by *Escherichia coli* in the piglet. Infect Immun 6:918

Keusch GT, Jacewicz M (1977) Pathogenesis of Shigella diarrhea. VII. Evidence for a cell membrane toxin receptor involving Beta 1→4-linked *N*-acetyl-D-glucosamine oligomers. J Exp Med 146:535–546

Keusch GT, Grady GF, Maja LJ, McIver J (1972) The pathogenesis of Shigella diarrhea. I. Enterotoxin production by *Shigella dysenteriae* 1. J Clin Invest 51:1212–1218

Kinsey MD, Dammin GJ, Formal SB, Giannella RA (1976) The role of altered intestinal permeability in the pathogenesis of Salmonella diarrhea in the rhesus monkey. Gastroenterology 71:429–434

Klipstein FA, Engert RF (1976) Partial purification and properties of *Enterobacter cloacae* haet-stable enterotoxin. Infect Immun 13:1307–1314

Klipstein FA, Horowitz IR, Engert RF, Schenk EA (1975) Effect of *Klebsiella pneumoniae* enterotoxin. J Clin Invest 56:799–807

Klipstein FA, Rowe B, Engert RF, Short HB, Gross RJ (1978) Enterotoxigenicity of enteropathogenic serotypes of *Escherichia coli* isolated from infants with epidemic diarrhea. Infect Immun 21:171–178

Kubota Y, Liu PV (1971) An enterotoxin of *Pseudomonas aeruginosa*. J Infect Dis 123:97–98

Lee JS, Silverberg JW (1976) Effect of histamine on intestinal fluid secretion in the dog. Am J Physiol 231:793–798

Levin MM, DuPont HL, Formal SB, Hornick RB, Takeuchi A, Gangarosa EJ, Snyder MJ, Libonati JP (1973) Pathogenesis of *Shigella dysenteriae* 1 (Shiga) dysentery. J Infect Dis 127:261–270

Levine MM, Naline DR, Hornick RB, Bergquist E, Waterman DH, Young CR, Sotman S, Rowe B (1978) *Escherichia coli* strains cause diarrhea but do not produce heat labile or heat stable enterotoxins and are non-invasive. Lancet I:1119–1122

Ligumsky M, Karmeli F, Sharon P, Zor U, Cohen F, Rachmilewitz D (1980) Enhanced thromboxane A_2 and prostacyclin production by cultured rectal mucosa in ulcerative colitis and its inhibition by steroids and sulfasalazine. Gastroenterology 78:1209

Ljungh A, Popoff M, Wadstrom T (1977) *Aeromonas hydrophila* in acute diarrheal disease: detection of enterotoxin and biotyping of strains. J Clin Microbiol 6:96–100

McDonel JL (1974) In vivo effects of *Clostridium perfringens* enteropathogenic factors on the rat ileum. Infect Immun 10:1156–1162
McDonel JL (1979) The molecular mode of action of *Clostridium perfringens* enterotoxin. Am J Clin Nutr 32:210–218
McDonel JL, Asano T (1975) Analysis of unidirectional fluxes of sodium during diarrhea induced by *Clostridium perfringens* enterotoxin in the rat terminal ileum. Infect Immun 11:526–529
McDonel JL, Duncan CL (1975) Histopathological effect of *Clostridium perfringens* enterotoxin in the rabbit ileum. Infect Immun 12:1214–1218
McDonel JL, Duncan CL (1977) Regional localization of activity of *Clostridium perfringens* Type A enterotoxin in the rabbit ileum, jejunum, and duodenum. J Infect Dis 136:661–666
McDonel JL, McClane BA (1979) Binding versus biological activity of *Clostridium perfringens*. Biochem Biophys Res Commun 87:497–504
Matuchansky C, Bernier J-J (1973) Effect of prostaglandin E_1 on glucose, water, and electrolyte absorption in the human jejunum. Gastroenterology 64:1111–1118
Mennie AT, Dalley V (1973) Aspirin in radiation induced diarrhea. Lancet I:1131
Molina NC, Peterson JW (1980) Cholera toxin-like toxin released by *Salmonella* species in the presence of Mitomycin C. Infect Immun 30:224–230
Moon HW, Isaacson RE, Pohlenz J (1979) Mechanisms of association of enteropathogenic *Escherichia coli* with intestinal epithelium. Am J Clin Nutr 32:119–127
Moss J, Richardson SH (1978) Activation of adenylate cyclase by heat-labile *Escherichia coli* enterotoxin. Evidence for ADP-ribosyltransferase activity similar to that of choleragen. J Clin Invest 62:281–285
O'Brien AD, Thompson MR, Gemski P, Doctor BP, Formal SB (1977) Biological properties of *Shigella flexneri 2A* toxin and its serological relationship to Shigella dysenteriae 1 toxin. Infect Immun 15:796–798
O'Brien AD, McClung HJ, Kapral FA (1978) Increased tissue conductance and ion transport in guinea pig ileum after exposure to *Staphylococcus aureus* delta-toxin in vitro. Infect Immun 21:102–113
O'Brien AD, Gentry MK, Thompson MR, Doctor BP, Gemski DP, Formal SB (1979) Shigellosis and *Escherichia coli* diarrhea: relative importance of invasive and toxigenic mechanisms. Am J Clin Nutr 32:229–233
Okamoto K, Inque T, Ichikawa H, Kawamoto Y, Miyama A (1981) Partial purification and characterization of heat-stable enterotoxin produced by *Yersinia enterocolitica*. Infect Immun 31:554–559
Olsnes S, Eiklid K (1980) Isolation and characterization of *Shigella Shigae* cytotoxin. J Biol Chem 255:284–289
Pai CH, Mors V (1978) Production of enterotoxin by *Yersinia enterocolitica*. Infect Immun 19:908–911
Peterson JW, Sandafeur PD (1979) Evidence of a role for permeability factors in the pathogenesis of Salmonellosis. Am J Clin Nutr 32:197–209
Pierce NF, Carpenter CCJ, Elliott HL, Greenough WB (1971) Effect of prostaglandins, theophylline, and cholera exotoxin upon transmucosal water and electrolyte movement in the canine jejunum. Gastroenterology 60:22–32
Pollack M (1980) *Pseudomonas aeruginosa* Exotoxin A. N Engl J Med 302:1360–1361
Powell DW, Plotkin GR, Maenza RM, Solberg LI, Catlin DH, Formal SB (1971) Experimental diarrhea. I. Intestinal water and electrolyte transport in rat salmonella enterocolitis. Gastroenterology 60:1053–1064
Racusen LC, Binder HJ (1980) Effect of prostaglandin on ion transport across isolated colonic mucosa. Dig Dis Sci 25:900–904
Rao MC, Guandalini S, Laird WJ, Field M (1979) Effects of heat-stable enterotoxin of *Yersinia enterocolitica* on ion transport and cyclic guanosine 3′,5′-monophosphate metabolism in rabbit ileum. Infect Immun 26:875–878
Ruiz-Palacios GM, Torres NI, Ruiz-Palacios BR, Torres J, Escamilla E, Tamayo J (1983) Lancet 2:250–252

Schmid WC, Phillips SF, Summerskill WHJ (1969) Jejunal secretion of electrolyte and water in non tropical sprue. J Lab Clin Med 73:772–783

Sellwood R, Gibbons RA, Jones GW, Rutter JM (1975) Adhesion of enteropathogenic *Escherichia coli* to pig intestinal brush borders: the existence of two pig phenotypes. J Med Microbiol 8:405–411

Sharon P, Ligumsky M, Rachmilewitz D, Zor U (1978) Role of prostaglandins in ulcerative colitis. Enhanced production during active disease and inhibition by sulfasalazine. Gastroenterology 75:638–640

Smith PL, Blumberg JB, Stoff JS, Field M (1981) Antisecretory effects on indomethacin on rabbit ileal mucosa in vitro. Gastroenterology 80:356–365

Spicer EK, Kavanaugh WM, Dallas WS, Falkow S, Konigsberg WH, Schafer DE (1981) Sequence homologies between A subunits of *Escherichia coli* and *Vibrio cholerae* enterotoxins. Proc Natl Acad Sci USA 78:50–54

Staples SJ, Asher SE, Giannella RA (1980) Purification and characterization of heat-stable enterotoxin produced by a strain of *E. coli* pathogenic for man. J Biol Chem 255:4716–4721

Sullivan R Sr (1969) Effects of enterotoxin B on intestinal transport in vitro. Proc Soc Exp Biol Med 131:1159–1162

Sullivan R, Asano T (1971) Effects of staphylococcal enterotoxin B on intestinal transport in the rat. Am J Physiol 220:1793–1797

Takeuchi A, Inman LR, O'Hanley PD, Cantey JR, Lushbaugh WB (1978) Scanning and transmission electron microscopic study of *Escherichia coli* 015 (RDEC-1) enteric infection in rabbits. Infect Immun 19:686–694

Tulloch EF Jr, Ryan KJ, Formal SB, Franklin FA (1973) Invasive enteropathic *Escherichia coli* dysentery. An outbreak in 28 adults. Ann Intern Med 79:13–17

Turnbull PCB (1976) Studies on the production of enterotoxins by *Bacillus cereus*. J Clin Pathol 29:941–948

Turnbull PCB, Kramer JM, Jorgensen K, Gilbert RJ, Melling J (1979) Properties and production characteristics of vomiting, diarrheal and necrotizing toxins of *Bacillus cereus*. Am J Clin Nutr 32:219–228

Ulshen MH, Rollo JL (1980) Pathogenesis of *Escherichia coli* gastroenteritis in man – another mechanism. N Engl J Med 302:99–101

Yablonski ME, Lifson N (1976) Mechanism of production of intestinal secretion by elevated venous pressure. J Clin Invest 57:904–915

CHAPTER 28

Mechanisms of Action of Laxative Drugs

G. W. GULLIKSON and P. BASS

A. Introduction

Laxatives are drugs which are used to increase the frequency of bowel movements in response to a real or perceived need. The number of stools per individual in a normal population ranges from three per day to three per week (CONNELL et al. 1965). While healthy gastrointestinal function lies within these wide limits, the belief of the laity that there is a need for a bowel movement a day is as prevalent now as it was several generations ago. The major use for laxatives is on a self-medicating basis. Use of such drugs is in response to this perceived need for a daily bowel movement, a change in the accustomed frequency, a vague feeling of malaise, or the constant exposure to various media advertisements. Sales of laxatives in the United States amounted to $ 306 million in 1979 (ANONYMOUS 1980). The major portion of this amount represented over-the-counter sales with the remaining consumption accounted for by direct use of these drugs in medical practice. Their use in medicine is most commonly in preparation for diagnostic procedures, before and after intestinal surgery, and in the prevention of complications in diseases in which straining at the stool is to be avoided.

Laxatives have been used throughout history in the form of herbal and folk remedies. Claims have been made for their efficacy in the treatment of numerous diseases unrelated to the gastrointestinal tract. These claims extend even to the present day in the belief that, because of its laxative action, dietary fiber will be useful in the prevention of diseases as diverse as diabetes and varicose veins (BURKITT and TROWELL 1975). The search for the mechanisms of laxative action have evolved throughout history from superstition to empiricism and in recent years to scientific evaluation.

The present concepts of laxative action are in contrast to the confusing traditional classification and subdivision of the laxatives derived from empirical observations. This classification mixes chemical jargon (wetting agent) with terms implying biologic activity (irritant) and in vitro physicochemical properties (osmotic). Unfortunately, this irrational nomenclature has been reinforced by standard textbooks (FINGL 1975; BONNYCASTLE 1965), handbooks (DARLINGTON 1973), and even advisory panels to the United States Food and Drug Administration (FDA) (OVER THE COUNTER DRUGS 1975). In recent years, however, a more scientific approach has been taken in an attempt to understand the mechanisms of laxative action.

An initial scientific approach was made by PHILLIPS et al. (1965). They noted that drugs like phenolphthalein, ricinoleic acid, and anthraquinone may alter specific cellular activity of the enzyme Na^+, K^+-ATPase. PHILLIPS suggested that "...the classical concept of cathartic action by a simple irritation with enhanced peristalsis must be re-evaluated and the probability of very specific mechanisms must be entertained." In Germany, FORTH, RUMMEL and colleagues independently recognized that the laxatives deoxycholate and oxyphenisatin exerted specific pharmacologic effects on the mucosa of the intestinal tract (FORTH et al. 1963, 1966 a, b; see Chap. 29).

The purpose of this chapter is to present the evidence for the modern theories of the actions of laxatives on the gastrointestinal tract. One of the key modern concepts is that laxatives can exert many of their actions on the small intestine in producing laxation. The development of supportive evidence has greatly accelerated in recent years and is frequently in conflict with preconceived ideas about laxative action which have evolved from their medical use.

The laxative group of drugs contains a wide variety of structurally dissimilar chemicals (Fig. 1) ranging from poorly absorbable inorganic electrolytes (e.g., magnesium sulfate) to plant and synthetic fiber and a variety of organic compounds which are either chemically synthesized or isolated from natural sources. In addition to exogenous laxatives, substances present in the gastrointestinal tract during pathologic malabsorption are implicated in several clinically observed syndromes characterized by diarrhea. These endogenous "laxatives" include the dihydroxy bile acids (WINGATE et al. 1973) and hydroxylated fatty acids (AMMON and PHILLIPS 1974), the latter structurally similar to ricinoleic acid, the active component of castor oil.

Recent evidence indicates that many of the laxatives or laxative-like agents are associated with two distinct effects on the gastrointestinal tract; an accumulation of fluid in the lumen of the small and large intestines and a laxative-induced smooth muscle electric and motor pattern in the small bowel. While data demonstrating these two effects have not been collected for all laxatives, evidence is substantial that many laxatives act by both of these mechanisms. Though it has been suggested (BINDER 1977) that fluid secretion is responsible for laxation, the specific contribution of motility to the movement of the fluid contents has not been studied to the same degree as the fluid-secretory processes. There is evidence that bacterial toxins can produce small intestinal smooth muscle electric and motor activity *before* eliciting fluid secretion (MATHIAS et al. 1980). It is not known whether laxatives may induce similar motor changes prior to their effects on fluid movement. In addition to these two distinct actions of laxatives on fluid movement and motility, laxatives may produce quantitatively different responses in these two parameters for the small and large intestines. Regional differences within either of the intestinal organs probably also exist adding further complexity in the response to laxative drugs.

B. Intestinal Tract Smooth Muscle Response to Laxatives

Laxatives alter the functions of the gastrointestinal tract, leading to diarrhea. One of these altered functions is the smooth muscle electric activity and therefore intestinal contractile activity. Intestinal smooth muscle is composed of an outer

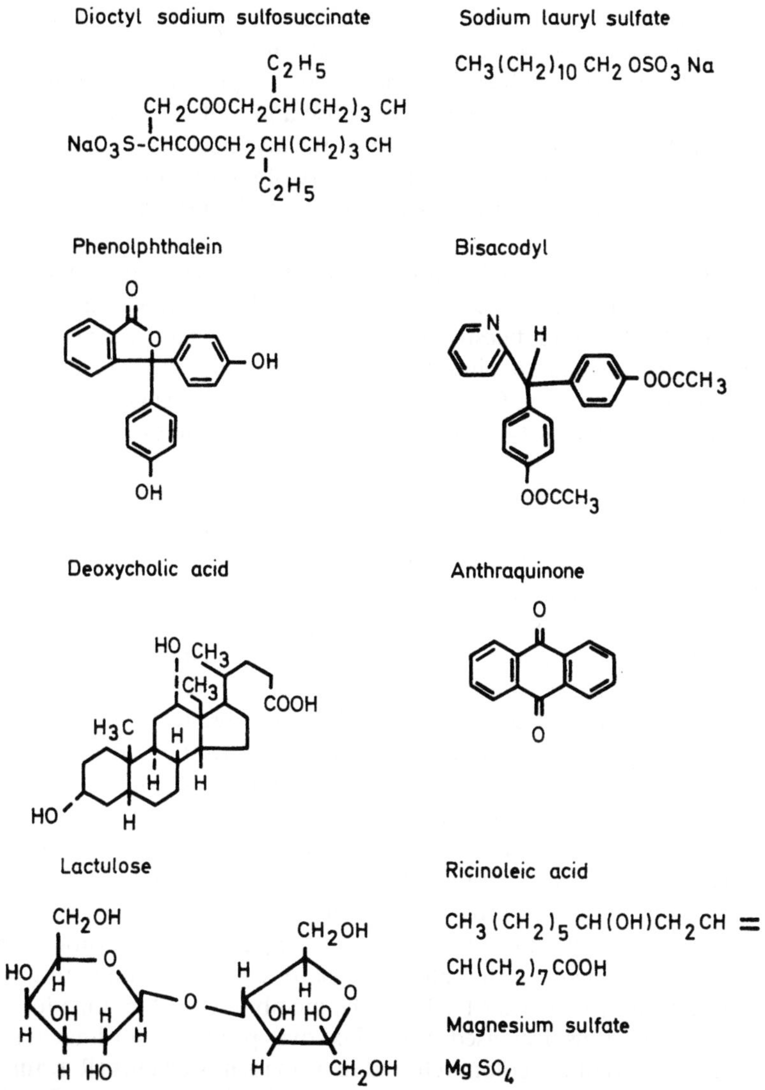

Fig. 1. Diverse structures of laxatives

(longitudinal) and inner (circular) layer. The longitudinal muscle generates a cyclic electric pattern referred to as the basic electric rhythm (BER). The frequency of the BER determines the maximal frequency of contractions which may occur on either the stomach or small intestine. A gradient in the BER rate exists along the intestine. Theoretically this gradient of BER creates a contractile gradient which permits the movement of luminal contents in the caudad direction. The rate of transit is dependent on the total contractile activity along the intestine. The percentage of BER potentials associated with spike potential bursts (contractions) or their organization into a discernible pattern can be altered by such factors as feeding state, nerve stimulation, or drug treatment.

The electric activity of the colon is qualitatively different from that of the small intestine. The myoelectric signals are extremely variable in frequency, amplitude, and the degree to which BER potentials are present with observed spike potentials. Studies to elucidate colonic electric and motor responses to laxative drugs are lacking owing to the complexity of the myoelectric and motor patterns. Further information concerning electric activity of the gastrointestinal tract may be found in several reviews (BASS 1967; DUTHIE 1974; BORTOFF 1976; WINGATE 1981).

Drug effects on intact small intestinal smooth muscle frequently depend on the feeding state of the animal. There are two physiologic states of muscle activity, interdigestive (fasted) and digestive (fed), each exhibiting distinctive electric and motor properties of the gastrointestinal tract in humans and several laboratory species (SZURSZEWSKI 1969; CARLSON et al. 1970; VAN TRAPPEN et al. 1977). In animals, this muscle activity may be recorded in the unanesthetized state with chronically implanted serosal electrodes and transducers (MCCOY and BASS 1963; BASS and WILEY 1972). In the interdigestive state in humans and dogs (Fig. 2), a distinctive pattern of approximately 40–60 min of quiescence (basal, phase I) is followed by intermittent activity (preburst, phase II) for 20–30 min which terminates in a high amplitude maximal activity (burst, phase III) for 10–20 min (CARLSON et al. 1970). This cycle repeats itself approximately every 2 h in the fasted state. It originates in the upper gastrointestinal tract and migrates down the small intestine. When the entire complex sweeps the tract, it is referred to as the migrating myoelectric complex (SZURSZEWSKI 1969). The digestive state is initiated by feeding and is characterized by its own distinctive electric and motor patterns (CARLSON et al. 1970). The spike potentials, the electric counterparts to contractile activity, occur randomly (Fig. 2) during the fed state. Laxatives will produce differing effects on muscle activity, depending on whether they are administered in basal interdigestive or the active digestive states (STEWART et al. 1975 b).

Traditionally, certain laxatives have been classified as having a stimulant effect on intestinal motility (BONNYCASTLE 1965). Implicit in this classification is the belief that laxatives increase the rate of transit of chyme by stimulating motility above that normally seen after feeding. The membrane contact time for the absorption of fluid is thus decreased. While laxatives produce coordinated motility patterns in portions of the colon, referred to as mass movements (RITCHIE 1972), recent evidence indicates that these drugs do not stimulate and may in fact depress motor activity elsewhere in the gastrointestinal tract.

Isolated intestinal smooth muscle studies verify that indeed laxatives like anthraquinones (LATVEN et al. 1952) and sodium ricinoleate (STEWART et al. 1975 a) or other surfactants (GAGINELLA et al. 1975 b) do depress contractility. Surprisingly, specificity of activity was obtained for the depressant effect of ricinoleate since its *trans* isomer, sodium ricinelaidate, was without activity. Similarly, the sodium salts of oleate (a common dietary fatty acid), linoleate, 12-hydroxystearate, and elaidate were nondepressant in the concentrations used. The structurally related abilities of fatty acid derivatives to inhibit smooth muscle activity paralleled their abilities to affect luminal fluid movement (GAGINELLA et al. 1975 a). Dioctylsodium sulfosuccinate (DSS), sodium dodecylsulfate (SDS), and several bile salts, can also depress the electrically driven guinea pig ileum over the same

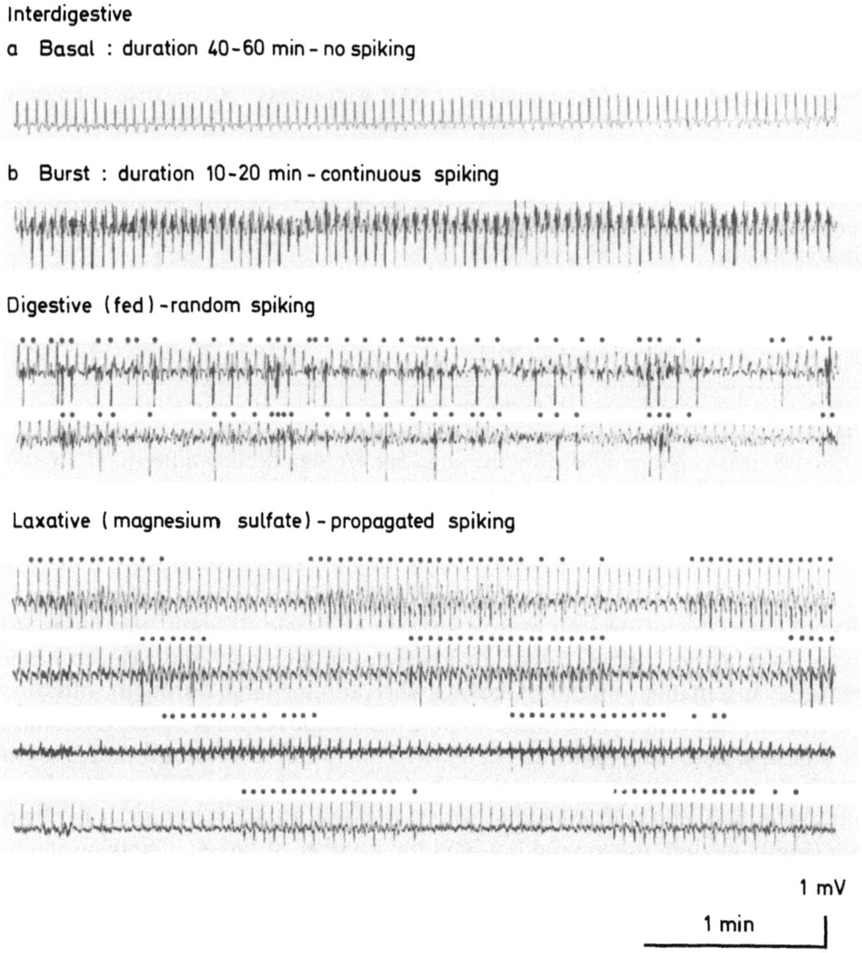

Fig. 2. Three electric patterns recorded from the canine small intestine. Each of the electromyograms consists of two electric components; the basic electric rhythm (BER), a cyclic depolarization of the muscle; and bursts of spike potentials, the intestinal muscle electric correlate of contraction. In several of the electromyograms, bursts of spike potentials are marked with *dots* to emphasize the patterns. Note the distinctive nature of the interdigestive (basal–burst) patterns, recorded on separate channels, digestive (fed) pattern recorded simultaneously from two sites 4 cm apart and laxative-induced pattern recorded simultaneously from four sites equally distanced over approximately 20 cm jejunum. Also note the random nature of the digestive pattern which contrasts with the progressive pattern induced by magnesium sulfate. Basal is also known as phase I and burst as phase III

narrow concentration range required for the depressant action of ricinoleate (GAGINELLA et al. 1975b). These latter smooth muscle depressants similarly caused luminal fluid accumulation. In addition to these laxatives, magnesium ion is also known to depress smooth muscle activity (BELESLIN 1970). In vitro depression of smooth muscle activity with a variety of laxatives is in contrast to the traditional idea of a direct stimulatory effect of these drugs on smooth muscle.

Table 1. The number of spike potentials produced during a 2-h interval: a comparison of interdigestive, digestive, and drug states (adapted from ATCHISON et al. 1978a)

Drug condition	Mean number of BER with bursts of spike potentials[a] generated in 2 h after dosing (± standard error)[b]	Comparison of means by Duncan's range test[c]		
Interdigestive (fasted)	413.6 ± 67.3	|		
Phenolphthalein[d]	478.3 ± 85.2	|	|	
NaCl (0.9%)[d]	565.4 ± 63.5	|	|	|
Magnesium sulfate[d]	623.0 ± 78.4	|	|	|
Castor oil[d]	707.8 ± 115.3		|	|
Digestive (fed)	846.5 ± 72.4			|

[a] Each burst of spike potentials is the electric counterpart of a contraction
[b] Each mean represents the average of two replicates at two sites for four animals
[c] Any two means not paralleled by the same line are significantly different ($P<0.05$)
[d] Administered during the start of the basal period of the interdigestive state

In vivo, drugs like the laxatives can be administered during either of the two physiologic states of smooth muscle activity and yield different responses. At a given dose, either castor oil or magnesium sulfate may increase contractile frequency in a manner similar to feeding when administered during the interdigestive (fasted) state and, yet, exhibit no pharmacologic response when given during the digestive (fed) state (STEWART et al. 1975b). Table 1 indicates the effect of simply counting the number of contractions (represented by the BER with spike potentials) at a given small intestinal site of the dog. In a 2-h period, it is obvious that simply feeding the animal doubled the number of bursts of spike potentials (413 versus 846). The data on the laxatives in Table 1 can thus be interpreted as: (a) an increase in activity when the drug is given during the interdigestive state; (b) a decrease in activity when compared with the digestive state; or (c) on a statistical basis, no significant change, especially if compared with dosing the animal with a saline solution.

In diarrheal states produced by laxatives, bacterial toxins, or prostaglandins, the absolute number of contractions may not be important. Rather, the *pattern* of contractile activity may be the key electric or motor component of diarrhea. A number of reports of migrating spike potential activity after diarrhea-inducing stimuli have been made (MATHIAS et al. 1976, 1977, 1978; ATCHISON et al. 1978 a, b; BURNS et al. 1978, 1980). The laxatives studied to date demonstrate this unique electric pattern which is shown in Fig. 2. This laxative-induced pattern consists of recurrent bursts of 3–15 spike potentials that presumably sweep the bowel of its contents. The pattern has been observed with laxatives of a diverse chemical nature, including magnesium sulfate, castor oil, and phenolphthalein. This recurring pattern has been recorded for up to 48 h for castor oil, disrupting normal fasted electric activity. This activity, organized as a caudad-directed pattern in the small intestine, presumably facilitates movement of fluid into the colon where absorptive capacity is exceeded or fluid secretion may be occurring. The reduced number of contractions (when compared with the fed state) combined with this propagative pattern would enhance transit since lowered resistance allows for unimpeded flow. The exact relationship between the depression of isolated smooth muscle function and the laxative-induced pattern observed in the intact preparation has not yet been established. However, it should be noted that both in the intact in vivo or the isolated tissue preparations, *no* stimulation of smooth muscle is observed after laxative treatment.

This same relationship between intestinal motor activity and laxative-induced diarrhea exists in disease states characterized by diarrhea and decreases in intestinal motility (KERN et al. 1951; CONNELL 1968). Conversely, treatment for diarrheal states consists of increasing circular muscle activity, increasing intraluminal resistance to flow, and slowing total transit time. Opiate derivatives such as morphine, codeine, and meperidine reduce the number of diarrheal stools, primarily through this mechanism (PLANT and MILLER 1926; BASS et al. 1961; BASS and WILEY 1965; NEILY 1969; RINALDO et al. 1971). Theoretically, stimulation of longitudinal muscle could lead to diarrhea through initiation of peristaltic movements, as has been demonstrated in vitro with several prostaglandins (BENNETT et al. 1968a, b). However, agents which depress both circular and longitudinal muscle contractility such as atropine or other anticholinergics have not been found to be effective in the treatment of diarrhea (CONNELL and KELLOCK 1959; IVEY 1975; REVES et al. 1983), suggesting that hypermotility or stimulated smooth muscle is not the cause of diarrhea. After considering motility data from diarrheal disease states, and responses to constipating and laxative agents, one cannot explain laxation by a "stimulant" action on the gastrointestinal smooth muscle.

C. Effects of Laxatives on Fluid and Electrolyte Movement

Luminal fluid accumulation may occur by effects of the laxatives on intestinal fluid absorption or secretory processes. While several laxatives have been postulated to act solely in the colon, owing to bacterial conversion to their active forms (see Sect. D), most produce effects on fluid movement in both the small and large intestines (Table 2).

The total volume of water excreted in the feces is the net result of absorptive and secretory processes occurring along the alimentary tract (Fig. 3). Diarrhea may result from either the delivery of large volumes of fluid into the colon (as from the inhibition of absorption or active secretion into the small bowel) or from a laxative-induced reduction in the capacity of the colon to absorb this fluid (DEBONGNIE and PHILLIPS 1978). Both small and large intestines are responsive to the antiabsorptive properties of the laxatives. Ricinoleic and deoxycholic acids, DSS, bisacodyl, and other laxatives are capable of producing net inhibition of fluid absorption and even secretion in the jejunum, ileum, and colon in a number of animal models and humans (MEKHJIAN and PHILLIPS 1970; MEKHJIAN et al. 1971; TEEM and PHILLIPS 1972; AMMON and PHILLIPS 1974; GAGINELLA et al. 1975a, b, 1977a; RACHMILEWITZ et al. 1976; SAUNDERS et al. 1977; GULLIKSON et al. 1977). The action on net absorption at any or all of these sites can lead to an increase in total fecal water content and subsequent diarrhea. The laxatives can exert these

Table 2. Laxatives producing antiabsorptive[a] effects

Laxative	Site of action[b]	Reference[c]
Anthraquinones	j	[3]
	i	[2]
	c	[3, 23]
Bile acids	j	[8, 19, 26]
	i	[7, 16]
	c	[4, 5, 12]
Bisacodyl	j	[3, 6, 27]
	i	[27]
	c	[3, 6, 15, 27]
Dioctyl sodium sulfosuccinate (DSS)	j	[19, 20, 26]
	i	[20]
	c	[17, 20]
Magnesium ion	j	[21, 24, 30]
	i	[1, 30]
	c	[1]
Oxyphenisatin	j	[29]
	c	[11]
Phenolphthalein	j	[28]
	i	[2, 28]
	c	[28]
Ricinoleic acid	j	[13, 18, 19, 22, 26]
	i	[2, 14, 18]
	c	[9, 10, 25]

[a] Antiabsorptive effects include inhibition of net absorption or induction of net secretion

[b] Abbreviations: j = jejunum; i = ileum; c = colon

[c] Numbers refer to: [1] LIUM and FLOREY (1939); [2] PHILLIPS et al. (1965); [3] FORTH et al. (1966a); [4] MEKHJIAN and PHILLIPS (1970); [5] MEKHJIAN et al. (1971); [6] EWE (1972); [7] SLADEN and HARRIES (1972); [8] TEEM and PHILLIPS (1972); [9] AMMON and PHILLIPS (1973); [10] BRIGHT-ASARE and BINDER (1973); [11] NELL et al. (1976); [12] WINGATE et al. (1973); [13] AMMON et al. (1974); [14] AMMON and PHILLIPS (1974); [15] EWE and HOLKER (1974); [16] KRAG and PHILLIPS (1974); [17] DONOWITZ and BINDER (1975); [18] GAGINELLA et al. (1975a); [19] GAGINELLA et al. (1975b); [20] SAUNDERS et al. (1975a); [21] STEWART et al. (1975b); [22] CLINE et al. (1976); [23] LEMMENS and BORJA (1976); [24] WANITSCHKE and AMMON (1976); [25] GAGINELLA et al. (1977a); [26] GULLIKSON et al. (1977); [27] RACHMILEWITZ et al. (1977); [28] SURAWICZ et al. (1977); [29] SUND and HILLESTAD (1978); [30] REICHELDERFER et al. (1979)

effects on fluid movement when administered either orally or rectally, though the latter route of administration has not been studied as thoroughly.

The net fluid and electrolyte absorption which is normally seen at any given site of the small and large intestine is the sum of absorptive and secretory processes (BINDER 1979). Active sodium absorption coupled with chloride ion movement is achieved in the small intestine through Na^+, K^+-ATPase located on the baso-

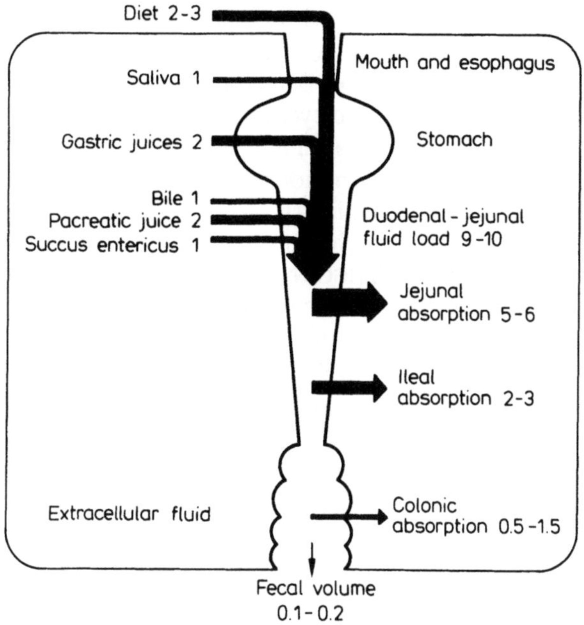

Fig. 3. Schematic view of fluid movement in the human gastrointestinal tract. Numbers represent 24-h volumes (l). *Width of arrow* is proportional to volume movement. Note the major absorption of fluid in the small intestine and limited absorptive capacity of the colon. Laxatives can alter the absorptive balance by acting in the small intestine, as well as the colon. Adapted from PHILLIPS (1973)

lateral membranes of the villus cells (FRIZZELL et al. 1979). Water then follows the movement of these ions. Active sodium and chloride absorption take place in the colon as well (FRIZZELL et al. 1976). Fluid and electrolyte absorption can be blocked in vivo by inhibitors of these active transport processes such as ouabain (CHARNEY and DONOWITZ 1978) and bile acids (GUIRALDES et al. 1975).

Small intestinal secretory processes are believed to reside in the crypt cells of the mucosal membrane (BAYLESS et al. 1971; SCHULTZ and CURRAN 1974; FIELD 1978), though there is some disagreement as to whether all fluid secretion takes place from these sites (DEJONGE 1975). The fluid secretion observed in classical secretory states such as after cholera enterotoxin or prostaglandin treatment is due to active secretion of chloride related to increases in intracellular levels of cAMP (KIMBERG et al. 1971; KIMBERG 1974). Anion secretion also occurs in the colon, but with a lesser response to the bacterial toxins and prostaglandins which cause secretion in the small intestine. These increases in cAMP leading to intestinal secretion may be produced either by direct stimulation of adenylate cyclase or by agents which inhibit the breakdown of cAMP (POWELL et al. 1974). In either case net fluid secretion will result.

The role of guanylate cyclase in intestinal transport has not been completely determined. In other physiologic processes guanylate cyclase activity can often produce an antagonism of effects elicited by adenylate cyclase activity (VOORHEES and DUELL 1975; LEE et al. 1972). Indeed, early evidence indicated that increased intracellular cGMP was associated with enhanced absorption (BRASITIS et al. 1976). Increases in cGMP levels in the intestine, however, have also been found to be associated with certain types of bacterially induced secretion (FIELD et al. 1978; RAO et al. 1979). In addition to cyclic nucleotides, secretion may be elicited directly by agents which raise intracellular levels of calcium. A calcium ionophore, A23187, is able to induce secretion without producing increases in cAMP (BOLTON and FIELD 1977; FRIZZELL 1977).

Secretion can also result from changes in passive forces such as the increase in plasma hydrostatic pressure (HIGGINS and BLAIR 1971) or a reduction in luminal pressure (HAKIM et al. 1977). The resulting filtration secretion is characterized by increases in the permeability of the intestine to plasma proteins and other macromolecules (DUFFY et al. 1978). WANITSCHKE (1980a) has postulated that intestinal filtration resulting from enhanced mucosal permeability is the driving force for secretion produced by laxatives. Passive forces may also contribute to intestinal secretion elicited by the laxatives by virtue of zones of local hyperosmolarity found in the regions of the microvilli (HALLBÄCK et al. 1978). Passive movement of fluid might occur in response to these osmotic forces (LUNDGREN and HAGLUND 1978) in combination with permeability alterations and thus lead to diarrhea. Laxatives can act to produce net fluid secretion by one or more of these mechanisms which decrease absorption or stimulate active or passive secretory processes. Evidence will be presented which demonstrates a potential contribution of these mechanisms to the actions of laxative drugs on secretion.

The mechanisms which bring about luminal fluid accumulation may be either specific or nonspecific. "Specific" is used in this chapter to describe a result which is mediated by one or a limited number of biologic processes, such as the stimulation or inhibition of a single enzyme or transport system. A drug–receptor interaction (e.g., cholinergic) is a highly specific mechanism in which structure–activity relationships are critical in determining the magnitude of the biologic event. The interaction of cholera toxin and GM1 gangliosides of the intestinal membrane is a pertinent example of this type of specific mechanism. In contrast, "nonspecific" may be used to describe a mechanism which leads to several distinctive results or a generalized alteration of biologic activity. Furthermore, a given effect may not be shared by structurally related compounds, but rather may be elicited by drugs of diverse structure which share a less apparent characteristic (e.g., lipid solubility or surface activity). The abilities of amphipaths and anesthetics to interact with biologic membranes (SEEMAN 1972) are examples of nonspecific activity.

A variety of structurally diverse laxative drugs have been shown to produce numerous effects, both on the gastrointestinal tract and on isolated enzymes. These include inhibiting the transport of amino acids and sugars (POPE et al. 1966), increasing the permeability of the gut to other drugs (GIBALDI 1970), inhibiting Na^+, K^+-ATPase (MITJAVILA et al. 1975), denaturing proteins (HELENIUS and SIMONS 1975), stimulating adenylate cyclase (PERKINS and MOORE 1971), and depressing intestinal smooth muscle contractility (GAGINELLA et al. 1975b). The diverse actions appear to be intimately related to the abilities of these compounds to interact nonspecifically with biologic membranes, rather than specific receptors. The following sections explore the effects of the nonspecific activity.

I. Cellular and Mucosal Damage

The ability to lower surface tension at an air–water, or oil–water, interface is an indirect measure of nonspecific interaction with membranes. A number of antiabsorptive compounds (ricinoleic acid, dihydroxy bile acids, DSS, and SDS) are surfactant and interact quite readily with cell membranes. The order of potency of these surfactant compounds to inhibit water absorption paralleled their abilities to lower surface tension (GULLIKSON et al. 1977). These same diverse chemicals were also potent lytic agents on a red blood cell membrane model, while trihydroxy bile salts, which had little effect on water absorption, did not have hemo-

Table 3. Actions of Laxatives on the intestinal mucosa[a]

Laxative	Inhibits Na^+, K^+ ATPase[b]	Stimulates adenylate cyclase or increases cAMP[c]	Causes mucosal injury[d]	Enhances mucosal permeability[e]
Anthraquinones	[8, 26, 41][f]	Not determined	[19]	[40]
Dihydroxy bile acids	[14, 20, 25]	+ [2, 10, 11, 38] − [18, 33]	[5, 7, 21, 22, 35] [31, 39]	[6, 7, 21, 24]
Bisacodyl	[8, 28a, 29]	+ [28a, 29] − [29]	[23, 28, 32]	Not determined
Castor oil (ricinoleic acid)	[26]	+ [1, 3] − [18]	[9, 12, 15, 16, 17]	[4, 9, 16]
Dioctyl sodium sulfosuccinate	[28a]	+ [13] − [34, 28a]	[30]	Not determined
Phenolphthalein	[8, 26, 27]	− [27]	[37]	Not determined
Oxyphenisatin	Not determined	− [36]	Not determined	[24]

[a] Adapted from GAGINELLA and BASS (1978)
[b] ATPase inhibition can reduce net fluid and electrolyte absorption
[c] Stimulation of adenylate cyclase or accumulation of cAMP leads to fluid secretion; + indicates increase in activity of cyclase or concentrations of cAMP; − indicates no change from control
[d] Mucosal injury determined from histologic evidence; related to impaired absorption and enhanced mucosal permeability
[e] Enhanced mucosal permeability to nonelectrolytes of various molecular weights
[f] Numbers refer to: [1] BINDER (1974); [2] BINDER et al. (1975); [3] BINDER (1977); [4] BRIGHT-ASARE and BINDER (1973); [5] CAMILLERI et al. (1980); [6] CASPARY and MEYNE (1980); [7] CHADWICK et al. (1979); [8] CHIGNELL (1968); [9] CLINE et al. (1976); [10] CONLEY et al. (1976); [11] COYNE et al. (1976); [12] DOBBINS and BINDER (1976); [13] DONOWITZ and BINDER (1975); [14] FAUST and WU (1967); [15] GADACZ et al. (1976); [16] GAGINELLA et al. (1977a); [17] GAGINELLA et al. (1977c); [18] GAGINELLA et al. (1978b); [19] GOERG et al. (1980b); [20] GUIRALDES et al. (1975); [21] GULLIKSON et al. (1977); [22] LOW-BEER et al. (1970); [23] MEISEL et al. (1977); [24] NELL et al. (1976); [25] PARKINSON and OLSEN (1964); [26] PHILLIPS et al. (1965); [27] POWELL et al. (1980); [28] RACHMILEWITZ et al. (1977); [28a] RACHMILEWITZ and KARMELI (1979); [29] RACHMILEWITZ et al. (1980); [30] SAUNDERS et al. (1975a); [31] SAUNDERS et al. (1975b); [32] SAUNDERS et al. (1977); [33] SIMON et al. (1978); [34] SIMON and KATHER (1980); [35] SLADEN and HARRIES (1972); [36] SUND and HILLESTAD (1978); [37] SURAWICZ et al. (1977); [38] TAUB et al. (1977); [39] TEEM and PHILLIPS (1972); [40] VERHAEREN et al. (1981); [41] WANITSCKE (1980b)

lytic activity. Similar to their effects on the red blood cell membrane, ricinoleate, deoxycholate, and DSS have produced dose-related cytotoxicity on isolated hamster small intestinal cells (GAGINELLA et al. 1977b). In vivo DSS, ricinoleic acid, bile salts, and magnesium sulfate produce jejunal cell loss in humans which is coincident with intestinal fluid secretion (BRETAGNE et al. 1981). In all of the studies cited the intestinal cytotoxicity of the surfactants and laxatives occurred over the same concentration ranges as the effects on water transport.

These effects of laxatives on the integrity of individual cells have been reflected in alterations of intestinal mucosal integrity in vivo (Table 3), as determined by scanning electron microscopy, light microscopy, or the use of an electron opaque tracer (lanthanum). The dramatic alterations in the villus tips after deoxycholate perfusion are shown in Fig. 4. Dihydroxy and unconjugated bile salts are more potent in producing histologic alterations than trihydroxy and conjugated bile salts (LOW-BEER et al. 1970; TEEM and PHILLIPS 1972; GULLIKSON et al. 1977; CHADWICK et al. 1979), reflecting a similar relationship existing for water transport effects. Ricinoleic acid, DSS, and bisacodyl also alter intestinal mucosal integrity and structure at concentrations which produce either net inhibition of fluid absorption or secretion (SAUNDERS et al. 1975a, 1977; CLINE et al. 1976; Gaginella et al. 1977a). Mucosal alterations as determined by mucus and DNA release appears prior to changes in fluid movement (CAMILLERI et al. 1980), indicating that secretion itself is not responsible for the development of damage.

The chief characteristics of the altered histology are shortened villus tips, enhanced permeability of villus cells to lanthanum, a "cracked clay" appearance of the villi, and an altered appearance of cytoplasmic organelles and cell nuclei. These histologic changes induced by laxatives are in contrast to the normal intestinal mucosa seen after cholera-induced active fluid secretion (ELLIOT et al. 1970; CLINE et al. 1976; GOERG et al. 1980a). An exact relationship between intestinal

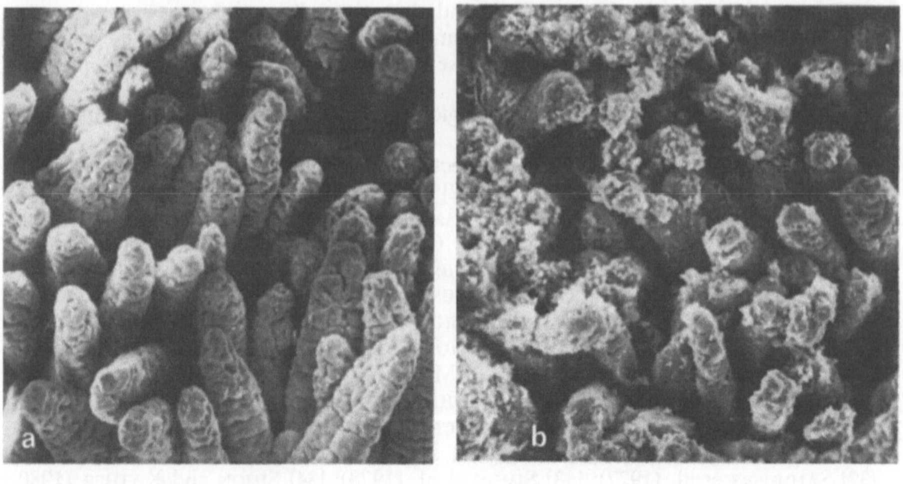

Fig. 4 a, b. Comparison of scanning electron microscope views of hamster small intestine after 30 min of perfusion. **a** after perfusion with 0.9% saline; **b** villus damage after exposure to 5 m*M* deoxycholic acid. Adapted from GULLIKSON et al. (1977) × 100

fluid accumulation in the lumen and histologic damage has been questioned (TEEM and PHILLIPS 1972). Water secretion was reversed, while histologic changes were irreversible during the experimental period. A later study from the same laboratory (GAGINELLA et al. 1977 c) demonstrated that alterations in structure produced by 10 m*M* ricinoleic acid could be at least partially reversed, as determined by changes in several criteria as observed with scanning electron microscopy. Similar attenuation of deoxycholate-induced damage has been demonstrated (GULLIKSON et al. 1981 a) when inhibition of secretion was achieved with the antidiarrheal drug lidamidine (MIR et al. 1978).

GULLIKSON et al. (1981 a, b) found that deoxycholate-related changes in histology and the release of mucosal membrane components could be attenuated by lidamidine, coincident with its antisecretory action. Histologic samples, taken from deoxycholate-perfused jejunal loops in dogs treated with lidamidine, showed that villi were not different in length from villi taken from dogs perfused with control buffer. Similarly, lidamidine, simultaneously with its antisecretory action, reduced the phospholipid and protein release caused by deoxycholate. Release of these two mucosal markers was also reduced when deoxycholate was removed from the perfusate solution and fluid absorption was returned to near normal. Mucosal damage then is associated with initiation of intestinal fluid secretion. Normal fluid transport returns when there is restoration of normal mucosal integrity.

II. Enhanced Mucosal Permeability

The alterations in structure produced by concentrations of ricinoleic and deoxycholic acids which are antiabsorptive can also be correlated with changes in mucosal permeability to tracer molecules of various sizes. Blood–lumen clearance of inulin (molecular weight 6,000) and dextran (molecular weight 16,000) in the small intestine were markedly enhanced by ricinoleic acid. Deoxycholate even produced a leakage of albumin (molecular weight 60,000) into the gut lumen (CLINE et al. 1976; GULLIKSON et al. 1977). Substances with low colonic permeability, such as urea, creatinine (Fig. 5), and polyethylene glycol (average molecular weight 400), were found to be readily permeable either in the blood–lumen or lumen–blood directions following exposure of the colon in a dose–response manner to ricinoleic acid (GAGINELLA et al. 1977 a). The alterations in permeability in the small intestine did not occur in response to either cholera toxin (CLINE et al. 1976) or taurocholate (GULLIKSON et al. 1977), the former acting by a cAMP mechanism and the latter not capable of inducing histologic or secretory effects. Further evidence of altered mucosal integrity in these studies were the losses of sucrase, a brush border marker enzyme and DNA from exfoliated cells. Similarly, bile acid-induced changes in the permeability of the small intestine and colon reflect the differential abilities of di- and trihydroxy bile acids to produce net fluid secretion (CHADWICK et al. 1979; CASPARY and MEYNE 1980). Thus, these laxatives produce histologic and permeability changes in the intestine within the concentration ranges for antiabsorptive effects (Table 3).

Evidence exists which directly correlates permeability changes and fluid secretion. Laxative-induced changes in intestinal permeability associated with secre-

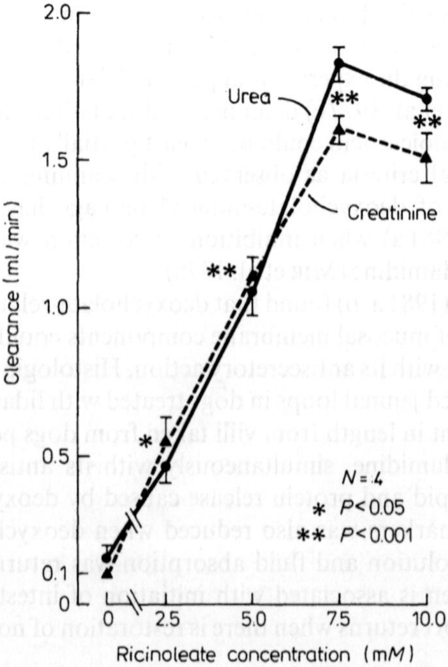

Fig. 5. Dose-dependent increase in the permeability of creatinine and urea in the rabbit colon perfused with ricinoleic acid. The drug enhanced blood–lumen clearance of these normally impermeable substances. The concentration range for effects on clearance is the same as that for effects on water movement. Adapted from GAGINELLA et al. (1977a)

tion are antagonized by the antisecretory agents lidamidine (GULLIKSON et al. 1981a) and loperamide (VERHAEREN et al. 1981). These results conflict with those of BINDER et al. (1978) who found intestinal permeability was not altered by propranolol, even though secretion was partially reversed. This contradiction may be due to different antisecretory mechanisms of the drugs used in each study. In addition, propranolol does not consistently produce antisecretory effects (GULLIKSON et al. 1981b; DONOWITZ and CHARNEY 1979b). Interpretive problems arise in using this β-blocker as a tool for studying intestinal secretion caused by laxatives (see Sect. C.III).

The question arises as to what forces cause the fluid movement if intestinal mucosal structure and permeability are the explanations for luminal fluid accumulation. It has been suggested (RUMMEL et al. 1975; WANITSCHKE 1980a) that loss of anisotropy of the fluid pump combined with vascular hydrostatic pressure are responsible for the secretion of water and electrolytes induced by laxatives. These authors have suggested that "leaky" tight junctions are the basis for the loss of the absorptive sodium gradient and the resulting passive paracellular water movement (see Chap. 29). Other studies have demonstrated that ricinoleic acid in concentrations as high as 8 mM in the hamster and 10 mM in the rabbit small intestines do not enhance the permeability of lanthanum at tight junctions (CLINE et al. 1976; GAGINELLA et al. 1976). Furthermore, the morphological studies cited previously suggest a more generalized alteration in structure being responsible for the plasma–lumen fluid movement than a specific structural effect on tight junctions only (see discussion of Fig. 5). Intestinal secretion may occur through denuded areas at the villous tips, across epithelial cells with enhanced permeability, and through more porous tight junctional areas. Vascular hydrostatic pressure may then act as the driving force for the observed secretion aided by the previously mentioned high osmotic pressure gradient which exists locally at the tips of the villi. Alternatively, laxative-induced permeability changes may lead to a reduction in active absorption because of the loss of efficiency of the sodium pump. This could be due to leakage of sodium back into the villous cells after active extrusion into basolateral extracellular spaces.

III. Role of cAMP in the Actions of Laxatives

There has been much speculation on the role of adenylate cyclase in the intestinal secretion of water and electrolytes by laxatives. Stimulation of this enzyme is believed to be responsible for the intestinal water secretion elicited by cholera toxin (SHARP and HYNIE 1971; KIMBERG et al. 1971; KIMBERG 1974), certain prostaglandins (KIMBERG et al. 1971; KIMBERG 1974), as well as vasoactive intestinal peptide (VIP) (SCHWARTZ et al. 1974; WALDMAN et al. 1977). Levels of cAMP are elevated by these agents, concurrently with their luminal fluid effects. This correlation has been reasonably interpreted as a cause and effect relationship. The probable common link between elevated cAMP levels and fluid secretion is calcium, which is known to be released by cAMP (BERRIDGE 1975) and produces active anion secretion (BOLTON and FIELD 1977).

A similar investigational approach has been used to determine the involvement of cAMP and the adenylate cyclase system in the fluid and electrolyte effects of the laxatives (see Table 3). The bile salts can alter ion permeabilities and increase short-circuit current in both small and large intestine (BINDER 1977a), in a manner similar to cholera toxin. A dihydroxy bile salt (taurochenodeoxycholate) was more effective than a trihydroxy bile salt (taurocholate), reflecting the potency relationship for water-secretory effects (VOLPE and BINDER 1975). Furthermore, agents such as DSS, bile acids, and ricinoleic acid, which increase short-circuit current, also significantly increase cAMP levels in the rat colon (DONOWITZ and BINDER 1975).

The manner in which laxatives increase cAMP is unknown. However, detergents, including deoxycholate and SDS, are known to stimulate adenylate cyclase in vitro in a nonspecific manner (PERKINS and MOORE 1971; HELENIUS and SIMONS 1975), which contrasts with the specificity of activation of adenylate cyclase by cholera toxin, VIP, and prostaglandins. Inhibition of phosphodiesterase could also account for the increases in cAMP and this effect has been reported for DSS (SIMON and KATHER 1980). Laxatives by their damaging effects may release prostaglandins which could also alter adenylate cyclase activity (BEUBLER and JUAN 1978; RACHMILEWITZ et al. 1980). It appears that the laxative-induced cAMP changes may be qualitatively different from those elicited by bacterial toxins and endogenous secretagogues.

This effect of laxatives on cAMP levels has been claimed to be specific for the colon rather than the small intestine (TAUB et al. 1977). Indeed GAGINELLA et al.

(1978 b) found that, while several hormones and prostaglandins (PGE_1 and PGE_2) stimulated adenylate cyclase in isolated hamster small intestinal villus cells, deoxycholate and ricinoleic acid were unable to stimulate cyclase activity above basal levels. Other reports have failed to substantiate a link between the secretion produced by phenolphthalein and oxyphenisatin and adenylate cyclase stimulation in the small intestine (SUND and HILLESTAD 1978; POWELL et al. 1980).

Use of inhibitors of cAMP formation such as RMI 12330A have demonstrated that there may be differences between the mechanisms by which cholera toxin and laxatives produce small intestinal secretion. RMI 12330A blocked ileal adenylate cyclase activity and intestinal secretion after exposure to cholera toxin (TAI et al. 1978; FARACK and NELL 1979), but was unable to inhibit deoxycholate or bisacodyl secretion (FARACK and NELL 1979). It appears that in the small intestine laxatives act by mechanisms other than adenylate cyclase stimulation.

In the colon, the role of cAMP in the secretory action of laxatives is also disputed (SIMON et al. 1978; SIMON and KATHER 1980). A series of studies relating the effects of deoxycholate to changes in cAMP have appeared in the literature (CONLEY et al. 1976; COYNE et al. 1976; TAUB et al. 1977). The common idea throughout these papers is that propranolol is able to block the secretory effects of deoxycholate by reducing cAMP concentrations.

CONLEY et al. (1976) have reported that deoxycholate produces an increase in colonic cAMP levels which accompanies the induction of fluid secretion. Propranolol, a β-blocker, was capable of inhibiting both the increases in cAMP and the fluid accumulation produced by deoxycholate. This action was not the result of β-blockade by propranolol, as epinephrine and norepinephrine were not capable of reversing the propranolol effect (COYNE et al. 1976).

Since the locus of action of deoxycholate is unknown, it is also unclear as to the potential sites at which propranolol is blocking the deoxycholate effect. These actions of propranolol in the rabbit colon reported by CONLEY et al. appear to bear some similarity to its effect on TSH-stimulated cAMP levels in the thyroid (MARSHALL et al. 1975). This blockade was of a nonspecific nature: occurring at relatively high concentrations, not isomerically specific, and not occurring with other β-blockers. The action of propranolol may be related to its local anesthetic properties since these drugs are known to produce increases in membrane fluidity (METCALFE and BURGEN 1968; AKIJAMA and IGISU 1979). These changes in membrane properties produced by propranolol affect the activity of intrinsic enzymes of membrane, such as adenylate cyclase (GORDON et al. 1980). In addition, the use of propranolol to demonstrate a role for cAMP in the secretory action of deoxycholate is further clouded by the uncertainty of propranolol's effect. Multiple pretreatments have at times been necessary to demonstrate an antisecretory activity (DONOWITZ and CHARNEY 1979 a). Other studies have shown propranolol to be devoid of antisecretory (GULLIKSON et al. 1981 b) or antidiarrheal activity (DONOWITZ and CHARNEY 1979 b), or actually to promote secretion (MORRIS and TURNBERG 1981). The meaning of reported increases in cAMP concentrations due to laxatives is unclear. They may merely represent another nonspecific membrane interaction, occurring simultaneously with effects on membrane structure and permeability.

IV. Effects of Laxatives on Na^+, K^+-ATPase and Energy Metabolism

The initial mechanism studies on the action of laxatives on fluid movement demonstrated an inhibitory effect on Na^+, K^+-ATPase (PHILLIPS et al. 1965). This enzyme, located on the basolateral membrane of the villus cells, is responsible for the active extrusion of Na^+ in the serosal direction. The creation of an electrochemical gradient results in the passive absorption of water through transcellular and intercellular pathways. Since the work of PHILLIPS et al., there have been numerous studies which have demonstrated an inhibitory effect on Na^+, K^+-ATPase by a variety of laxatives (see Table 3). The potential of this action in producing intestinal fluid accumulation is obvious in light of the absorptive function of both the small and large intestines (see Fig. 3). Additionally, the inhibition of active absorption may uncover latent secretory processes which lead to a net secretory state (BINDER 1979) without the direct stimulation of secretion.

In addition to the inhibition of the enzyme Na^+, K^+-ATPase, laxatives may reduce absorptive function by inhibiting cellular metabolic functions involved in ATP production. Reduced tissue levels of ATP have been correlated with impaired intestinal fluid absorption after treatment with taurocholate and glycocholate (FAUST and WU 1965). These reductions in ATP were in part due to the ability of these bile salts to inhibit oxygen consumption and uncouple oxidative phosphorylation (FAUST and WU 1967). Agents which elicit intestinal fluid accumulation (ricinoleic, deoxycholic, and oleic acids and SDS) are known to inhibit the enzyme adenine nucleotide translocase (ANT) (GAGINELLA et al. 1975c; WOJTCZAK and ZALUSKA 1967; DUSZYNSKI and WOJTCZAK 1974). ANT transports ADP across the mitochondrial membrane in exchange for ATP which may be used as substrate for Na^+, K^+-ATPase. Inhibition of ANT then represents another mechanism by which laxatives may inhibit the function of Na^+, K^+-ATPase. While this section summarizes the biochemical evidence for the inhibitory effect of laxatives on electrolyte movement through Na^+, K^+-ATPase, laxatives also produce generalized inhibition of transport processes (PARKINSON and OLSEN 1964).

V. Hormones as Mediators of Laxative Action

A number of hormones found in the gastrointestinal tract are capable of altering intestinal motility (PARKER and BENEVENTANO 1970; DINOSO et al. 1973; STEWART and BASS 1976b) and inducing net fluid secretion in the small or large intestines (GARDNER et al. 1967; BARBEZAT and GROSSMAN 1971a, b; MORITZ et al. 1973; WALDMAN et al. 1977). Because of these dual actions, a role for these substances in the effects of laxatives has been evoked.

Cholecystokinin (CCK) is known both to induce a laxative-like effect on intestinal fluid movement and to alter gastrointestinal motility and myoelectric activity (MORITZ et al. 1973; STEWART and BASS 1976b). CCK has been implicated in the actions of at least two laxative drugs, ricinoleic acid and magnesium sulfate. Similar effects on intestinal motility were obtained by ricinoleate and by CCK (STEWART and BASS 1976b). Either intraduodenal infusion of ricinoleic acid or an intravenous bolus injection of COOH terminal octapeptide of CCK produced similar marked alterations in the digestive pattern of the small intestine of the dog. The initial contractile responses to both CCK and ricinoleate could be prevented by atropine. These similar actions for CCK and ricinoleate may apply only to motor activity, however, since ricinoleate does not appear to produce a hormonally mediated effect on fluid secretion. Perfusion of ricinoleate in jejunal loops did not effect fluid movement in ileal loops in the same animal (GADACZ et al. 1976).

The mechanism of action of magnesium ion in producing intraluminal fluid accumulation and altered motility also has been attributed to CCK release (STEWART and BASS 1976b; HARVEY and READ 1973). In human and animal models, isotonic magnesium sulfate solutions can produce net fluid secretion (WANITSCHKE and AMMON 1976; REICHELDERFER et al. 1979), suggesting that the magnesium ion possesses intrinsic pharmacologic activity, in addition to its osmotic properties. While plasma determinations of CCK in response to magnesium and other laxatives have not been made, MALAGELADA et al. (1978) have utilized an in vivo bioassay for CCK in response to intraluminal magnesium sulfate. $MgSO_4$ produced a decided laxative effect on fluid movement, but only weak stimulation of pancreatic and gallbladder secretion. CCK may then explain at most only a small part of the effects of magnesium ion on fluid movement. The secretory effects of magnesium may be elicited through calcium (REICHELDERFER et al. 1979), a candidate as the final mediator of intestinal ion secretion. Release of calcium by isotonic magnesium sulfate has been seen concurrently with intestinal secretion. This release of calcium could not be accounted for in terms of intestinal damage and permeability changes.

While several clinically observed types of diarrhea are associated with elevated plasma levels of hormones such as VIP (BLOOM et al. 1973; SAID and FALOONA 1975; KREJS et al. 1977), gastrin, and glucagon (BARBEZAT and GROSSMAN 1971b), there is only fragmentary evidence that any of these hormones released during diarrheal disease are associated with laxative-induced secretory effects. VIP has been shown to be depleted from isolated enterocytes by ricinoleic acid (KERZNER et al. 1979). Determination of the release of such hormones needs to be made in order to verify their involvement in laxative-induced fluid secretion. VIP has been quantified in hamster intestine and is in greatest abundance in smooth muscle and denuded villi (GAGINELLA et al. 1978a). It appears to be associated with nerve fibers, rather than villus or crypt cells. One of the functions of VIP may be as a neural transmitter which stimulates intestinal secretion in response to various stimuli. Any definitive actions of laxatives on these neural plexuses, however, have yet to be determined.

The prostaglandins are candidate autocoids which may mediate the effects of laxatives on motor and secretory activities of the gastrointestinal tract. Prostaglandin $F_2\alpha$ infusion produces an electric pattern associated with fluid secretion, similar to that observed with cholera enterotoxin (MATHIAS et al. 1977), several bacterial toxins (BURNS et al. 1978, 1980; MATHIAS et al. 1978), and the laxatives (ATCHISON et al. 1978a, b; MATHIAS et al. 1978). Indomethacin, an inhibitor of prostaglandin cyclooxygenase, is capable of blocking the electric patterns after cholera exposure (MATHIAS et al. 1977), implying that prostaglandins may function in the motor responses observed during diarrheas of various etiologies.

The discovery of a role for prostaglandins in the altered motility associated with certain types of diarrhea gives rise to the possibility that the mucosal membrane alterations and damage elicited by laxatives (CLINE et al. 1976; GAGINELLA et al. 1977a; GULLIKSON et al. 1977) may result in a prostaglandin-mediated effect on fluid absorption (RACHMILEWITZ 1980). Prostaglandins of the E and F series are potent stimulants of intestinal secretion, and the effectiveness of prostaglandin cyclooxygenase inhibitors (bismuth subsalicylate and aspirin) in the treatment of various types of diarrhea (DUPONT et al. 1977; MENNIE et al. 1975) suggests that prostaglandins may play a role in their etiology. In addition, tissue prostaglandin levels have been observed to be elevated in diseases characterized by diarrhea (SANDLER et al. 1968; GOULD 1975). Laxative agents such as aloe and phenolphthalein (COLLIER et al. 1976) stimulate the formation of E and F prostaglandins from arachidonic acid. Similarly, bisacodyl, an agent which has been shown to alter intestinal morphology, increases jejunal and colonic levels of PGE_2 (RACHMILEWITZ and KARMELI 1979; RACHMILEWITZ et al. 1980). It has further been shown that laxatives such as bisacodyl and phenolphthalein lead to the enhanced release of PGE activity in the rat colon (BEUBLER and JUAN 1978). This release and the concomitant fluid accumulation could be blocked by pretreatment with indomethacin, while the luminal fluid effects of an osmotic laxative (mannitol) could not be inhibited. Administration of indomethacin similarly prevented increases in intestinal PGE_2 content and adenylate cyclase activity brought about by bisacodyl (RACHMILEWITZ et al. 1980). These effects of indomethacin on fluid movement, adenylate cyclase activity, and prostaglandin content are similar to those previously described for laxative-induced motility patterns and further suggest a role for prostaglandins in the action of laxatives.

While there is evidence linking enhanced release and mucosal content of prostaglandins to the actions of laxatives, the effect on fluid transport cannot be explained entirely by prostaglandins. The mucosal damage which occurs after exposure of the intestinal mucosa to various laxatives would be expected to increase prostaglandin release as part of the inflammatory process. It is not known whether prostaglandins are in sufficient local concentrations to account for the fluid secretion produced by laxatives which damage the mucosa. RAMPTON et al. (1981) showed that while indomethacin blocked colonic release of PGE_2 caused by deoxycholate, the fluid transport effects and DNA release remained. Similarly, further studies by BEUBLER and JUAN (1979) had demonstrated a differential effect of laxatives on prostaglandin release and fluid transport. Indomethacin reduced the effects of DSS and sennoside A and B on PGE release, but did not decrease their effects on fluid movement. Furthermore, indomethacin attentuated, but did not completely abolish, the effects of ricinoleic, oleic, and deoxycholic acids on fluid movement. Other mechanisms of action must be evoked to explain the entirety of the effects of laxatives on fluid transport.

Laxatives of several distinct chemical entities have been described here in terms of their effects on motility and fluid secretion in the gastrointestinal tract. A large subgroup of laxatives consists of a heterogeneous class of macromolecules known as the bulk laxatives. These polysaccharides also exert effects on fluid content of the feces and motor activity of the intestinal tract. Their effects, however, appear to be quite different from those previously discussed.

D. Bulk and Dietary Fibers

A major subgroup of laxatives consists of a heterogeneous group of polysaccharides (glycans). These laxatives act by mechanisms which are different from those described in previous sections of this chapter. In the past, dietary fiber has been thought to act entirely by hydration and swelling. This simple property of in vitro water imbibition does not directly correlate with the pharmacologic effects of various fibers (STEPHEN and CUMMINGS 1980). Indeed, as a group, these chemicals have a wide variety of biologic actions which may account for their laxative properties. It may be helpful first to understand the chemical nature of these materials before considering their effects on gastrointestinal function.

Carbohydrates are subgrouped as homoglycans which consist of unsubstituted six-carbon units, or heteroglycans such as the mucopolysaccharides with sulfate or amino group attachments. Examples of homoglycans are starch, cellulose, inulin, agar, and dextrans, the latter possessing heparin-like properties. The heteroglycans like pectins, gum acacia, tragacanth, or carrageenans are often used as demulcents, suspending agents, and laxatives.

Dietary fiber consisting of these homo- or heteroglycans has recently gained much attention for its role in gastrointestinal function. Dietary fiber is a generic term for the remnants of ingested plant cells that are resistant to alimentary enzyme digestion, though fiber may be broken down by bacteria, especially in the colon (TROWELL 1974). Dietary fiber consists of homoglycans (celluloses), heteroglycans (pectins, gums), lignins (polymers of hydroxyphenylpropyl units), indigestible lipids (waxes, cutins), trace elements, and plant enzymes. Dietary fiber, which can be defined by its biologic breakdown, contrasts with crude fiber, the plant residue remaining after harsh chemical treatment. Crude fiber is thus a classification based on chemical degradation, which bears no apparent relationship to biologic breakdown of dietary fiber. Terms such as residue, roughage, fiber, and bulk are also imprecise, though they have not been replaced by specific scientific terms (HELLENDOORN 1978). As a group, these substances represent mixed ratios of macromolecular polymers which possess different physical and chemical properties that affect gastrointestinal function. Whether the fiber is plant or synthetic in origin, small changes in structure may affect its pharmacologic properties. Thus, we are left with no simple measurement for a dosage of an active component.

In a review of laxative drugs, an advisory panel to the FDA classified the following substances as "bulk forming" laxatives: dietary bran, karaya (sterculia gum), malt soup extract, various psyllium preparations, cellulose derivatives, semisynthetic substances (methylcellulose, sodium carboxymethylcellulose) and polycarbophil (OVER THE COUNTER DRUGS 1975). The various actions of bulk or dietary fiber laxatives are presented in Table 4 and are described in Sects. D.I–V. In addition, the topic has been discussed in several symposia (REILLY and KIRSNER 1975; INGLETT and FALKEHAG 1979), in reviews (CUMMINGS 1973; SPILLER 1978; ANDERSON and CHEN 1979; LEVIN and HORWITZ 1979; CONNEL 1981), on television and by the press, as well as in books for lay consumption (GALTON 1976; FLATH 1976), and the scientific community (BURKITT and TROWELL 1975).

Table 4. Biological actions of dietary fiber

Stomach
Delay in stomach emptying
Small intestine
Osmotic effect (probably minimal) or not quantified
Interaction with water, bile salts, nutrients, and drugs
Accelerated intestinal transit
Colon[a]
Proliferation of bacteria
Short-chain (C_2–C_5) fatty acid production by bacteria
Gas (CO_2, H_2) formation (flatulence) by bacteria
Bacterial or mucosal metabolism and alteration of substances delivered to the colon, e. g., fiber, bile salts
Alteration in intestinal transit, decrease in circular muscle activity
Interaction of above factors may contribute to increase in fecal bulk and water output

[a] Activity is dependent on whether the fiber is completely or partially altered by gastrointestinal bacteria

Both the scientific literature and the media have championed the virtues of bulk laxation.

I. Water-Retaining Properties

Certain plant materials have the capacity to swell when placed in water. For example, pectins are used in jam making because of their ability to form gels. Several studies have reported the water-holding capacity of fiber in vitro (Gray and Tainter 1941; Blythe et al. 1949; Monaco and Dehner 1955; Ireson and Leslie 1970; McConnell et al. 1974) and in turn have attempted to relate these actions to the in vivo laxation properties of fecal bulking agents (Ivy and Isaacs 1938; Gray and Tainter 1941; McConnell et al. 1974). In evaluating the published data, it is clear that several of these investigators could not demonstrate a direct relationship for in vitro water-holding effects and fecal water and solid output. Rather, these studies suggest that some of the breakdown products of bulk fibers may act as "irritant" laxatives (Tainter and Buchanan 1954), or the gas released into the stools may help contribute to the bulk and softness (Hoppert and Clark 1945). A careful study by Stephen and Cummings (1980) established the in vitro water-holding properties of 17 dietary fiber substances varying from food (carrot, apple) and bulk laxatives (sodium carboxymethylcellulose, bran) to gel-forming polysaccharides (pectin). In contrast to the expected results, an inverse relationship between water holding and fecal bulking was found. Clinically, in this series, pectin had the highest water-holding capacity (56 g water in 1 g pectin) but produced only a minimal change in fecal weight. In contrast, bran with a low water-holding capacity (4 g water in 1 g bran) markedly increased fecal weight. Clearly, in vitro water imbibition does not correlate with laxation.

Dietary fiber in addition may possess different properties in the small and large intestine. In the small intestine, dietary fiber may indeed hold water, as well as adsorb bile acids, and act as an ion exchanger (Eastwood and Kay 1979). In the colon, however, bacterial enzyme degradation of fiber may markedly alter the in vitro physical and chemical character of fiber. Thus, any action of fiber exerted in the small intestine may not occur in the colon, owing to bacterial alteration of the fiber. The metabolism of the fiber and pH changes in the colon generated by this metabolism raise serious questions about whether water binding is the only mechanism for bulk laxatives. Indeed, the colonic bacteria may play a major role in the mechanism of action of the fiber.

II. Role of Bacteria in the Action of Bulk Laxatives

The idea that the water-retaining property of fiber causes the increased volume in stools is inconsistent with the fact that fiber material is degraded in the colon. This degradation alters the chemical and physical properties of the fiber so that the remaining material in the stool has a lower water-holding capacity than that of the ingested intact fiber (HELLENDOORN 1978). This fact confirms WILLIAMS and OLMSTED (1936) who concluded "... that some factor in addition to the hydroscopic properties of the stool residue must account for the increment in stool weight." It is well established that bacteria in the cecum and stomach of ruminants readily break down plant constituents. As early as 1936, WILLIAMS and OLMSTED showed clinically that as much as 56% of a portion of the heteroglycans was degraded, while the lignans were least affected. These authors indicated that the products of the glycans might be short-chain fatty acids which may cause laxation. The digestibility of certain glycans in both humans and animals has been confirmed (MANGOLD 1934; SEALOCK et al. 1941; HUMMEL et al. 1943; HOPPERT and CLARK 1945). In a preliminary report, MILTON-THOMPSON and LEWIS (1971) showed in a balanced dietary study that 57% (13%–85%) of an 8.5 g/day intake of cellulose is metabolized by the gut.

In humans, both cellulose and pectin (completely bacteria degradable) produce increases in the total amount of fecal volatile fatty acids (SPILLER et al. 1980) when compared with a control (sucrose) diet. Cellulose, however, is a laxative while pectin is not. Cellulose, in contrast to pectin, shortens transit time and increases fecal weight. This differential action between cellulose and pectin may be due to a slower rate of dietary fiber digestion of the cellulose. The latter may be carried further down the tract and exert a quantitatively different effect on the descending or sigmoid area of the colon. The kinetics of colonic and rectal absorption of short-chain fatty acids, such as those released by fiber digestion, have been reported in humans (MCNEIL et al. 1978; RUPPIN et al. 1980). At concentrations up to 90 mM, these substances are readily absorbed along with water. An effect of these fatty acids on fluid absorption appears to be doubtful since there must be either a colonic accumulation of fatty acids to produce fluid secretion or delayed absorption of fatty acids to hold water osmotically and thus produce an increase in fecal water content, leading to diarrhea. However, the bacterial effects on dietary fiber could yield other products that affect the stool. In addition, the effect of fiber products on bacteria may also be a factor.

The idea that certain types of indigestible matter in the colon foster the growth of bacteria was made by HOPPERT and CLARK (1945). This increase in bacterial population was quantified by FUCHS et al. (1976). Subjects on wheat bran obtained the expected laxative effect, which was accompanied by a significant increase in the fecal anaerobic bacterial population. A clinical comparison between relatively indigestible (wheat) and digestible (cabbage) fibers has lead to the hypothesis that dietary fibers may have two distinctive actions in the colon; hydration of undigested fiber and stimulation of bacterial growth (STEPHEN and CUMMINGS 1980). Using wheat fiber in which only 36% of the fiber is digested in the gut, they obtained a laxative effect characterized by a fourfold increase in fecal fiber content, a doubling of the daily stool weight and solid content, and only a slight increase in bacterial mass. In contrast, digestible cabbage fiber produced less laxation with only a 40% increase in fecal fiber, a 69% increase in stool weight, and a 25% increase of solid content. However, bacterial mass was significantly higher (63%) than seen with wheat fiber (15%). Since fecal solids normally consist of 55% bacteria, this increase in bacterial mass can lead to greater fecal output. Thus the fecal weight can be enhanced by increases in bacterial mass due to the products of digestible fiber. Fecal water content increases (150 ml for wheat fiber and 107 ml for cabbage fiber versus a mean of 64 ml for control) were also significant in both cases and proportional to the daily stool weight. It was speculated that the water is derived from two sources, hydration of the residual undigested fiber and from the water content of the increased bacterial mass.

Bacteria may also be the causative agent of gas production in the colon, a further action related to laxation. As demonstrated by STEGERTA (1968) and HELLENDOORN (1978) with bean diets and in certain grain cereals (HICKEY et al. 1972), one can markedly increase flatus output. This was attributed to the presence of sugars, possibly raffinose and stachyose, that were not digested in the small bowel. These substances appear to be substrates for bacteria in the colon and lead to the formation of CO_2, hydrogen, and possibly methane. This intestinal gas could then travel quickly through the tract (BENNETT and BASS 1972). Gas produced by bacteria may explain HOPPERT and CLARK's (1945) suggestion that colonic gas accumulation may contribute to defecation.

Bacteria can also act to convert laxative prodrugs into their active forms. Sulisatin is a laxative with two of its phenolic groups esterified with sulfate. The lack of arylsulfatase activity in the small intestinal mucosa allows the drug to pass unaltered to the colon (MORETO et al. 1979). Colonic bacteria are capable of converting this drug to hydroxy and dihydroxy derivatives which can alter motility and produce colonic secretion in a manner previously described. This is in contrast to acetate ester derivatives of similar diphenolic laxatives (bisacodyl, oxyphenisatin) which are readily cleaved by the esterases in the small intestine. Thus, the phenolic laxatives may be synthesized to be dependent on hydrolysis by colonic bacterial enzymes before they can be active as laxatives. The carbohydrate laxative drugs, psyllium and lactulose (described in Sect. D.V), also are dependent for activation on colonic bacteria.

In summary, bacterial action on fiber can lead to several results. Presumably, these effects are determined by the composition of the dietary fiber, and interactions with the pH, ionic and organic constituents of the gastrointestinal tract. Thus several mechanisms for the laxative effect of fiber are possible: (a) water-holding capacity of undigested dietary fiber; (b) fiber digestion products, like short-chain fatty acids, which may cause fluid accumulation in the colon; (c) increased fecal mass due to fiber products enhancing the bacterial population in the colon; and (d) increased gas production leading to distension and the urge to defecate.

III. Altered Transit Time

Transit times of the entire gastrointestinal tract are shortened by several dietary fibers. With the development of radiolabeled cellulose fiber (MALAGELADA et al. 1980), it is now possible to quantitate transit time. In their first study using this technique, MALAGELADA et al. showed that cellulose empties very slowly from the stomach of the dog, when compared with a liquid test meal. This technical development of labeled fiber should lead to more accurate studies of gastric emptying and gut transit times of dietary fibers in health and disease. Until now, one was dependent on X-ray or inert solids for monitoring total transit time. Roentgenographic studies have not been informative (FANTUS et al. 1940; STRETCHER and QUIRK 1943), though one of these earlier studies did lead to the suggestion that bran may reduce "spasm" in the colon.

Several outstanding physicians in Britain have popularized the concept that high dietary fiber intake accompanied by rapid transit times and large volumes of soft stools may reduce the incidence of certain diseases (CLEAVE et al. 1969; BURKITT et al. 1972). Several African cultures which consume a high fiber diet have markedly reduced incidences of certain large bowel diseases such as cancer and diverticulitis. These studies lack epidemiologic verification which would require a multifactorial approach. Certainly, the hypothesis is worthy of a proper experimental study (MENDELOFF 1977). Several studies (HARVEY et al. 1973; PAYLER et al. 1975) have shown that unprocessed or wheat bran can lead to a "normalizing" effect by shortening (e.g., from 3.8 to 2.4 days) or delaying (e.g., from 1 to 1.7 days) the time for the appearance of inert markers in the feces. Both the chemical and physical state of the high residue substance may be important since these shortened transit times could not be confirmed for various samples of wheat bran, cellulose (EASTWOOD et al. 1973; KIRWAN et al. 1974), ground oat flakes (PAYLER et al. 1975), or corn flakes (CONNELL and SMITH 1974). These variable results could be due to particle size (BRODRIBB and GROVES 1978), method of cooking (WYMAN et al. 1976), or altered composition from milling. To date, clinical transit studies have been done only for the entire gastrointestinal tract. Studies determining the comparative effects of a dietary fiber on small or large bowel transit times of comparative contractile activity in various segments have not been undertaken in a systematic manner.

Objective monitoring of colonic smooth muscle activity in primates on low and high dietary fiber intake has been reported (BRODRIBB et al. 1979, 1980). There was a differential effect on frequency and force of smooth muscle contractions and electric activity of the cecum, and transverse and sigmoid colon. In only 3 weeks, the cecal area of animals on zero or low fiber diet had markedly higher muscle activity which decreased caudally along the bowel. This gradient of activity was present both during the fasted and fed states. Transit time was also twice as long in the animals receiving a zero dietary fiber intake. Thus, increased circular muscle activity associated with low dietary fiber prolongs transit time and leads to small stool weight. Unfortunately, the monkey studies were not designed to detect motility pattern changes over short distances of the bowel. This defect in experimental design was corrected in a study on electric properties of pigs' cecal–colon area (FIORAMONTI and BUENO 1980). In the comparison of a high dietary fiber with a milk diet there was a differential effect on electric activity. More propulsive and less rhythmic segmental electric patterns were generated with the bran than with the milk diet. Thus, as shown with other laxatives (see Sect. B) not only the number, but the organization of muscle activity is important for propulsion. The electric activity of the cecal–ascending colon area may be conducive for this area to act as a reservoir for colonic contents. This potential reservoir may be the site where bacteria–dietary fiber interaction produces the by-products that exert the biologic effects of the dietary fibers.

Rats or rabbits placed on a low dietary fiber intake experienced changes in the colon leading to the production of diverticula which could be minimized and/or prevented with psyllium seed or other dietary fiber diets, but not with karaya gum (CARLSON and HOELZEL 1949; HODGSON 1975). Low dietary fiber intake by rabbits for 30 weeks may also increase the contractile responsiveness of the duodenum and colon to prostigmine and CCK (MCLEISH and JOHNSON 1978). WARD et al. (1979) reported the effects of feeding two groups of rats low and high dietary fiber for a year. Surprisingly, the animals on the high residue diet developed a significantly thicker muscle and mucosal layer of the colon. In contrast to these acquired changes in intestinal structure produced by fiber, a 10% cellulose diet in mice has no effect on the renewal rate of epithelial cells of the colon (STRAGAND and HAGEMAN 1977). Thus, fiber can affect transit, diverticula formation and, at least experimentally, the thickness of the muscle. The mechanism for these effects has not been elucidated.

IV. Fiber Interaction

The heterogeneous chemical nature of dietary fiber can lead to additive or antagonistic influences on each other or on other substances present in the gastrointestinal tract. The active constituents of the fiber may act as ion exchange resins which bind and enhance the fecal excretion of certain ions (REINHOLD et al. 1976; EASTWOOD and KAY 1979). The consumption of 16 g purified cellulose for 30 days caused an increase in fecal content of calcium and magnesium accompanied by a negative balance of these ions (SLAVIN and MARLETT 1978). The ability of fiber to adsorb bile salts in the small intestine could deliver them to the colon. Bile salts produce fluid secretion in both organs (see Sect. C). Normally, bile salts are actively absorbed in the ileum with negligible amounts passing into the colon. Dietary fiber could alter this process.

The adsorptive capacity of organic solvent extracts of various foods such as celery, lettuce, and beans, as well as fractions of dietary fiber has been demonstrated (BIRKNER and KERN 1974; STORY and KRITCHEVSKY 1976). EASTWOOD and HAMILTON (1968) showed that a grain mixture consisting of corn and barley bound di- and trihydroxy bile acids in vitro. This binding was affected by the pH of the media with less adsorption occurring as pH increased. Various fiber fractions were separated, and it was demonstrated that lignin was the major binding substance. Another study demonstrated that lignins in vitro have a 3:1 preferential affinity for dihydroxy versus trihydroxy bile acids (KAY et al. 1979). It is also well established that these primary trihydroxy bile acids which do enter the colon are readily transformed to dihydroxy bile salts by colonic bacteria. Dihydroxy bile acids produce greater effects on intestinal fluid absorption than the trihydroxy acids (GULLIKSON et al. 1977). Thus, these laxative bile acids may be accumulated in larger amounts in the colon. Again, the extrapolation from in vitro tests to the gut lumen may not be really meaningful. Extrapolation of the data from extracted food preparations to the original food substances indicates the need for a very large amount of a given food to adsorb a small amount of bile acid.

Clinically, 15 g/day psyllium (Metamucil) or cellulose were modest binders of radiolabeled cholate when compared with cholestyramine, a potent bile salt chelator (STANLEY et al. 1973). Cholestyramine's well-documented laxative side effects may be due to this mechanism (HOFMANN 1978). Animal studies indicate that psyllium added to diets can decrease bile acid half-life by 40% by increasing the rate of bile acid excretion, as well as the turnover rate and pool size (BEHER and CASAZZA 1971). Other studies on the interactions between bile salts and cellulose have also been reported (VAN BERESTEYN et al. 1979; SCHNEEMAN and GALLAHER 1980). Clinically, 10 g/day intake of psyllium seed for 3 or 6 weeks may increase total fecal bile acid output and decrease serum cholesterol by approximately 15% (FORMAN et al. 1968; GARVIN et al. 1965). A comparison between wheat bran and bagasse (sugar cane residue) showed that the latter increased fecal steroid loss while the bran did not (WALTERS et al. 1975). Steroid levels in the liver, blood, and gastrointestinal tract may be influenced by dietary fibers (SPILLER et al. 1978; KRITCHEVSKY 1978; STORY and KRITCHEVSKY 1978; TAPILA et al. 1978; VAN BERESTEYN et al. 1979). These agents may alter bile salt micelle formation, affect transit time, or change the microflora. Fiber may vary as to its efficacy in producing these laxative effects because of its heterogeneous chemical nature.

Dietary fibers may alter the digestion of nutrients and other substances. The relationship of dietary fiber and carbohydrate and lipid metabolism has been reviewed (ANDERSON and CHEN 1979; REISER 1979). For example, the addition of sucrose to wheat flour causes a malabsorption of the products of this disaccharide. Sucrose, normally hydrolyzed and absorbed in the small intestine, is carried into the colon and altered by the bacteria (ANDERSON et al. 1980). In contrast, the absorption of vitamin A is enhanced if given with guar flour and apple pectin (KASPER et al. 1979a). Alternately, carboxymethylcellulose, in humans, can reduce the acute toxicity of digitoxin (FEINBLATT et al. 1950), as well as delay and impair the absorption of nitrofurantoin (SEAGER 1968). In other studies, the blood levels of digoxin in normal individuals were not altered when the drug was taken with cellulose, pectin, or wheat bran (KASPER et al. 1979b). There was, however, a delay in the time needed to reach peak blood levels. These changes in drug activity and blood levels are probably due to the dietary fiber causing a slowing of stomach emptying. Wheat bran has also been shown to reduce dimethylhydrazine-induced colon tumors in rats (WILSON et al. 1977). Other information on chemical and drug-dietary fiber interactions is not available as this topic has not been extensively studied.

Clinical trials have been conducted with various dietary fibers for treatment of diverticular disease (TAYLOR and DUTHIE 1976; BRODRIBB 1977; EASTWOOD et al. 1978) and relief of symptoms of hemorrhoids (WEBSTER et al. 1978). Fiber has even been suggested to be useful for treating hypertension (DODSON 1980). The topic has been reviewed (CUMMINGS 1973; ALMY and HOWELL 1980). The latter review is an excellent objective summary of the epidemiology, animal models, and treatment of diverticular disease. It emphasizes the difficulty in objectively evaluating the role of the various dietary fibers and laxatives. To date, no definitive evidence has been gathered that dietary fiber is prophylactic or therapeutic for any disease. As concluded by CONNELL (1976) "a great deal of further work requires to be done to justify the claims that have been made on the role of fiber in altering normal or abnormal bowel habit."

V. Carbohydrate Laxative Drugs

There is not a sharp distinction between the chemical nature of the carbohydrates, such as bran, that are used as dietary supplements and psyllium seed that is utilized as a "drug" dietary supplement. Several carbohydrate derivatives and other macromolecules have been specifically used or developed for clinical use as laxatives. In their review, TAINTER and BUCHANAN (1954) described seven categories of polysaccharides which were used as laxatives, ranging from the natural substances like tragacanth, gums, and psyllium seed to the synthetic derivatives of methylcellulose and sodium carboxymethylcellulose. Their review adequately presents the history, pharmacology, and clinical trials of the glycans.

A wider choice in the form of delivery of dietary fiber is possible. A 70% cellulose and 30% pectin mixture (Phybrex) was evaluated clinically as a powder mixed with water or baked into biscuits and compared with psyllium powders and a placebo of corn syrup solids (SPILLER et al. 1979). The similar laxative effects among the two powders and the biscuits indicate that different delivery forms of fecal bulking agents could be made available. This would permit a wider choice of consumption as a baked food, stew, or other recipe form. In addition, two other substances have been described as laxatives, polycarbophil and lactulose.

Polycarbophil is a hydrophilic polyacrylic resin with a high water-binding capacity of 4:1, when compared with psyllium (GROSSMAN et al. 1957; PIMPARKER et al. 1961; RULEDGE et al. 1963). It has been demonstrated to be clinically effective in treating both constipation and diarrhea. This dual action may be related to the water-retaining properties of the resin and its lack of biodegradability. The data in these references were sufficient to warrant the advisory panel on laxatives to the FDA to recommend approval for marketing of polycarbophil (OVER THE COUNTER DRUGS 1975) and it is available on the American market as Mitrolan.

The synthetic disaccharide lactulose has galactose and fructose units as its two hexose components. Its history, biologic actions, and medical use are critically presented in a book (CONN and LIEBERTHAL 1979). Synthesized in the late 1920s, it was not studied for biologic activity until the 1950s, when it was shown to increase the colonic anaerobic bacterial population, an action shared with other carbohydrates. Its major use in medicine is in the treatment of portal-systemic encephalopathy with soft stools being one of the end points of therapeutic effectiveness.

Laxation is predictive of a disaccharide, like lactulose, that is not metabolized by the enzymes of the small intestine to monosaccharides that are absorbed. Typical of the carbohydrate laxatives, lactulose may exert an osmotic effect in the small intestine, since it would act as an intact, minimally absorbed molecule. Interestingly, in humans, lactulose in a dose range of 5–20 g shortens the mouth–colon transit time (BOND and LEVITT 1975). This suggests that the larger volume of water osmotically retained by the lactulose in the small intestine may enhance propulsive motor patterns. Quantification and objective measurements of the osmotic action in the small intestine for this or any other carbohydrate laxative has not been performed. Lactulose administered chronically (4 months) to rabbits does prevent certain effects of a low residue diet such as prolongation of transit time, decrease in fecal output, and the increase in mean colonic luminal pressure (HODGSON 1975). It is well documented that bacterial degradation of lactulose in the colon (BOND and LEVITT 1975) yields various gases (H_2, CO_2) and short-chain fatty acids, the major one being lactate (PELED and GILAT 1979). It has been suggested that the lowering of the colonic pH (from 7.05 to 4.85), or the increase of intraluminal colonic osmolarity owing to the increased presence of short-chain fatty acids is the mechanism for laxation. As with the other carbohydrates, lactulose's capacity to cause proliferation of bacteria, increase gas and fatty acid production, along with other actions, does not permit determination of a primary mechanism of action for laxation.

Clinically, a statistically valid model for evaluating lactulose as a laxative has been described (BASS and DENNIS 1981). A response was generated in normal subjects to 20 g and 40 g lactulose (Chronulac) for stool frequency, volume, consistency, and wet and dry weight. In addition, effective laxation was demonstrated in a constipated population (Table 5). Objective clinical trials were instrumental in permitting laxative claims for lactulose in the United States. Other clinical trials have also been described (CONN and LIEBERTHAL 1979). It is also the first laxative to be made available in the United States on a prescription only basis.

Table 5. Mean treatment response in constipated subjects

Stool response variable	Treatment group (40 g medication)				P^a
	Lactulose ($N=10$)		Placebo ($N=14$)		
	Pretreatment	Treatment	Pretreatment	Treatment	
Frequency (per week)	1.6	4.5*	1.4	2.8*	0.08
Volume (ml/day)	13.8	54.4*	15.8	38.6*	0.06
Wet weight (g/day)	17.7	65.7*	20.5	46.9*	0.05
Dry weight (g/day)	5.3	15.0*	6.6	13.3*	0.26
Moisture (%)	64.2	73.2*	67.6	69.8	0.02
Consistency score[b]	4.9	3.8*	4.7	4.3	0.01

* Significantly different from respective pretreatment value ($P<0.05$)

[a] P value associated with the lactulose–placebo treatment difference from a covariance analysis

[b] Stool consistency score: 1 = liquid ... 7 = very hard

A comparison among bran, psyllium seed, and lactulose in patients with diverticular disease revealed equal effectiveness in alleviating intestinal pain and increasing stool output (EASTWOOD et al. 1978). However, no consistent effects were obtained on the colonic motor activity. Several simple sugars like sorbitol and mannitol are also capable of laxation. Poorly absorbed, they have been assumed to act by exerting an osmotic pressure in the small intestine. Their possible action in the colon has largely been ignored. Certainly, in vitro they are readily metabolized by fecal bacteria (VINCE et al. 1978). Thus, mono-, di-, or polysaccharides may lead to laxation by a series of complex processes in both the small and large intestines. Details of mechanisms are only now being described.

E. Summary

Evidence has been presented which questions the traditional terms associated with several of the mechanisms of laxative action. The mechanisms of action described in this chapter would suggest that "stimulant and wetting agent" type laxatives have a common modality, unrelated to their usual classifications – the ability to induce net fluid and electrolyte secretion into the lumens of the small or large intestine. Specific control mechanisms for secretion which operate for hormonally or bacterially induced secretion, however, do not appear to apply to the actions of the secretory laxatives. This laxative-induced fluid accumulation is not due solely to one mechanism, as laxatives produce a variety of nonspecific effects on the intestinal mucosal membrane which could account for laxation. In addition, a common motor or electrical *pattern* may be associated with the effects of several laxatives, rather than a stimulant effect on motility. The misconception that fluid-induced swelling is the only mechanism of bulk laxatives has also been challenged. The actions of these bulk laxatives appear to be due to interrelated factors which are dependent on the action of colonic bacteria on their complex carbohydrate structure.

Terms which describe the efficacy of laxative action – aperient, purgative, cathartic, or drastic – also must be reevaluated. The fluid effects of secretagogue laxatives are dose-related phenomenon in experimental models. Clinically, a "mild" laxative, such as DSS (Colace), must be considered in terms of its low dose (100 mg), compared to a "harsh" laxative, such as castor oil (30–60 g). Harshness of action of any of the intestinal secretagogues in humans will be directly proportionate to dose. In contrast, the nature and diversity of the polysaccharides contained in bulk laxatives do not permit the development of classical dose–response relationships.

References

Akiyama S, Igisu H (1979) Effects of D-L-propanolol and other beta adrenergic receptor blocking agents on membrane fluidity of erythrocytes. Jpn J Pharmacol 29:144–146

Almy TP, Howell DA (1980) Diverticular disease of the colon. N Eng J Med 302:324–331

Ammon HV, Phillips SF (1973) Inhibition of colonic water and electrolyte absorption by fatty acids in man. Gastroenterology 65:744–749

Ammon HV, Phillips SF (1974) Inhibition of ileal water absorption by intraluminal fatty acids. J Clin Invest 53:205–210

Ammon HV, Thomas PJ, Phillips SF (1974) Effects of oleic and recinoleic acids on net jejunal water and electrolyte movement. Perfusion studies in man. J Clin Invest 53:374–379

Anderson JW, Chen WL (1979) Plant fiber. Carbohydrate and lipid metabolism. Am J Clin Nutr 32:346–363

Anderson I, Levine A, Levitt MD (1980) Use of breath H_2 excretion to study absorption of wheat flour. Gastroenterology 78:1131

Anonymous (1980) Annual drugstore sales survey. Drug Topics 124:22–75

Atchison WD, Klasek GJ, Bass P (1978a) Laxative effects on small intestinal electric activity of the conscious dog. In: Duthie HL (ed) Gastrointestinal motility in health and disease. 6th International symposium on gastrointestinal motility. MTP, Lancaster, pp 73–81

Atchison WD, Stewart JJ, Bass P (1978b) A unique distribution of laxative-induced spike potentials from the small intestine of the dog. Am J Dig Dis 23:513–520

Barbezat GO, Grossman MI (1971a) Intestinal secretion: stimulation by peptides. Science 174:422–424

Barbezat GO, Grossman MI (1971b) Cholera-like diarrhea induced by glucagon plus gastrin. Lancet 1:1025–1026

Bass P (1967) In vivo electrical activity of the small bowel. In: Code CF, Heidel W (eds) Handbook of physiology, sect 6 alimentary canal, vol IV motility. Williams and Wilkins, Baltimore, p 2051

Bass P, Dennis S (1981) The laxative effects of lactulose in normal and constipated subjects. J Clin Gastroenterol 3 [Suppl 1]:23–29

Bass P, Wiley JN (1965) Effects of ligation and morphine on electric and motor activity of dog duodenum. Am J Physiol 208:908–913

Bass P, Wiley JN (1972) Contractile force transducer for recording muscle activity in unanesthetized animals. J Appl Physiol 32:567–570

Bass P, Code CF, Lambert EH (1961) Motor electric activity of the duodenum. Am J Physiol 201:287–291

Bayless TM, Luebbers E, Elliot HL (1971) Immature jejunal crypts: absence of response to stimulus for fluid secretion. Gastroenterology 60:762

Beher WT, Casazza KK (1971) Effects of psyllium hydrocolloid on bile acid metabolism in normal and hypophysectomized rats. Proc Soc Exp Biol Med 136:253–256

Beleslin DB (1970) Nature of the peristaltic block produced by magnesium. Nature 225:383–384

Bennett A, Eley KG, Scholes GB (1968a) Effect of prostaglandins E_1 and E_2 on intestinal motility in the guinea pig and rat. Br J Pharmacol 34:639–647

Bennett A, Eley KG, Scholes GB (1968b) Effects of prostaglandin E_1 and E_2 on human guinea pig and rat isolated small intestine. Br J Pharmacol 34:630–638

Bennett DR, Bass P (1972) The action of inhalation anesthetics on the gastrointestinal tract. In: Chenoweth MB (ed) Modern inhalation anesthetics. Springer, Berlin Heidelberg New York, p 318

Berridge M (1975) The interaction of cyclic nucleotides and calcium in the control of cellular activity. Adv Cyclic Nucleotide Res 6:1–98

Beubler E, Juan H (1978) PGE-mediated laxative effects of diphenolic laxatives. Naunyn Schmiedebergs Arch Pharmacol 305:241–246

Beubler E, Juan H (1979) Effect of ricinoleic acid and other laxatives on net water flux and prostaglandin E release by the rat colon. J Pharm Pharmacol 31:681–685

Binder HJ (1974) Cyclic adenosine monophosphate controls bile salt and hydroxy fatty acid-induced colonic electrolyte secretion. J Clin Invest 53:7–8A

Binder HJ (1977) Pharmacology of laxatives. Ann Rev Pharmacol Toxicol 17:355–367

Binder HJ (1979) Net fluid and electrolyte secretion: the pathophysiologic basis for diarrhea. In: Binder HJ (ed) Mechanisms of intestinal secretion. Liss, New York, p 1

Binder HJ, Filburn C, Volpe BT (1975) Bile salt alteration of colonic electrolyte transport: role of cyclic adenosine monophosphate. Gastroenterology 68:503–508

Binder HJ, Dobbins JW, Racusen LC, Whiting DS (1978) Effect of propranolol on ricinoleic acid – and deoxycholic acid – induced changes of intestinal electrolyte movement and mucosal permeability. Evidence against the importance of altered permeability in the production of fluid and electrolyte accumulation. Gastroenterology 75:668–673

Birkner HJ, Kern F (1974) In vitro adsorption of bile salts to food residues, salicylazosulfapyridine and hemicellulose. Gastroenterology 67:237–244

Bloom SR, Polak JM, Pearse AGE (1973) Vasoactive intestinal polypeptide and watery diarrhea syndrome. Lancet 2:14–16

Blythe RH, Gulesich JJ, Tuthill HL (1949) Evaluation of hydrophic properties of bulk laxatives including the new agent, sodium carboxymethylcellulose. J Am Pharm Assoc 38:59–64

Bolton JE, Field M (1977) Ca ionophore-stimulated ion secretion in rabbit ileal mucosa; relation to actions of cyclic 3′,5′ AMP and carbamylcholine. J Membr Biol 35:159–173

Bond JH Jr, Levitt MD (1975) Investigation of small bowel transit time in man utilizing pulmonary hydrogen (H_2) measurements. J Lab Clin Med 85:546–555

Bonnycastle DD (1965) Cathartics and laxatives. In: Di Palma JR (ed) Drill's pharmacology in medicine, 3rd edn. McGraw-Hill, New York, p 747

Bortoff A (1976) Myogenic control of intestinal motility. Physiol Rev 56:418–434

Brasitis TA, Field M, Kimberg DV (1976) Intestinal mucosal cyclic GMP: regulation and relation to ion transport. Am J Physiol 231:275–282

Bretagne JF, Vidon N, L'Hirondel C, Bernier JJ (1981) Increased cell loss in the human jejunum induced by laxatives (ricinoleic acid, dioctyl sodium sulphosuccinate, magnesium sulphate, bile salts). Gut 22:264–269

Bright-Asare P, Binder HJ (1973) Stimulation of colonic secretion of water and electrolytes by hydroxy fatty acids. Gastroenterology 64:81–88

Brodribb AJM (1977) Treatment of symptomatic diverticular disease with a high-fiber diet. Lancet 1:664–666

Brodribb AJM, Groves C (1978) Effect of bran particle size on stool weight. Gut 19:60–63

Brodribb AJM, Condon RG, Cowles V, De Cosse JJ (1979) Effect of dietary fiber on intraluminal pressure and myoelectrical activity of left colon in monkeys. Gastroenterology 77:70–74

Brodribb J, Condon RE, Cowles V, De Cosse JJ (1980) Influence of dietary fiber on transit time, fecal composition and myoelectrical activity of the primate right colon. Dig Dis Sci 25:260–266

Burkitt DP, Trowell HC (1975) Refined carbohydrate foods and disease some implications of dietary fiber. Academic, London, p 356

Burkitt DP, Walker ARP, Painter NS (1972) Effect of dietary fiber on stools and transit time, and its role in the causation of disease. Lancet 2:1408–1412

Burns TW, Mathias JR, Carlson GM, Martin JL, Shields RP (1978) Effect of toxigenic Escherichia coli on myoelectric activity of small intestine. Am J Physiol 235:E311–E315

Burns TW, Mathias JR, Martin JL, Carlson GM, Shields RP (1980) Alteration of myoelectric activity of small intestine by invasive Escherichia coli. Am J Physiol 238:G57–G62

Camilleri M, Murphy R, Chadwick VS (1980) Dose-related effects of chenodeoxycholic acid in the rabbit colon. Dig Dis Sci 25:433–438

Carlson AJ, Hoelzel F (1949) Relation of diet to diverticulosis of the colon in rats. Gastroenterology 12:108–115

Carlson GM, Ruddon RW, Hug CC Jr, Bass P (1970) Effects of nicotine on gastric antral and duodenal contractile activity in the dog. J Pharmacol Exp Ther 172:367–376

Caspary WF, Meyne K (1980) Effects of chenodeoxy- and ursodeoxycholic acid on absorption, secretion and permeability in rat colon and small intestine. Digestion 20:168–174

Chadwick VS, Gaginella TS, Carlson GL, Debongnie J-C, Phillips SF, Hofmann AF (1979) Effect of molecular structure on bile acid-induced alterations in absorptive function, permeability, and morphology in the perfused rabbit colon. J Lab Clin Med 94:661–674

Charney AN, Donowitz M (1978) Functional significance of intestinal Na-K-ATPase: in vivo ouabain inhibition. Am J Physiol 234:E629–E636

Chignell CF (1968) The effect of phenolphthalein and other purgative drugs on rat intestinal ($Na^+ + K^+$) adenosine triphosphatase. Biochem Pharmacol 17:1207–1212

Cleave TL, Campbell GD, Painter NS (1969) Diabetes coronary thrombosis and the saccharin disease, 2nd edn. Wright, Bristol

Cline WS, Lorenzsonn V, Benz L, Bass P, Olsen WA (1976) The effects of sodium ricinoleate on small intestinal function and structure. J Clin Invest 58:380–390

Collier HOJ, McDonald-Gibson WJ, Saeed SA (1976) Stimulation of prostaglandin biosynthesis by drugs: effects in vitro of some drugs affecting gut function. Br J Pharmacol 58:193–199

Conley D, Coyne M, Chung A, Bonorris G, Schoenfield L (1976) Propranolol inhibits adenylate cyclase and secretion stimulated by deoxycholic acid in the rabbit colon. Gastroenterology 71:72–75

Conn HO, Lieberthal MM (1979) The hepatic coma syndrome and lactulose. William and Wilkins, Baltimore, p 419

Connell AM (1968) The irritable colon syndrome. Postgrad Med J 44:668–671

Connell AM (1976) Natural fiber and bowel dysfunction. J Clin Nutr 29:1427–1431

Connell AM (1981) Dietary Fiber. In: Johnson LR (ed) Physiology of the gastrointestinal tract. Raven, New York, p 1291

Connell AM, Kellock TD (1959) Treatment of chronic non-specific diarrhoea. A clinical comparison. Br Med J 1:151–153

Connell AM, Smith CL (1974) The effect of dietary fiber on transit time. In: Daniel EE (ed) 4th International symposium on gastrointestinal motility. Mitchell, Vancouver, pp 365–368

Connell AM, Hilton C, Irvine G, Lennard-Jones JE, Misiewicz JJ (1965) Variation of bowel habit in two population samples. Br Med J 2:1095–1099

Coyne M, Bonorris G, Chung A, Conley D, Croke J, Schoenfield L (1976) Inhibition by propranolol of bile acid stimulation of rabbit colonic adenylate cyclase in vitro. Gastroenterology 71:68–71

Cummings JH (1973) Progress report dietary fiber. Gut 14:69–81

Darlington RC (1973) Laxatives. In: Griffenhagen AB, Hawkins LB (eds) Handbook of non-prescription drugs. Am Pharm Assoc, Washington, DC, p 62

Debongnie JC, Phillips SF (1978) Capacity of the human colon to absorb fluid. Gastroenterology 74:698–703

Dejonge HR (1975) The response of small intestinal villous and crypt epithelium to cholera toxin in rat and guinea pig. Evidence against a specific role of the crypt cells in choleragen-induced secretion. Biochem Biophys Acta 381:128–143

Dinoso VP, Meshkinpour H, Lorber SH, Gutierrez JG, Chey WY (1973) Motor responses of the sigmoid colon and rectum to exogenous cholecystokinin and secretin. Gastroenterology 65:438–444

Dobbins JW, Binder HJ (1976) Effect of bile salts and fatty acids on the colonic absorption of oxalate. Gastroenterology 70:1096–1100

Dodson PM (1980) Dietary fiber, sodium and blood pressure. Br Med J 1:564

Donowitz M, Binder HJ (1975) Effect of dioctyl sodium sulfosuccinate on colonic fluid and electrolyte movement. Gastroenterology 69:941–950

Donowitz M, Charney AN (1979 a) Propranolol prevention of cholera enterotoxin-induced intestinal secretion in the rat. Gastroenterology 76:482–491

Donowitz M, Charney AN (1979 b) No effect of propranolol on chronic diarrhea. N Engl J Med 300:201

Duffy PA, Granger DN, Taylor AE (1978) Intestinal secretion induced by volume expansion in the dog. Gastroenterology 75:413–418

Dupont HL, Sullivan P, Pickering LK, Haynes G, Ackerman PB (1977) Symptomatic treatment of diarrhea with bismuth subsalicylate among students attending a Mexican university. Gastroenterology 73:715–718

Duszynski J, Wojtczak L (1974) Effect of detergents on ADP translocation on mitochondria. FEBS Lett 40:72–76

Duthie HL (1974) Electrical activity of gastrointestinal smooth muscle. Gut 15:669–681

Eastwood MA, Hamilton D (1968) Studies on the adsorption of bile salts to non-absorbed components of diet. Biochem Biophys Acta 152:165–173
Eastwood MA, Kay RM (1979) An hypothesis for the action of dietary fiber along the gastrointestinal tract. Am J Clin Nutr 32:364–367
Eastwood MA, Kirkpatrick JR, Mitchell WD, Bone A, Hamilton T (1973) Effects of dietary supplements of wheat bran and cellulose on feces and bowel function. Br Med J 4:392–394
Eastwood MA, Smith AN, Brydon WG, Pritchard J (1978) Comparison of bran, ispaghula, and lactulose on colon function in diverticular disease. Gut 19:1144–1147
Elliot HL, Carpenter CC, Sack RB (1970) Small bowel morphology in experimental canine cholera. A light and electron microscopic study. Lab Invest 22:112–120
Ewe K (1972) Effect of laxatives on intestinal water and electrolyte transport. Eur J Clin Invest 2:283
Ewe K, Holker B (1974) Einfluß eines diphenolischen Laxans (Bisacodyl) auf den Wasser- und Elektrolyte-Transport im menschlichen Kolon. Klin Wochenschr 52:827–833
Fantus B, Kopstein G, Schmidt HR (1940) Roentgen study of intestinal motility as influenced by bran. JAMA 114:404–408
Farack UM, Nell G (1979) The influence of an adenylcyclase inhibitor on the cholera toxin-desoxycholic acid- and bisacodyl-induced intestinal secretion in the rat. Naunyn Schmiedebergs Arch Pharmacol 308 [Suppl]:R27
Faust RG, Wu SL (1965) The action of bile salts on fluid and glucose movement by rat and hamster jejunum in vitro. J Cell Comp Physiol 65:435–448
Faust RG, Wu SL (1967) The effect of bile salts on oxygen consumption, oxidative phosphorylation and ATPase activity of mucosal homogenates from rat jejunum and ileum. J Cell Physiol 67:149–158
Feinblatt HM, Feinblatt TM, Ferguson EA Jr (1950) Modification of digitoxin action by sodium carboxymethylcellulose. NY State J Med 50:2461–2464
Field M (1978) Some speculation on the coupling between sodium chloride transport processes in mammalian and teleost intestine. In: Hoffman JF (ed) Membrane transport processes. Raven, New York, p 277
Field M, Graf LH, Laird WJ, Smith PL (1978) Heat stable enterotoxin of Escherichia coli: In vitro effects of guanylate cyclase activity, cyclic GMP concentration, and ion transport in small intestine. Proc Natl Acad Sci USA 75:2800–2804
Fingl E (1975) Laxatives and cathartics. In: Goodman LS, Gilman A (eds) The pharmacological basis of therapeutics, 5th edn. MacMillan, New York, p 976
Fioramonti J, Bueno L (1980) Motor activity in the large intestine of the pig related to dietary fibre and retention time. Br J Nutr 43:155–162
Flath CI (1976) The miracle nutrient. How dietary fibers can save your life. Bantam, New York
Forman DT, Garvin JE, Forestner JE, Taylor CB (1968) Increased excretion of fecal bile acids by an oral hydrophilic colloid. Proc Soc Exp Biol Med 127:1060–1063
Forth W, Baldauf J, Rummel W (1963) Ein Beitrag zur Klärung des Wirkungsmechanismus einiger Laxantien. Naunyn Schmiedebergs Arch Pharmacol Exp Path 246:91–92
Forth W, Rummel W, Baldauf J (1966a) Wasser- und Elektrolytebewegung am Dünn- und Dickdarm unter dem Einfluß von Laxantien, ein Beitrag zur Klärung ihres Wirkungsmechanismus. Naunyn Schmiedebergs Arch Pharmacol Exp Path 254:18–32
Forth W, Rummel W, Glasner H, Andres H (1966b) Zur resorptionshemmenden Wirkung von Gallensäuren. Naunyn Schmiedebergs Arch Pharmacol Exp Path 254:364–380
Frizzell RA (1977) Active chloride secretion by rabbit colon: calcium-dependent stimulation by ionophore A23187. J Membr Biol 35:175–187
Frizzell RA, Koch MJ, Schultz SG (1976) Ion transport by rabbit colon. I. Active and passive components. J Membr Biol 35:297–316
Frizzell RA, Field M, Schultz SG (1979) Sodium-coupled chloride transport by epithelial tissues. Am J Physiol 236:F1–F9
Fuchs HM, Dorfman S, Floch MH (1976) The effect of dietary fiber supplementation in man: II. Alteration in fecal physiology and bacterial flora. Am J Clin Nutr 29:1443–1447

Gadacz TR, Gaginella TS, Phillips SF (1976) Inhibition of water absorption by ricinoleic acid. Evidence against hormonal mediation of the effect. Am J Dig Dis 21:859–862

Gaginella TS, Bass P (1978) Laxatives: an update on mechanism of action. Life Sci 23:1001–1010

Gaginella TS, Stewart JJ, Olsen WA, Bass P (1975a) Actions of ricinoleic acid and structurally related fatty acids on the gastrointestinal tract. II. Effects on water and electrolyte absorption in vitro. J Pharmacol Exp Ther 195:355–361

Gaginella TS, Stewart JJ, Gullikson GW, Olsen WA, Bass P (1975b) Inhibition of small intestinal mucosal and smooth muscle cell function by ricinoleic acid and other surfactants. Life Sci 16:1595–1606

Gaginella TS, Bass P, Olsen W, Shug A (1975c) Fatty acid inhibition of water absorption and energy production in the hamster jejunum. FEBS Lett 53:347–350

Gaginella TS, Lewis JC, Phillips SF (1976) Ricinoleic acid effects on rabbit intestine. Mayo Clin Proc 51:569–573

Gaginella TS, Chadwick VS, Debongnie JC, Lewis JC, Phillips SF (1977a) Perfusion of rabbit colon with ricinoleic acid: dose related mucosal injury, fluid secretion and increased permeability. Gastroenterology 73:95–101

Gaginella TS, Haddad AC, Go VLW, Phillips SF (1977b) Cytotoxicity of ricinoleic acid (castor oil) and other intestinal secretagogues on isolated intestinal epithelial cells. J Pharmacol Exp Ther 201:259–266

Gaginella TS, Lewis JC, Phillips SF (1977c) Rabbit ileal mucosa exposed to fatty acids, bile acids and other secretogogues. Scanning electron microscopic appearances. Am J Dig Dis 22:781–790

Gaginella TS, Mekhjian HS, O'Dorisio TM (1978a) Vasoactive intestinal peptide: quantitation by radioimmunoassay in isolated cells, mucosa, and muscle of the hamster intestine. Gastroenterology 74:718–721

Gaginella TS, Phillips SF, Dozois RR, Go VLW (1978b) Stimulation of adenylate cyclase in homogenates of isolated intestinal epithelial cells from hamsters. Effects of gastrointestinal hormones, prostaglandins, and deoxycholic and ricinoleic acid. Gastroenterology 74:11–15

Galton L (1976) The truth about fiber in your food. Crown, NY, p 246

Gardner JD, Peskin GW, Cerda JJ, Brooks FP (1967) Alterations of in vitro fluid and electrolyte absorption by gastrointestinal hormones. Am J Surg 113:57–64

Garvin JE, Forman DT, Eiseman WR, Phillips CR (1965) Lowering of human serum cholesterol by an oral hydrophilic colloid. Proc Soc Exp Biol Med 120:744–746

Gibaldi M (1970) Role of surface active agents in drug absorption. Fed Proc 29:1343–1349

Goerg KJ, Gross M, Nell G, Rummel W, Schultz L (1980a) Comparative study of the effect of cholera toxin and sodium deoxycholate on the paracellular permeability and on net fluid and electrolyte transfer in the rat colon. Naunyn Schmiedebergs Arch Pharmacol 312:91–97

Goerg KJ, Wanitschke R, Schulz L (1980b) Scanning electron microscopic study of the effect of rhein on the surface morphology of the rat colonic mucosa. Pharmacology [Suppl 1] 20:36–42

Gordon LM, Sauerheber RD, Esgate JA, Dipple I, Marchmount RJ, Houslay MD (1980) The increase in bilayer fluidity of rat liver plasma membranes achieved by the local anesthetic benzyl alcohol affects the activity of intrinsic membrane enzymes. J Biol Chem 255:4519–4527

Gould SR (1975) Prostaglandins, ulcerative colitis and sulphasalazine. Lancet 2:988

Gray H, Tainter ML (1941) Colloid laxatives available for clinical use. Am J Dig Dis 8:130–139

Grossman AJ, Batterman RC, Leifer P (1957) Polyacrylic resin: effective hydrophylic colloid for the treatment of constipation. J Am Geriatr Soc 5:187–192

Guiraldes E, Lamabadusuriya SP, Oyesiku JE, Whitfield TE, Harries JT (1975) A comparative study on the effects of different bile salts on mucosal ATPase and transport in the rat jejunum in vivo. Biochem Biophys Acta 389:495–505

Gullikson GW, Cline WS, Lorenzsonn V, Benz L, Olsen WA, Bass P (1977) Effects of anionic surfactants on hamster small intestinal membrane structure and function: relationship to surface activity. Gastroenterology 73:501–511
Gullikson GW, Jasty V, Dajani EZ (1981 a) Effect of lidamidine on deoxycholate-induced histological and permeability changes in canine jejunum. Pharmacologist 23:122
Gullikson GW, Dajani EZ, Bianchi RG (1981 b) Inhibition of intestinal secretion in the dog: a new approach for the management of diarrheal states. J Pharmacol Exp Ther 219:591–597, 1981
Hakim AA, Papeleux CB, Lane JB, Lifson N, Yablonski ME (1977) Mechanism of production of intestinal secretion by negative luminal pressure. Am J Physiol 233:E416–E421
Hallbäck D-A, Hultén L, Jodal M, Lindhagen J, Lundgren O (1978) Evidence for the existence of a countercurrent exchanger in the small intestine in man. Gastroenterology 74:683–690
Harvey RF, Read AE (1973) Saline purgatives act by releasing cholecystokinin. Lancet 2:185–187
Harvey RF, Pomare EW, Heaton KW (1973) Effects of increased dietary fibre on intestinal transit. Lancet 1:1278–1280
Helenius A, Simons K (1975) Solubilization of membranes by detergents. Biochem Biophys Acta 415:29–79
Hellendoorn EW (1978) Fermentation as the principal cause of the physiological activity of indigestible food residue. In: Spiller GA, Amen RJ (eds) Topics in dietary fiber research. Plenum, New York, p 127
Hickey CA, Murphy EL, Calloway DH (1972) Intestinal gas production following ingestion of commercial wheat cereals and milling fractions. Cereal Chem 49:276–281
Higgins JT, Blair NP (1971) Intestinal transport of water and electrolytes during extracellular volume expansion in dogs. J Clin Invest 50:2569–2579
Hodgson J (1975) Effect of lactulose in rabbits fed on a low residue diet. Am J Gastroenterol 64:115–121
Hofmann AF (1978) The enterohepatic circulation of bile acids. In: Sleisenger MH, Fordtran JS (eds) Gastrointestinal disease, 2nd edn. Saunders, Philadelphia, p 92
Hoppert CA, Clark AJ (1945) Digestibility and effect on laxation of crude fiber and cellulose in certain common foods. J Am Diet Assoc 21:157–160
Hummel FC, Shepherd MC, Macy IG (1943) Disappearance of cellulose and hemicellulose from the digestive tracts of children. J Nutr 25:59–70
Inglett GE, Falkehag SI (1979) Dietary fibers: chemistry and nutrition. Academic, New York, p 285
Ireson JD, Leslie GB (1970) An in vitro investigation of colloidal bulk-forming laxatives. Pharmaceutical J 205:540
Ivey KJ (1975) Are anticholinergics of use in the irritable colon syndrome? Gastroenterology 68:1300–1307
Ivy AC, Isaacs BL (1938) Karaya gum as a mechanical laxative. An experimental study on animals and man. Am J Dig Dis 5:315–321
Kasper H, Rabast U, Fassl H, Fehle F (1979 a) The effect of dietary fiber on the postprandial serum vitamin A concentration in man. Am J Clin Nutr 32:1847–1849
Kasper H, Zilly W, Fassl H, Fehle F (1979 b) The effect of dietary fiber on postprandial serum digoxin concentration in man. Am J Clin Nutr 32:2436–2438
Kay RM, Strasberg SM, Petrunka CN, Wayman M (1979) Differential adsorption of bile acids by lignins. In: Inglett GE, Falkehag SI (eds) Dietary fiber chemistry and nutrition. Academic, New York, p 57
Kern F Jr, Almy TP, Abbot FK, Bogdonoff MD (1951) The motility of the distal colon in non-specific ulcerative colitis. Gastroenterology 19:492–502
Kerzner B, O'Dorisio T, Gaginella T, Mekhjian H, Super D, Frye T, Ailabouni A, McClung HJ (1979) Ricinoleic acid: mechanism of action in isolated enterocytes. Gastroenterology 76:1168
Kimberg DV (1974) Cyclic nucleotides and their role in gastrointestinal secretion. Gastroenterology 67:1023–1064

Kimberg DV, Field M, Johnson J, Henderson A, Gershon E (1971) Stimulation of intestinal mucosal adenyl cyclase by cholera enterotoxin and prostaglandin. J Clin Invest 50:1218–1230

Kirwan WO, Smith AN, McConnell AA, Mitchell WD, Eastwood MA (1974) Action of different bran preparations on colonic function. Br Med J 4:187–189

Krag E, Phillips SF (1974) Effect of free and unconjugated bile acids on net water, electrolyte, and glucose movement in the perfused human ileum. J Lab Clin Med 83:947–956

Krejs GJ, Walsh JH, Morawski SG, Fordtran JS (1977) Intractable diarrhea. Intestinal perfusion studies and plasma VIP concentrations in patients with pancreatic cholera syndrome and surreptitious ingestion of laxatives and diuretics. Am J Dig Dis 22:280–292

Kritchevsky D (1978) Influence of dietary fiber on bile acid metabolism. Lipids 13:982–985

Latven AR, Sloane AB, Munch JC (1952) Bioassay of cathartics. I. Emodin type. J Am Pharm Assoc 41:548–552

Lee T-P, Kuo JF, Greengard P (1972) Role of muscarinic cholinergic receptors in regulation of guanosine-3′:5′-cyclic monophosphate content in mammalian brain, heart muscle, and intestinal smooth muscle. Proc Natl Acad Sci USA 69:3287–3291

Lemmens L, Borja E (1976) The influence of dihydroxyanthracene derivatives on water and electrolyte movement in rat colon. J Pharm Pharmacol 28:498–501

Levin B, Horwitz D (1979) Dietary Fiber. Med Cl North Am 63:1043–1055

Lium R, Florey HW (1939) The action of magnesium sulfate on the intestine of the cat. Q J Exp Physiol 29:303–319

Low-Beer TS, Schneider RE, Dobbins WO (1970) Morphological changes of the small intestinal mucosa of guinea pig and hamster following incubation in vitro and perfusion in vivo with unconjugated bile salts. Gut 11:486–492

Lundgren O, Haglund U (1978) The pathophysiology of intestinal countercurrent exchanger. Life Sci 23:1411–1422

Malagelada JR, Holtermuller KH, McCall JT, Go VLW (1978) Pancreatic, gallbladder and intestinal responses to intraluminal magnesium salts in man. Am J Dig Dis 23:481–484

Malagelada JR, Carter SE, Brown ML, Carlson GL (1980) Radiolabeled fiber. A physiologic marker for gastric emptying and intestinal transit of solids. Dig Dis Sci 25:81–87

Mangold E (1934) The digestion and utilization of crude fibre. Nutr Abstr Rev 3:647–656

Marshall NJ, Von Borcke S, Malan PG (1975) Studies on inhibition of TSH stimulation of adenyl cyclase activity in thyroid plasma membrane preparations by propranolol. Endocrinology 96:1513–1519

Mathias JR, Carlson GM, DiMarino AJ, Bertiger G, Morton HE, Cohen S (1976) Intestinal myoelectric activity in response to live vibrio cholerae and cholera enterotoxin. J Clin Invest 58:91–96

Mathias JR, Carlson GM, Bertiger G, Martin JL, Cohen S (1977) Migrating action potential complex of cholera: a possible prostaglandin-induced response. Am J Physiol 232:E529–E534

Mathias JR, Martin JL, Burns TW, Carlson GM, Shields R (1978) Ricinoleic acid effect on the electrical activity of the small intestine in rabbits. J Clin Invest 61:640–644

Mathias JR, Carlson GM, Martin JL, Shields RP, Formal S (1980) Shigella dysenteriae 1 entertoxin: proposed role in the pathogenesis of shigellosis. Am J Physiol 239:G382–G386

McConnell AA, Eastwood MA, Mitchell WD (1974) Physical characteristics of vegetable food stuffs that could influence bowel function. J Sci Food Agric 25:1457–1464

McCoy EJ, Bass P (1963) Chronic electric activity of gastroduodenal area: effects of food and certain catecholamines. Am J Physiol 205:439–445

McLeish JA, Johnson AG (1978) Low residue diet affects motility of the duodenum as well as the colon. In: Duthie HL (ed) Gastrointestinal motility in health and disease. MTP, Lancaster, p 185

McNeil NI, Cummings JH, James WPT (1978) Short chain fatty acid absorption by the human large intestine. Gut 19:819–822

Meisel JL, Bergman D, Saunders DR, Rubin CE (1977) Human rectal mucosa: proctoscopic and morphologic changes caused by laxatives. Gastroenterology 72:1274–1279
Mekhjian HS, Phillips SF (1970) Perfusion of the canine colon with unconjugated bile acids. Gastroenterology 59:120–129
Mekhjian HS, Phillips SF, Hofmann A (1971) Colonic secretion of water and electrolytes induced by bile acids: perfusion studies in man. J Clin Invest 50:1569–1577
Mendeloff AI (1977) Dietary fiber and human health. N Eng J Med 297:811–814
Mennie AT, Dalley VM, Dinneen LC, Collier HOJ (1975) Treatment of radiation-induced gastrointestinal distress with acetyl salicylate. Lancet 2:942–943
Metcalfe JC, Burgen ASV (1968) Relaxation of anesthetics in the presence of cyto-membranes. Nature 220:587–588
Milton-Thompson GJ, Lewis B (1971) The breakdown of dietary cellulose in man. Gut 12:853–854
Mir GN, Alioto RL, Sperow JW, Eash JR, Krebs JB, Yelnosky J (1978) In vivo antimotility and antidiarrheal activity of lidamidine hydrochloride (WHR-1142A), a novel antidiarrheal agent. Arzneimittelforsch Drug Res 28:1448–1454
Mitjavila MT, Mitjavila S, Gas N, Derache R (1975) Influence of various surface-active agents on the activity of several enzymes in the brush border of enterocytes. Toxicol Appl Pharmacol 34:72–82
Monaco AL, Dehner EJ (1955) An in vitro evaluation of some hydrophilic colloids as bulking agents. J Am Pharm Assoc 44:237–241
Moretó M, Goñalons E, Mylonakes N, Goráldez A, Torralba A (1979) 3,3-Bis-(4-hydroxyphenyl)-7-methyl-2-indolinone (BHMI), the active metabolite of the laxative sulisatin. Arzneimittelforsch 29:1561–1564
Moritz M, Finkelstein G, Meshkinpour H, Fingerut J, Lorber SH (1973) Effect of secretin and cholecystokinin on the transport of electrolyte and water in human jejunum. Gastroenterology 64:76–80
Morris AI, Turnberg LA (1981) Influence of isoproterenol and propranolol on human intestinal transport in vivo. Gastroenterology 81:1076–1079
Neily J (1969) The effects of analgesic drugs on gastrointestinal motility in man. Br J Surg 56:925–930
Nell G, Forth W, Rummel W, Wanitschke R (1976) Pathway of sodium moving from blood to intestinal lumen under the influence of oxyphenisatin and deoxycholate. Naunyn Schmiedebergs Arch Pharmacol 293:31–37
Over the counter drugs (1975) Proposed establishment of monographs for OTC laxative, antidiarrheal, emetic and antiemetic products. Federal Register 40: part II, p 12902–12944
Parker JG, Beneventano TC (1970) Acceleration of small bowel contrast study by cholecystokinin. Gastroenterology 58:679–684
Parkinson TM, Olsen JA (1964) Inhibitory effects of bile acids on adenosine triphosphatase, oxygen consumption, and the transport and diffusion of water soluble substances in the small intestine of the rat. Life Sci 3:107–112
Payler DK, Pomare EW, Heaton KW, Harvey RF (1975) The effect of wheat bran on intestinal transit. Gut 16:209–213
Peled Y, Gilat T (1979) The metabolism of lactulose by the fecal flora. Gastroenterology 77:821–822
Perkins JP, Moore MM (1971) Adenyl cyclase of rat cerebral cortex. J Biol Chem 246:62–68
Phillips RA, Love AHG, Mitchell TG, Neptune EM (1965) Cathartics and the sodium pump. Nature 206:1367–1368
Phillips SF (1973) Fluid and electrolyte fluxes in the gut. Hosp Pract 8:137–146
Pimparker BD, Paustian FF, Roth JLA, Bockus HL (1961) Effect of polycarbophil on diarrhea and constipation. Gastroenterology 40:397–404
Plant OH, Miller GH (1926) Effects of morphine and some other opium alkaloids on the muscle activity of the alimentary canal. I. Action on the small intestine in unanesthetized dogs and man. J Pharmacol Exp Ther 27:361–383

Pope JL, Parkinson TM, Olson JA (1966) Action of bile salts on the metabolism and transport of water soluble nutrients by perfused rat jejunum in vitro. Biochem Biophys Acta 130:218–232

Powell DW, Farris RK, Carbonetto ST (1974) Theophylline, cyclic AMP, choleragen and electrolyte transport by rabbit ileum. Am J Physiol 227:1428–1435

Powell DW, Lawrence BA, Morris SM, Etheridge DR (1980) Effect of phenolphthalein on in vitro rabbit ileal electrolyte transport. Gastroenterology 78:454–463

Rachmilewitz D (1980) Prostaglandins and diarrhea. Dig Dis Sci 25:897–898

Rachmilewitz D, Karmeli F (1979) Effect of bisacodyl (BIS) and dioctyl sodium sulfosuccinate on rat intestinal prostaglandin E_2 (PGE_2) content, Na-K ATPase and adenyl cyclase activity. Gastroenterology 76:1221

Rachmilewitz D, Saunders DR, Rulein CE, Tytgat GN (1976) Pharmacology of laxatives: effects of bisacodyl (BIS) on structure and function of intestinal mucosa. Gastroenterology 70:928

Rachmilewitz D, Saunders DR, Rubin CE, Tytgat GN (1977) Effect of bisacodyl on the structure and function of rodent and human intestine. Gastroenterology 72:849–856

Rachmilewitz D, Karmeli F, Okon E (1980) Effects of bisacodyl on c-AMP and prostaglandin E_2 contents, (Na+K) ATPase, adenyl cyclase, and phosphodiesterase activities of rat intestine. Dig Dis Sci 25:602–608

Rampton DS, Breuer NF, Vaja SG, Sladen GE, Dowling RH (1981) Role of prostaglandins in bile salt-induced changes in rat colonic structure and function. Clin Sci 61:641–648

Rao MC, Guandalini S, Laird WJ, Field M (1979) Effects of heatstable enterotoxin of Yersinia enterocolitica on ion transport and c-GMP metabolism in rabbit ileum. Infect Immun 268:875–878

Reichelderfer M, Pero B, Lorenzsonn V, Olsen WA (1979) Is magnesium-induced intestinal secretion mediated by changes in intracellular calcium? Gastroenterology 76:1224

Reilly RW, Kirsner JB (1975) Fiber deficiency and colonic disorders. Plenum, New York, p 185

Reinhold JG, Faradji B, Abaidi P, Ismaei-Beige F (1976) Decreased absorption of calcium, magnesium, zinc, and phosphorus by humans due to increased fiber and phosphorus consumptions as white bread. J Nutr 106:493–503

Reiser S (1979) Effect of dietary fiber on parameters of glucose tolerance in humans. In: Inglett GE, Falkehag SI (eds) Dietary fiber chemistry and nutrition. Academic, NY, p 173

Reves R, Bass P, DuPont HL, Sullivan P, Mendiola J (1983) Failure to demonstrate effectiveness of an anticholinergic drug in the symptomatic treatment of acute traveler's diarrhea. J Clin Gastroenterol 5:223–227

Rinaldo JA Jr, Orinion EA, Simpelo RV, Check FE, Beauregard W (1971) Differential response of longitudinal and circular muscles of intact canine colon to morphine and bethanechol. Gastroenterology 60:438–444

Ritchie J (1972) Mass peristalsis in the human colon after contact with oxyphenisatin. Gut 13:211–219

Ruledge ML, Willner MM, King JT (1963) Calcium polycarbophil in acute childhood diarrhea. Clin Pediatr (Phila) 2:61–63

Rummel W, Nell G, Wanitschke R (1975) Action mechanisms of antiabsorptive and hydragogue drugs. In: Csáky TZ (ed) Intestinal absorption and malabsorption. Raven, New York, p 209

Ruppin H, Bar-Meir S, Soergel KH, Wood CM, Schmitt MG Jr (1980) Absorption of short-chain fatty acid by the colon. Gastroenterology 78:1500–1507

Said SI, Faloona GR (1975) Elevated plasma and tissue levels of vasoactive intestinal polypeptide in watery diarrhea syndrome due to pancreatic, bronchogenic and other tumors. N Eng J Med 293:155–160

Sandler M, Karim SMM, Williams ED (1968) Prostaglandins in amine-peptide-secretory tumor. Lancet 2:1053–1054

Saunders DR, Sillery J, Rachmilewitz D (1975 a) Effect of dioctyl sodium sulfosuccinate on structure and function of rodent and human intestine. Gastroenterology 69:380–386

Saunders DR, Hedges JR, Sillery J, Esther L, Matsumura K, Rubin CE (1975 b) Morphological and functional effects of bile salts on rat colon. Gastroenterology 68:1236–1245
Saunders DR, Sillery J, Rachmilewitz D, Rubin CE, Tytgat GN (1977) Effect of bisacodyl on the structure and function of rodent and human intestine. Gastroenterology 72:849–856
Schneeman BO, Gallaher D (1980) Changes in small intestinal digestive enzyme activity and bile acids with dietary cellulose in rats. J Nutr 110:584–590
Schultz SG, Curran PF (1974) Sodium and chloride transport across isolated rabbit ileum. Curr Top Membr Transport 5:225–281
Schwartz CJ, Kimberg DV, Sheerin HE, Field M, Said SI (1974) Vasoactive intestinal peptide stimulation of adenylate cyclase and active electrolyte secretion in intestinal mucosa. J Clin Invest 54:536–544
Seager H (1968) The effect of methylcellulose on the absorption of nitrofurantoin from the gastrointestinal tract. J Pharm Pharmacol 20:968–969
Sealock RR, Basinski DH, Murlin JR (1941) Apparent digestability of carbohydrates, fats and "indigestible residue" in whole wheat and white bread. J Nutr 22:589–596
Seeman P (1972) The membrane actions of anesthetics and tranquilizers. Pharmacol Rev 24:583–655
Sharp GWG, Hynie S (1971) Stimulation of intestinal adenyl cyclase by cholera toxin. Nature 229:266–268
Simon B, Kather H (1980) Laxatives and human colonic mucosal cyclic AMP. Dig Dis Sci 25:155–156
Simon B, Czygan P, Stiehl A, Kather H (1978) Human colonic adenylate cyclase: effects of bile acids. Eur J Clin Invest 8:321–323
Sladen GE, Harries JT (1972) Studies on the effects of unconjugated dihydroxy bile salts on rat small intestinal function in vivo. Biochem Biophys Acta 288:443–456
Slavin JL, Marlett JA (1978) The effect of purified cellulose on human bowel function. Fed Proc 37:756
Spiller GA (1978) Topics on dietary fiber research. Plenum, New York, p 221
Spiller GA, Chernoff MC, Hill RA, Gates JE, Nassar JJ, Shipley EA (1978) Effect on transit time, fecal weight and volatile fatty acids of purified cellulose, pectin and low residue diets in humans. Fed Proc 37:755
Spiller GA, Shipley EA, Chernoff MC, Cooper WC (1979) Bulk laxative efficacy of a psyllium seed hydrocolloid and of a mixture of cellulose and pectin. J Clin Pharmacol 19:313–320
Spiller GA, Chernoff MC, Hill RA, Gates JE, Nassar JJ, Shipley EA (1980) Effect of purified cellulose, pectin and a low-residue diet on fecal volatile fatty acids, transit time and fecal weight in humans. Am J Clin Nutr 33:754–759
Stanley MM, Paul D, Gacke D, Murphy J (1973) Effect of cholestyramine, metamucil and cellulose on fecal bile salt excretion in man. Gastroenterology 65:889–894
Steggerta FR (1968) Gastrointestinal gas following food consumption. Ann NY Acad Sci 150:57–66
Stephen AM, Cummings JH (1980) Mechanisms of action of dietary fibre in the human colon. Nature 284:283–284
Stewart JJ, Bass P (1976 a) Effects of ricinoleic and oleic acids on the digestive contractile activity of the canine small and large bowel. Gastroenterology 70:371–376
Stewart JJ, Bass P (1976 b) Effect of intravenous C-terminal octapeptide of cholecystokinin and intraduodenal ricinoleic acid on contractile activity of the dog intestine. Proc Soc Exp Biol Med 152:213–217
Stewart JJ, Gaginella TS, Bass P (1975 a) Actions of ricinoleic acid and structurally related fatty acids on the gastrointestinal tract. I. Effects on smooth muscle contractility in vitro. J Pharmacol Exp Ther 195:347–354
Stewart JJ, Gaginella TS, Olsen WA, Bass P (1975 b) Inhibitory actions of laxatives on motility and water and electrolyte transport in the gastrointestinal tract. J Pharmacol Exp Ther 192:458–467
Story JA, Kritchevsky D (1976) Comparison of the binding of various bile acids and bile salts in vitro by several types of fibers. J Nutr 106:1292–1294

Story JA, Kritchevsky D (1978) Bile acid metabolism and fiber. Am J Clin Nutr 31:S199–S202

Stragand JJ, Hagemann RF (1977) Dietary influence on colonic cell renewal. Am J Clin Nutr 30:918–923

Stretcher MH, Quirk L (1943) Constipation: clinical and roentgenologic evaluation of the use of bran. Am J Dig Dis Nutr 10:179

Sund RB, Hillestad B (1978) Diphenolic laxatives and intestinal c-AMP: experiments with oxyphenisatin in the rat in vivo. Acta Pharmacol Toxicol 42:321–322

Surawicz C, Saunders DR, Rubin CE, Tytgat GN (1977) Pharmacology of laxatives: effects of phenolphthalein (PHE) on structure and function of intestinal mucosa. Gastroenterology 72:1137

Szurszewski JH (1969) A migrating electric complex of the canine small intestine. Am J Physiol 217:1757–1773

Tai YH, Wong R, Decker RA, Wright JA, Marnane WG (1978) Inhibitory effects of RMI 12330A on ileal total ionic transport and mucosal adenylate cyclase and Na-K-ATPase activities in normal tissues and tissues treated with purified cholera toxin from the rabbit. Gastroenterology 74:1101

Tainter ML, Buchanan OH (1954) Quantitative comparisons of colloidal laxatives. Ann NY Acad Sci 58:438–454

Tapila S, Miettinen TA, Metsäranta L (1978) Effects of bran on serum cholesterol, faecal mass, fat, bile acids and neutral sterols, and biliary lipids in patients with diverticular disease of the colon. Gut 19:137–145

Taub M, Bonorris G, Chung A, Coyne MJ, Schoenfield LJ (1977) Effect of propranolol on bile acid and cholera enterotoxin-stimulated c-AMP and secretion in rabbit intestine. Gastroenterology 72:101–105

Taylor I, Duthie HL (1976) Bran tablets and diverticular disease. Br Med J 1:988–990

Teem MV, Phillips SF (1972) Perfusion of the hamster jejunum with conjugated and unconjugated bile acids: inhibition of water absorption and effects on morphology. Gastroenterology 62:261–267

Trowell H (1974) Definitions of fibre. Lancet 1:503

Van Beresteyn ECH, Van Schaik M, Kerkhof Mogot MF (1979) Effect of bran and cellulose on lipid metabolism in obese female zucker rats. J Nutr 109:2085–2097

Van Trappen G, Janssens J, Hellemans J, Ghoos Y (1977) The interdigestive motor complex of normal subjects and patients with bacterial overgrowth of the small intestine. J Clin Invest 59:1158–1166

Verhaeren EHC, Dreessen MJ, Lemli JA (1981) Influence of 1,8-dihydroxy-anthraquinone and loperamide on the paracellular permeability across colonic mucosa. J Pharm Pharmacol 33:526–528

Vince A, Killingley M, Wrong OM (1978) Effect of lactulose on ammonia production in a fecal incubation system. Gastroenterology 74:544–549

Volpe BT, Binder HJ (1975) Bile salt alteration of ion transport across jejunal mucosa. Biochem Biophys Acta 394:597–604

Voorhees JJ, Duell EA (1975) Imbalanced cyclic AMP-cyclic GMP levels in psoriasis. In: Drummond GI, Greengard P, Robison GA (eds) Advances in cyclic nucleotide research, vol 5, Raven, New York, p 735

Waldman DB, Gardner JD, Zfass AM, Makhlouf GM (1977) Effects of vasoactive intestinal peptide, secretin, and related peptides on rat colonic transport and adenylate cyclase activity. Gastroenterology 73:518–523

Walters RL, McLean Baird I, Davis PS, Hill MJ, Drasar BS, Southgate DAT, Green J, Morgan B (1975) Effects of two types of dietary fiber on faecal steroid and lipid excretion. Br Med J 2:536–538

Wanitschke R (1980 a) Intestinal filtration as a consequence of increased mucosal hydraulic permeability. A new concept for laxative action. Klin Wochenschr 58:267–278

Wanitschke R (1980 b) Influence of rhein on electrolyte and water transfer in the isolated rat colonic mucosa. Pharmacology [Suppl 1] 20:21–26

Wanitschke R, Ammon HV (1976) Effects of magnesium sulfate on transit time and water transport in the human jejunum. Gastroenterology 70:949

Ward MWN, Lewin MR, Clark CG (1979) The influence of dietary fiber on colonic muscle. Eur Surg Res 11:360–365
Webster DJT, Gough DCS, Craven JL (1978) The use of bulk evacuant in patients with hemorrhoids. Br J Surg 65:291–292
Williams RD, Olmsted WH (1936) The effect of cellulose, hemicellulose and lignin on the weight of the stool: a contribution to the study of laxation in man. J Nutr 11:433–449
Wilson RB, Hutcheson DP, Wideman L (1977) Dimethyhydrazine-induced colon tumors in rats fed diets containing beef fat or corn oil with and without wheat bran. Am J Clin Nutr 30:176–181
Wingate DL (1981) Backwards and forwards with the migrating complex. Dig Dis Sci 26:641–666
Wingate DL, Krag E, Mekhjian HS, Phillips SF (1973) Relationships between ion and water movement in the human jejunum, ileum and colon during perfusion with bile acids. Clin Sci Mol Med 45:593–606
Wojtczak L, Zaluska H (1967) The inhibition of translocation of adenine nucleotides through mitochondrial membranes by oleate. Biochem Biophys Res Commun 28:76–81
Wyman JB, Heaton KW, Manning AP, Wicks ACB (1976) The effect on intestinal transit and the feces of raw and cooked bran in different doses. Am J Clin Nutr 29:1474–1479

CHAPTER 29

Action Mechanisms of Secretagogue Drugs

G. NELL and W. RUMMEL

A. Introduction

A large number of agents with laxative or diarrheal effects have been shown to influence intestinal fluid and electrolyte transfer. They inhibit the absorption of electrolytes and water and they can also cause an accumulation of fluid within the intestinal lumen. Depending on the administered dose or concentration of the agent and on the particular experimental conditions, inhibition of absorption may result, either on its own or accompanied by secretion. In order to characterize the pharmacodynamic properties of these agents to influence intestinal fluid transfer, they have been named secretagogue (GAGINELLA et al. 1977a), antiabsorptive and hydragogue (RUMMEL et al. 1975), or hydrophoric agents (GAGINELLA and BASS 1978). In this chapter the term "secretagogue" is used, since this expression seems to be the most widely accepted one. It is a phenomenological term without implications with regard to the action mechanisms. This restriction appears reasonable, particularly if one takes into account that, owing to the cytologic heterogeneity of the intestinal epithelium, different types of cells might be involved to different degrees in secretion. Confusion with the term "active secretion", i.e., active transport of electrolytes and fluid from the blood to the intestinal lumen should be avoided (see Sect. B). Table 1 gives a list of diarrheal agents with secretagogue effects. In the case of the so-called laxatives (triarylmethane derivatives, anthraquinones, drastic purgatives, and surfactants) those references are given in which to our knowledge the secretagogue effect of the substance under consideration was described first. With regard to the other classes of agents, current reviews are quoted (see Chap. 28). Some of the agents listed in Table 1 are of endogenous origin (e.g., bile acids and several hormones) or normally present in the gut lumen (e.g., oleic acid). It is commonly accepted that the secretagogue effect is an important factor in the diarrheal action of the agents listed in Table 1 (for references see BINDER 1979).

Table 1 shows that a large number of substances can cause net transfer of fluid from the blood to the intestinal lumen. It is to be expected that they may act via different mechanisms leading to the common final result, namely fluid accumulation within the gut lumen. In this chapter, current views about the action mechanisms of the so-called laxative drugs (triarylmethane derivatives, anthraquinones, and surfactants) are discussed. The drastic purgatives are not taken into account because they are obsolete. A summary of the early literature in this field is given by MAGNUS (1924b). Neither are the "osmotic" or "saline" laxatives included because there has been essentially no new information since the investi-

Table 1. Diarrheal agents with secretagogue effects

Agent	References
Triarylmethane derivatives (e.g., bisacodyl, phenolphthalein)	FORTH et al. (1963, 1966a); PHILLIPS et al. (1965)
Anthraquinone derivatives	CARNOT and GLÉNARD (1913); MCCALLUM (1906); cited by MAGNUS (1924a)
Drastic purgatives (colocynth and similar drugs)	LAUDÉR-BRUNTON (1874)
Surfactants:	
Anionic: ricinoleic acid and other C_{18} fatty acids	MEYER-BETZ and GEBHARDT (1912); SCHMID (1952); PHILLIPS et al. (1965); AMMON and PHILLIPS (1973); BRIGHT-ASARE and BINDER (1973)
Bile salts	BUGLIA (1909)
Dioctylsodium sulfosuccinate	DONOWITZ and BINDER (1974, 1975); SAUNDERS et al. (1975b)
Cationic: trimethylhexadecyl-ammonium stearate	NISSIM (1960a, b)
Bacterial enterotoxins and infectious agents which invade the tissue (e.g., enterotoxins from *Vibrio cholerae, Escherichia coli*)	For references see reviews by BANWELL and SHERR (1973); BINDER (1979)
Hormonal agents	For references see reviews by BINDER (1979); DONOWITZ et al. (1979); GAGINELLA and O'DORISIO (1979)
Cholinergic drugs	For references see POWELL and TAPPER (1979)

gations around the turn of the century. Since then it has commonly been held that these drugs act solely by exerting an osmotic force on fluid transfer (for reference see HEYMANN 1927a, b). However, in the reviews cited, the question remained unsettled whether some of the saline laxatives (e.g., $MgSO_4$) may also produce intestinal fluid accumulation by stimulating active secretion. This question has still not been answered definitely. It has been hypothesized that $MgSO_4$ may act via release of cholecystokinin (for references see GAGINELLA and BASS 1978). This problem needs further investigation.

This chapter is focused on the action mechanisms of the secretagogue effects of these drugs and does not deal with their influence on intestinal motility since the role of motility in causing laxative effects is at present rather poorly understood (for references see Gaginella and BASS 1978). Because of limitations of space only the main features of concepts established within the last 10 years are described. For further references the reader is referred to a number of reviews of this field (FORTH and RUMMEL 1975; RUMMEL et al. 1975; BINDER 1977; GAGINELLA and BASS 1978; PHILLIPS and GAGINELLA 1979; EWE 1980b; WANITSCHKE 1980b).

B. Theoretical Considerations

The reversal of fluid absorption to secretion can be caused by changes of different factors which determine the size of unidirectional fluxes. The scheme (Fig. 1) ex-

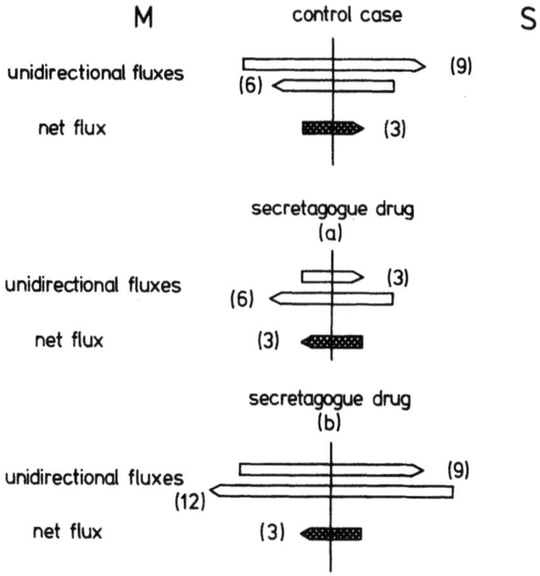

Fig. 1. Theoretical possibilities of converting the direction of the net flux of an ion from the mucosal to the serosal side (absorption) to net flux from the serosal to the mucosal side (secretion). *M*, mucosal side; *S*, serosal side; *open arrows*, unidirectional fluxes; *full arrows*, net fluxes; numbers in parentheses indicate fluxes in arbitrary units

emplifies two types of secretagogue action. The membrane represents the total epithelial layer as a black box. In the control case, the unidirectional flux from the mucosal to the serosal side exceeds that in the opposite direction. The net flux is the difference between the two opposing unidirectional fluxes. Therefore, the net flux occurs in the absorptive direction. Under the influence of secretagogue drugs, the direction of the next flux is reversed to secretion. In (a) only the unidirectional flux from the mucosal to the serosal side is reduced. Since the unidirectional flux in the contrary direction remains constant, net transfer from the serosal to the mucosal side results. In (b) the same is true if the unidirectional flux from the serosal to the mucosal side is increased sufficiently in spite of an unchanged unidirectional flux from the mucosal to the serosal side. For a more detailed discussion of intermediate cases the reader is referred to HAKIM and LIFSON (1969) and BINDER (1979). It should be borne in mind that conclusions from measurements of the unidirectional fluxes with regard to the driving forces can be only tentative because several factors can affect the magnitude of the flux: e.g., concentration gradients, electrical potential differences, energy supply for pumps, permeability, hydrostatic and osmotic pressure; more than one factor might be changed by a secretagogue drug. The following possible action mechanisms of secretagogue drugs have been discussed.

I. Inhibition of Active Absorption

This topic comprises the inhibition of active absorption of sodium (and chloride). Parenthetically, active absorption or active secretion mean net transfer either from the mucosal to the serosal side of the epithelium or in the contrary direction, which occurs in the absence of an external driving force (e.g., hydrostatic pressure in the case of filtration) and depends on metabolism. Most attention has been focused on the inhibition of Na^+, K^+-ATPase which plays a key role in active sodium transport in the intestine (e.g., S. G. SCHULTZ et al. 1974). Because of the inhibition of sodium chloride absorption the solute-dependent water flow will also cease. For references to coupling of solute and solvent flows see the review by DIAMOND (1979). If one assumes a mechanism of active secretion (i.e., active transport of ions from the contraluminal to the luminal side) which persists after inhibition of active absorption, then inhibition of the latter suffices to explain net movement of fluid and electrolytes from the blood into the intestinal lumen. The secretory mechanism may be located either in the same cells as the active absorption device or in a different part of the cell population.

II. Active Secretion

Inducing or increasing active secretion to a sufficient magnitude would cause net movement from the blood to the lumen even if active absorption were to persist unchanged. This effect may be either a direct action of the particular secretagogue or brought about by an intermediate reaction, e.g., an increase in concentration of some endogenous substances with secretagogue action (e.g., prostaglandins, BEUBLER and JUAN 1979). An intermediate step in the events leading ultimately to active secretion may be a change in the cellular level of cyclic nucleotides. Most attention has been focused on an increase in the cellular content of cAMP in analogy to the commonly accepted model for explaining the action of cholera enterotoxin (see review by GILL 1977). However, indications exist which allow one to locate the site of action of some secretagogues in the chain of events distal to the cAMP. One hypothesis is concerned with a possible role of Ca^{2+} as a further mediator of intestinal secretion (for references see BOLTON and FIELD 1977; FRIZZELL 1977 a, b).

III. Filtration

The basis of this concept is the assumption that some secretagogue drugs elicit the flow from blood to lumen of a fluid whose composition approximately equals that of an ultrafiltrate. This result may be achieved by an increase in the subepithelial hydrostatic pressure and/or an increase in permeability of the mucosal epithelium, i.e., an increased leakage of the junctions between the epithelial cells. Of course, an increase in permeability alone could possibly result in a standstill of absorption, but never cause noteworthy net movement from the serosal to the mucosal side. There may be some net movement of fluid from blood to lumen due only to an increase in permeability if a compound leaks out which is not present in the lumen, thereby dragging some water with it. Thus, all hypotheses which are centered around an increase in permeability by secretagogue drugs have necessarily to assume a driving force, namely the aforementioned subepithelial hydrostatic pressure.

C. Triarylmethane and Anthraquinone Derivatives

I. Effect on Intestinal Fluid and Electrolyte Transfer

As early as 1913 CARNOT and GLÉNARD showed that senna glycosides can induce fluid secretion in the rabbit intestine. About 10 years after the introduction of the triarylmethane derivatives of the bisacodyl type into therapy FORTH et al. (1963) demonstrated the ability of bisacodyl to inhibit intestinal fluid absorption and to reverse it to secretion when applied in higher concentrations. These findings have been extensively confirmed with different experimental designs and species (Table 2). One exception should be mentioned; POWELL et al. (1980) found secretion of sodium and chloride only after addition of phenolphthalein to the mucosal side of a short-circuited Ussing chamber preparation of the rabbit ileum, whereas absorption of these ions was stimulated after administration to the serosal side. Therefore, they explained their finding that this drug caused secretion of fluid only during the first hour in the in vivo perfused rabbit ileum whereas absorption was reestablished afterwards, with the assumption that after absorption the drug stimulated fluid absorption from the serosal side. However, a more plausible explanation may be the disappearance of the drug from the perfusion fluid since it can be calculated from their methodological details (recirculating perfusion) that, after 1 h, at least 50% of the drug had left the intestinal lumen.

Triarylmethane derivatives stimulate potassium secretion, especially in the colon of rat and human (FORTH et al. 1966a; EWE and HÖLKER 1974; SCHREINER et al. 1980). The same is true for anthraquinone derivatives (LEMMENS and BORJA 1976; EWE 1980a; LENG-PESCHLOW 1980). In principle, potassium secretion can be assumed to contribute to fluid secretion for osmotic reasons, but this effect is far too small to account for the whole amount of secreted fluid.

II. Chemistry, Structure–Activity Relationship, and Pharmacokinetics

With regard to chemistry and structure–activity relationship of the triarylmethane derivatives, the reader is referred to the reviews by O. E. SCHULTZ et al. (1974) and FORTH and RUMMEL (1975). In order to provoke a secretagogue and laxative action, two free hydroxyl groups in *para* positions on the two benzene rings are necessary. Therefore, the whole group of triarylmethane derivatives is also called "diphenolic laxatives". This configuration is, however, not sufficient since, in addition, the secretagogue efficacy of the molecule depends on the structure of the third aryl group. If this aromatic ring contains nitrogen, then the distance of the nitrogen atom from the central carbon atom of the methyl group, and the dissociation constant of the nitrogen group influences the secretagogue activity. For data and further references on pharmacokinetics the publications of FERLEMANN and VOGT (1965), VOGT et al. (1965), FORTH et al. (1972), EWE and HÖLKER (1974), WEIST and BIRKNER (1974), JAUCH et al. (1975, 1977), NAITO et al. (1976), SUND et al. (1979, 1981, 1982), SUND and HILLESTAD (1982), and HILLESTAD et al. (1982) should be consulted.

The pharmacokinetic behavior of a trimethylmethane derivative depends on whether the two phenolic hydroxyl groups are esterified or not. If the ester linkage

Table 2. Effect of triarylmethane and anthraquinone derivatives on intestinal fluid, sodium, and chloride transfer

Substance	Species	Effect	Experimental conditions in vivo	References
Bisacodyl, oxyphenisatin, and related compounds	Rat	Inhibition of fluid absorption and/or secretion	Tied-off loops	[1, 8]
			Perfusion	[3, 4, 9, 10
		Inhibition of sodium absorption and/or secretion	Tied-off loops	[1, 2, 7, 11
		Inhibition of chloride absorption	Tied-off loops	[8]
	Human	Inhibition of fluid absorption and/or secretion	Perfusion	[10, 12]
		Inhibition od sodium absorption and/or secretion	Perfusion	[12]
Phenolphthalein	Rat	Inhibition of fluid absorption and/or secretion	Tied-off loops	[4, 5]
			Perfusion	[4, 5, 13]
	Rabbit	Inhibition of fluid absorption and/or secretion	Perfusion	[14]
		Sodium secretion	Tied-off loops	[15]
Anthraquinone derivatives	Rat	Inhibition of fluid absorption and/or secretion	Tied-off loops	[16, 17]
			Perfusion	[18]
		Inhibition of sodium absorption and/or secretion	Tied-off loops	[16]
			Perfusion	[18]
		Inhibition of chloride absorption and/or secretion	Perfusion	[18]
	Mouse		Enteropooling	[19]
	Rabbit	Sodium secretion	Tied-off loops	[15]
	Cat	Inhibition of fluid absorption	Perfusion	[20]
	Human	Secretion of water, sodium, and chloride	Perfusion	[21]
Bisacodyl, oxyphenisation, and related compounds	Rat	Inhibition of fluid absorption	Fisher–Parsons method, in vitro tied-off loops	[22, 23]
			Everted sacs	[24]
		Inhibition of sodium absorption	Everted sacs	[24]
			Short-circuited everted sacs	[25]
Phenolphthalein	Rabbit	Inhibition or stimulation of absorption or secretion of sodium and chloride [a]	Short-circuited Ussing chamber preparation	[14]
Anthraquinone derivatives	Rat	Inhibition of absorption of water, sodium, and chloride	Everted sacs	[26]
	Rabbit	Fluid secretion	Vascular perfused intestine	[27]

[1] FORTH et al. (1963); FORTH et al. (1966a); [3] FORTH et al. (1972); [4] BEUBLER and JUAN (1977); [5] BEUBLER and JUAN (1978); [6] BEUBLER and LEMBECK (1979); [7] SUND et al. (1979); [8] SCHREINE et al. (1980); [9] HART and MCCOLL (1968); [10] SAUNDERS et al. (1977); [11] NELL et al. (1973a) [12] EWE and HÖLKER (1974); [13] SAUNDERS ET AL. (1978); [14] POWELL et al. (1980); [15] PHILLIPS et al (1965); [16] LEMMENS and BORJA (1976); [17] BEUBLER and JUAN (1979); [18] LENG-PESCHLOW (1980) [19] SCHMID (1952); [20] STRAUB and TRIENDL (1934); [21] EWE (1980A); [22] FORTH and RUMME (1975); [23] RACHMILEWITZ et al. (1980); [24] WANITSCHKE et al. (1977a); [25] WANITSCHKE and SOERGEL (1975); [26] WANITSCHKE (1980a); [27] CARNOT and GLÉNARD (1913)

[a] POWELL et al. (1980) found secretion of sodium and chloride after mucosal application and enhancement of sodium and chloride absorption after serosal application

is easily split off in the small intestine, as in the case of bisacodyl, then the substance with the free hydroxyl groups is absorbed and excreted mainly as glucuronide with bile. The glucuronide cannot be absorbed and moves down to the colon, where it is split again and becomes pharmacodynamically effective. Clearly, the lag time between peroral application and laxative effect is mainly determined by the enterohepatic cycle. This was confirmed with sulfated derivatives, for instance picosulfate, which differs from bisacodyl only in that the two hydroxyl groups are not esterified with acetyl, but with sulfate groups. In the latter case, the ester linkage cannot be split in the small intestine. The substance reaches the colon largely unchanged and unabsorbed. There the sulfate group is split off by bacterial enzymes and the resulting diphenol – the same as yielded by hydrolysis of bisacodyl – induces laxation. The latency time is very much shorter in this case since the enterohepatic cycle is circumvented (FORTH et al. 1972). This difference between bisacodyl and picosulfate may, however, depend on the dose (SUND et al. 1981).

Structure–activity relationships and pharmacokinetics of the anthraquinone derivatives are less well understood. For references the reader is referred to the papers of VAN OS (1976) on chemistry and of LEMLI and LEMMENS (1980), KOBASHI et al. (1980), and DREESEN et al. (1981) on pharmacokinetics and metabolism. In analogy to the triarylmethane group, two phenolic hydroxyl groups are essential for purgative action. This is the reason that the action mechanisms of anthraquinones are discussed together with the diphenolic laxatives.

III. Proposed Action Mechanisms

1. Inhibition of Active Sodium and Sodium Coupled Solute Transport

The discussion is centered on the question whether inhibition of the key enzyme of active sodium transport, namely Na^+, K^+-ATPase, by diphenolic laxatives is responsible or at least contributes to the observed effects on sodium and fluid transfer. It has been reported by several authors (CHIGNELL 1968; IM et al. 1980; RACHMILEWITZ et al. 1980; SCHREINER et al. 1980; WANITSCHKE 1980a) that diphenolic laxatives and anthraquinone derivatives inhibit Na^+, K^+-ATPase of rat intestinal mucosa in vivo and in vitro. VERHAEREN (1980) showed that these drugs are also able to uncouple oxidative phosphorylation in isolated vegetable mitochondria and in those of colonic mucosa of the guinea pig. The author speculated that this action may contribute to the laxative effect.

It has been shown repeatedly that diphenolic compounds inhibit glucose absorption in the small intestine in vivo (HART and MCCOLL 1967, 1968) and in vitro (FORTH et al. 1963; HAND et al. 1966; ADAMIC and BIHLER 1967). These observations have been extended to senna derivatives (LENG-PESCHLOW 1980; EWE 1980a). This effect may be due in part to the inhibition of Na^+, K^+-ATPase. According to present concepts this would lead to an increase of intracellular sodium concentration and therefore diminish the sodium gradient across the brush border membrane. Thus, the essential driving force for sugar uptake into the epithelial cells would be decreased (for references see S. G. SCHULTZ 1977). In addition, a direct effect of phenolphthalein on the carrier-mediated entry mechanism through the luminal membrane of the intestinal epithelial cell has been shown quite conclusively (HAND et al. 1966; ADAMIC and BIHLER 1967; IM et al. 1980).

This is not unexpected in view of the chemical similarity with compounds like phloretine. The transport of methionine and 2-aminoisobutyric acid is also inhibited (HAND et al. 1966; ADAMIC and BIHLER 1967). However, it seems unlikely that inhibition of nutrient absorption would contribute significantly to the effect on intestinal fluid transfer, since the drugs are also effective in parts of the intestine lacking transfer mechanisms for glucose and amino acids, e.g., the rat colon. The latter is even more sensitive to diphenolic laxatives than the small intestine (FORTH et al. 1966a; NELL et al. 1973a).

2. Stimulation of Active Secretion

There are only very few investigations in which the effects of triarylmethane derivatives and anthraquinones on ion transfer were measured under clear-cut in vitro conditions. WANITSCHKE and SOERGEL (1975) and WANITSCHKE et al. (1977a) demonstrated inhibition of fluid and sodium transfer in everted sacs of the rat colon under short- and open-circuit conditions, respectively, in the presence of oxyphenisatin. They were unable to demonstrate secretion. The same result was obtained later by WANITSCHKE (1980a) with rhein in open-circuited everted sacs of rat colon. POWELL et al. (1980), using an Ussing chamber preparation, showed that phenolphthalein induced sodium and chloride secretion under short-circuit conditions in the rabbit ileum, when applied to the mucosal side.

Since it is commonly accepted that cholera enterotoxin induces active fluid secretion via stimulation of the adenylate cyclase system, this possibility has also been tested in the case of diphenolic laxatives. SUND and HILLESTAD (1978) found no influence of oxyphenisatin on cAMP content in rat small intestine in vivo. POWELL et al. (1980) found either no influence or even a decrease in cAMP and cGMP in rabbit ileal mucosa in vitro in the presence of phenolphthalein. RACHMILEWITZ et al. (1980) described in rats an increase of the activity of adenylate cyclase, and, in the jejunum, of phosphodiesterase 18 h after oral administration of bisacodyl, but not after 4 h. The mucosal cAMP levels were not altered. Obviously, the changes in the rates of synthesis and degradation balance each other. SCHREINER et al. (1980), using tied-off colonic loops of the rat, described an increase in cAMP levels in acute experiments and no influence after chronic administration of bisacodyl, whereas the cGMP content was diminished in acute and enhanced in long-term experiments.

The question was also raised whether the proposed stimulation of active secretion is mediated by an endogenous secretagogue compound. BEUBLER and coworkers showed that diphenolic laxatives and sennosides A and B released prostaglandins into the intestinal lumen (BEUBLER and JUAN 1977, 1978, 1979). RACHMILEWITZ et al. (1980) found an increased content of prostaglandin E_2 within the intestinal mucosa in the rat after oral delivery of bisacodyl and speculated that prostaglandin E_2 may induce active secretion via stimulation of adenylate cyclase.

3. Increase in Permeability

It was shown that diphenolic laxatives increase the permeability of the rat colon when tested by nonelectrolyte molecules of graded size in vivo and in vitro (NELL et al. 1976a, b, 1977). WANITSCHKE and SOERGEL (1975) demonstrated a decrease in electrical resistance in rat colonic mucosa in vitro. NATAF et al. (1981) showed that dihydroxyanthraquinone and phenolphthalein caused an increase in stool output of α-1-antitrypsin, a plasma protein, in humans. VERHAEREN et al. (1981) showed that dihydroxyanthraquinone increased the permeability of guinea pig colonic mucosa to the complex TcEDTA in vivo. This effect was abolished by the antidiarrheal agent loperamide. These findings raised the question where the site in the epithelium might be at which the increase in permeability develops. In principle, two sites exist where the changes might occur: the cell membranes of the enterocytes, or the intercellular junctions.

Damage of the mucosa of the small and large intestine has been reported after administration of diphenolic laxatives (MEISEL et al. 1977; SAUNDERS et al. 1977). Thus, the passage of even large molecules may occur across destroyed or denuded areas of the intestinal mucosa. However, destruction of the epithelium is a dose-related phenomenon. It is possible to induce fluid secretion without morphologically demonstrable damage within a certain range of concentrations (NELL et al. 1973a; SAUNDERS et al. 1978; GOERG et al. 1980a). It was concluded that under these conditions the paracellular pathway through the lateral intercellular space and the so-called tight junction is changed by the drug for the following reasons.

First, some of the applied test molecules are unable to penetrate cell membranes because of their size and polarity; these include the anion, ^{51}CrEDTA, and the nonelectrolytes mannitol, lactose, inulin, and polyethylene glycol (PEG) 4000 (NELL et al. 1976a, b, 1977). Second, the mucosal content of sodium and potassium was not altered concomitantly (NELL et al. 1976a, b; WANITSCHKE et al. 1977a). Therefore, it is unlikely that the sodium and potassium permeability of the membranes of the intestinal epithelial cells might have been altered since in this case an influence on intracellular concentrations of sodium and potassium is to be expected because of the change of the pump : leak ratio. Examples for such a change are the effects of vasopressin (for references see ANDREOLI and SCHAFER 1976) and amphotericin B (GRAF and GIEBISCH 1979; REUSS et al. 1980) on epithelial cells in amphibia.

The third line of argument is based on the following considerations. Oxyphenisatin causes a massive increase in the unidirectional sodium flux from blood to lumen in rat colon in vivo. If this occurred via the transcellular route then radioactively labeled sodium would be expected to enter rapidly both the intra- and extracellular sodium pools (the former amounts to 40% of total mucosal sodium). Thus, oxyphenisatin would cause a more rapid uptake of ^{22}Na into the mucosal tissue from the serosal side. There is, however, no difference in the time course of ^{22}Na uptake by the mucosa between 1 and 5 min after intravenous administration of ^{22}Na in spite of the concomitantly increased transfer of ^{22}Na from blood to lumen. The distribution volume of ^{22}Na did not exceed the extracellular space on the serosal side at 5 min after intravenous administration. The tissue uptake of ^{22}Na from the luminal side was not influenced at all (NELL et al. 1976a, b). These findings are in agreement with the assumption that sodium moves from blood to lumen on the paracellular pathway in the presence of oxyphenisatin. Further confirmation was obtained by other experiments. Sodium net movement from the blood to the lumen was independent of osmotically induced water flow in both directions caused by the administration of hypo- and hypertonic solutions of choline chloride into tied-off colonic loops of rats (NELL et al. 1973b). It has to be postulated that a superimposed osmotic water flow may have influenced sodium movement by solvent drag if both movements occurred along the same pathway. Since this was not the case it was concluded that, according to present hypotheses concerning the gallbladder (VAN OS et al. 1979), the osmotic flow crosses the epithelium along the transcellular pathway whereas the sodium movement caused by oxyphenisatin prefers the paracellular pathway.

In concentrations which exhibit maximal effects on fluid transfer, diphenolic laxatives enhance the rate of cell shedding within the physiologic extrusion zones of the mucosal epithelium (NELL 1973a; SPECHT 1977). Therefore, it may be speculated that the increased leakage of the test molecules may be confined to these zones. However, it was shown that the continuity of the epithelial layer is maintained under these circumstances (Fig. 2). In order to see if the apparently normal pathway across the tight junctions of the epithelial layer is rendered more permeable by diphenolic laxatives, lanthanum ions were used as a probe. It was shown morphologically and by flux measurements that oxyphenisatin enhances the permeation of ionic lanthanum from the serosal to the mucosal side of everted sacs of the rat colon with apparently intact epithelium. Lanthanum ions were never detected within the cytoplasm (NELL et al. 1977; SPECHT 1977).

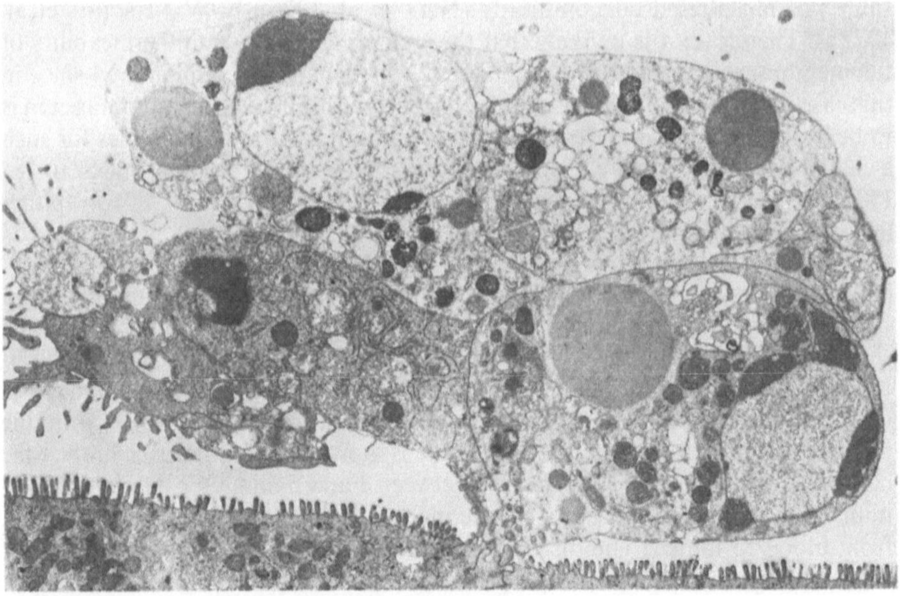

Fig. 2. Influence of diphenolic laxative on rat colonic mucosa. Everted sac preparation. Incubation medium: Tris-buffered, modified Krebs-Henseleit solution containing 10^{-5} mol/l oxyphenisatin on mucosal side. Incubation time, 20 min. TEM, 9,250 : 1. Clusters of damaged cells are extruded on the free surface. Nevertheless, the continuity of the epithelial sheet is maintained

In summary, triarylmethane derivatives increase the permeability of the paracellular pathway across the epithelium by rendering the tight junctions more leaky, enhance shedding of epithelial cells in the extrusion zones, and, in higher concentrations, cause epithelial damage. The question remains to be answered, how the increase in permeability may be related causally to the reversal of the direction of net transfer of fluid.

The descending colon of the rat absorbs water and sodium in such a way that a hypertonic solution appears on the contraluminal side (PARSONS and PATERSON 1965). Accordingly, an increase of the hydrostatic pressure on the serosal side influences the net absorption of sodium and water in an everted sac of stripped colonic mucosa differently (Fig. 3). The scales for sodium and water are related in such a manner that equal distances from the X-axis mean net transfer of sodium and water in the same relation as the sodium concentration in the bathing solution. The regression lines for sodium and water differ significantly with respect to the slope and the intercept with the abscissa ($p<0.05$). The epithelium absorbs sodium and water against a pressure gradient of up to 5 cm H_2O. At pressures between 6 and 11 cm H_2O, the net movement of water is directed from the serosal to the mucosal side while sodium still undergoes net absorption. At a hydrostatic pressure of approximately 11 cm H_2O, net sodium absorption also ceases. At pressures higher than 11 cm H_2O, a hypotonic fluid appears on the mucosal side.

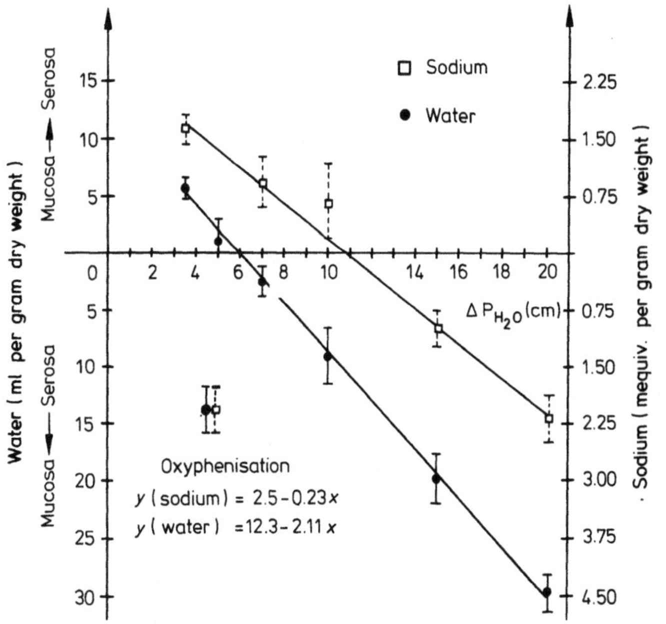

Fig. 3. Influence of hydrostatic pressure on the rate and direction of sodium and water movement in the stripped rat colon. Mean ± standard error, N for each point varies between 5 and 17. Composition of the solution according to PARSONS and PATERSON (1965); experimental duration 2 h. Modified from WANITSCHKE et al. (1977b)

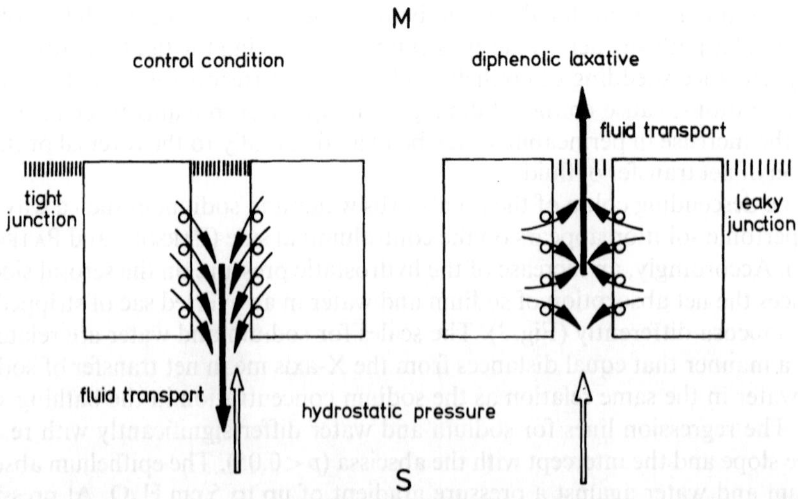

Fig. 4. A model for explaining the effects of diphenolic laxatives on intestinal epithelium. *M*, mucosal side; *S*, serosal side. Modified from RUMMEL (1976)

This means that the colonic epithelium discriminates between sodium and water. In the presence of oxyphenisatin, this discriminating capacity of the colonic mucosa is abolished and an isotonic fluid moves along the hydrostatic pressure gradient (WANITSCHKE et al. 1977 b).

On the basis of these results, the following model has been postulated in order to explain the secretagogue action of diphenolic laxatives (Fig. 4). In the control case, the anisotropy of the pumping system, which is responsible for a vectorial transepithelial flow of sodium and water across the intestinal epithelium in the absorptive direction, is due to the localization of Na^+, K^+-ATPase in the basolateral membrane (for references see WRIGHT et al. 1979) and the relative tightness of the tight junctions whereby the backflux of sodium to the luminal side is impeded. Sodium ions move across the luminal membrane into the epithelial cell and are then extruded into the intercellular space. A passive water movement occurs on the transcellular and also on the intercellular pathways. The efficiency of the net absorption of sodium and water depends on the pump : leak ratio. Under normal conditions, the system is able to overcome an opposing hydrostatic pressure of about 5 cm H_2O. Diphenolic laxatives make junctions more leaky and thereby render the system ineffective. The anisotropy is lost and the direction of fluid and sodium transfer is mainly a function of the transepithelial hydrostatic pressure gradient (for further details the reader is referred to the reviews by RUMMEL et al. 1975; RUMMEL 1976; WANITSCHKE 1980 b). This hypothesis resembles the hypothesis which has ben proposed to explain the effect of extracellular volume expansion on intestinal fluid transfer (for references see DUFFY et al. 1978). The difference between the two models is that in the case of volume expansion the change of the interstitial hydrostatic pressure is the primary event with a consecutive increase in permeability, whereas in the presence of the diphenolic laxatives, the increase in permeability is the first event. The hydrostatic pressure need not change.

IV. Conclusion

Three models for the effects of diphenolic and chemically related laxatives have been presented so far. None of these models can be rejected completely on the basis of present knowledge. It remains to evaluate their advantages and drawbacks.

1. Inhibition of Na^+, K^+-ATPase

Several authors have demonstrated an inhibition of this key enzyme of active sodium transport under in vivo and in vitro conditions. The question remains open whether this inhibition is sufficient in a quantitative sense to explain the observed effects. On the one hand, there is no doubt that Na^+, K^+-ATPase is an essential part of the sodium pumping system of the intestinal mucosa (S.G. SCHULTZ et al. 1974). On the other hand, it is not known whether the activity of this enzyme is rate limiting under in vivo conditions. In other words, the quantitative relation between enzyme activity and sodium transport rate is unknown. There are few publication concerning this issue. SCHIFFL and LOESCHKE (1977) reported a strictly parallel time course for the stimulation of Na^+, K^+-ATPase activity and net sodium absorption in the rat cecum adapting to a poorly absorbable diet containing PEG 4000. CHARNEY and DONOWITZ (1978) described an inhibition of Na^+, K^+-ATPase associated with a reversal of sodium and water absorption to secretion in rabbit ileum perfused in vivo with high ouabain concentrations on the mucosal side. On the other hand, READ et al. (1979) found no change in transepithelial sodium transport despite an inhibition of the activity of Na^+, K^+-ATPase by ouabain administered into the mesenteric artery in dog ileum in vivo. In addition, NELLANS and SCHULTZ (1976) failed to detect a correlation between transepithelial sodium transport and the (probably Na^+, K^+-ATPase-mediated) potassium exchange across the basolateral cell membrane under different experimental conditions in rabbit ileum in vivo.

Thus, on the basis of our present knowledge, the significance of a partial inhibition of Na^+, K^+-ATPase by diphenolic laxatives as a determining factor for the inhibition or even the reversal of the sodium and fluid net transfer cannot be established. At least, over a certain concentration range, the inhibition of Na^+, K^+-ATPase seems not to play an important role since NELL et al. (1976a, b) found no change in sodium and potassium content of the rat colonic mucosa in vivo in the presence of oxyphenisatin in a concentration which caused maximal fluid secretion. WANITSCHKE et al. (1977a) confirmed this result under in vitro conditions. The results of MORETO et al. (1981) are no contradiction to the arguments of NELL et al. (1976a, b) and WANITSCHKE et al. (1977a). These authors found that the diphenolic laxative bisacodyl increased K^+ efflux across the mucosal and serosal border of epithelial cells of rabbit colon mucosa in vitro. However, they reported a concomitant decrease in tissue potassium content of more than 50% in 100 min. Thus, it has to be concluded, that under conditions in which a significant increase of potassium permeability of the cell membranes is demonstrated, a decrease of tissue content of potassium is readily shown.

A decrease in transepithelial electrical potential difference has been reported with bisacodyl by EWE (1977) in the case of human rectum and by SCHREINER et al. (1980) in the rat colon. The same result was achieved with oxyphenisatin

(WANITSCHKE and SOERGEL 1975; SCHREINER et al. 1980). This finding is compatible with an inhibition of Na^+, K^+-ATPase, but no proof of it because it can also be explained by an increase of the leak permeability.

2. Stimulation of Active Secretion

This possibility is even more difficult to evaluate. The first prerequisite in order to accept this hypothesis is clearly the demonstration of secretion under in vitro conditions in the absence of an external driving force. WANITSCHKE and co-workers were not able to demonstrate secretion in everted sacs of rat colonic mucosa with oxyphenisatin and rhein (WANITSCHKE et al. 1977a, 1980a). Also in the short-circuited everted sac, only inhibition of sodium absorption was found (WANITSCHKE and SOERGEL 1975). Only POWELL et al. (1980) demonstrated secretion of sodium and chloride in the presence of phenolphthalein on the mucosal side in an Ussing chamber in rabbit ileal mucosa. Amazingly, these authors demonstrated the reverse effect, namely stimulation of absorption of sodium and chloride after addition of the drug to the serosal side. Thus, in order to clarify this question, a systematic investigation of the in vitro effects of triarylmethane derivatives and anthraquinones on intestinal fluid and electrolyte transfer is needed, taking into account the possible influences of different experimental conditions, before final conclusions can be drawn.

Several authors have tried to answer this question by measuring mucosal levels of cAMP and cGMP and/or the activities of their synthesizing and degrading enzymes. The basic assumption of this approach is the inference by analogy from the effects of cholera enterotoxin on cAMP on the one hand and on fluid transfer on the other. The results are conflicting, probably depending on the particular experimental conditions. In addition, this type of inference may be fallacious in a twofold manner, since: (a) the effects of a drug on the levels of cyclic nucleotides may be an epiphenomenon; and (b) even in the case of cholera enterotoxin, under certain conditions a dissociation of the effects on cAMP and electrolyte transfer has been shown (FIELD et al. 1975; SHEERIN and FIELD 1977; FORSYTH et al. 1979). The results of FARACK and NELL (1979) and FARACK et al. (1983) indicate a fundamental difference between the mode of action of bisacodyl and cholera enterotoxin. An inhibitor of the adenylate cyclase (RMI 12330A, a lactamimide), almost abolished the secretagogue effect of cholera enterotoxin on rat intestine, but not of the diphenolic laxative.

BEUBLER and JUAN (1977, 1978, 1979) showed a release of prostaglandin E-like material into the luminal fluid in the presence of diphenolic laxatives and sennosides A and B in the rat intestine. RACHMILEWITZ et al. (1980) found an increase of the prostaglandin E_2 content of the intestinal mucosa after oral administration of bisacodyl in rats. Both groups speculated that laxatives of this type may elicit fluid secretion via this mechanism. In other words, it is assumed that certain prostaglandins, whose production is increased by laxative drugs, cause active secretion. This is an intriguing possibility, but its quantitative significance cannot be evaluated at present since after pretreatment with indometacin, an inhibitor of prostaglandin synthesis, there is no obligatory correlation between the effect of the inhibitor on prostaglandin release and fluid secretion caused by diphenolic laxatives and senna derivatives (BEUBLER and JUAN 1978, 1979).

3. Increase in Permeability Resulting in Filtration

The crucial question for the application of this model to in vivo conditions has not yet been examined adequately. It is not known whether there exists a subepithelial hydrostatic pressure in excess of the luminal one under in vivo conditions with and without laxatives. These experiments have not been performed because of obvious methodological difficulties. However, there exists some indirect evidence that a hydrostatic pressure gradient from the serosal to the mucosal side of the epithelium may exist (for references see HAKIM and LIFSON 1969; MORTILLARO and TAYLOR 1976; LEE 1979). In addition, the model has been constructed on the basis of experimental results in the rat colon. It remains to be tested whether it is possible to extrapolate to other parts of the intestine which are much more leaky under normal conditions. A comprehensive review of the relationship between hydrostatic pressure and fluid secretion in the small intestine has recently been made by LIFSON (1979).

It can be stated that the assumption of a stimulation of active secretion by secretagogue laxatives is the less well supported model experimentally. Models, however, which are based on the inhibition of active sodium transport and on a filtrative movement of fluid into the gut lumen owing to an increase of epithelial permeability fit much better with the experimental results. They are not mutually exclusive and both mechanisms may contribute causally to the observed effects in a presently unknown quantitative manner.

D. Surfactants

I. Effect on Intestinal Fluid and Electrolyte Transfer

BUGLIA (1909) was the first to report that bile salts and sodium soap inhibit fluid absorption in dog intestine and reverse it to secretion at higher concentrations. His findings that surfactants may interfere with intestinal fluid absorption has been extended and confirmed in several species and under different in vivo and in vitro conditions, especially during the last 20 years (Table 3). The main interest has focused on the effects of bile salts because of possible physiologic and pathophysiologic implications. Fatty acids were investigated because the most effective agent within this group, ricinoleic acid, is the active principle of castor oil (GAGINELLA and PHILLIPS 1975) and because of pathophysiologic reasons (see the end of this section). Synthetic surfactants have been studied since dioctylsulfosuccinate is used as a laxative and a variety of others have attracted some interest, because they are used widely in pharmaceutical preparations designed for peroral applications (for references see, e.g., BRISEID et al. 1974).

As far as it has been investigated, all parts of the intestine of several species are sensitive to the effects of surfactants on fluid and sodium chloride transfer. One exception is the finding of TAUB et al. (1977) that, in the rabbit, deoxycholic acid is effective in the colon only, not in the jejunum. However, HAJJAR et al. (1975) reported that deoxycholic acid causes fluid secretion along the entire small intestine of rabbits. The apparent discrepancy of these results seems to depend on

Table 3. Effect of surfactants on intestinal fluid, sodium, and chloride transfer

Substance	Species	Effect	Experimental conditions in vivo	References
Anionic surfactants				
Bile salts	Rat	Inhibition of fluid absorption and/or secretion	Tied-off loops	[1–9]
			Perfusion	[5, 10–19, 19a–c]
		Inhibition of sodium absorption and/or secretion	Tied-off loops	[1–3, 5, 6, 8, 10, 11, 20]
			Perfusion	[5, 10, 11, 15–19, 19b, 19c]
		Inhibition of chloride absorption and/or secretion	Tied-off loops	[3, 5]
			Perfusion	[5, 10, 11, 17–19, 19b]
	Rabbit	Inhibition of fluid absorption and/or secretion	Tied-off loops	[21–24]
			Perfusion	[25–27, 27a]
		Inhibition of sodium absorption and/or secretion	Perfusion	[27, 27a]
	Hamster	Inhibition of fluid absorption and/or secretion	Perfusion	[28, 29]
	Dog	Inhibition of fluid absorption and/or secretion	Tied-off loops	[30, 31]
			Perfusion	[32, 32a)
		Inhibition of sodium chloride absorption and/or secretion	Perfusion	[32, 32a, 32b]
	Human	Inhibition of fluid absorption and/or secretion	Perfusion	[33–39, 39a, 40]
		Inhibition of sodium chloride absorption and/or secretion	Perfusion	[33, 34, 36, 38 39, 39a]
Saponins	Dog	Inhibition of fluid and sodium chloride absorption	Tied-off loops	[31]
Long-chain fatty acids	Rat	Inhibition of fluid absorption and/or secretion	Tied-off loops	[7]
			Perfusion	[14–16, 41]
		Inhibition of sodium absorption and/or secretion	Perfusion	[15, 41]
		Inhibition of sodium absorption and/or secretion	Perfusion	[41]
	Rabbit	Inhibition of fluid absorption and/or secretion	Perfusion	[42, 43]
		Inhibition of sodium absorption and/or secretion	Tied-off loops	[44]
	Hamster	Inhibition of fluid and sodium absorption and/or secretion	Perfusion	[45]
	Dog	Inhibition of fluid absorption and/or secretion	Thirty–Vella loops	[46, 47]
		Inhibition of sodium chloride absorption	Thirty–Vella loops	[46]
	Human	Inhibition of fluid absorption and/or secretion	Perfusion	[40, 48–50]
		Inhibition of sodium chloride absorption and/or secretion	Perfusion	[48, 49]
Sodium soap	Dog	Inhibition of fluid absorption and/or secretion		[30]

Table 3 (continued)

Substance	Species	Effect	Experimental conditions in vitro	References
Synthetic surfactants				
Dioctylsulfo-succinate	Rat	Inhibition of fluid absorption and/or secretion	Tied-off loops	[6, 7, 51]
			Perfusion	[52]
		Inhibition of sodium absorption and/or secretion	Tied-off loops	[6, 51]
		Inhibition of chloride absorption and/or secretion	Tied-off loops	[51]
	Human	Inhibition of fluid absorption and/or secretion	Perfusion	[52]
Dodecylsulfate	Rat	Inhibition of fluid absorption and/or secretion	Tied-off loops	[6, 53–55]
		Inhibition of sodium absorption and/or secretion	Tied-off loops	[54]
p-*n*-Decylbenzene sulfonate	Dog	Inhibition of fluid absorption	Thirty–Vella loop	[46]
Cationic surfactants				
Cetrimonium bromide	Rat	Inhibition of fluid absorption and/or secretion	Tied-off loops	[6]
			Perfusion	[56]
		Inhibition of sodium absorption and/or secretion	Tied-off loops	[6]
	Rabbit	Inhibition of fluid absorption and/or secretion	Perfusion	[56]
Trimethylhexa-decylammonium stearate	Rat	Inhibition of fluid absorption	Perfusion	[56]
Benzalkonium chloride	Rat	Inhibition of fluid and sodium absorption and or secretion	Tied-off loops	[6]
Nonionic surfactants				
Triton X-100, Lubrol WX	Rat	Inhibition of fluid and sodium absorption and/or secretion	Tied-off loops	[6]
Anionic surfactants				
Bile salts	Rat	Inhibition of fluid absorption and/or secretion	Fisher–Parsons method	[1, 2, 57]
			Everted sacs	[58, 59]
			Fisher–Parsons method	[1, 2] [59]
			Everted sacs	[59]
		Inhibition of sodium absorption	Short-circuited everted sacs	[60]
			Short-circuited Ussing chamber preparation	[61, 62]
		Inhibition of chloride absorption	Fisher–Parsons method	[1, 2]
			Short-circuited Ussing chamber preparation	[61]
	Rabbit	Secretion of sodium chloride	Short-circuited Ussing chamber preparation	[63]
	Hamster	Inhibition of fluid absorption and/or secretion	Everted sacs	[29, 58, 64]

Table 3 (continued)

Substance	Species	Effect	Experimental conditions in vitro	References
Long-chain fatty acids	Rat	Inhibition of fluid absorption	Everted sacs	[65]
		Inhibition of sodium absorption	Short-circuited Ussing chamber preparation	[66]
		Chloride secretion	Short-circuited Ussing chamber preparation	[66]
	Hamster	Inhibition of fluid absorption	Everted sacs	[29, 64, 67–69]
		Inhibition of sodium chloride absorption	Everted sacs	[68, 69]
Synthetic surfactants				
Dioctylsulfo-succinate	Rat	Inhibition of sodium absorption	Short-circuited Ussing chamber preparation	[51]
	Hamster	Inhibition of fluid absorption	Everted sacs	[29, 64]
		Inhibition of sodium chloride absorption	Everted sacs	[64]
Dodecylsulfate	Hamster	Inhibition of fluid absorption	Everted sacs	[29, 64]
Cationic surfactants				
Cetrimonium bromide and related compounds	Rat	Inhibition of fluid absorption	Everted sacs	[70]
Nonionic surfactants				
Polysorbate 80	Hamster	Inhibition of fluid absorption	Everted sacs	[64]

[1] FORTH et al. (1966b); [2] FORTH and RUMMEL (1967); [3] HARRIES and SLADEN (1972); [4] NELL et al. (1972); [5] LAMABADUSURIYA et al. (1975); [6] SUND and JACOBSEN (1978); [7] BEUBLER and JUAN (1979); [8] GORDON et al. (1979); [9] TAKAGI and TAKEDA (1979); [10] SLADEN and HARRIES (1972); [11] GUIRALDES et al. (1975); [12] SAUNDERS (1975); [13] SAUNDERS et al. (1975a); [14] DOBBINS and BINDER (1976); [15] BINDER et al. (1978); [16] SCARPELLO et al. (1978); [17] KONDER et al. (1979); [18] CASPARY and MEYNE (1980); [19] GEORG et al. (1980b); [19a] KARLSTRÖM et al. (1983); [19b] KONDER et al. (1981); [19c] RAMPTON et al. (1981); [20] NELL et al. (1976b); [21] CONLEY et al. (1976a); [22] CONLEY et al. (1976b); [23] TAUB et al. (1977); [24] TAUB et al. (1978); [25] HAJJAR et al. (1975); [26] CHADWICK et al. (1979); [27] CAMILLERI et al. (1980); [27a[CAMILLARY et al. (1982); [28] TEEM and PHILLIPS (1972); [29] GULLIKSON et al. (1977); [30] BUGLIA (1909); [31] PETERS (1942); [32] MEKHJIAN and PHILLIPS (1970); [32a] GULLIKSON et al. (1981); [32b] KELLY et al. (1981); [33] MEKHJIAN et al. (1971); [34] RUSSEL et al. (1973); [35] WINGATE et al. (1973a); [36] KRAG and PHILLIPS (1974); [37] FAIRCLOUGH et al. (1977); [38] ODDSSON et al. (1977a); [39] ODDSSON et al. (1977b); [39a] BROWN and AMMON (1981); [40] WANITSCHKE and AMMON (1978); [41] BRIGHT-ASARE and BINDER (1973); [42] GAGINELLA et al. (1977b); [43] HAJJAR et al. (1979); [44] PHILLIPS et al. (1965); [45] CLINE et al. (1976); [46] AMMON and PHILLIPS (1974); [47] GADACZ et al. (1976); [48] AMMON and PHILLIPS (1973); [49] AMMON et al. (1974); [50] AMMON et al. (1977); [51] DONOWITZ and BINDER (1975); [52] SAUNDERS et al. (1975b); [53] BRISEID et al. (1974); [54] SUND (1975); [55] BRISEID et al. (1976); [56] NISSIM (1960b); [57] WINGATE (1974);

the experimental conditions. HAJJAR et al. (1975) used a perfusion technique in vivo whereas TAUB et al. (1977) measured fluid transfer in tied-off loops after 5 h. Thus, the latter group may not have been able to recognize the effect on fluid transfer because the duration of the experiment was too long. In rats, it has been reported repeatedly that bile acids are more effective in the jejunum than in the ileum (HARRIES and SLADEN 1972; SLADEN and HARRIES 1972; SAUNDERS 1975). In contradistinction to the results obtained with triarylmethane derivatives (see Sect. C.I), FORTH et al. (1966b) found no difference in the susceptibility of jejunum and colon. CASPARY and MEYNE (1980) reported that the effects of bile salts were more pronounced in the colon than in the ileum. TAKAGI and TAKEDA (1979) reported that fluid absorption in the ileum was less affected than in the jejunum and colon. Thus, it seems that the action of bile salts on fluid transfer is more marked in the rat jejunum and colon than in the ileum.

In addition to the effects compiled in Table 3, surfactants have also been reported to influence potassium movement under in vivo conditions. Bile acids stimulate potassium secretion in the rat colon (FORTH et al. 1966b; BINDER et al. 1978; SUND and MATHESON 1978; CASPARY and MEYNE 1980; GOERG et al. 1980b) and in the rat small intestine (FORTH et al. 1966b; HARRIES and SLADEN 1972; SLADEN and HARRIES 1972; SUND and JACOBSEN 1978; SUND and MATHESON 1978; KONDER et al. 1979, 1981). In the rat cecum, GORDON et al. (1979) found no influence on the potassium movement and, in the canine colon, MEKHJIAN and PHILLIPS (1970) found no influence on potassium net movement. In the canine jejunum, inhibition of potassium absorption has been reported (GULLIKSON et al. 1981; KELLY et al. 1981). In humans, bile acids caused inhibition of potassium absorption or secretion in the jejunum (ODDSSON et al. 1977b; BROWN and AMMON 1981), in the ileum (ODDSSON et al. 1977a), and in the colon (MEKHJIAN et al. 1971).

In the human and rat colon, long-chain fatty acids also increased potassium secretion (AMMON and PHILLIPS 1973; BINDER et al. 1978). Potassium secretion is elicited by oleate in the human jejunum (BROWN and AMMON 1981). DONOWITZ and BINDER (1975) found no influence of dioctylsulfosuccinate on potassium transfer in the rat cecum. In the small intestine of rats, an increase in potassium secretion has been reported (SUND and JACOBSEN 1978; SUND and MATHESON 1978). For the nonionic group of detergents, the same effect was found in the presence of Lubrol WX in rat small and large intestine (SUND and JACOBSEN 1978; SUND and MATHESON 1978). The cationic detergents cetrimonium bromide and benzalkonium chloride increased potassium secretion in the rat small intestine (SUND 1978; SUND and JACOBSEN 1978). This has also been shown for cetrimonium bromide in the large intestine of the rat (SUND 1978).

---

[58] FAUST and WU (1965a); [59] WANITSCHKE et al. (1977a); [60] WANITSCHKE and SOERGEL (1975); [61] BINDER and RAWLINS (1973); [62] BINDER et al. (1975); [63] VOLPE and BINDER (1975); [64] GAGINELLA et al. (1975a); [65] YAU and MEKHLOUF (1974); [66] RACUSEN and BINDER (1979); [67] GAGINELLA et al. (1975b); [68] GAGINELLA et al. (1975c); [69] STEWART et al. (1975); [70] TAYLOR (1963)

Under in vitro conditions, deoxycholic acid inhibited the serosal appearance of potassium in the rat jejunum (FORTH et al. 1966b). In one report, ricinoleic acid had no effect on potassium transfer in everted sacs of hamster small intestine (STEWART et al. 1975), in another, it caused slight inhibition of absorption (GAGINELLA et al. 1975c).

In conclusion, it is quite obvious that detergents elicit or enhance potassium secretion, or at least may inhibit potassium absorption, in the small and large intestine of several species under in vivo conditions. The few exceptions seem to be due to different experimental conditions (e.g., different concentrations). Under in vitro conditions the effect of surfactants on potassium transport has not been studied adequately. The in vivo studies cited do not allow one to draw inferences about the action mechanism of surfactants on potassium transfer. The dose dependence of the effect of detergents on potassium transfer seems to differ from that on sodium and fluid transfer. At least in rat colon, potassium secretion is maximally stimulated by deoxycholate in concentrations, which do not influence fluid transfer (GOERG et al. 1978; FARACK et al. 1981; 1982). As stated for the triarylmethane derivatives (see Sect. C.I), potassium secretion is too small to contribute significantly to the observed fluid movements in the presence of detergents.

As we have indicated, interest has been drawn to the effects of bile salts and long-chain fatty acids on intestinal fluid and electrolyte transfer not merely for pharmacologic reasons. It has been shown that bile salts and fatty acids play an important role in the pathophysiology of certain diarrheal diseases. Bile salts may also contribute to the regulation of water content of the feces under physiologic conditions (for references see the reviews of FORTH and RUMMEL 1975; RUMMEL 1976; PHILLIPS and GAGINELLA 1977, 1979).

II. Structure–Activity Relationship

It is supposed that some common property of detergents is responsible for their effects on intestinal fluid and electrolyte transfer since substances of unrelated chemical structure (see Table 3) display more or less similar effects. In that sense the effects of surfactants are called “nonspecific”. This is the reason why a variety of these substances with the only common feature of altering surface tension has been combined in this chapter. Comparative studies with chemically different surfactants have been carried out, above all by NISSIM (1960b), GAGINELLA et al. (1975a), GULLIKSON et al. (1977), and SUND and JACOBSON (1978). No systematic study of the correlation of the effects of surfactants of different types (cationic, anionic, nonionic) on fluid transfer on the one hand and surface tension on the other has been reported so far. Only GULLIKSON et al. (1977) have published a comparative study regarding some anionic surfactants. They found a rough agreement between the effects on water transport in everted sacs of hamster jejunum and on surface tension. However, within distinct groups of anionic surfactants, e.g., bile salts, there was no satisfactory correlation of these parameters. Thus, the authors concluded that the influence on surface tension “...is only a partial predictor of membrane interaction. Equally important is the charge distribution and structural properties of the molecule.”

More extensive studies of structure–activity relationships have been performed in some chemically related groups of surfactants. The bile salts have been studied most thoroughly in this respect. The results are not unequivocal, but some features can already be stated. There is no ambiguity that dihydroxy bile salts are more effective than trihydroxy ones in all species so far examined (FORTH et al. 1966 b; MEKHJIAN and PHILLIPS 1970; MEKHJIAN et al. 1971; HARRIES and SLADEN 1972; TEEM and PHILLIPS 1972; RUSSEL et al. 1973; WINGATE et al. 1973 a; KRAG and PHILLIPS 1974; WINGATE 1974; BINDER et al. 1975; HAJJAR et al. 1975; VOLPE and BINDER 1975; GULLIKSON et al. 1977; WANITSCHKE and AMMON 1978; CHADWICK et al. 1979; GORDON et al. 1979; KONDER et al. 1979). The question whether conjugated bile salts are less effective than free ones has been answered less clearly. In the rat, it was reported that conjugated bile salts are distinctly less effective than free bile salts, at least when using chromatographically pure substances (FORTH et al. 1966 b; HARRIES and SLADEN 1972; FORTH and RUMMEL 1975). The same was found for rabbit (HAJJAR et al. 1975) and hamster intestine (TEEM and PHILLIPS 1972; GULLIKSON 1977). In dogs (MEKHJIAN and PHILLIPS 1970), no influence of conjugation was found. In humans, MEKHJIAN et al. (1971) and RUSSEL et al. (1973) reported that conjugated and free bile salts were equally effective. However, KRAG and PHILLIPS (1974) and WANITSCHKE and AMMON (1978) showed that free dihydroxy bile salts were more effective than conjugated derivatives in humans.

FORTH et al. (1966 b) were the first to point out that dihydroxy bile salts with the hydroxyl groups in the α position are the most effective. This finding was later confirmed and extended by CHADWICK et al. (1979) and GORDON et al. (1979). These authors showed clearly that the two hydroxyl groups have to be in the 3α, 7α, or 12α position in order to guarantee the greatest efficacy. GORDON et al. (1979) stated that in these cases the distance between the groups amounts to 5 Å. These findings also explain the result of CASPARY and MEYNE (1980) that chenodeoxycholic acid (3α,7α-dihydroxycholanic acid) is more effective than ursodeoxycholic acid (3α,7β-dihydroxycholanic acid).

In summary, the main structural requirements of bile salts in order to influence intestinal fluid transport are two hydroxyl groups in the 3α, 7α, or 12α position, respectively, which guarantee a distance of 5 Å. Whether free bile salts are more effective than conjugated ones may depend on the species.

Considerable attention has also been focused on the structure–activity relationships of long-chain fatty acids. However, at present, only one point seems to be clear, namely that ricinoleic acid is the most effective substance of this group in several species (AMMON and PHILLIPS 1973, 1974; AMMON et al. 1974; GAGINELLA et al. 1975 b, c; DOBBINS and BINDER 1976; WANITSCHKE and AMMON 1978). With respect to the other open questions, namely the influence of chain length, hydroxylation, *cis*/*trans* configuration at the $\Delta 9,10$ double bond, significance of the carboxyl group, either controversial results have been reported, or the investigation was done in a single species under one set of experimental conditions only. Thus, definite conclusions cannot be drawn as yet.

In summary, detergents are usually treated as a uniform group regarding their effects on intestinal fluid and electrolyte transfer, because of the common feeling that their action on these parameters is due to a nonspecific effect on membranes, which is related to their physicochemical properties. However, as far as is known, there is no satisfactory correlation between their ability to lower surface tension on the one hand and influence intestinal fluid transfer on the other. This is especially evident when chemically similar homologous substances such as the bile salts are considered. It is obvious that properties like charge distribution and distance between hydroxyl groups, and other structural requirements which influence solubility in the aqueous phase and the interactions with biologic membranes, play an important role.

III. Proposed Action Mechanisms

1. Inhibition of Active Transport Processes

As in the case of triarylmethane derivatives (Sect. C.III.1), it has also been investigated in considerable detail whether surface active agents interfere with ATP metabolism. PARKINSON and OLSON (1964), POPE et al. (1966), GRACEY et al. (1972, 1973), GUIRALDES et al. (1975), LAMABADUSURIYA et al. (1975), HAFKENSCHEID (1977), and FERARD et al. (1980) reported an inhibition of Na^+, K^+-ATPase. FAUST and WU (1965c) found a stimulation. HEPNER and HOFMANN (1973) and MITJAVILA et al. (1975) reported an increase or decrease in the activity of this enzyme depending on the intestinal preparation, the particular bile salt, and its concentration. FAUST and WU (1965a, b) and ROSENBERG and HARDISON (1965) described a decrease in ATP content of intestinal tissue in the presence of bile salts which is, of course, easier to reconcile with an increase than with a decrease in the activity of Na^+, K^+-ATPase.

Other anionic surfactants, like oleic acid and dodecylic acid (HEPNER and HOFMANN 1973) were reported to have no effect on the activity of Na^+, K^+-ATPase whereas dioctylsulfosuccinate was shown to decrease the activity of this enzyme (RACHMILEWITZ and KARMELI 1979; RACHMILEWITZ et al. 1981). Nonionic surfactants (Triton X-100, Tween 20, 60, 80) increased the activity of Na^+, K^+-ATPase at low and decreased it at higher concentrations (MITJAVILA et al. 1975). The cationic detergent cetrimonium bromide has little influence on Na^+, K^+-ATPase activity (TAYLOR 1963). With regard to fatty acids, it was proposed by GAGINELLA et al. (1975b) that they may limit the availability of ATP for intestinal transport processes by inhibiting the activity of adenine nucleotide translocase, the carrier responsible for mitochondrial ADP and ATP transport.

Some of the earlier reports that oxygen consumption of intestinal preparations is inhibited by bile salts (PARKINSON and OLSEN 1964; FAUST and WU 1965c; ROSENBERG and HARDISON 1965; POPE et al. 1966; MITJAVILA et al. 1973) are in keeping with the hypothesis of inhibition of active, i.e., metabolically driven, transport processes. FAUST and WU (1965c) showed that bile acids may uncouple oxidative phosphorylation.

It has been shown repeatedly that surfactants impair not only intestinal electrolyte transport, but interfere also with the active transport of monosaccharides and amino acids.

Bile salts inhibit monosaccharide absorption in vivo and in vitro in several species in acute experiments (DAWSON and ISSELBACHER 1960; NUNN et al. 1963; PARKINSON and OLSON 1963; FAUST 1964; FAUST and WU 1965a; FORTH et al.

1966b; LACK and WEINER 1966; POPE et al. 1966; FORTH and RUMMEL 1967; GRACEY et al. 1971a, 1973; HARRIES and SLADEN 1972; SLADEN and HARRIES 1972; TOMKIN and LOVE 1972; WINGATE et al. 1973a; CASPARY 1974; KRAG and PHILLIPS 1974; WINGATE 1974; GUIRALDES et al. 1975; LAMABADUSURIYA et al. 1975; SUND and JACOBSEN 1978; SUND and MATHESON 1978; WANITSCHKE and AMMON 1978; CASPARY and MEYNE 1980; FERARD et al. 1980; et al.Brown and AMMON 1981). In animals with chronic bile fistulae, intestinal 3-*O*-methylglucose transport was increased (ROY et al. 1970).

Bile salts also inhibit intestinal absorption of several amino acids (PARKINSON and OLSON 1963; LACK and WEINER 1966; POPE et al. 1966; CASPARY 1974; BURKE et al. 1975; HAJJAR et al. 1975). Long-chain fatty acids have been reported to decrease monosaccharide absorption (REYNELL and SPRAY 1958; AMMON and PHILLIPS 1974; AMMON et al. 1977; WANITSCHKE and AMMON 1978; BROWN and AMMON 1981; KELLY et al. 1981). The same effect has been reported regarding amino acids (AMMON et al. 1977; HAJJAR et al. 1979).

In principle, the same results have been reported in the case of synthetic anionic surfactants, namely dodecylsulfate and dioctylsulfosuccinate (NISSIM 1962; HART and MCCOLL 1967; SUND and JACOBSEN 1978; SUND and MATHESON 1978; SUND and OLSEN 1981). NISSIM (1962) reported that at low concentrations dodecylsulfate increased glucose absorption. Nonionic surfactants also interfere with monosaccharide absorption (Triton X-100, Lubrol WX: SUND and JACOBSEN 1978; SUND and MATHESON 1978). The same is true for cationic detergents (cetrimonium bromide, benzalkonium chloride, and similar compounds: NISSIM 1960b, 1961, 1962; TAYLOR 1963; ZATZMANN and MOORE 1968; SUND 1978; SUND and MATHESON 1978). Like dodecylsulfate, cetrimonium bromide increased glucose absorption at low concentrations (NISSIM 1962). Probably, the enhancement of glucose absorption in these in vivo experiments was due to an increase of the passive component of glucose transfer since the glucose concentration in the luminal fluid was 200 mg-%.

In addition, a variety of surfactants have been shown to inhibit cellular uptake mechanisms of hexoses and amino acids (ROSENBERG and HARDISON 1965; GRACEY et al. 1971b, 1972, 1973; BURKE et al. 1976; GAGINELLA et al. 1977c). It is generally thought that interference with nutrient transport is a nonspecific interaction of surfactants with biologic membranes, related somehow to their detergent properties (e.g., SUND and MATHESON 1978) and not due to a specific reaction with some receptor molecule as was for instance speculated by NISSIM (1964).

With regard to the site of action of surfactants on nutrient transport, several hypotheses have been discussed. Detergents have been shown to inhibit influx across the brush border membrane (FRIZZELL and SCHULTZ 1970; HAJJAR et al. 1975, 1979; FELDMAN et al. 1977). In addition, sodium-dependent solute flux may be inhibited by surfactants via an increase in cellular sodium content caused by an inhibition of Na^+, K^+-ATPase (see discussion in HAJJAR et al. 1979). Furthermore, passive permeability of the intestinal tissue may be increased by these substances leading to an increase in backflux of solutes from the serosal to the mucosal side (e.g., HAJJAR et al. 1979; SUND and JACOBSEN 1978). Of course, gross damage of the epithelium may occur with higher concentrations of surfactants (see Sect. D.III.3).

As stated for the triarylmethane derivatives, it is unlikely that inhibition of nutrient absorption contributes significantly to the effect of intestinal fluid transfer, since detergents also interfere with fluid movements in parts of the intestine lacking transport mechanisms for monosaccharides and amino acids, like the colon of several species.

2. Stimulation of Active Secretion

There have been only three publications which demonstrate active fluid and electrolyte secretion in the presence of surfactants under distinct in vitro conditions. FAUST and WU (1965a) reported that bile salts elicited fluid secretion in everted sacs of rat and hamster small intestine in the absence but not in the presence of glucose in the bathing solution. VOLPE and BINDER (1975) showed secretion of sodium and chloride in a short-circuited preparation of rabbit intestine in the presence of bile salts. RACUSEN and BINDER (1979) demonstrated chloride secretion during a period of 15 min after addition of ricinoleic acid to an Ussing chamber preparation of rat colon also under short-circuit conditions. BINDER and coworkers also used glucose-free solutions (VOLPE and BINDER 1975; RACUSEN and BINDER 1979). In all other publications mentioned in Table 3, only inhibition of absorption and no secretion was found under in vitro conditions.

BINDER was the first to put forward the hypothesis that, as in the case of cholera enterotoxin and theophylline, the mechanism by which secretion is elicited by surfactants is mediated by cAMP (BINDER and RAWLINS 1973). BINDER and coworkers showed that, under in vitro conditions, there was a good correlation between an increase in cAMP on the one hand and an increase in short-circuit current, which was supposed to represent anion secretion, on the other. These authors showed this relationship for bile acids (BINDER et al. 1975) and ricinoleic acid (RACUSEN and BINDER 1979). The time course of the increase in cAMP and short-circuit current is similar too for bile salts (BINDER 1975) and ricinoleic acid (RACUSEN and BINDER 1979). An increase in cAMP was also demonstrated in vivo in the presence of bile salts (BINDER et al. 1975) and dioctylsulfosuccinate (DONOWITZ and BINDER 1975). The same authors stressed an additional argument in order to prove that surfactant-induced alteration of intestinal electrolyte transfer is cAMP mediated. They compared the effects of bile salts, dioctylsulfosuccinate, and ricinoleic acid with those of theophylline. They showed that the effects are similar regarding short-circuit current and net ionic transfer. The effects of both surfactants and theophylline were abolished after substitution of bicarbonate and chloride by the nonpermeating anion isoethionate. The effect of theophylline on short-circuit current could be inhibited by prior addition of bile salts to the bathing solution and vice versa. The addition of dibutyryl-cAMP produced effects on short-circuit current and ion fluxes similar to those of the surfactants (BINDER and RAWLINS 1973; BINDER et al. 1975; DONOWITZ and BINDER 1975; VOLPE and BINDER 1975; RACUSEN and BINDER 1979).

This hypothesis was supported by the findings of SCHOENFIELD and co-workers. These authors found, in rabbit colon, that deoxycholic acid causes fluid secretion dose dependently and stimulates adenylate cyclase activity. Both effects could be abolished by propranolol (COYNE et al. 1976; CONLEY et al. 1976a, b). Later, these findings were extended to human colon mucosa in vitro. Under these conditions, 9,10-hydroxystearic acid had the same effects (COYNE et al. 1977). The same group showed that this secretagogue effect of deoxycholic acid and its inhibition by propranolol is specific to the colon (TAUB et al. 1977, 1978). Their finding that deoxycholic acid did not alter fluid movement in rabbit small intestine is at variance with the results of HAJJAR et al. (1975), see Sect. D.I.

The findings of these groups were confirmed and extended by MERTENS et al. (1976) for rabbit ileum in vitro, by SCARPELLO et al. (1978) who reported that deoxycholic acid increased cAMP levels in rat colon in vivo, and by CORAZZA et al. (1979) who found an increase in cAMP levels after peroral treatment with chenodeoxycholate in human colonic mucosa; cGMP levels were also increased. BRISEID et al. (1976, 1977) reported that dodecylsulfate increased cAMP levels in rat jejunal mucosa in vivo. RACHMILEWITZ et al. (1981) showed that dioctylsulfosuccinate increased the activity of both the colonic adenylate cyclase and of the cAMP degrading enzyme, phosphodiesterase, in rats in vivo. Therefore, the mucosal cAMP level was not influenced.

However, contradictory results have also been published. SUND and HILLESTAD (1981) found no effect of deoxycholic acid on cAMP levels in rat jejunal mucosa. GAGINELLA et al. (1978) reported no stimulation of adenylate cyclase activity in isolated intestinal cells of hamster intestine and SIMON et al. (1978) demonstrated that bile salts over a wide concentration range are not able to stimulate human colonic adenylate cyclase activity. SCARPELLO et al. (1978) found no influence of ricinoleic acid on cAMP in rat colon. GAGINELLA et al. (1978) and SIMON and KATHER (1980) reported that ricinoleic acid did not influence adenylate cyclase activity in hamster and human intestine, respectively. SUND and HILLESTAD (1981) showed that dioctylsulfosuccinate did not influence cAMP levels. SIMON and KATHER (1980) demonstrated that dioctylsulfosuccinate did not stimulate adenylate cyclase in human colonic mucosa. However, in contrast to bile salts and ricinoleic acid, it inhibits phosphodiesterase activity. SUND and HILLESTAD (1981) showed that cetrimonium bromide and Lubrol WX do not influence cAMP levels of rat jejunal mucosa. Dodecylsulfate only causes a short transitory increase.

As in the case of triarylmethane derivatives, it has also been investigated whether secretion induced by surfactants may be secondary to the liberation of an endogenous substance by the drugs. BEUBLER and JUAN (1979) showed that deoxycholic acid, ricinoleic and oleic acid, and dioctylsulfosuccinate induced fluid secretion and release of prostaglandin-like material in rat colon concomitantly. Indometacin, an inhibitor of prostaglandin synthesis, reduced both effects in the presence of ricinoleic, oleic, and deoxycholic acid. With dioctylsulfosuccinate, indometacin diminished only the effect on prostaglandin release, but not on water transfer. A good correlation was shown between prostaglandin release and effect on water flux with fatty acids, but not with deoxycholate and dioctylsulfosuccinate. RAMPTON et al. (1981) also demonstrated that deoxycholate increases the output of immunoreactive prostaglandin in the rat in vivo. Indometacin reduced this output significantly, but did not influence fluid secretion. LUDERER et al. (1980) speculated that ricinoleic acid may serve as an exogenous substrate for intestinal prostaglandin synthesis. RACHMILEWITZ et al. (1981) reported that dioctylsulfosuccinate increased jejunal and colonic prostaglandin E_2 content in the rat in vivo.

3. Increase in Permeability

The effect of surfactants on the permeability of epithelia has been tested with two different methodological approaches. First, the mucosal transfer has been measured of molecules known to permeate the mucosa by simple diffusion, at least after some pharmacologic manipulation (e.g., inhibition of active glucose transport by phlorhizin). Second, the effect of detergents on electrical conductivity has been estimated. Bile salts have been shown to increase the permeation of passively transported hydrophilic molecules (see Sect. C.III.3) of different size (POPE et al. 1966; FELDMAN et al. 1970, 1973; FRIZZELL and SCHULTZ 1970; KAKEMI et al. 1970; NELL et al. 1975, 1976a, b, 1981; DOBBINS and BINDER 1976; CHADWICK et al. 1977, 1979; GULLIKSON et al. 1977; BINDER et al. 1978; GOERG et al. 1980b, 1983; WINNE and GÖRIG 1982). SLADEN and HARRIES (1972) were the only group to find no increase in intestinal permeability in the presence of bile salts.

The long-chain fatty acids also increase intestinal permeability as measured by test molecules (BRIGHT-ASARE and BINDER 1973; CLINE et al. 1976; DOBBINS and BINDER 1976; GAGINELLA et al. 1977b; BINDER et al. 1978; NATAF et al. 1981; WINNE and GÖRIG 1982). The same has been shown for dioctylsulfosuccinate and dodecylsulfate (LISH and WEIKEL 1959). Other anionic surfactants exerted similar effects (alkylbenzene sulfonate, linear alkylate sulfonate, MOORE et al. 1971) and the same was found with the cationic surfactant cetrimonium bromide and the nonionic Triton X-100 (MOORE et al. 1971). A review of the earlier results in this field was published by GIBALDI and FELDMANN (1970). Bile salts also increase the permeability for ions in the intestinal mucosa which leads to an increase in electrical conductivity (BINDER and RAWLINS 1973; WALL and BAKER 1974; SCHWITER et al. 1975; VOLPE and BINDER 1975; WANITSCHKE and SOERGEL 1975; SUND et al. 1980). On the contrary, FELDMAN et al. (1971) reported a decrease in electrical conductivity in the presence of bile salts. This seems to be a dose-dependent phenomenon since NELL et al. (1981) showed that deoxycholate decreases the electrical conductivity at low and increases it at higher concentrations. Ricinoleic acid and dioctylsulfosuccinate have also been shown to increase electrical conductance (RACUSEN and BINDER 1979; DONOWITZ and BINDER 1975). With regard to other surfactants, FELDMAN et al. (1975) reported that the anionic detergent dodecylsulfate and the neutral Tween 80 increased electrical conductivity whereas cetrimonium bromide was found to decrease it. Whether the latter finding points to a different action of anionic/nonionic, and cationic surfactants, respectively, on intestinal conductivity can be decided only if the dose–response relationship is studied.

Several groups have demonstrated that the effect of surfactants on fluid movement on the one hand and on permeability on the other hand displays a similar dose–response relationship (CLINE et al. 1976; GAGINELLA et al. 1977b; GULLIKSON et al. 1977; GOERG et al. 1978; GOERG 1979; GOERG et al. 1983).

At this point, the question arises whether the increase in permeability is due to damage of the mucosal epithelium in the sense that the continuity of the epithelium is disrupted and ultimately the basal membrane or the underlying tissue is exposed directly to the luminal fluid. One argument against the possibility that permeability changes are the consequence of gross epithelial damage comes from reversibility studies. It has been shown that the effect of surfactants on permeability is reversible, at least within a certain concentration range. This has been shown with regard to the effect of deoxycholate in vivo and in vitro (GOERG et al. 1980b, 1983; SUND et al. 1980), for ricinoleic acid (BRIGHT-ASARE and BINDER 1973) and for dioctylsulfosuccinate (GOERG 1979). These findings correspond to the demonstration of reversibility of the effects of surfactants on fluid movement. This has been shown for bile salts (MEKHJIAN and PHILLIPS 1970; MEKHJIAN et al. 1971; TEEM and PHILLIPS 1972; RUSSELL et al. 1973; WINGATE et al. 1973a; GOERG et al. 1978, 1980b, 1983; GOERG 1979; KONDER et al. 1979; GULLIKSON et al. 1981), for ricinoleic acid (AMMON and PHILLIPS 1973, 1974; BRIGHT-ASARE and BINDER 1973; AMMON et al. 1974; GAGINELLA et al. 1975a; KELLY et al. 1981), for dioctylsulfosuccinate (DONOWITZ and BINDER 1975; GAGINELLA et al. 1975a; SAUNDERS et al. 1975b; GOERG 1979), and for the nonionic surfactant polysorbate 80 (GAGINELLA et al. 1975a).

The effect of detergents on intestinal morphology has also been studied by histologic methods. In principle, it was shown, that, depending on the dose of the surfactant, a variety of morphological changes, from minimal alterations to severe damage, may occur. Clustering of microvilli, appearance of knob-like particles in the microvilli, shortening and disappearance of microvilli, "ballooning" of enterocytes, loss of normal structure of cellular organelles (Golgi apparatus, mitochondria, endoplasmic reticulum, nuclei), increase in shedding of epithelial cells, disruption of the continuity of the epithelial cell layer with appearance of patchy defects, and inflammatory infiltration of the mucosa have been shown.

The most extensive work has been done with bile salts (DAWSON and ISSELBACHER 1960; FRY and STAFFELDT 1964; LOW-BEER et al. 1970; MEKHJIAN and PHILLIPS 1970; HARRIES and SLADEN 1972; TEEM and PHILLIPS 1972; TOMKIN and LOVE 1972; GRACEY et al. 1973; NADAI et al. 1975; SAUNDERS et al. 1975a; GAGINELLA et al. 1977a; GULLIKSON et al. 1977; WANITSCHKE et al. 1977a; YONEZAWA 1977; CHADWICK et al. 1979; GOERG 1979; GORDON et al. 1979; GOERG et al. 1980b, 1983; FAGUNDES-NETO et al. 1981). Long-chain fatty acids induce similar alterations (REYNELL and SPRAY 1958; CLINE et al. 1976; GAGINELLA and PHILLIPS 1976; GAGINELLA et al. 1976, 1977a, b). A mixture of bile and oleic acid caused "clefts" in villus tips (KVIETYS et al. 1981). The same findings have been reported for dioctylsulfosuccinate (MOFFAT et al. 1975; SAUNDERS et al. 1975b; GAGINELLA et al. 1977a; GOERG 1979). A variety of synthetic surfactants of the anionic, nonionic, and cationic type, namely dodecylsulfate (NADAI et al. 1972, 1975; SUGIMURA 1974a, b; YONEZAWA 1977), sarcosinate (YONEZAWA 1977), polysorbate 80, HCO-50, and benzathonium chloride (NADAI et al. 1975), pluronic F68 (NADAI et al. 1975; YONEZAWA 1977), Tween 80 and BRIJ 35 (YONEZAWA 1977), cetrimonium bromide (NISSIM 1960b; TAYLOR 1963), and cetrimonium stearate (NISSIM 1960a, b).

The morphological effects of surfactants are reversible (HARRIES and SLADEN 1972; NADAI et al. 1975; GAGINELLA and PHILLIPS 1976; GAGINELLA et al. 1977a; GOERG 1979; GOERG et al. 1982). The findings of several authors that one of the first effects of surfactants at relatively low concentrations is discharge of mucus from mucus-producing cells has been corroborated by direct measurement of mucus output from the intestinal mucosa in perfusion experiments in the presence of bile salts (LEWIN et al. 1979; CAMILLERI et al. 1980; FARACK et al. 1982). The speculation of CAMILLERI et al. (1980, 1982) that the bile acid-induced mucus depletion of the intestinal mucosa with loss of its cytoprotection effect may lead to mucosal damage which is associated with changes in fluid transfer seems to be questionable since WANITSCHKE et al. (1977a) and SPECHT (1977) showed that, in the presence of bile salts, the epithelial surface is covered by a thick mucous film in contrast to the controls. GAGINELLA et al. (1977a) also reported that sometimes surface mucus is augmented in the presence of secretagogues. Thus, in order to maintain the argument of CAMILLERI et al. (1980, 1982), one has to assume that the mucus discharged in the presence of bile salts differs qualitatively from that produced normally.

The dose-dependent influence of surfactants on the integrity of biologic membranes is reflected by the liberation of constituents of cell membranes and other cell organelles. Several authors showed that surfactants liberate surface bound enzymes, proteins, and phospholipids (FRIZZELL and SCHULTZ 1970; HADORN et al. 1971; NORDSTRÖM 1972; FELDMAN et al. 1973; CLINE et al. 1976; FELDMAN and REINHARD 1976; GULLIKSON et al. 1977; VASSEUR et al. 1978, 1980; WHITMORE et al. 1979). Of course, it is difficult to decide what part of the liberated material (proteins, phospholipids) is derived from mucus or from cell membranes of the enterocytes. DNA appearance in the gut lumen has also been demonstrated and may indicate increased cell shedding and gross mucosal damage with higher concentrations of the surfactant (CLINE et al. 1976; GAGINELLA et al. 1977b; GULLIKSON et al. 1977; BERNIER et al. 1979; CHADWICK et al. 1979; CAMILLERI et al. 1980, 1982; RAMPTON et al. 1981).

Some authors reported a correlation between mucosal alterations on the one hand and on fluid movement on the other (TAYLOR 1963; SAUNDERS et al. 1975a, b; GAGINELLA 1977b; GORDON et al. 1979). In contrast, it was reported that water and electrolyte movement is influenced by surfactants in concentrations which do not cause demonstrable morphological alterations (MEKHJIAN et al. 1970; HARRIES and SLADEN 1972; TEEM and PHILLIPS 1972; DONOWITZ and BINDER 1975; SAUNDERS et al. 1975a, b; RAMPTON et al. 1981). SPECHT (1977), WANITSCHKE et al. (1977a), GOERG et al. (1978, 1980b, 1982, 1983), and GOERG (1979) found that, under conditions in which fluid movement was profoundly influenced by deoxycholate, no disruption of the continuity of the epithelial cell layer occurs. Thus, it can be stated that an influence on intestinal fluid transfer is not regularly accompanied by mucosal epitheliolysis as has been assumed for instance by CHADWICK et al. (1979).

Attempts at answering the question whether surfactants, in concentrations which induce large changes in fluid movement, cause mucosal epitheliolysis encounter some technical problems in handling the tissue samples for scanning electron microscopy. Obviously, the detergents cause an increase in cell shedding connected with a loosening of the coherence of the epithelial cells. Thus, depending for instance on the degree of rinsing, which is necessary in order to wash away the mucous layer which is augmented in presence of surfactants, the risk of artificially removing parts of the loosened epithelium is very high. Figure 5a shows the normal appearance of rat colonic mucosa. In the presence of 8 mmol/l deoxycholate the surface of border cells protrudes (Fig. 5b). The border lines between the single cells are clearly visible. Around the crypts swollen cells can be seen; these cells have lost their microvilli. Patchy defects or discontinuities of the epithelial layer, however, were not observed. Figure 5c shows that these alterations are largely reversible. The mucosal surface is flat again. As a residue of the deoxycholate effect, the extrusion of enterocytes in the area between the crypts, i.e., the physiologic extrusion zone, is still enhanced. Figure 5d shows denudation of the lamina propria after too vigorous rinsing.

Thus, the conclusion can be drawn that on the one hand there is overwhelming evidence that changes in fluid movement induced by surfactants are associated with an increase in intestinal permeability. On the other hand, it has been shown that surfactants are capable of inducing a series of morphological alterations of the intestinal mucosa, from subtle changes of surface appearance to severe damage. However, secretagogue effects are not necessarily correlated with gross epithelial damage.

At this stage of the discussion the question arises: what is the site of the increase in permeability of the intestinal mucosa caused by surfactants under conditions where no disintegration of the epithelial continuity occurs? The answer is the same as already given in Sect. C.III.3, namely that it is the barrier of the paracellular way, the matrix of the junctional complex. The first argument supporting this answer is the increase in permeability with regard to test molecules which are unable to penetrate the cellular membranes (NELL et al. 1975, 1976a, b, 1981; GOERG et al. 1980, 1983). Second, the mucosal distribution of sodium and potassium is not altered by deoxycholate with concentrations which already display maximal effects on fluid transfer (NELL et al. 1976a, b; WANITSCHKE et al. 1977a). Thus, it seems unlikely that the integrity of the cell membranes has been disturbed to an appreciable extent. The third line of argument is based on that for oxyphenisatin, namely the ^{22}Na distribution in the mucosal epithelium (NELL et al. 1976a, b). It has been shown that the specific activity of the tracer ^{22}Na within the mucosal tissue is not increased by deoxycholate in concentrations which cause a large increase of sodium flow from the serosal to the mucosal side. In addition, the distribution volume of ^{22}Na did not exceed the serosal extracellular space. These findings indicate that the site of the increase in sodium permeability is the paracellular pathway.

In the light of these results and interpretations it seems clear that the site of the permeability change in the presence of relatively low concentrations of surfactants is the junctional matrix. It seems improbable that holes which are created temporarily by increased cell shedding are the locus of increased permeability since such holes have never been detected in the concentration range in question (WANITSCHKE et al. 1977a; GOERG et al. 1980b, 1982). On the contrary, SPECHT (1977; Fig. 10) has demonstrated that, during the extrusion process, the epithelial lining remains intact. Thus, the only remaining sites of action are the intercellular junctions.

It has been argued that this interpretation is not tenable because, morphologically, lanthanum and ruthenium red, which are extracellular tracers, are excluded from the tight junctions even after exposure to ricinoleic acid in electron microscopic studies (CLINE et al. 1976; GAGINELLA et al. 1976). However, this argument

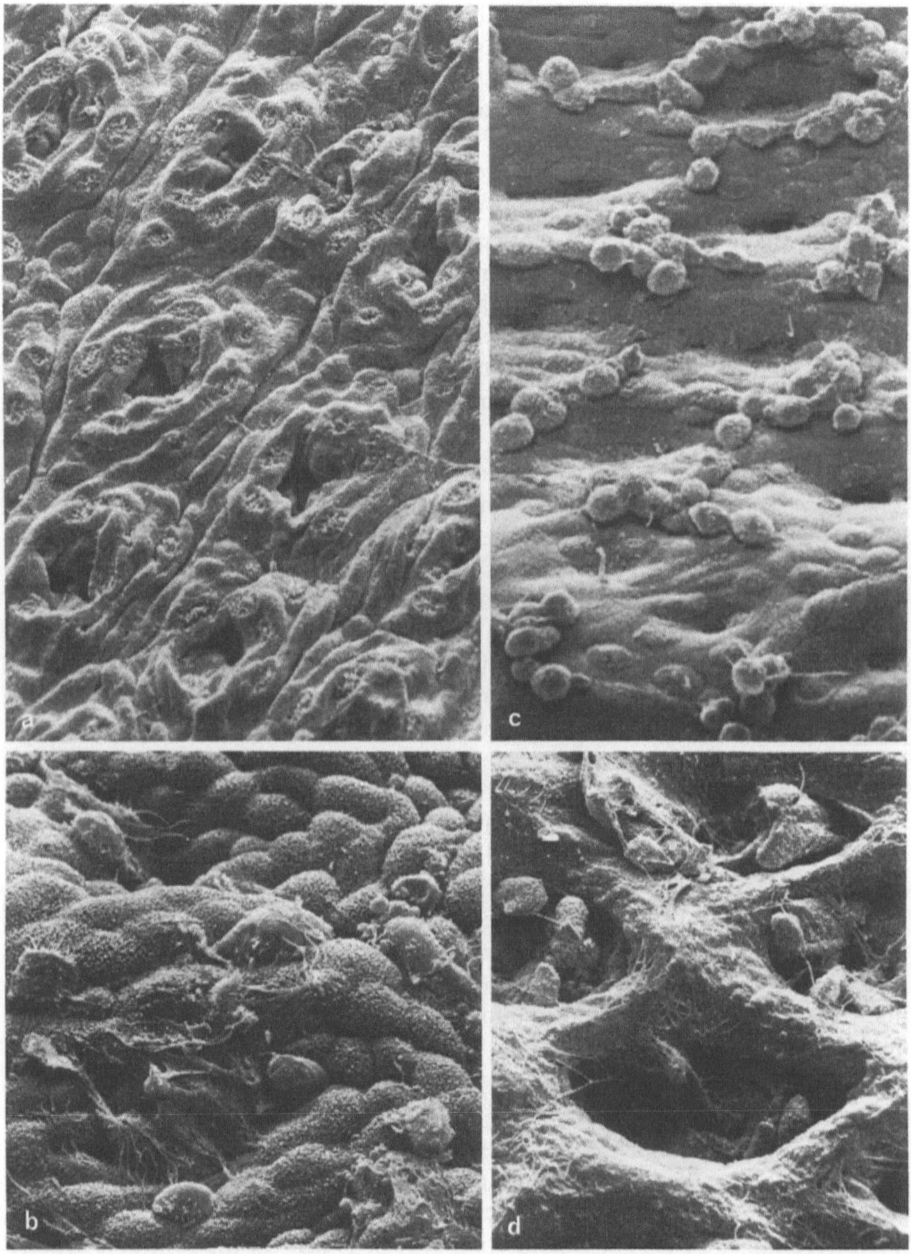

Fig. 5a–d. Effect of deoxycholate on perfused rat colon. Mucosal surface pictures obtained by scanning electron microscopy. **a** Control specimen. Perfusion with buffer solution for 60 min. 1,000:1. **b** Deoxycholate-treated colonic mucosa. Perfusion with 8 mmol/l for 90 min. 1,800:1. **c** Recovered mucosa. Treatment with 8 mmol/l deoxycholate for 120 min, followed by perfusion with buffer solution for 90 min. 900:1. **d** Colonic mucosa artificially denuded of surface epithelial cells. Treatment with 8 mmol/l deoxycholate for 90 min, followed by vigorous rinsing with buffer solution before tissue preparation for microscopy. 1,100:1. For further details see text and GOERG et al. (1982)

does not hold since it has been demonstrated that lanthanum permeability of the mucosal epithelium when using ionic lanthanum is increased by oxyphenisatin, as determined by morphological means and isotopic measurements, in spite of the fact that the junctional areas are not stained with the tracer under these conditions (NELL et al. 1977; SPECHT 1977). With regard to bile salts, FAGUNDES-NETO et al. (1981) have presented some morphological evidence that the passage of horseradish peroxidase across the junctions is increased by bile salts. Therefore, at present an increase of the permeability of the junctional area by surfactants remains at least a useful working hypothesis. Probably, the question can be answered definitely by freeze-fracture studies of the junctional area.

In summary, surfactants cause a broad range of functional and morphological changes, including mucosal epitheliolysis, depending on concentration. In a certain concentration range, in which both fluid movement and permeability are affected, they seem to increase the permeability of the paracellular pathway by rendering the tight junctions more leaky. The question of how the increase in paracellular permeability may be related to the secretagogue effect has been discussed fully in Sect. C.III.3.

IV. Conclusions

1. Inhibition of Na^+, K^+-ATPase

As discussed in Sect. D.III.1, results have been published about the influence of surfactants on Na^+, K^+-ATPase which are partially at variance. This is not surprising in view of the very different experimental conditions which have been employed. For instance, some experiments were done in vivo and others in vitro. In some reports, surfactants have been added to the intestinal preparation during a transport study and afterwards the enzyme activity was measured, whereas in other investigations the surfactants have been added to the incubation medium of the enzyme assay solely. Beyond that, it has to be recalled that it has been reported with preparations of Na^+, K^+-ATPase from other sources that, in principle, surfactants are to increase or decrease the activity of this enzyme, depending on concentration (e.g., CHAN 1967).

In some experiments, the activity of Na^+, K^+-ATPase was measured under in vivo conditions after addition of bile salts to the perfusion fluid (GRACEY et al. 1973; GUIRALDES et al. 1975; LAMABADUSURIYA et al. 1975). Regarding the interpretation of these results, the quantitative considerations outlined in Sect. C.IV.1 should be remembered. There seems to exist a concentration range where the inhibition of this enzyme seems not to play an important role since no change in mucosal distribution of sodium and potassium was found in the presence of maximal effect on fluid transfer (NELL et al. 1976b, WANITSCHKE et al. 1977a) as was the case when using ouabain (S. G. SCHULTZ et al. 1966). At present, it seems impossible to arrive at quantitative estimates of a possible contribution of the inhibition of Na^+, K^+-ATPase or other influences on ATP metabolism (see Sect. D.III.1) to the overall effect of surfactants on intestinal fluid and electrolyte transfer.

As mentioned for triarylmethane derivatives and related compounds, it has been reported repeatedly that surfactants are able to decrease the transmural potential difference in vivo and in vitro. This has been described for bile salts (SLADEN and HARRIES 1972; WINGATE 1974; GUIRALDES et al. 1975; LAMABADUSURIYA et al. 1975; WANITSCHKE and SOERGEL 1975; BINDER et al. 1978; CASPARY and MEYNE 1980; SUND et al. 1980; FARACK et al. 1982), for long-chain fatty acids (BRIGHT-ASARE and BINDER 1973; BINDER et al. 1978), for cetrimonium bromide (TAYLOR 1963; SUND et al. 1980), and for dioctylsulfosuccinate, dodecylsulfate, and Triton X-100 (SUND et al. 1983). This finding however, does not point to an obligatory inhibition of active transport processes. It may also be interpreted in connection with the increase of the paracellular permeability.

2. Stimulation of Active Secretion

As stated in Sect. D.III.2, secretion of fluid and electrolytes has been shown only three times under well-controlled in vitro conditions. The applicability of these results to in vivo conditions remains questionable since, for instance, in all three cases glucose-free solutions have been used. In the short-circuited mucosa in an Ussing chamber preparation in one instance controls did not absorb sodium and chloride (VOLPE and BINDER 1975) and in the other report ricinoleic acid caused only a short-lived effect (RACUSEN and BINDER 1979). In several other publications, especially with everted sacs, the authors were able to show as the maximal effect inhibition of absorption, but no secretion. This result was achieved with bile salts (WANITSCHKE and SOERGEL 1975; GULLIKSON et al. 1977; WANITSCHKE et al. 1977a), with long-chain fatty acids (YAU and MAKHLOUF 1974; GAGINELLA et al. 1975c; GULLIKSON et al. 1977), with the synthetic anionic surfactants dodecylsulfate and dioctylsodium sulfosuccinate (GULLIKSON et al. 1977), and with cetrimonium bromide (TAYLOR 1963).

Based on the assumption that surfactants may cause secretion of electrolytes in the same manner as is commonly accepted for the action of cholera enterotoxin, the content and metabolism of cyclic nucleotides in the intestinal mucosa in the presence of surfactants has been investigated to a considerable extent. However, the results are conflicting as outlined in Sect. D.III.2. The most convincing results in favor of such a hypothesis have been published by BINDER and co-workers. They showed a similar dose–response relationship and time course for the effects on mucosal cAMP levels and short-circuit current as an estimate of ion transport under in vitro conditions. However, there is some doubt whether the results of in vitro experiments of this type can be extrapolated to in vivo conditions in every respect. SCHWITER et al. (1975) presented some objections, e.g., that the effect of bile salts in an Ussing chamber in vitro was much larger when applied to the serosal rather than to the mucosal side, whereas in vivo bile salts are applied to the mucosal side. In particular, one of the main pillars of the cAMP hypothesis, namely the similarity and nonadditivity of the effects of surfactants and theophylline on intestinal electrolyte transport, has been challenged by SUND and OLSEN (1981). These authors showed that surfactants cause an increase in the equilibrium concentration of sodium, but that it never exceeds the plasma concentration. In contrast, theophylline augments the equilibrium concentration of sodium to values above 200 mmol/l. Thus, the effects of surfactants on sodium transfer are most plausibly explained by an increase in permeability of the paracellular pathway whereas theophylline obviously causes secretion by the transcellular pathway.

The striking differences of the results of SCHOENFIELD and co-workers (e.g., COYNE et al. 1976, 1977) on the one hand and of GAGINELLA et al. (1978) and SIMON et al. (1978, 1980) on the other have lacked a plausible interpretation till now. The experiments of SCHOENFIELD and co-workers, who showed that propranolol inhibits both deoxycholate-induced fluid secretion and stimulation of adenylate cyclase (CONLEY et al. 1976b; TAUB et al. 1977, 1978) are difficult to interpret. The experimental model of these authors was the tied-off loop of rabbit colon and they measured fluid transport and the activity of adenylate cyclase 5 h after the beginning of the experiment once only. Obviously, "...dose–response and time course studies are needed for a more definite explanation of our findings" (TAUB et al. 1978). Others were not able to reproduce their findings, even with maximally tolerated doses of propranolol (CHADWICK et al. 1976).

In conclusion, in view of the variance of results concerning the effect of surfactants on cyclic nucleotide metabolism, one should bear in mind the findings of ØYE and SUTHERLAND (1966) that deoxycholate may increase or decrease the activity of adenylate cyclase from avian erythrocytes, depending on the particular experimental conditions.

Regarding the inference from measurements of cyclic nucleotide metabolism that surfactants act like cholera enterotoxin on intestinal fluid and electrolyte transfer, the reader is referred to the discussion in Sect. C.III.2. In addition to the fundamental objections outlined there, characteristic differences have been shown between the effect of cholera enterotoxin and surfactants. FARACK and NELL (1979) and FARACK et al. (1979; 1983a, b) reported that it is possible to inhibit the effects of cholera enterotoxin on fluid transport in rat jejunum with chlorpromazine and the lactamide RMI 12330A (in the latter case probably by an inhibition of the stimulation of the activity of adenylate cyclase), whereas the secretagogue effect of deoxycholate was not influenced by these drugs.

Several authors have shown some evidence that the secretagogue effect of surfactants may be mediated by an increased prostaglandin synthesis (BEUBLER and JUAN 1979; RACHMILEWITZ and KARMELI 1979; RACHMILEWITZ et al. 1981). However, it is difficult to estimate the quantitative contribution of such an effect since there is only a partial correlation between the inhibitory effects of indometacin on prostaglandin synthesis and fluid secretion in the presence of several surfactants. The hypothesis of LUDERER et al. (1980) that ricinoleic acid may serve as substrate for prostaglandin synthesis cannot be extended to all surfactants because of their different chemical structure. It has been speculated that the effect of diluted bile on fluid transfer may include a cholinergic mechanism since it can be inhibited partially by atropine (KVIETYS et al. 1981). However, the results with atropine were equivocal. CAMILLERI et al. (1982) also reported an inhibition of bile salt-induced fluid secretion by atropine (and an enhancement by carbachol). TAKAGI and TAKEDA (1979) and KARLSTRÖM et al. (1983) did not find an effect for atropine.

Another mechanism of active secretion caused by surfactants has been proposed recently by MAENZ and FORSYTH (1982). These authors showed that deoxycholate and ricinoleate increased the permeability to Ca^{2+} of brush border vesicles of pig jejunum by acting as a calcium ionophore. They speculated that these substances may thus elevate intracellular Ca^{2+} which in turn may stimulate active secretion in the same manner as the Ca^{2+} ionophore A23187.

In summary, it has been shown that surfactants are able to induce electrolyte secretion and interfere with cyclic nucleotide metabolism under particular experimental conditions. The contribution of these effects to the action of surfactants on intestinal fluid transfer cannot be evaluated in a quantitative manner at present.

3. Increase in Permeability

It was shown in Sect. D.III.3 that the effects of surfactants on intestinal fluid transfer and permeability are similar with respect to dose–response relationship, time course, and reversibility. The increase in permeability is not inevitably correlated with mucosal epitheliolysis. This seems to be a question of concentration of the respective surfactant and the exposure time. Evidence has been presented that, at least in a certain concentration range, probably the paracellular pathway is mainly affected. Of course, with higher concentrations an increase in cell membrane permeability also occurs (e.g., ROSENBERG and HARDISON 1965). WINGATE (1974) observed that bile salts abolish the normal preference of lactate release of the intestinal mucosa to the serosal side under in vitro conditions. The author interpreted this result to mean an increase of the permeability of the luminal cell membrane of the enterocytes. However, it could also be caused by an increase of the permeability of the paracellular pathway.

BINDER and co-workers tried to show that permeability changes cannot be a determining parameter in influencing fluid transfer by surfactants. First, these authors demonstrated that, in the presence of amphotericin B, the permeability of the rat colon is enhanced, but fluid absorption is not only not inhibited, but even increased (BINDER et al. 1978). However, this result does not argue against the importance of the increase of permeability of paracellular pathways in inhibiting fluid absorption since, as far as is known at present, amphotericin B enhances the permeability of the luminal cell membrane (e.g., GRAF and GIEBISCH 1979), thereby increasing the amount of sodium available to the basolateral sodium pump. Thus, it may lead to quite contrary effects on fluid absorption if one applies a substance which acts preferentially on the permeability of the intercellular connections or the cell membrane. Second, these authors demonstrated that it is possible to inhibit fluid secretion caused either by deoxycholate or ricinoleic acid by treatment with propranolol in the rat colon in vivo. The concomitant increase in permeability, however, was not influenced. Thus, they concluded that changes in mucosal permeability are not primarily responsible for the effects of these surfactants on fluid transfer. However, one has to take into account that a treatment with high doses of propranolol (10 mg/kg over a 3-day period) may cause hemodynamic changes of the mucosal microcirculation. Thus, since a driving force is needed for fluid secretion in the presence of enhanced permeability, the loss of this driving force may modify fluid transport in the presence of surfactants without changing permeability itself. It should be remembered that other authors were unable to show an effect of propranolol on bile salt-induced fluid secretion (CHADWICK et al. 1976; GULLIKSON et al. 1981).

Therefore, taking those considerations and the data outlined in Sect. D.III.3 together, the authors of this chapter conclude that at present the change in permeability is the most plausible hypothesis in explaining the effect of surfactants on intestinal fluid transfer. The reversal of fluid absorption to secretion may occur according to the model described in Sect. C.III.3.

WINGATE et al. (1973 b) showed that, in the presence of bile salts, the correlation between water and sodium flow did not change, in spite of a large variation in net fluxes from absorption to secretion in human intestine in vivo. They interpreted their results to indicate that bulk flow on the intercellular pathway is influenced by bile salts. This conclusion is in agreement with the model presented.

However, as discussed in Sect. C.IV.3, the question remains open whether the postulated driving force, namely the subepithelial hydrostatic pressure is sufficient to account for the observed effects in vivo. Another point should also be mentioned. In explaining both the effects of triarylmethane derivatives and related compounds on the one hand and of surfactants or the other with the filtration model one should bear in mind that the influence of the latter substances, e.g., deoxycholate, on intestinal permeability is larger than the effect of the former by at least one order of magnitude whereas the effect on fluid transfer is similar (NELL et al. 1976 a, b). Thus, the relative contribution of the possible mechanisms discussed here could well be very different.

E. General Summary and Concluding Remarks

A variety of reasons have been given for the secretagogue effects of drugs: stimulation of adenylate cyclase, inhibition of Na^+, K^+-ATPase, and increase of epithelial permeability. Secretagogue drugs stimulate adenylate cyclase, but not under all conditions. A temporal and quantitative conformity between the stimulation of secretion and the activation of adenylate cyclase or the increase of cAMP does not exist in every case.

With respect to the potential role of Na^+, K^+-ATPase, similar statements can be made. No doubt, under certain conditions, secretagogues inhibit this enzyme which is responsible for several active intestinal transport processes. It is, however, also true that, in some cases, in spite of a remarkable inhibition not only does stimulation of secretion fail to take place, but no change of absorption can be observed. Furthermore, the reversal from absorption to secretion, e.g., as caused by triarylmethane derivatives and deoxycholate, is not associated with a change of Na/K distribution in the epithelial tissue as can be seen when ouabain is administered on concentrations which inhibit absorption.

With regard to the role of an increase of the epithelial permeability caused by secretagogues, a very good temporal and quantitative conformity, at least for deoxycholate and ricinoleate, exists between the development and restoration of the reversal from absorption to secretion on the one hand and the change of the epithelial permeability on the other. But also in this case it remains to be seen why no quantitative correlation exists between the degree of increase of epithelial permeability, as measured by test molecules of different size, and the degree of stimulation of the secretion when comparing oxyphenisatin with deoxycholate.

Finally, two very trivial conclusions can be drawn when surveying the great variety of the reported results: first that no single explanation fits with reality and second that it is difficult to distinguish between "caused by" and "associated with".

Acknowledgments. The authors work was supported by grants for the Sonderforschungsbereich 38, Membranforschung, DFG.

References

Adamic S, Bihler I (1967) Inhibition of intestinal sugar transport by phenolphthalein. Mol Pharmacol 3:188–194

Ammon HV, Phillips SF (1973) Inhibition of colonic water and electrolyte absorption by fatty acids in man. Gastroenterology 65:744–749

Ammon HV, Phillips SF (1974) Inhibition of ileal water absorption by intraluminal fatty acids. Influence of chain length, hydroxylation, and conjugation of fatty acids. J Clin Invest 53:205–210

Ammon HV, Thomas PJ, Phillips SF (1974) Effects of oleic and ricinoleic acid on net jejunal water and electrolyte movement. Perfusion studies in man. J Clin Invest 53:374–379

Ammon HV, Thomas PJ, Phillips SF (1977) Effects of long chain fatty acids on solute absorption. Perfusion studies in the human jejunum. Gut 18:805–813

Andreoli TE, Schafer JA (1976) Mass transport across cell membranes: the effects of antidiuretic hormone on water and solute flows in epithelia. Annu Rev Physiol 38:451–500

Banwell JG, Sherr H (1973) Effect of bacterial enterotoxins on the gastrointestinal tract. Gastroenterology 65:467–477

Bernier JJ, L'Hirondel C, Bretagne JF (1979) Cell loss under laxatives in human jejunum. Gastroenterology 76:1099

Beubler E, Juan H (1977) Is the effect of diphenolic laxatives mediated via release of prostaglandin E? Experientia 34:386–387

Beubler E, Juan H (1978) PGE-mediated laxative effect of diphenolic laxatives. Naunyn Schmiedebergs Arch Pharmacol 305:241–246

Beubler E, Juan H (1979) Effect of ricinoleic acid and other laxatives on net water flux and prostaglandin E release by the rat colon. J Pharm Pharmacol 31:681–685

Beubler E, Lembeck F (1979) Inhibition of stimulated fluid secretion in the rat small and large intestine by opiate agonists. Naunyn Schmiedebergs Arch Pharmacol 306:113–118

Binder HJ (1975) Bile salt stimulation of colonic cyclic AMP: mechanism of bile salt induced electrolyte secretion? In: Matern S, Hackenschmidt J, Back P, Gerok W (eds) Advances in bile acid research. Schattauer, Stuttgart, pp 425–428

Binder HJ (1977) Pharmacology of laxatives. Annu Rev Pharmacol Toxicol 17:355–367

Binder HJ (1979) Net fluid and electrolyte secretion: the pathophysiologic basis for diarrhea. In: Binder HJ (ed) Mechanisms of intestinal secretion. Liss, New York, pp 1–15

Binder HJ, Rawlins CL (1973) Effect of conjugated dihydroxy bile salts on electrolyte transport in rat colon. J Clin Invest 52:1460–1466

Binder HJ, Filburn C, Volpe BT (1975) Bile salt alteration cf colonic electrolyte transport: role of cyclic adenosine monophosphate. Gastroenterology 68:503–508

Binder HJ, Dobbins JW, Racusen LC, Whiting DS (1978) Effect of propranolol on ricinoleic acid- and deoxycholic acid-induced changes of intestinal electrolyte movement and mucosal permeability. Evidence against the importance of altered permeability in the production of fluid and electrolyte accumulation. Gastroenterology 75:668–673

Bolton JE, Field M (1977) Ca ionophore-stimulated ion secretion in rabbit ileal mucosa: relation to actions of cyclic 3'-5' AMP and carbamylcholine. J Membr Biol 35:159–173

Bright-Asare D, Binder HJ (1973) Stimulation of colonic secretion of water and electrolytes by hydroxy fatty acids. Gastroenterology 64:81–88

Briseid G, Briseid K, Bergersen B (1974) Studies on the increased absorption cf ouabain, phenolsulphonphthalein, and pralidoxime caused by sodium lauryl sulfate from single loop preparations in the rat. Naunyn Schmiedebergs Arch Pharmacol 282:45–47

Briseid G, Briseid K, Kirkevold K (1976) Increased intestinal absorption in the rat caused by sodium lauryl sulfate, and its possible relation to the cAMP system. Naunyn Schmiedebergs Arch Pharmacol 292:137–144

Briseid G, Øye I, Briseid K (1977) Increased level of cAMP in the rat intestinal mucosa caused by sodium lauryl sulfate. Naunyn Schmiedebergs Arch Pharmacol 298:263–266

Brown BD, Ammon HV (1981) Effect of glucose on jejunal water and solute absorption in the presence of glycodeoxycholate and oleate in man. Dig Dis Sci 26:710–717

Buglia G (1909) Hängt die Resorption von der Oberflächenspannung der resorbierten Flüssigkeit ab? Biochem Z 22:1–23

Burke V, Gracey M, Thomas J, Malajczuk A (1975) Inhibition of intestinal amino acid absorption by unconjugated bile salt in vivo. Aust NZ J Med 5:430–432

Burke V, Gracey M, Thomas J, Malajczuk A (1976) Inhibition of intestinal uptake of amino acids by unconjugated bile salt. AJEBAK 54:391–402

Camilleri M, Murphy R, Chadwick VS (1980) Dose-related effects of chenodeoxycholic acid in the rabbit colon. Dig Dis Sci 25:433–438

Camilleri M, Murphy R, Chadwick VS (1982) Pharmacological inhibition of chenodeoxychate-induced fluid and mucus secretion and mucosal injury in the rabbit colon. Dig Dis Sci 27:865–868

Carnot P, Glénard R (1913) De l'action du séné sur les mouvements de l'intestin perfusé. C R Soc Biol (Paris) 4:120–122

Caspary WF (1974) Inhibition of active hexose and amino acid transport by conjugated bile salts in rat ileum. Eur J Clin Invest 4:17–24

Caspary WF, Meyne K (1980) Effects of chenodeoxy- and ursodeoxycholic acid on absorption, secretion and permeability in rat colon and small intestine. Digestion 20:168–174

Chadwick VS, Gaginella TS, Debongnie JC, Carlson GL, Phillips SF, Hofmann AF (1976) Mucosal epitheliolysis: a mechanism for the increased colonic permeability induced by dihydroxy bile acids. Gut 17:816

Chadwick VS, Phillips SF, Hofmann AF (1977) Measurements of intestinal permeability using low molecular weight polyethylene glycols (PEG 400). II. Application to normal and abnormal permeability states in man and animals. Gastroenterology 73:247–251

Chadwick VS, Gaginella TS, Carlson GL, Debongnie JC, Phillips SF, Hofmann AF (1979) Effect of molecular structure on bile acid-induced alterations in absorptive function, permeability, and morphology in the perfused rabbit colon. J Lab Clin Med 94:661–674

Chan PC (1967) Reversible effect of sodium dodecyl sulfate on human erythrocyte membrane adenosine triphosphatase. Biochim Biophys Acta 135:53–60

Charney AN, Donowitz M (1978) Functional significance of intestinal Na^+-K^+-ATPase: in vivo ouabain inhibition. Am J Physiol 234: E629–E636

Chignell CF (1968) The effect of phenolphthalein and other purgative drugs on rat intestinal ($Na^+ + K^+$) adenosine triphosphatase. Biochem Pharmacol 17:1207–1212

Cline WS, Lorenzsonn V, Benz L, Bass P, Olsen WA (1976) The effects of sodium ricinoleate on small intestinal function and structure. J Clin Invest 58:380–390

Conley DR, Coyne MJ, Bonorris GG, Chung A, Schoenfield LJ (1976a) Bile acid stimulation of colonic adenylate cyclase and secretion in the rabbit. Dig Dis Sci 21:453–458

Conley D, Coyne M, Chung A, Bonorris G, Schoenfield L (1976b) Propranolol inhibits adenylate cyclase and secretion stimulated by deoxycholic acid in the rabbit colon. Gastroenterology 71:72–75

Corazza GR, Ciccarelli R, Caciagli F, Gasbarrini G (1979) Cyclic AMP and cyclic GMP levels in human colonic mucosa before and during chenodeoxycholic acid therapy. Gut 20:489–492

Coyne MJ, Bonorris GG, Chung A, Conley DR, Corke J, Schoenfield LJ (1976) Inhibition by propranolol of bile acid stimulation of rabbit colonic adenylate cyclase in vitro. Gastroenterology 71:68–71

Coyne MJ, Bonorris GG, Chung A, Conley D, Schoenfield LJ (1977) Propranolol inhibits bile acid and fatty acid stimulation of cyclic AMP in human colon. Gastroenterology 73:971–974

Dawson AM, Isselbacher KJ (1960) Studies on lipid metabolism in the small intestine with observation on the role of bile salts. J Clin Invest 39:730–740

Diamond JC (1979) Osmotic water flow in leaky epithelia. J Mebr Biol 51:195–216
Dobbins JW, Binder HJ (1976) Effect of bile salts and fatty acids on the colonic absorption of oxalate. Gastroenterology 70:1096–1100
Donowitz M, Binder HJ (1974) Dioctyl sodium sulfosuccinate stimulates large intestinal water and electrolyte secretion: mechanism of laxative action? Gastroenterology 66:A-184/838
Donowitz M, Binder HJ (1975) Effect of dioctyl sodium sulfosuccinate on colonic fluid and electrolyte movement. Gastroenterology 69:941–950
Donowitz M, Charney AN, Tai YH (1979) A comprehensive picture of serotonin-induced ileal secretion. In: Binder HJ (ed) Mechanisms of intestinal secretion. Liss, New York, pp 217–230
Dreesen M, Eyssen H, Lemli J (1981) The metabolism of sennosides A and B by the intestinal microflora: in vitro and in vivo studies on the rat and the mouse. J Pharm Pharmacol 33:679–681
Duffy PA, Granger DN, Taylor AE (1978) Intestinal secretion induced by volume expansion in the dog. Gastroenterology 75:413–418
Ewe K (1977) Influence of diphenolic laxatives on water and electrolyte permeation in man. In: Kramer M, Lauterbach F (eds) Intestinal permeation. Excerpta Medica, Amsterdam, pp 420–426
Ewe K (1980a) Effect of rhein on the transport of electrolytes, water and carbohydrates in the human jejunum and colon. Pharmacology 20 [Suppl 1]:27–35
Ewe K (1980b) The physiological basis of laxative action. Pharmacology 20 [Suppl 1]:2–20
Ewe K, Hölker B (1974) Einfluß eines diphenolischen Laxans (Bisacodyl) auf den Wasser- und Elektrolyttransport im menschlichen Colon. Klin Wochenschr 52:827–833
Fagundes-Neto V, Teichberg S, Bayne MA, Morton B, Lifshitz F (1981) Bile salt-enhanced rat jejunal absorption of a macromolecular tracer. Lab Invest 44:18–26
Fairclough PD, Feest TG, Chadwick VS, Clark ML (1977) Effect of sodium chenodeoxycholate on oxalate absorption from the excluded human colon- a mechanism for "enteric" hyperoxaluria. Gut 18:240–244
Farack UM, Nell G (1979) The influence of an adenylcyclase inhibitor on the cholera-toxin-, desoxycholic acid- and bisacodyl-induced intestinal secretion in the rat. Naunyn Schmiedebergs Arch Pharmacol 308 [Suppl]:R27
Farack UM, Nell G, Rummel W (1979) Der Einfluß von Chlorpromazin auf die durch Choleratoxin und Desoxycholsäure induzierte Flüssigkeitssekretion am Rattenjejunum. Z Gastroenterol 17:664–665
Farack UM, Nell G, Lueg O (1981) Untersuchungen zum Mechanismus der Kaliumsekretion am Rattencolon unter dem Einfluß von Natriumdesoxycholat. Verh Dtsch Ges Inn Med 87:875–877
Farack UM, Nell G, Lueg O, Rummel W (1982) Independence of the activation of mucus and potassium secretion on the inhibition of sodium and water absorption by deoxycholate in rat colon. Naunyn Schmiedebergs Arch Pharmacol 321:336–340
Farack UM, Nell G, Loeschke K, Rummel W (1983a) Is the secretagogue effect of deoxycholic acid mediated by the adenylate cyclase-cAMP system. Digestion 28:170–175
Farack UM, Nell G, Rummel W (1983b) Differentiation of secretagogue drugs by chlorpromazine in rat intestine in vivo. Naunyn-Schmiedeberg's Arch Pharmacol 324:70–74
Faust RG (1964) Effects of bile salts, sodium deoxycholate, strophantin-G and metabolic inhibitors on the absorption of D-glucose by the rat jejunum, in vitro. J Cell Comp Physiol 63:55–64
Faust RG, Wu SML (1965a) The action of bile salts on fluid and glucose movement by rat and hamster jejunum, in vitro. J Cell Comp Physiol 65:435–448
Faust RG, Wu SML (1965b) The effect of bile salts on tissue ATP levels of everted sacs of rat and hamster ileum. J Cell Physiol 65:449–451
Faust RG, Wu SML (1965c) The effect of bile salts on oxygen consumption, oxidative phosphorylation, and ATP-ase activity of mucosal homogenate from rat jejunum and ileum. J Cell Physiol 67:149–158

Feldman S, Reinhard M (1976) Interaction of sodium alkyl sulfates with everted rat small intestinal membrane. J Pharm Sci 65:1460–1462

Feldman S, Salvino M, Gibaldi M (1970) Physiologic surfaceactive agents and drug absorption. VII. Effect of sodium deoxycholate on phenol red absorption in the rat. J Pharm Sci 59:705–707

Feldman DS, Rabinovitch S, Feldman EB (1971) Effects of bile salts and detergents on ion transport of absorbing ileum. J Clin Invest 50:29a

Feldman S, Reinhard M, Willson C (1973) Effect of sodium taurodeoxycholate on biological membranes: release of phosphorus, phospholipid, and protein from everted rat small intestine. J Pharm Sci 62:1961–1964

Feldman DS, Rabinovitch S, Feldman EB (1975) Surfactants and bioelectric properties of rat jejunum. Dig Dis Sci 20:866–870

Feldman EB, Watt R, Feldman DS (1977) Conjugated dihydroxy bile salt inhibition of glucose influx in rat jejunum in vitro. Dig Dis Sci 22:415–418

Ferard G, Galluser M, Sall I, Pousse A (1980) Effect of sodium deoxycholate on intestinal glucose absorption and $(Na^{+}K^{+})$-ATPase in the rat. Enzyme 25:387–393

Ferlemann G, Vogt W (1965) Entacetylierung und Resorption von phenolischen Laxantien. Naunyn Schmiedebergs Arch Pharmacol 250:479–487

Field M, Sheerin HE, Henderson A, Smith PL (1975) Catecholamine effects on cyclic AMP levels and ion secretion in rabbit ileal mucosa. Am J Physiol 229:86–92

Forsyth GW, Hamilton DL, Scoot A, Goertz KE, Kapitany RA (1979) Failure to reverse choleratoxin induced intestinal secretion by agents which decrease mucosal cAMP. Can J Physiol Pharmacol 57:1004–1010

Forth W, Rummel W (1967) Resorptionshemmung, eine physiologische Wirkung von Gallensäuren? In: Hoffmann G, Delaloye B (eds) Radioisotope in der Gastroenterologie. Schattauer, Stuttgart, pp 141–146

Forth W, Rummel W (1975) Activation and inhibition of intestinal absorption by drugs. In: Forth W, Rummel W (eds) Gastrointestinal absorption of drugs. Pergamon, Oxford, pp 171–244 (International encyclopedia of pharmacology and therapeutics, sec 39B: pharmacology of intestinal absorption, vol 1)

Forth W, Baldauf J, Rummel W (1963) Ein Beitrag zur Klärung des Wirkungsmechanismus einiger Laxantien. Naunyn Schmiedebergs Arch Pharmacol 246:91

Forth W, Rummel W, Baldauf J (1966a) Wasser- und Elektrolytbewegung am Dünn- und Dickdarm unter dem Einfluß von Laxantien, ein Beitrag zur Klärung ihres Wirkungsmechanismus. Naunyn Schmiedebergs Arch Pharmacol 254:18–32

Forth W, Rummel W, Glasner H (1966b) Zur resorptionshemmenden Wirkung von Gallensäuren. Naunyn Schmiedebergs Arch Pharmacol 254:364–380

Forth W, Nell G, Rummel W, Andres H (1972) The hydragogue and laxative effect of the sulfuric acid ester and the free diphenol of 4,4′-dihydroxydiphenyl(pyridyl-2)-methane. Naunyn Schmiedebergs Arch Pharmacol 274:46–53

Frizzell RA (1977a) Active chloride secretion by rabbit colon: Calcium dependent stimulation by ionophore A23187. J Membr Biol 35:175–187

Frizzell RA (1977b) Interaction between cyclic AMP and cell calcium in the stimulation of electrolyte secretion by mammalian colon. In: Bonfils et al. (eds) First International Symposium on Hormonal Receptors in Digestive Tract Physiology. INSERM Symposium No. 3. Biomedical Press, Elsevier/North Holland, pp 455–468

Frizzell RA, Schultz SG (1970) Effect of bile salts on transport across brush border of rabbit ileum. Biochim Biophys Acta 211:589–592

Fry RJM, Staffeldt E (1964) Effect of diet containing sodium deoxycholate on the intestinal mucosa of the mouse. Nature 203:1396–1398

Gadacz TR, Gaginella TS, Phillips SF (1976) Inhibition of water absorption by ricinoleic acid. Evidence against hormonal mediation of the effect. Dig Dis Sci 21:859–862

Gaginella TS, Bass P (1978) Laxatives: an update on mechanism of action. Life Sci 23:1001–1010

Gaginella TS, Phillips SF (1975) Ricinoleic acid: current view of an ancient oil. Am J Dig Dis 20:1171–1177

Gaginella TS, Phillips SF (1976) Ricinoleic acid (castor oil) alters surface structure. A scanning electron microscopic study. Mayo Clin Proc 51:6–12

Gaginella TS, O'Dorisio TM (1979) Vasoactive intestinal polypeptide: neuromodulator of intestinal secretion? In: Binder HJ (ed) Mechanisms of intestinal secretion. Liss, New York, pp 231–247

Gaginella TS, Stewart JJ, Gullikson GW, Olsen WA, Bass P (1975a) Inhibition of small intestinal mucosa and smooth muscle cell function by ricinoleic acid and other surfactants. Life Sci 16:1595–1606

Gaginella TS, Bass P, Olsen W, Shug A (1975b) Fatty acid inhibition of water absorption and energy production in the hamster jejunum. FEBS Lett 53:347–350

Gaginella TS, Stewart JJ, Olsen WA, Bass P (1975c) Actions of ricinoleic acid and structurally related fatty acids on the gastrointestinal tract. II. Effects on water and electrolyte absorption in vitro. J Pharmacol Exp Ther 195:355–361

Gaginella TS, Lewis JC, Phillips SF (1976) Ricinoleic acid effects on rabbit intestine. An ultrastructural study. Mayo Clin Proc 51:569–573

Gaginella TS, Lewis JC, Phillips SF (1977a) Rabbit ileal mucosa exposed to fatty acids, bile acids and other secretagogues. Dig Dis Sci 22:781–790

Gaginella TS, Chadwick VS, Debongnie JC, Lewis JC, Phillips SF (1977b) Perfusion of rabbit colon with ricinoleic acid: dose related mucosal injury, fluid secretion, and increased permeability. Gastroenterology 73:95–101

Gaginella TS, Haddad AC, Go VLW, Phillips SF (1977c) Cytotoxicity of ricinoleic acid (castor oil) and other intestinal secretagogues on isolated intestinal epithelial cells. J Pharmacol Exp Ther 201:259–266

Gaginella TS, Phillips SF, Dozois RR, Go VLW (1978) Stimulation of adenylate cyclase in homogenates of isolated intestinal epithelial cells from hamster. Gastroenterology 74:11–15

Gibaldi M, Feldman S (1970) Mechanisms of surfactant effects on drug absorption. J Pharm Sci 59:579–589

Gill DM (1977) Mechanism of action of cholera toxin. In: Greengard P, Robinson GA (eds) Advances in cyclic nucleotide research. Raven, New York, pp 86–118

Goerg KJ (1979) Relationship between fluid production, mucosal permeability and changes of the mucosal morphology in the rat colon under the influence of deoxycholate and dioctylsulfosuccinate. Gastroenterol Clin Biol 3:169–170

Goerg KJ, Nell G, Specht W (1978) Correlation between the ^{51}CrEDTA clearance and the secretion of fluid and electrolytes under the influence of deoxycholate in the rat colon. Naunyn Schmiedebergs Arch Pharmacol 302 [Suppl]:R1

Goerg KJ, Wanitschke R, Schulz L (1980a) Scanning electron microscopic study of the effect of rhein on the surface morphology of the rat colonic mucosa. Pharmacology 20 [Suppl 1]:36–42

Goerg KJ, Gross M, Nell G, Rummel W, Schulz L (1980b) Comparative study of the effect of cholera toxin and sodium deoxycholate on the paracellular permeability and on net fluid and electrolyte transfer in the rat colon. Naunyn Schmiedebergs Arch Pharmacol 312:91–97

Goerg KJ, Specht W, Nell G, Rummel W, Schulz L (1982) Effect of deoxycholate on the perfused rat colon. Scanning and transmission electron microscopic study of the morphological alterations occurring during the secretagogue action of deoxycholate. Digestion 25:145–154

Goerg KJ, Nell G, Rummel W (1983) Effect of deoxycholate on the perfused rat colon. Concentration dependence of the effect on net fluid and electrolyte transfer and the correlation with paracellular permeability. Digestion 26:105–113

Gordon SJ, Kinsey MD, Magen JS, Joseph RE, Kowlessar OD (1979) Structure of bile acids associated with secretion in the rat cecum. Gastroenterology 77:38–44

Gracey M, Burke V, Oshin A (1971a) Influence of bile salts on intestinal sugar transport in vivo. Scand J Gastroenterol 6:273–276

Gracey M, Burke V, Oshin A (1971b) Reversible inhibition of intestinal active sugar transport by deconjugated bile salt in vitro. Biochim Biophys Acta 225:308–314

Gracey M, Burke V, Storrie M, Oshin A (1972) Dissociation of intestinal active sugar transport from ($Na^+ + K^+$) ATPase activity. Clin Chim Acta 36:555–560

Gracey M, Papadimitriou J, Burke V, Thomas J, Bower G (1973) Effects on small intestinal function and structure by feeding a conjugated bile salt. Gut 14:519–528

Graf J, Giebisch G (1979) Intracellular sodium activity and sodium transport in Necturus gall bladder epithelium. J Membr Biol 47:327–355

Guiraldes E, Lamabadusuriya SP, Oyesiku JEJ, Whitfield AE, Harries JT (1975) A comparative study on the effects of different bile salts on mucosal ATPase and transport in the rat jejunum in vivo. Biochim Biophys Acta 389:495–505

Gullikson GW, Cline WS, Lorenzsonn V, Benz L, Olsen WA, Bass P (1977) Effects of anionic surfactants on hamster small intestinal membrane structure and function: relationship to surface activity. Gastroenterology 73:501–511

Gullikson GW, Dajani EZ, Bianchi RG (1981) Inhibition of intestinal secretion in the dog: a new approach for the management of diarrheal states. J Pharmacol Exp Ther 219:591–597

Hadorn B, Steiner N, Sumida C, Peters TJ (1971) Intestinal enterokinase. Mechanisms of its "secretion" into the lumen of the small intestine. Lancet I:165–166

Hafkenscheid JCM (1977) Influence of bile acids on the ($Na^+ + K^+$) activated and Mg^{2+} -activated ATPase of rat colon. Pfluegers Arch 369:203–206

Hajjar JJ, Khuri RN, Bikhazi AB (1975) Effect of bile salts on amino acid transport by rabbit intestine. Am J Physiol 229:518–523

Hajjar JJ, Murphy DM, Scheig RL (1979) Mechanism of inhibition of alanine absorption by Na ricinoleate. Am J Physiol 236:E534–E538

Hakim AA, Lifson N (1969) Effects of pressure on water and solute transport by dog intestinal mucosa in vitro. Am J Physiol 216:276–284

Hand DW, Sanford PA, Smyth DH (1966) Polyphenolic compounds and intestinal transfer. Nature 209:618

Harries JT, Sladen GE (1972) The effects of different bile salts on the absorption of fluid, electrolytes, and monosaccharides in the small intestine of the rat in vivo. Gut 13:596–603

Hart SL, McColl I (1967) The effect of purgative drugs on the intestinal absorption of glucose. J Pharm Pharmacol 19:70–71

Hart SL, McColl I (1968) The effect of the laxative oxyphenisatin on the intestinal absorption of glucose in rat and man. Br J Pharmacol Chemother 32:683–686

Hepner GW, Hofmann AF (1973) Different effects of free and conjugated bile acids and their keto derivatives on (Na^+, K^+)-stimulated and Mg^{2+} ATPase of rat intestinal mucosa. Biochim Biophys Acta 291:237–245

Heymann P (1927a) Schwer resorbierbare Salze. In: Heffter A, Heubner W (eds) Handbuch der experimentellen Pharmakologie, vol 3/1. Springer, Berlin, pp 40–81

Heymann P (1927b) Zuckerarten und Verwandtes. In: Heffter A, Heubner W (eds) Handbuch der experimentellen Pharmakologie, vol 3/1. Springer, Berlin, pp 82–132

Hillestad B, Sund RB, Buajordet M (1982) Intestinal handling of bisacodyl and picosulphate by everted sacs of the rat jejunum and stripped colon. Acta Pharmacol Toxicol 51:388–394

Im WB, Misch DW, Powell DW, Faust RG (1980) Phenolphthalein- and harmaline-induced disturbances in the transport functions of isolated brush border and basolateral membrane vesicles from rat jejunum and kidney cortex. Biochem Pharmacol 29:2307–2317

Jauch R, Hammer R, Busch U, Kopitar Z, Ohnuma N, Niki T (1977) Pharmakokinetik und Metabolismus von Na-Picosulfat bei der Ratte. Arzneimittelforsch 27:1045–1050

Jauch R, Hankwitz R, Beschke K, Pelzer H (1975) Bis-(p-hydroxyphenyl)-pyridil-2-methane: The common laxative principle of bisacodyl and sodium picosulphate. Arzneimittelforsch 25:1796–1800

Kakemi K, Sezaki H, Konishi R, Kimura T, Murakami M (1970) Effect of bile salts on the gastrointestinal absorption of drugs. Chem Pharm Bull (Tokyo) 18:275–280

Karlström L, Cassuto J, Jodal M, Lundgren O (1983) The importance of the enteric nervous system for the bile-salt-induced secretion in the small intestine of rat. Scand J Gastroenterol 18:117–123

Kelly DG, Kerlin P, Sarr MG, Phillips SF (1981) Ricinoleic acid causes secretion in autotransplated (extrinsically denervated) canine jenunum. Dig Dis Sci 26:966–970

Kobashi K, Nishimura T, Kusaka M, Hattori M, Namba T (1980) Metabolism of sennosides by human intestinal bacteria. Planta medica 40:225–236

Konder H, Dennhardt R, Haberich FJ (1979) Die Wirkung unkonjugierter Gallensäuren auf die Elektrolyt- und Wasserabsorption im proximalen Jejunum. Res Exp Med (Berl) 175:37–49

Konder H, Dennhardt R, Haberich FJ (1981) Die Wirkung von Desoxycholat auf die Elektrolyt- und Wasserabsorption im terminalen Ileum. Res Exp Med (Berl) 178:141–150

Krag E, Phillips SF (1974) Effect of free and conjugated bile acids on net water, electrolyte, and glucose movement in the perfused human ileum. J Lab Clin Med 83:947–955

Kvietys PR, Wilborn W, Granger DN (1981) Effect of atropine on bile-oleic acid-induced alterations in dog jejunal hemodynamics, oxygenation, and net transmucosal water movement. Gastroenterology 80:31–38

Lack L, Weiner IM (1966) Intestinal bile salt transport: structure activity relationships and other properties. Am J Physiol 210:1142–1152

Lamabadusuriya SP, Guiraldes E, Harries JT (1975) Influence of mixtures of taurocholate, fatty acids, and monolein or the toxic effects of deoxycholate in rat jejunum in vivo. Gastroenterology 69:463–469

Lauder-Brunton T (1874) On the action of purgative medicines. Practitioner 12:342–350

Lee JS (1979) Lymph capillary pressure of rat intestinal villi during fluid absorption. Am J Physiol 237:E301–E307

Lemli J, Lemmens L (1980) Metabolism of sennosides and rhein in the rat. Pharmacology 20 [Suppl 1]:50–57

Lemmens L, Borja E (1976) The influence of dihydroxyanthracene derivatives on water and electrolyte movement in rat colon. J Pharm Pharmacol 28:498–501

Leng-Peschlow E (1980) Inhibition of intestinal water and electrolyte absorption by senna derivatives in rats. J Pharm Pharmacol 32:330–335

Lewin MR, El Masri SH, Clark CG (1979) Effects of bile acids on mucus secretion in the dog colon. Eur Surg Res 11:392–398

Lifson N (1979) Fluid secretion and hydrostatic pressure relationships in the small intestine. In: Binder HJ (ed) Mechanisms of intestinal secretion. Liss, New York, pp 249–261

Lish PM, Weikel JH (1959) Influence of surfactants on absorption from the colon. Toxicol Appl Pharmacol 1:501–504

Low-Beer TS, Schneider RE, Dobbins WO (1970) Morphological changes of the small-intestinal mucosa of guinea pig and hamster following incubation in vitro and perfusion in vivo with unconjugated bile salts. Gut 11:486–492

Luderer JR, Demers LM, Nomides CT, Hayes AH (1980) Mechanism of action of castor oil: a biochemical link to the prostaglandins. In: Samuelson B, Ramwell PW, Paoletti R (eds) Advances in prostaglandin and thromboxane research, vol 8. Raven, New York, pp 1633–1635

Maenz DD, Forsyth GW (1982) Ricinoleate and deoxycholate are calcium ionophores in jejunal brush border vesicles. J Membr Biol 70:125–133

Magnus R (1924a) Allgemeines über Abführmittel. Anthrachinonderivate, Chrysarobin, Phenolphthalein. In: Heffter A (ed) Handbuch der experimentellen Pharmakologie, vol 2/2. Springer, Berlin, pp 1592–1644

Magnus R (1924b) Drastische Abführmittel. Allgemeines. Koloquinten (Colocynthin). Elaterin. Podophyllin. Podophyllotoxin. Convolvulin, Jalapin (Scammonin), Turpathin, Ipomoein. Gummi-Gutti, Cambogiasäure, Euphorbium. Lärchenschwamm, Agaricinsäure. In: Heffter A (ed) Handbuch der experimentellen Pharmakologie, vol 2/2. Springer, Berlin, pp 1645–1676

Meisel JL, Bergman D, Gracey D, Saunders DR, Rubin CE (1977) Human rectal mucosa: proctoscopic and morphological changes caused by laxatives. Gastroenterology 72:1274–1279

Mekhjian HS, Phillips SF (1970) Perfusion of the canine colon with unconjugated bile acids. Gastroenterology 59:120–129

Mekhjian HS, Phillips SF, Hofmann AF (1971) Colonic secretion of water and electrolytes induced by bile acids: perfusion studies in man. J Clin Invest 50:1569–1577

Mertens RB, Mayer SE, Wheeler HO (1976) Effect of conjugated bile acids on cyclic AMP levels in rabbit ileal mucosa. Gastroenterology 70:919

Meyer-Betz F, Gebhardt T (1912) Röntgenuntersuchungen über den Einfluß der Abführmittel auf die Darmbewegungen am gesunden Menschen. Münch Med Wochschr 59:1793–1797

Mitjavila MT, Mitjavila S, Derache R (1973) Mesures du métabolisme et de la lyse de cellules épithéliales isolées de l'intestin du rat incubées en présence de divers détergents. Toxicology 1:237–248

Mitjavila MT, Mitjavila S, Gas N, Derache R (1975) Influence of various surface-active agents on the activity of several enzymes in the brush-border of enterocytes. Toxicol Appl Pharmacol 34:72–82

Moffatt RE, Kramer LL, Lerner D, Jones R (1975) Studies on dioctyl sodium sulfosuccinate toxicity: clinical, gross and microscopic pathology in the horse and guinea pig. Can J Comp Med 39:434–441

Moore JD, Zatzmann ML, Overack DE (1971) Effects of synthetic surfactants on intestinal permeability. Proc Soc Exp Biol Med 137:1135–1139

Moreto M, Planas JM, Naftalin RJ (1981) Effects of secretagogues on the K^+ permeability of mucosal and serosal borders of rabbit colonic mucosa. Biochim Biophys Acta 648:215–224

Mortillaro N, Taylor AE (1976) Interaction of capillary and tissue forces in the cat small intestine. Circ Res 39:348–358

Nadai T, Kondo R, Tatematsu A, Sezaki H (1972) Drug-induced histological changes and its consequences on the permeability of the small intestinal mucosa. I. EDTA, tetracycline and sodium laurylsulfate. Chem Pharm Bull (Tokyo) 20:1139–1144

Nadai T, Kume M, Tatematsu A, Sezaki H (1975) Drug induced histological changes and its consequences on the permeability of the small intestinal mucosa. Chem Pharm Bull (Tokyo) 23:543–551

Naito SI, Shioda K, Sawada M, Niki S, Awataguchi M, Mizutani M (1976) Hydrolysis of bis(p-hydroxyphenyl) pyridyl-2-nathane disulphate. I. Presence of arylsulphatase and laxative activity. Chem Pharm Bull 24:1943–1947

Nataf C, Desmazures C, Bernier JJ (1979) Mesure de l'entéropathie exsudative provoquée par les laxatifs. Gastroenterol Clin Biol 3:594

Nataf C, Desmazures C, Giraudeaux V, Bernier JJ (1981) Etude des pertes intestinales de proteines provoquées par les laxatifs chez l'homme normal. Gastroenterol Clin Biol 5:187–192

Nell G, Forth W, Rummel W, Wanitschke R (1972) Abolition of the apparent Na^+ impermeability of the colon mucosa by deoxycholate. In: Back P, Gerok W (eds) Bile acids in human diseases. Schattauer, Stuttgart, pp 263–267

Nell G, Overhoff H, Forth W, Kulenkampff H, Specht W, Rummel W (1973 a) Influx and efflux of sodium in jejunal and colonic segments of rats under the influence of oxyphenisatin. Naunyn Schmiedebergs Arch Pharmacol 277:53–60

Nell G, Overhoff H, Forth W, Rummel W (1973 b) The influence of water gradients and oxyphenisatin on the net transfer of sodium and water in the rat colon. Naunyn Schmiedebergs Arch Pharmacol 277:363–372

Nell G, Forth W, Freiberger T, Rummel W, Wanitschke R (1975) Characterization of permeability changes by test molecules in rat colonic mucosa under the influence of sodium deoxycholate. In: Matern S, Hackenschmidt J, Back P, Gerok W (eds) Advances in bile acid research. Schattauer, Stuttgart, pp 419–424

Nell G, Forth W, Rummel W, Wanitschke R (1976a) Pathway of sodium moving from blood to intestinal lumen under the influence of oxyphenisatin and deoxycholate. Naunyn Schmiedebergs Arch Pharmacol 293:31–37
Nell G, Forth W, Rummel W, Wanitschke R (1976b) Pathway of sodium moving from blood to intestinal lumen under influence of oxyphenisatin and deoxycholate. In: Robinson JWL (ed) Intestinal ion transport. MTP Press, Lancaster, pp 189–196
Nell G, Rummel W, Wanitschke R (1977) Characterization of the paracellular pathway by test molecules in colonic mucosa. In: Kramer M, Lauterbach F (eds) Intestinal permeation. Excerpta Medica, Amsterdam, pp 413–418
Nell G, Goerg KJ, Rummel W (1981) Effect of bile acids on the permeability of the colon. In: Demling L, Soergel KH, Ruppin H, Domschke W (eds) Diarrhea. Thieme, Stuttgart
Nellans HN, Schultz SG (1976) Relations among transepithelial sodium transport, potassium exchange, and cell volume in rabbit ileum. J Gen Physiol 68:441–463
Nissim JA (1960a) Reduction of intestinal absorption by a synthetic chemical. Nature 185:222–224
Nissim JA (1960b) Reduction of the intestinal absorption of glucose, methionine and sodium butyrate by the cation trimethylhexadecylammonium. Nature 187:308–310
Nissim JA (1961) Enhancement of inhibition of intestinal absorption by cetrimide-phloridzin combination. Nature 191:37–39
Nissim JA (1962) Enhancement of the intestinal absorption of glucose by small doses of cetrimide and sodium lauryl sulphate. Nature 196:1106–1107
Nissim JA (1964) Mechanism of intestinal absorption: the concept of a spectrum of intracellular plasma. Nature 204:148–151
Nordström C (1972) Enzymic release of enteropepdidase from isolated rat duodenal brush borders. Biochim Biophys Acta 268:711–718
Nunn AS, Baker RA, Searle GW (1963) Inhibition of intestinal glucose absorption by bile salt. Life Sci 2:646–650
Oddsson E, Rask-Madsen J, Krag E (1977a) Effect of glycochenodeoxycholic acid on unidirectional transepithelial fluxes of electrolytes in the perfused human ileum. Scand J Gastroenterol 12:199–204
Oddson E, Rask-Madsen J, Krag E (1977b) Transmural ionic fluxes and electrical potential difference in the human jejunum during perfusion with a dihydroxy bile acid. Scand J Gastroenterol 12:453–456
Øye I, Sutherland EW (1966) The effect of epinephrine and other agents on adenyl cyclase in cell membrane of avian erythrocytes. Biochim Biophys Acta 127:347–354
Parkinson TM, Olson JA (1963) Inhibitory effects of bile acids on the uptake metabolism and transport of water soluble substances in the small intestine of the rat. Life Sci 2:393–398
Parkinson TM, Olson JA (1964) Inhibitory effects of bile acids on adenosine triphosphatase, oxygen consumption, and the transport and diffusion of water soluble substances in the small intestine of the rat. Life Sci 3:107–112
Parsons DS, Paterson CR (1965) Fluid and solute transport across rat colonic mucosa. Q J Exp Physiol 50:220–231
Peters HC (1942) The influence of bile salts on active intestinal absorption of chloride. Am J Physiol 136:340–345
Phillips SF, Gaginella TS (1977) Intestinal secretion as a mechanism in diarrheal disease. In: Glass GBJ (ed) Progress in gastroenterology, vol 3. Grune and Stratton, New York, pp 481–518
Phillips SF, Gaginella TS (1979) Effects of fatty acids and bile acids on intestinal water and electrolyte transport. In: Binder HJ (ed) Mechanisms of intestinal secretion. Liss, New York, pp 287–294
Phillips RA, Love AHG, Mitchell TG, Neptune EM Jr (1965) Cathartics and the sodium pump. Nature 206:1367–1368
Pope JL, Parkinson TM, Olson JM (1966) Action of bile salts on the metabolism and transport of water soluble nutrients by perfused rat jejunum in vitro. Biochim Biophys Acta 130:218–232

Powell DW, Tapper EJ (1979) Intestinal ion transport: cholinergic-adrenergic interactions. In: Binder HJ (ed) Mechanisms of intestinal secretion. Liss, New York, pp 175–192
Powell DW, Lawrence BA, Morris SM, Etheridge DR (1980) Effect of phenolphthalein on in vitro rabbit ileal electrolyte transport. Gastroenterology 78:454–463
Rachmilewitz D, Karmeli F (1979) Effect of bisacodyl and dioctyl sodium sulfosuccinate on rat intestinal prostaglandin E_2 content/Na-K-ATPase and adenyl cyclase activities. Gastroenterology 76:1221
Rachmilewitz D, Karmeli F, Okon E (1980) Effects of bisacodyl on cAMP and prostaglandin E_2 contents, (Na+K) ATPase, adenyl cyclase, and phosphodiesterase activities of rat intestine. Dig Dis Sci 25:602–608
Rachmilewitz D, Karmeli F, Okon E (1981) Effect of dioctyl sodium sulfosuccinate on cyclic AMP and prostaglandin E_2 contents, and Na, K, -ATPase, adenylate cyclase and phosphodiesterase activities in rat intestine. Isr J Med Sci 17:28–35
Racusen LC, Binder HJ (1979) Ricinoleic acid stimulation of active anion secretion in colonic mucosa of the rat. J Clin Invest 63:743–749
Rampton DS, Breuer NF, Vaja SG, Sladen GE, Dowling RH (1981) Role of prostaglandines in bile salt-induced changes in rat colonic structure and function. Clin Sci 61:641–648
Read NW, Krejs GJ, Jones VE, Fordtran JS (1979) Effect of ouabain on Na, K-ATPase and electrolyte transport in the dog ileum in vivo. Gut 20:356–365
Reuss L, Weinman SA, Grady TP (1980) Intracellular K^+-activity and its relation to basolateral ion transport in Necturus gall bladder epithelium. J Gen Physiol 76:33–52
Reynell PC, Spray GH (1958) Chemical gastroenteritis in the rat. Gastroenterology 34:867–873
Rosenberg IH, Hardison WG (1965) Mechanism of bile salt inhibition of intestinal transport. Fed Proc 24:375
Roy CC, Dubois RS, Phillipon F (1970) Inhibition by bile salts of the jejunal transport of 3-*O*-methyl glucose. Nature 225:1055–1056
Rummel W (1976) Biologische Membranfunktionen in Gesundheit und Krankheit, Wirkungen von Gallensäuren und Laxantien auf den mucosalen Transfer. Bull Schweiz Akad Med Wiss 32:233–250
Rummel W, Nell G, Wanitschke R (1975) Action mechanisms of antiabsorptive and hydragogue drugs. In: Csaky TZ (ed) Intestinal absorption and malabsorption. Raven, New York, pp 209–227
Russel RI, Allan JG, Gerskowitch VP, Cochran KM (1973) The effect of conjugated and unconjugated bile acids on water and electrolyte absorption in the human jejunum. Clin Sci Mol Med 45:301–311
Saunders DR (1975) Regional differences in the effect of bile salts on absorption by rat small intestine in vivo. J Physiol (Lond) 250:373–383
Saunders DR, Hedges JR, Sillery J, Esther L, Matsumura K, Rubin CE (1975a) Morphological and functional effects of bile salts on rat colon. Gastroenterology 68:1236–1245
Saunders DR, Sillery J, Rachmilewitz D (1975b) Effect of dioctyl sodium sulfosuccinate on structure and function of rodent and human intestine. Gastroenterology 69:380–386
Saunders DR, Sillery J, Rachmilewitz D, Rubin CE, Tytgat GN (1977) Effect of bisacodyl on the structure and function of rodent and human intestine. Gastroenterology 72:849–856
Saunders DR, Sillery J, Surawica C, Tytgat GN (1978) Effect of phenolphthalein on the function and structure of rodent and human intestine. Dig Dis Sci 23:909–913
Scarpello JHB, Cary BA, Sladen GE (1978) Effects of ileol and caecal resection on the colon of the rat. Clin Sci Mol Med 54:241–249
Schiffl H, Loeschke K (1977) Induction of Na-K-ATPase in plasma membranes of rat cecum mucosa by diet: time course and kinetics. Pfluegers Arch 372:83–90
Schmid W (1952) Zum Wirkungsmechanismus diätetischer und medikamentöser Darmmittel. Arzneimittel-Forsch 2:6–20
Schreiner J, Nell G, Loeschke K (1980) Effect of diphenolic laxatives on Na^+-K^+-activated ATPase and cyclic nucleotide content of rat colon mucosa in vivo. Naunyn Schmiedebergs Arch Pharmacol 313:249–255

Schultz OE, Fedders S, Holm WD, Schulze V (1974) Zusammenhänge zwischen Konstitution und laxativer Wirkung bei Triarylmethanderivaten. Arzneimittel-Forsch 24:1933–1941

Schultz SG (1977) Sodium-coupled solute transport by small intestine: a status report. Am J Physiol 233:E249–E254

Schultz SG, Frizzell RA, Nellans HN (1974) Ion transport by mammalian small intestine. Annu Rev Physiol 36:51–91

Schultz SG, Fuisz RE, Curran PF (1966) Amino acid and sugar transport in rabbit ileum. J Gen Physiol 49:849–866

Schwiter EJ, Hepner GW, Rose RC (1975) Effect of bile acids on electrical properties of rat colon: evaluation of an in vitro model for secretion. Gut 16:477–481

Sheerin HE, Field M (1977) Ileal mucosal cyclic AMP and Cl secretion: serosal vs. mucosal addition of cholera toxin. Am J Physiol 232:E210–E215

Simon B, Kather H (1980) Interaction of laxatives with enzymes of cyclic AMP metabolism from human colonic mucosa. Eur J Clin Invest 10:231–234

Simon B, Cyzgan P, Stiehl A, Kather H (1978) Human colonic adenylate cyclase: effects of bile acis. Eur J Clin Invest 8:321–323

Sladen GE, Harries JT (1972) Studies on the effects of unconjugated dihydroxy bile salts on rat small intestinal function in vivo. Biochim Biophys Acta 288:443–456

Specht W (1977) Morphology of the intestinal wall. Its mucosa membrane under normal and experimental conditions. In: Kramer M, Lauterbach F (eds) Intestinal permeation. Excerpta Medica, Amsterdam, pp 4–40

Stewart JJ, Gaginella TS, Olsen WA, Bass P (1975) Inhibitory actions of laxatives on motility and water and electrolyte transport in the gastrointestinal tract. J Pharmacol Exp Ther 192:458–467

Straub W, Triendl E (1934) Über die Wirkung des Senna-Infuses auf den Dickdarm der Katze. Naunyn Schmiedebergs Arch Pharmacol 175:528–535

Sugimura F (1974a) Studies of intestinal absorption under pathological conditions. I. Light microscopic studies of intestinal damage caused by sodium lauryl sulfate. Nihon Univ J Med 16:25–37

Sugimura F (1974b) Studies of intestinal absorption under pathological conditions. II. Electron microscopic studies of intestinal damage caused by sodium lauryl sulfate. Nihon Univ J Med 16:39–50

Sund RB (1975) The effect of dodecylsulphate upon net sodium and water transport from tied jejunal loops in anaesthetized rats. Acta Pharmacol Toxicol (Copenh) 37:282–296

Sund RB (1978) Glucose and cation transport in rat jejunum, ileum and colon in vivo: control experiments, and effect of cationic surfactant. Acta Pharmacol Toxicol (Copenh) 42:117–124

Sund RB, Hillestad B (1978) Diphenolic laxatives and intestinal cAMP: experiments with oxyphenisatin in the rat in vivo. Acta Pharmacol Toxicol (Copenh) 42:321–322

Sund RB, Hillestad B (1981) Studies on hydragogue drugs: effect of surfactants on cAMP levels in the rat jejunal mucosa in short time experiments in vivo. Acta Pharmacol Toxicol (Copenh) 49:110–115

Sund RB, Hillestad B (1982) Uptake, conjugation and transport of some laxative diphenoles by everted sacs of the rat jejunum and stripped colon. Acta Pharmacol Toxicol (Copenh) 51:377–387

Sund RB, Jacobsen DN (1978) In vivo reversibility of the jejunal glucose and cation-transport alteration caused by intraluminal surfactants in the rat. Acta Pharmacol Toxicol (Copenh) 43:339–345

Sund RB, Matheson I (1978) Glucose and cation transport in rat jejunum, ileum and colon in vivo: effects of anionic and nonionic surfactants, and of desoxycholate. Acta Pharmacol Toxicol (Copenh) 42:253–258

Sund RB, Olsen G (1981) Net sodium and glucose transport in the jejunum, ileum and colon of anaesthetized rats in response to intraluminal theophylline and anionic surfactants. Acta Pharmacol Toxicol (Copenh) 49:65–71

Sund RB, Hol L, Storbråten A (1979) Studies in the rat on the absorption, biliary excretion, laxative action and interference with intestinal transport of some oxyphenisatin derivatives. Acta Pharmacol Toxicol (Copenh) 44:251–259

Sund RB, Nell G, Andres H, Rummel W (1980) Deoxycholic acid and synthetic surfactants: effect on net sodium and water transport, ^{51}Cr EDTA permeability and bioelectrical parameters in the isolated colonic mucosa of the rat. Gastroenterol Biol Clin 5:124

Sund RB, Songedal K, Harestad T, Salvesen B (1981) Enterohepatic circulation, urinary excretion and laxative action of some bisacodyl derivatives after intragastric administration in the rat. Acta Pharmacol Toxicol (Copenh) 48:73–80

Sund RB, Roland M, Kristiansen S, Salvesen B (1982) Biliary excretion of bisacodyl and picosulphate in man: studies in gallstone patients after biliary tract surgery. Acta Pharmacol Toxicol (Copenh) 50:50–57

Takagi T, Takeda M (1979) Chenodeoxycholic acid-induced diarrhea in rats: effects of atropine and codeine. Arch Int Pharmacodyn Ther 240:328–339

Taub M, Bonorris G, Chung A, Coyne MJ, Schoenfield LJ (1977) Effect of propranolol on bile acid- and cholera enterotoxin-stimulated cAMP and secretion in rabbit intestine. Gastroenterology 72:101–105

Taub M, Coyne MJ, Bonorris GG, Chung A, Coyne B, Schoenfield LJ (1978) Inhibition by propranolol of bile acid- and PGE_1-stimulated cAMP and intestinal secretion. Am J Gastroenterol 70:129–135

Taylor CB (1963) The effect of cetyltrimethylammonium bromide and some related compounds on transport and on metabolism in the intestine of the rat in vitro. J Physiol (Lond) 165:199–218

Teem MV, Phillips SF (1972) Perfusion of the hamster jejunum with conjugated and unconjugated bile acids: inhibition of water absorption and effects on morphology. Gastroenterology 62:261–267

Tomkin GH, Love AHG (1972) Investigation of glucose transport and ^{57}Co Vitamin B_{12} uptake using the everted sac technique with histological examination of the sacs after suspension in bile salts and indole. Digestion 6:129–138

van Os FHL (1976) Anthraquinone derivatives in vegetable laxatives. Pharmacology 14 [Suppl 1]:7–17

van Os CH, Wiedner G, Wright EM (1979) Volume flows across gall bladder epithelium induced by small hydrostatic and osmotic gradients. J Membr Biol 49:1–20

Vasseur M, Ferard G, Pousse A (1978) Rat intestinal brush border enzymes release by deoxycholate in vivo. Pfluegers Arch 373:133–138

Vasseur M, Pousse A, Ferard G (1980) The relationship between surface tension and release of rat jejunal brush border membrane hydrolases induced by sodium deoxycholate. Reprod Nutr Develop 20 (5A):1461–1466

Verhaeren E (1980) Mitochondrial uncoupling activity as a possible base for a laxative and antipsoriatic effect. Pharmacology 20:43–49

Verhaeren EHC, Dreesen MJ, Lemli JA (1981) Influence of 1,8-dihydroxyanthraquinone and loperamide on the paracellular permeability across colonic mucosa. J Pharm Pharmacol 33:526–528

Vogt W, Schmidt G, Dakhil T (1965) Die Bedeutung der Glucuronidbildung und -spaltung für das Schicksal von Dihydroxy-diphenylpyridylmethan. Naunyn Schmiedebergs Arch Pharmacol 250:488–495

Volpe BT, Binder HJ (1975) Bile salt alteration of ion transport across jejunal mucosa. Biochim Biophys Acta 394:597–604

Wall MJ, Baker RD (1974) Intestinal transmural electrical properties: effects of conjugated bile salt in vitro. Am J Physiol 227:499–506

Wanitschke R (1980a) Influence of rhein on electrolyte and water transfer in the isolated rat colonic mucosa. Pharmacology 20 [Suppl 1]:21–26

Wanitschke R (1980b) Intestinal filtration as a consequence of increased mucosal hydraulic permeability. Klin Wochenschr 58:267–278

Wanitschke R, Ammon HV (1978) Effects of dihydroxy bile acids and hydroxy fatty acids on the absorption of oleic acid in the human jejunum. J Clin Invest 61:178–186

Wanitschke R, Soergel KH (1975) Effect of deoxycholate and oxyphenisatin on isolated rat colonic mucosa. Clin Res 23:520A

Wanitschke R, Nell G, Rummel W, Specht W (1977a) Transfer of sodium and water through isolated rat colonic mucosa under the influence of deoxycholate and oxyphenisatin. Naunyn Schmiedebergs Arch Pharmacol 297:185–190

Wanitschke R, Nell G, Rummel W (1977b) Influence of hydrostatic pressure gradients on net transfer of sodium and water across isolated rat colonic mucosa. Naunyn Schmiedebergs Arch Pharmacol 297:191–194

Weist FR, Birkner H (1974) Zur Pharmakokinetik von Bisacodyl (Dulcolax) nach oraler und rektaler Applikation. Therapiewoche 24:2281–2283

Whitmore DA, Brookes LG, Wheeler KP (1979) Relative effects of different surfactants on intestinal absorption and the release of proteins and phospholipids from the tissue. J Pharm Pharmacol 31:277–283

Wingate DL (1974) The effect of glycin-conjugated bile acids on net transport and potential difference across isolated rat jejunum and ileum. J Physiol (Lond) 242:189–207

Wingate DL, Phillips SF, Hofmann AF (1973a) Effect of glycine-conjugated bile acids with and without lecithin on water and glucose absorption in perfused human jejunum. J Clin Invest 52:1230–1236

Wingate DL, Krag E, Mekhjian HS, Phillips SF (1973b) Relationship between ion and water movement in the human jejunum, ileum and colon during perfusion with bile acids. Clin Sci Mol Med 45:593–606

Winne D, Görig H (1982) Appearance of ^{14}C-polyethylene glycol 4000 in intestinal venous blood: influence of osmolarity and laxatives, effect on net water flux determination. Naunyn Schmiedebergs Arch Pharmacol 321:149–156

Wright EM, Mircheff AK, Hanna SD, Harms V, van Os CH, Walling MW, Sachs G (1979) The dark side of the intestinal epithelium: the isolation and characterisation of basolateral membranes. In: Binder HJ (ed) Mechanisms of intestinal secretion. Liss, New York, pp 117–130

Yau WM, Makhlouf GM (1974) Different effects of hormonal peptides and cyclic adenosine 3′,5′-monophosphate on colonic transport in vitro. Gastroenterology 67:662–667

Yonezawa M (1977) Basic studies of the intestinal absorption. I. Changes in the rabbit intestinal mucosa after exposure to various surfactants. Nihon Univ J Med 19:125–141

Zatzmann ML, Moore JD (1968) Time to achieve steady state luminal glucose concentration during intestinal lavage. J Appl Physiol 25:95–97

CHAPTER 30

Use and Abuse of Cathartics

K. J. MORIARTY and A. M. DAWSON

A. Introduction

Much of the confusion regarding these drugs surrounds the use of a number of different terms for what are essentially the same type of drug. The terms laxative (*Latin laxare*, to loosen) and aperient (*Latin aperire*, to open) describe their action with reasonable accuracy (JONES and GODDING 1972). However, cathartic (*Greek katharsis*, cleansing) and purgative (*Latin purgare*, to purify) have more emotive overtones and more accurately reflect Victorian concepts of the necessity for regular ingestion to ensure "inner cleanliness" (ANONYMOUS 1962) and maintain good health, the dire consequences of "intestinal autointoxication" resulting if ingestion ceased and constipation occurred (ALVAREZ 1924; DONALDSON 1922). Indeed, a prelude to modern chemical warfare was the embargo placed on the export of cathartics from Britain to Europe during the Napoleonic Wars (S. SMITH, cited in ANONYMOUS 1973c). The resulting constipation in the French troops, deprived of their regular purge, is thought to have greatly contributed to their ultimate defeat.

The Sydenham Society recognised three types of purgative (TRAVELL 1954). A laxative produced a formed movement, a cathartic a semiformed one and a drastic caused watery diarrhoea. More recently, a laxative has been defined as a drug that promotes the excretion of a soft, formed stool and a cathartic as one producing a more fluid stool (BRUCKSTEIN 1978; FINGL 1980). However the terms are often used interchangeably and obviously it is mainly a question of degree, in that a laxative has a cathartic action at higher dosage. No distinction will be attempted in this chapter, cathartic and laxative being used interchangeably.

Cathartics are widely used in western society. In 1973, it is estimated that more than 130 million dollars were spent on cathartics in the United States (BINDER and DONOWITZ 1975), while in the same year the cost of laxative prescribing to the National Health Service in the United Kingdom was £7 million. In 1971, 1% of all prescriptions issued in the United States were for laxatives (ANONYMOUS 1973 b). Of even greater concern, however, is the uncontrolled over-the-counter purchase of laxatives, which is widespread on both sides of the Atlantic.

The purpose of this chapter is to define indications for the appropriate use of these drugs and to emphasise the problems resulting from inappropriate use. Before doing this, it is helpful to discuss what is understood by a normal stool habit. Wider recognition of the range of normal by both the lay public and the medical profession may help to reduce the disturbingly high prevalence of laxative ingestion, particularly among healthy people (CONNELL et al. 1965; THOMPSON and HEATON 1980).

There is considerable geographical and racial variation in bowel habit. For instance, the African stool is four times as large and passed twice as quickly through the gut as its western counterpart (BURKITT et al. 1972). Over 98% of an English population passed between three bowel movements per day and three per week (CONNELL et al. 1965). In this study, 16% of a normal industrial population and 29% of patients without known organic disease who were attending their general practitioner took laxatives. Of the laxative takers, only 20% of these actually considered themselves to be constipated. In all, 4% of the industrial population and 16% of those seen in general practice felt they suffered from constipation. By this, some meant that they passed hard stools, others that the bowel movements were infrequent, while with others the meaning of constipation bore no relationship to stool consistency or bowel frequency. On the other hand, there was a correlation between increasing bowel frequency and the subject's opinion that their stools were "loose".

For what is largely a subjective sensation, there is no universally accepted definition of constipation. One eminent author suggested that it was that condition in which the residue of food ingested in one day was not excreted within the next 48 h (HURST 1937). However, this definition makes no allowance for the elderly, in whom a transit time of about 72 h is normal (BROCKLEHURST and KAHN 1969).

B. Classification

The current classification will doubtless be revised when the mechanism of action of different cathartics is better understood (BINDER and DONOWITZ 1975). At present they are divided into bulking agents, which include dietary fibre and the bulk laxatives, contact cathartics, stool softeners, osmotic laxatives and per rectum evacuants.

I. Bulking Agents

Dietary fibre is defined as the portion of plant food which is not digested in the small intestine. It comprises cellulose, lignin, gums, pectins, hemicelluloses, and other polysaccharides. There are four other types of hydrophilic bulking agent, namely wheat bran, the cellulose derivatives, the mucilagenous gums and the mucilagenous seeds and seed coats. The water-holding properties of these agents enable them to increase stool bulk and they are fully discussed in Chap. 28.

Occasionally, bulk laxatives may cause intestinal obstruction if there is existing partial obstruction of the bowel (SOUTER 1965). Obstruction to the oesophageal outlet may also occur if too little fluid is taken with these preparations (GOLDMAN 1937; VOINCHET and MOUCHET 1974). Flatulence and griping abdominal pains may result if too high a dose is used.

A by-product of the milling of wheat, bran contains about 20% fibre comprising lignin and celluloses. It may be taken as a cereal, All Bran, Prewett's miller's bran or as muffins. Large doses are required for efficacy. In one study, 12 g daily (4 tablespoonsful) of miller's bran was used as a dietary supplement in diverticular disease (PAINTER et al. 1972) to achieve symptomatic improvement.

The cellulose derivatives include methylcellulose and sodium carboxymethylcellulose. The former is available as tablets, an oral solution or a syrup and the latter as a powder. Examples of mucilagenous gums are karaya gum (sterculia) and Indian tragacanth. Sterculia gum is obtained from *Sterculia urens* and other species of *Sterculia*. It comprises a polysaccharide containing acetic acid. The commercial preparation, Normacol, is available as flavoured granules. Immediate hypersensitivity reactions to karaya gum with asthma, rhinitis, urticaria, and eczema are described (FINGL 1980).

The mucilagenous seeds and seed coats are derivatives of the Indian flowering plant genus, *Plantago*, which has been used in Hindu medicine for over 3,000 years (BLOCK 1947). The main constituents are psyllium and ispaghula husk, commercial preparations including Fybogel, Isogel, and Metamucil. These drugs are well tolerated (CASS and WOLF 1952), particularly if taken with fruit juice. Dextrose is used to disperse psyllium. Adverse reactions include renal pigmentation following long-term ingestion of whole psyllium seeds (FISHER 1938) and asthma (BUSSE and SCHOENWETTER 1975).

II. Contact Cathartics

It has been suggested that the description "contact" is preferable to "irritant" or "stimulant", in that these laxatives have an effect on both water and electrolyte transport and motility in the intestine, rather than purely on motility (FINGL 1980). Included in this group are the diphenylmethane derivatives, the anthraquinones, castor oil and dioctylsodium sulphosuccinate.

1. Diphenylmethane Derivatives

The members of this group are phenolphthalein, bisacodyl, and oxyphenisatin. They are best taken at night so as to produce a bowel movement the following morning. There are two kinds of phenolphthalein, white and yellow. The latter is the more potent, contains more impurities and is included in a number of over-the-counter preparations, often in combination with other laxatives. The former is better standardised. The laxative action of phenolphthalein was initially recognised when VON VÁMOSSY (1900) was commissioned by the Hungarian government to investigate the artificial colouring of wine with phenolphthalein. From the evidence available, it seems most likely that there is virtually complete intestinal absorption of a dose of the highly lipid-soluble phenolphthalein. This has an enterohepatic circulation, being conjugated by the liver to the glucuronide, about 15% of which is excreted by the kidney (FANTUS and DYNIEWICZ 1938), the rest in the bile. Because phenolphthalein is ineffective as a laxative in patients with obstructive jaundice (STEIGMANN et al. 1938), it has been suggested that the glucuronide is responsible for the laxative action. However, in a recent study on rat ileum and colon, it was shown that whereas unconjugated phenolphthalein reduced water absorption, the conjugated form actually enhanced it (SHARAIHA and GRAHAM 1981). The authors hypothesised that the highly water-soluble glucuronide is not absorbed by the small intestine, but is deconjugated by colonic bacteria to free phenolphthalein which then causes water and electrolyte secretion in the colon and hence laxation. Adverse effects include an allergic skin reaction, a fixed drug eruption and a Stevens–Johnson syndrome, all thought to be due to hypersensitivity (ABRAMOWITZ 1950). A potentially fatal encephalitis, also due to a hypersensitivity reaction has been described following phenolphthalein ingestion (KENDALL 1954).

Bisacodyl is available both as an oral and rectal preparation. The tablet has an enteric coating (Dulcolax) to prevent neutralisation by gastric acid. Like phenolphthalein, it is metabolised by the liver to the glucuronide and has an enterohepatic circulation (CUMMINGS 1974). As with phenolphthalein, it is the unconjugated form which is the active agent (THOMPSON 1979). Suppositories are usually effective within 1 h, but may produce a burning sensation in the rectum or proctitis if used chronically (MEISEL et al. 1977).

Oxyphenisatin is no longer available in the United States, having been withdrawn after reports of jaundice, chronic active hepatitis and cirrhosis following its use (ANONYMOUS 1972; DELCHIER et al. 1979; GOLDSTEIN et al. 1973; MACHARDY and BALART 1970; NAESS 1970; PEARSON et al. 1971; REYNOLDS et al. 1970, 1971). These side effects have been noticed particularly when oxyphenisatin has been used in combination with the detergent, dioctylsodium sulphosuccinate, which enhances its absorption.

2. Anthraquinones

These include the senna glycosides, senna, cascara, aloes, rhubarb, frangula, and the free anthraquinone, danthron. The primary glycosides of rhein dianthrone, namely 10,10-bis(9,10-dihydro-1,8-dihydroxy-9-oxoanthracene-3-carboxylic acid), are the main active constituents of senna pod and leaf. Standardised preparations of senna such as Senokot have been produced (FAIRBAIRN and MICHAELS 1950; LOU 1949) and validated in humans (BROWNE et al. 1957). The senna glycosides are poorly absorbed from the small intestine, unlike danthron (FAIRBAIRN and MOSS 1970; SCHMID 1952). First used by American Indians, the active ingredients of cascara are cascarosides A, B, C, and D. A and B are glycosides of barbaloin [10(1)-deoxyglycosyl aloe-emodin anthrone], whereas C and D are glycosides of chrysaloin [10(1)-deoxyglucosyl chrysophanol anthrone]. Senna is more potent than cascara, in that the former produces a bowel action within 6 h of ingestion, whereas the latter is effective after about 8 h (DUNCAN 1957). They are both more potent than phenolphthalein (HUBACHER and DOERNBERG 1964).

Danthron (1,8-dihydroxyanthraquinone) is a breakdown product of the senna glycosides and is much less effective than senna or cascara. Its laxative action is usually observed 6–8 h after ingestion. It is absorbed from the intestine and detoxified by the liver, but has been incriminated in causing hepatotoxicity when used in combination with dioctylsodium sulphosuccinate (TOLMAN et al. 1976).

It has been suggested that the anthraquinones may be excreted in breast milk and thus produce laxation in suckling infants (ILLINGWORTH 1953). However, there is no objective evidence for this view (FINGL 1980; JONES and GODDING 1972). They are known to impart a pink or orange colour to urine and to cause melanosis coli (WITTOESCH et al. 1958).

3. Castor Oil

Castor oil is derived from the seeds of *Ricinus communis* and contains the triglycerides of ricinoleic acid. This is hydrolysed to the active ingredient, ricinoleic acid and also glycerol by intestinal lipases. It is a rapidly acting cathartic, producing a semiformed to liquid stool usually within 2–3 h of ingestion. Because of its rapid action, castor oil has been used to rid the gut of worms after a course of anthelminthics and also in the treatment of overdose of fat-soluble drugs.

4. Dioctylsodium Sulphosuccinate

Dioctylsodium sulphosuccinate is an anionic detergent whose ability to soften the stool within 24–72 h of administration helps to prevent straining at stool in patients with cardiovascular disease or who have undergone anorectal or abdominal surgery. It is generally well tolerated, but nausea and abdominal cramps may occur. Following its administration to humans, disruption of the gastric mucosal barrier (COCHRAN et al. 1977) and increased cell loss from the jejunum (BRETAGNE et al. 1981) have been described, but whether these phenomena are of practical importance is doubtful. Certainly, the effect of dioctylsodium sulphosuccinate on water and electrolyte transport in human jejunum has been shown to be completely reversible (MORIARTY et al. 1982). It also has a cytotoxic effect on cultured liver cells (DUJOVNE and SHOEMAN 1972). If used in combination with other laxatives, it may facilitate their absorption as well as being absorbed itself. Thus, it has been incriminated in the hepatotoxicity associated with oxyphenisatin (GOLDSTEIN et al. 1973; NAESS 1970) and danthron (TOLMAN et al. 1976).

It is available as a tablet, syrup or solution. The usual adult dosage is 50–500 mg daily. Administration with fruit juice or milk improves the bitter taste. It has been shown to be effective in a dosage of 300 mg daily in the treatment of constipation in the elderly (HYLAND and FORAN 1968).

III. Stool Softeners

Liquid paraffin is a mixture of hydrocarbons derived from petroleum. Its use as a stool softener depends on its ability to penetrate the stool and render it soft. However, a number of serious adverse effects have been recognised following its administration. Its action as a lipid solvent may interfere with the absorption of the fat-soluble vitamins (JAVERT and MACRI 1941) and it has been incriminated as a carcinogen (BOYD and DOLL 1954). Recurrent inhalation of small amounts gave rise to lipid pneumonia (BUECKNER and STRUG 1956; FORBES and BRADLEY 1958; FREIMAN et al. 1940; LAUGHLEN 1925; SALM and HUGHES 1970; ZURROW and SERGAY 1966). This complication is potentially fatal especially in the elderly and in childhood (ELSTON 1966), although it has been successfully treated with prednisolone (AYVAZIAN et al. 1967). Leakage of oil through the anal sphincter may cause incontinence (JONES and GODDING 1972), pruritus ani and delayed healing of perianal wounds. Liquid paraffin alone is now obsolete, but in combination with magnesium hydroxide as Mil-Par, it is a popular proprietary remedy.

IV. Osmotic Laxatives

Nonabsorbed solute retains fluid in the gut lumen. This is propelled into the lumen of the colon, where it softens stool and stimulates intestinal contraction. Such solutes are the saline cathartics, mannitol, and lactulose. The saline cathartics are the sulphate and phosphate salts of sodium and magnesium. Magnesium sulphate is available as the well-known Epsom salts. It has been suggested that an additional action could be mediated through the magnesium-induced release of cholecystokinin (Harvey and Read 1973a, b), which increases intestinal motility and water and electrolyte secretion. Magnesium-containing laxatives are effective within 3 h of ingestion, but should be used with caution in patients with uraemia, because about 20% of magnesium administered is absorbed (Godding 1975a). Sodium-containing laxatives may exacerbate or precipitate congestive cardiac failure. If excessive dosage is used, these laxatives are particularly likely to cause dehydration.

Mannitol is a nonabsorbed hexahydric alcohol and has been used in large doses for the preparation of the bowel for colorectal surgery and colonoscopy. However, a fatal colonic explosion during colonoscopic polypectomy has been reported after bowel preparation with mannitol (Bigard et al. 1979), for colonic bacteria degrade mannitol to hydrogen and methane, which are potentially explosive in the presence of oxygen (Taylor et al. 1981).

Lactulose (4-*O*-β-D-galactopyranosyl-D-fructose) is a synthetic disaccharide, whose use in the treatment of portosystemic encephalopathy is described in Chap. 28. It is available as a syrup (Duphalac). Nausea, vomiting, cramping abdominal pain and flatulence have been described following its use. Overdosage may lead to dehydration (Kaupke et al. 1977) and water and electrolyte disturbances.

V. Per Rectum Evacuants

These include both suppositories and a variety of enemas which work by a combination of a direct physical and a contact effect on the large intestine, leading to increased colonic motility and water and electrolyte secretion. In simple constipation, bisacodyl or glycerine suppositories may suffice. When the patient is more impacted, a large volume soap and water enema is often effective. If used judiciously, it is well tolerated, but occasionally serious complications including hypovolaemic shock (Pike et al. 1971), hyperkalaemia due to absorption from potassium-containing soap solution (Young and Brooke 1968) and anaphylactic shock (D. Smith 1967) may occur. Olive oil, arachis oil or dioctylsodium sulphosuccinate are used in retention enemas to soften the stool and are especially useful if faecal impaction occurs after perineal surgery or barium enema. Hypertonic phosphate (sodium phosphate–diphosphate) is available as a small volume disposable pack and is especially useful when rapid evacuation of the rectum and sigmoid colon is required, as in sigmoidoscopy or fibre sigmoidoscopy. However, hypocalcaemic tetany, sometimes fatal, due to phosphate absorption has been reported following the use of these preparations (Honig and Holtzapple 1975; McConnell 1971; Swerdlow et al. 1974). Damage to the rectal mucosa is described following enema use (Meisel et al. 1977), as have lacerations and perforations of the anorectal region (LARGE and MUKHEIBER 1956; PIETSCH et al. 1977; ROWLAND and ROGERS 1959; TURELL 1960).

C. Indications for Use

The use of laxatives in the preparation of the bowel for colorectal surgery, radiological and endoscopic procedures has been mentioned, as has their role in the treatment of hepatic encephalopathy, drug poisoning and helminthic infections. They are also effective in the treatment of constipation, diverticular disease, the irritable bowel syndrome, haemorrhoids, anal fissure, acute diarrhoea and the management of ileostomy and colostomy effluent (ANONYMOUS 1973a; FINGL 1980; GODDING 1975b). A discussion of the role of dietary fibre and bulk laxatives in the treatment of diverticular disease and anorectal disorders is included in Chap. 28. Laxatives such as magnesium sulphate may prove helpful in right-sided faecal stasis associated with left-sided proctocolitis (JALAN et al. 1970; LENNARD-JONES et al. 1962). When prescribed, the smallest effective dose of cathartic should be used. If the bowels become regular, every effort should be made gradually to reduce this dosage. Although highlighted many years ago (HURST 1919), this rationale to therapy is still as valid as ever.

I. Constipation

Simple constipation is infrequent or irregular defaecation which may be painful and is not secondary to an underlying cause. It has been suggested that the substitution of wholemeal bread for white bread and the use of bran or another fibre-containing breakfast cereal sufficient to provide a fibre intake of between 6 and 10 g daily would go a long way to preventing constipation (BURKITT and MEISNER 1979). Psyllium is also effective in the treatment of constipation (BLOCK 1947). If treatable factors such as lack of dietary fibre or exercise, ignoring the call to stool, irregular meals, shift work or poor toilet facilities have been excluded, contact laxatives such as bisacodyl or Senokot may prove helpful in the management of constipation (JONES and GODDING 1972).

Pregnancy and the puerperium are frequently complicated by constipation and the laxative most favoured for its treatment is Senokot (DUNCAN 1957; HERLAND and LOWENSTEIN 1957; LENNON 1957), in that it has been shown to reduce straining during defaecation (HALPERN et al. 1960) and thus decrease the propensity to haemorrhoids (GRAHAM-STEWART 1963). Particular care of the bowels is important in the management of paraplegic patients (CONNELL et al. 1963). Stool softeners such as dioctylsodium sulphosuccinate may be useful, as also may Senokot or glycerine suppositories. Enemas are sometimes required.

Megacolon and megarectum may occur due to organic lesions such as Hirschsprung's disease, but are most frequently due to functional constipation. Faecal incontinence due to impaction with overflow ensues. Enemas may be necessary to empty the colon prior to attempted retraining of the bowel. Alternatively, magnesium sulphate or a contact laxative such as Senokot or bisacodyl may be helpful (NIXON 1961). When these measures fail, repeated enemas may be required.

Regarding the management of faecal impaction, a particular hazard in the elderly, obviously prevention is the ideal. This can be achieved by proper attention to the care of the patient's bowels and the administration of prophylactic laxatives. Senokot, dioctylsodium sulphosuccinate and glycerine suppositories may be appropriate in this context. In established impaction, olive oil enemas may be effective, but if not, manual disimpaction should not be unduly delayed.

II. The Irritable Bowel Syndrome

The irritable bowel syndrome is an extremely common condition characterised by abdominal pain and alteration of bowel habit (CHAUDHARY and TRUELOVE 1962). Symptoms may be improved by dietary fibre and bulk laxatives (MANNING et al. 1977; PAINTER 1972; PIEPMEYER 1974). The frequent passage of small, hard scybala or a painful, irregular stool passed every few days may be replaced by the more even and regular passage of a formed stool following the addition of fibre or a bulk laxative to the diet. Occasionally the symptoms of gas and pain are aggravated by an increase in dietary fibre and a decrease in fibre intake may prove beneficial. Ispaghula husk has been claimed to be superior to bran in the treatment of this condition (RITCHIE and TRUELOVE 1980).

D. Laxative Abuse

There are two types of laxative abuse, namely habitual abuse and surreptitious abuse.

I. Habitual Abuse

These patients usually freely admit to their laxative consumption on enquiry, for it is regarded as entirely natural. The laxative habit is often enforced in childhood by parents who instill in their child the necessity of a daily bowel action for "inner cleanliness" and good health (ANONYMOUS 1962). A lifelong obsession with the bowels develops, especially when a neurotic personality trait predominates. In this group, the metabolic consequences of laxative abuse are rare.

While these patients are generally fit, they may develop a variety of gastrointestinal complaints, particularly if a cathartic colon results. In one series (SOPER 1938), phenolphthalein was consumed by 177 out of 1,000 consecutive gastrointestinal patients. In 152 of these, the diagnosis of "catarrhal colitis" had been made, but diarrhoea stopped when ingestion ceased. A change in cultural mores with rejection of Victorian concepts of "inner cleanliness" has ensured that these practices are dying. This may account for the observation that laxative consumption is more common with increasing age. In one study, 15% of patients aged 20–50 years consumed laxatives, as compared with more than 50% in those aged over 60 years (CONNELL et al. 1965). This increase does not relate to the presence or absence of constipation, because in another survey in people over the age of 70 years, about 55% of those interviewed took laxatives, whilst only 20% felt they were constipated (EXTON-SMITH 1972).

However, a number of habitual laxative abusers do suffer from the "spastic constipation" variety of the irritable bowel syndrome (CHAUDHARY and

TRUELOVE 1962), opening their bowels every few days. They become dependent on laxatives to achieve an effective catharsis. When evacuation occurs, it may take several days before the faecal mass is again adequate to stimulate defaecation. Rather than wait for this to occur, they again resort to laxatives, which become less effective with increasing usage. They become addicted, gradually increasing the dose over the years as the bowel becomes less responsive. The laxatives most used have been phenolphthalein and the anthraquinones. Detection of anthraquinone use may be made following the recognition of melanosis coli at sigmoidoscopy and thickening of the muscularis mucosa (GOULSTON and MCGOVERN 1969) on rectal biopsy. Eventually, a cathartic colon, recognisable on barium enema, may result.

1. Melanosis Coli

Melanosis coli has long been recognised as a brown–black melanin-like pigmentation in the large bowel (L. PICK 1911; WILLIAMS 1867) and its presence on sigmoidoscopy or rectal biopsy suggests laxative consumption (BARTLE 1928). The pigmentation has been shown to be due to lipofuscin, both from its staining properties (PEARSE 1972) and electron microscopic studies (GHADIALLY and PARRY 1966; SCHRODT 1963). Lipofuscin is found in macrophages in the lamina propria of the muscularis mucosa. The macrophages contain cytolysosomes formed by the incorporation of damaged organelles into lysosomes. Lipofuscin is produced by hydrolysis of these organelles by lysosomal enzymes.

Melanosis is found in the large bowel and appendix, but not in the rest of the small intestine. The right side of the colon is first affected, but the condition can spread to involve the whole colon. The regional lymph nodes may also contain pigment. Lymphoid follicles, adenomas and carcinomas in the large bowel do not take up the pigment, a feature which can prove useful in colonoscopic identification. It is most commonly associated with ingestion of the anthraquinone laxatives, senna, aloes, and cascara (BOCKUS et al. 1933). Although there are no recent supportive studies, it seems that the post-mortem incidence of melanosis coli, which was as high as 11% in one study (STEWART and HICKMAN 1931) is decreasing owing to the diminishing popularity of the anthraquinones (MORSON and DAWSON 1979). Thus no case of melanosis was found in 200 consecutive sigmoidoscopies (ABUNASSAR and THOMPSON 1979, unpublished work) as compared with an incidence of 4.7% in an earlier study (BOCKUS et al. 1933).

The evidence incriminating anthraquinone usage in the causation of melanosis is first that the pigmentation usually appears 1 year or more after commencing anthraquinone ingestion (BOCKUS et al. 1933), second that it disappears on withdrawal of the laxative, usually within 4–12 months (BOCKUS et al. 1933; WITTOESCH et al. 1958) and finally that it can be produced in monkeys by the administration of cascara (SPEARE 1951). It is not specific for anthraquinones because it has been reported following heavy metal poisoning, particularly lead (N. PICK 1891) and after the ingestion of laxatives containing mercurous chloride (WANDS et al. 1974; WILLIAMS 1867). In the latter cases, it was not possible to exclude simultaneous ingestion of anthraquinones. In WITTOESCH's study, 850 of 887 patients with melanosis coli admitted to habitual use of laxatives.

2. Cathartic Colon

If anthraquinones are regularly consumed for 30 years or so (B. SMITH 1972), irreversible colonic damage, resulting in cathartic colon can result (JONES 1967; MARSHAK and GERSON 1960; MISIEWICZ and WALLER 1966). However, severe damage can also occur following shorter periods of ingestion. Melanosis is usually present. The anthraquinones are neurotoxins and are concentrated in the colon. Initially, they cause overstimulation of the neurones of the myenteric plexus which become pale and swollen (B. SMITH 1968). Schwann cell proliferation develops with depletion due to death of the overstimulated neurones and axons.

The neurones remaining are weakly argentophilic (B. SMITH 1967), dark and shrunken. Both they and the axons are irregular. The end stage is reached with atrophy of the intestinal smooth muscle cells. The unusual mucosal appearance has been likened to the "skin on a toad's back" (MORSON 1971) and the combination of thinning of the muscularis propria, hypertrophy of the muscularis mucosa (GOULSTON and MCGOVERN 1969) and submucosal deposition of adipose tissue gives rise to an inert dilated aperistaltic colon.

The radiological changes at barium enema of the dilated, cathartic colon were first described by HEILBRUN in 1943. Other reports followed (HEILBRUN and BERNSTEIN 1955; JEWELL and KLINE 1954). PLUM et al. (1960) summarised the abnormal radiological features in a review of 27 cases at the Mayo Clinic, Rochester, Minnesota. Their findings were confirmed in a further report (RAWSON 1966). The right side of the colon and usually the terminal ileum also are first affected, the rest of the colon being involved later. There is loss of the normal colonic haustral pattern, but the bowel wall is smooth and regular, unlike ulcerative colitis, where there is mucosal irregularity. The bowel is dilated and distensible which contrasts with the thickened, shortened colon in ulcerative colitis. When the large bowel is dilated in ulcerative colitis the patient is usually in a toxic state (KORELITZ and JANOWITZ 1960), but a dilated colon due to laxative usage may occur with minimal symptoms.

A characteristic feature is the presence of pseudostrictures in the colon, best visualised and assessed by fluoroscopy to distinguish them from strictures due to other colonic pathology. They represent smooth contractions, quite unlike the normal physiological contractions and are due to neuromuscular incoordination in the presence of a hypertrophied muscularis mucosa. They appear and disappear, reappearing elsewhere and thus dilated and constricted segments of colon coexist. Colonoscopy with colonic biopsies may prove helpful in evaluating any radiological abnormality and also in the recognition of melanosis coli affecting the proximal colon. Improvement of abnormalities on cessation of laxative consumption has been demonstrated (HEILBRUN 1943; JEWELL and KLINE 1954). Dilation of the terminal ileum with disturbance of the normal mucosal pattern (HEILBRUN 1943; PLUM et al. 1960) may be visualised on a small bowel meal. It should be remembered that characteristic radiological abnormalities may well be absent both in habitual and surreptitious laxative abusers (CUMMINGS et al. 1974).

3. Management

Successful management will depend on the cooperation of the patient, which is more likely to be forthcoming if the clinician gains the confidence of the patient by offering an effective and less harmful alternative to the laxative habit. That habit plays a large role in the continued use of laxatives was shown in an elegant study in psychiatric patients (HAWARD and HUGHES-ROBERTS 1962). These workers withdrew all laxatives, added Senokot to a morning drink and then took the patients to the toilet 9 h later until defaecation occurred. When this behaviour pattern had been established, the Senokot was gradually withdrawn from the drink. After 3 months on this regime, the proportion of patients requiring laxatives fell from 44% to 8%.

The diphenylmethane or anthraquinone laxatives should be withdrawn and replaced by a high fibre diet together with liberal amounts of a bulk laxative, sufficient to establish regular defaecation. This period of bowel retraining may take some months or even longer, the dosage of the bulk laxative being adjusted according to response. In the early stages, a saline laxative such as magnesium sulphate may also prove helpful (JONES and GODDING 1972). Encouragement and close supervision of both the pharmacological and the psychological aspects of care will improve the chances of a successful outcome. If a dilated, aperistaltic cathartic colon has developed, this may prove refractory to the measures described. In these patients, colectomy with caecorectal or ileorectal anastomosis may be beneficial and lead to a more regular bowel habit (JONES 1967; PLUMLEY 1973; TODD 1973).

II. Surreptitious Abuse

This is analogous to other factitious illnesses and the patient presents with intractable diarrhoea, often having been investigated in a number of hospitals, when no cause has been found. In addition there may be abdominal pain, hypokalaemia, thirst, muscular weakness, melanosis coli and characteristic radiological changes in the bowel (AITCHISON 1958; COGHILL et al. 1959; KRAMER and POPE 1964; LITCHFIELD 1959; RAWSON 1966; WOLFF et al. 1968). Over 90% of patients are women (CUMMINGS 1974).

Initially, they often fool their regular medical attendants and psychiatrists, but disturbed psychiatric behaviour may become manifest when the patient has been found out. The overwhelming female predominance of surreptitious laxative abusers has served to focus attention on underlying psychosexual disturbances. Some patients display stong psychoneurotic traits (DE GRAEFF 1961; HEIZER et al. 1968) and others hysterical behaviour (CUMMINGS et al. 1974; WOLFF et al. 1968) and paranoid, obsessional (COGHILL et al. 1959) and psychopathic tendencies have also been reported. Interestingly, the latter was suggested as being the underlying cause in one of the rare cases described in the male (FRENCH et al. 1956). The emotional detachment and almost total lack of concern (KRAMER and POPE 1964) about their illness, which are characteristic of surreptitious laxative abusers, is further supportive evidence that psychogenic factors are operant in the pathogenesis of this condition.

A large proportion of patients work in the nursing or paramedical services (CUMMINGS et al. 1974; KRAMER and POPE 1964; LOVE et al. 1971). The environment affords them the opportunity to learn how better to deceive the medical profession and the same is true of patients who have had multiple hospital admissions. Other factitious illnesses such as factitious fever and self-inflicted injury (KRAMER and POPE 1964) have been described in association. These patients are extremely devious and will go to great lengths to conceal their purgative consumption (FLEISCHER et al. 1969; FRENCH et al. 1956; GOSSAIN and WERK 1972; GRAUWELS 1962; LOVE et al. 1971; VAN ROOYEN and ZIADY 1972; SCHWARTZ and RELMAN 1953). They sometimes persuade friends or relatives to bring further supplies of laxatives into the hospital, unknown to the unsuspecting staff.

The development of surreptitious laxative abuse in patients who suffered from anorexia nervosa in early life has been noted (CUMMINGS et al. 1974). This suggests that the two conditions may have a similar psychopathological basis. Laxative abuse and anorexia nervosa may also coexist (AITCHISON 1958; DE GRAEFF 1961; LOVE et al. 1971; VECHT-VAN DEN BERGH 1979) and this combination has a particularly poor prognosis (ASBECK et al. 1972; HALMI et al. 1973).

These patients exhibit many of the features of Münchausen's syndrome (ASHER 1951), namely chronic factitious illness (or illnesses), a desire to manipulate and deceive the medical profession to the point of being prepared to undergo multiple painful investigative procedures including surgery, and secondary gain from their action in the form of attention, sympathy and removal from conflict either at home or work.

It has been suggested that Baron von Münchausen may well have contributed to the death of his only son, Polle, at the age of 1 year (BURMAN and STEVENS 1977). Polle syndrome, also known as Münchausen's syndrome by proxy (KURLANDSKY et al. 1979; MEADOW 1977; PICKERING and KOHL 1981) is factitious illness in children induced by their parents, themselves sufferers from Münchausen's syndrome. It was as late as 1977 before FLEISCHER and AMENT described three cases of chronic diarrhoea in children owing to the parental administration of phenolphthalein-containing laxatives. These cases were diagnosed fortuitously by the observation of pink-stained diapers caused by the phenolphthalein in alkaline conditions. Undoubtedly, this is not a new practice, and one can only speculate on the possible dire consequences in previously unrecognised cases. The children had been extensively investigated with frequent hospital attendances and admissions. Lack of concern and emotional detachment of the mother were described (ACKERMAN and STROBEL 1981).

The children of Münchausen are still at risk today (LEE 1979; PICKERING and KOHL 1981; VAISRUB 1978; VERITY et al. 1979). It is most probable that the mother in one report (ACKERMAN and STROBEL 1981) was herself a laxative abuser in that she had an undiagnosed diarrhoea. An established diagnosis of factitious illness in one member of the family should therefore alert the clinician to the possibility that symptoms in other family members may also have a factitious origin.

1. Diarrhoea

The deliberate self-administration of laxatives causing factitious diarrhoea has only been recognised in recent years (COGHILL et al. 1959; FRENCH et al. 1956; GASTARD and GOIFFON 1960; KRAMER and POPE 1964; SCHWARTZ and RELMAN 1953). The importance of surreptitious laxative ingestion as a cause of chronic diarrhoea of unknown origin (CUMMINGS 1974; READ et al. 1980) and associated faecal incontinence (READ et al. 1979) has been reported.

Normal daily stool weight varies with race and diet (BURKITT et al. 1972). The daily stool weight on a western diet is not usually greater than 225 g (READ et al. 1980). Surreptitious laxative ingestion is characterised by large volume diarrhoea, as distinct from the usual form of the irritable bowel syndrome, in which there is frequency of defaecation, but the total daily stool weight is not increased. Daily faecal weight should be measured accurately. While this should be undertaken with metabolic ward zeal, it can be done on any well-run ward. Occasionally the stool volume is spurious owing to the factitious addition of water to the stool. If this is suspected, the patient should be closely supervised when at stool.

In a patient presenting with diarrhoea, sigmoidoscopy and rectal biopsy are essential. As with habitual abuse of anthraquinones, surreptitious abuse may coexist, and the latter patients may eventually also develop a cathartic colon. The next step in the investigation of an unexplained diarrhoea is to look for evidence of malabsorption, and many tests used for this purpose may give misleading results when there is excessive ingestion of laxatives. Finding steatorrhoea can put one off one's guard, but it has been described in association with phenolphthalein (COGHILL et al. 1959; FRENCH et al. 1956; HEIZER et al. 1968) and bisacodyl (HEIZER et al. 1968) ingestion. The ingestion of magnesium-containing laxatives may also cause steatorrhoea in normal subjects (HEIZER et al. 1968) by forming insoluble magnesium salts of fatty acids.

Other tests of absorption may give misleading results. An abnormal xylose tolerance test (BENSON et al. 1957) has been reported following surreptitious laxative abuse (CUMMINGS et al. 1974; FRAME et al. 1971; HEIZER et al. 1968). It is a test of limited use in that patients have been known either to dilute their urine or to dispose of it, leading to inadequate collections. The Lundh test of pancreatic function may also be deranged (CUMMINGS et al. 1974). An abnormal glucose tolerance test has been described (CUMMINGS et al. 1974; HEIZER et al. 1968) and is attributed to depletion of total body potassium (CONN 1965; SAGILD et al. 1961).

Failure of absorption of the fat-soluble vitamins, A, D (STAFFURTH and ALLOTT 1962), E and K occurs and osteomalacia (FRAME et al. 1971; MEULENGRACHT 1938, 1939) and tetany (GOLDFINGER 1969; CUMMINGS et al. 1974) may ensue. Reduced intestinal absorption of calcium and magnesium (HEIZER et al. 1968) and the metabolic alkalosis increase the risk of tetany (STAFFURTH and ALLOTT 1962). Deficiency of vitamin K leads to a bleeding diathesis and easy bruising. A protein-losing enteropathy in association with malabsorption, following in one case phenolphthalein and in the other bisacodyl ingestion (HEIZER et al. 1968), has also been described. Excessive loss of albumin from the gastrointestinal tract is best demonstrated by the use of ^{51}Cr-labelled albumin (WALDMANN 1961) and if severe causes peripheral oedema.

Intestinal perfusion may help to distinguish surreptitious laxative ingestion from the pancreatic cholera syndrome, often the main differential diagnosis. There is no difference in intestinal transport of glucose, water and electrolytes in the jejunum, ileum or colon between normal subjects and those with diarrhoea due to surreptitious laxative abuse (KREJS et al. 1977; READ et al. 1980), presumably because the effect of laxatives on the intestinal mucosa is transient and consumption ceases during perfusion. However in patients with the pancreatic cholera syndrome, there is greater jejunal secretion of water and electrolytes (KREJS et al. 1977) than in normal subjects and laxative takers.

2. Water and Electrolyte Depletion

The excessive gastrointestinal losses of sodium and water (COGHILL et al. 1959; FORDTRAN and INGELFINGER 1968) in diarrhoea lead to dehydration, hypotension, uraemia and thirst. Increased renin secretion and secondary hyperaldosteronism results (ANONYMOUS 1966; FLEISCHER et al. 1969; DE GRAEFF and SCHUURS 1960; LOVE et al. 1971; VAN ROOYEN and ZIADY 1972; WOLFF et al. 1968), thus conserving sodium at the expense of potassium. Therefore, the hypokalaemia typically associated with surreptitious ingestion of laxatives is multifactorial (HOUGHTON and PEARS 1958; MÅRTENSSON 1953; SCHWARTZ and RELMAN 1953). The secondary hyperaldosteronism results in increased losses of potassium from the colon (SHIELDS et al. 1966) and kidney (SLADEN 1972). There is faecal loss of potassium per se in diarrhoea and self-induced vomiting and reduced dietary intake of potassium may also contribute (AITCHISON 1958). Metabolic alkalosis occurs in association with the hypokalaemia (DARROW et al. 1948), but a metabolic acidosis (GOLDFINGER 1969) has also been described. Hypokalaemia is responsible for a number of the clinical features associated with surreptitious laxative ingestion.

MAHLER and STANBURY (1956) drew attention to polydipsia as a cardinal symptom of severe total body potassium deficiency. The polydipsia and polyuria (WOLFF et al. 1968) have led to the erroneous diagnosis of diabetes insipidus (RAWSON 1966), which can be distinguished from thirst associated with laxative ingestion by measurement of the plasma and urinary osmolalities. Patients with a past history of unexplained weakness, areflexic paralysis (COGHILL et al. 1959; HOUGHTON and PEARS 1958) and even quadriplegia (BERNING and FISCHER 1961), all due to potassium deficiency are described, their attacks occurring over a number of years prior to the recognition of their laxative consumption. Paralysis of the respiratory muscles is potentially life threatening. Cardiac arrhythmias occur most frequently due to hypokalaemia, but hypocalcaemia may also contribute. The typical ECG changes of hypokalaemia are depression of the ST segment, lowered T waves, and prominent U waves, which are especially seen in the left chest leads. In severe deficiency, extrasystoles may occur, as may potentially fatal ventricular arrhythmias. In severe hypokalaemia, paralytic ileus may develop and cause vomiting, resulting in further fluid depletion due to intestinal loss of water and electrolytes.

The patient may present to the renal physician for investigation of renal failure. A nephropathy, which in the early stages is reversible, develops in response to prolonged severe hypokalaemia (ANONYMOUS 1966; COGHILL et al. 1959; DE GRAEFF and SCHUURS 1960; HOUGHTON and PEARS 1958; LINQUETTE et al. 1964; PERKINS et al. 1950; SCHWARTZ and RELMAN 1953). Ammonium urate stones may form (COGHILL et al. 1959) and are attributed to the reduced urinary citrate excretion, alkaluria and metabolic alkalosis (STANBURY 1958). They may cause haematuria and pyelonephritis (HEIZER et al. 1968). Irreversible renal damage may eventually occur (DE GRAEFF and SCHUURS 1960) leading to further potassium loss (MAHLER and STANBURY 1956; PERKINS et al. 1950).

3. Other Features

Central, epigastric, lower and generalised abdominal pain (CUMMINGS et al. 1974) have been described. Pain may be colicky, associated with abdominal distension or proptosis and be eased by bowel action or the passage of flatus. Alternatively, it may radiate from the epigastrium to the back, suggesting peptic ulceration or pancreatic disease, the latter particularly if steatorrhoea is present. Abdominal tenderness with rebound may be found on examination.

Poor appetite is a well-recognised feature. This can be compounded by food fads (COGHILL et al. 1959; DE GRAEFF 1961) and vomiting, which is frequently self-induced. Weight loss, weight-related amenorrhoea and the development of thin downy hair covering the skin (CUMMINGS et al. 1974) suggest the diagnosis of anorexia nervosa. The diarrhoea and hypokalaemia should alert the clinician to the fact that the anorexia and other features are consequences of laxative ingestion.

Finger clubbing associated with chronic Senokot ingestion has been described (SILK et al. 1975). That the clubbing was due to Senokot was confirmed by its reversibility when ingestion ceased and its recurrence when laxative consumption was resumed. A subsequent case associated with hypoalbuminaemia and protein-losing enteropathy has been described (LEVINE et al. 1981). Other unusual manifestations associated with surreptitious laxative abuse are pancreatic islet cell hyperplasia (LESNA et al. 1977) and skin pigmentation (COGHILL et al. 1959; DE GRAEFF and SCHUURS 1960; HEIZER et al. 1968; RAMIREZ and MARIEB 1970; VAN ROOYEN and ZIADY 1972).

4. Diagnosis

It cannot be emphasised enough that the single most important factor in establishing the diagnosis of surreptitious laxative ingestion is a high index of suspicion on the part of the clinician (CUMMINGS et al. 1974). However, the only definite way to diagnose this condition is to demonstrate laxatives in the urine or stool and to find a large supply of them in the patient's possession.

a) Chemical Detection

α) Diphenolic, Anthraquinone and Vegetable Laxatives. On the ward, the presence of phenolphthalein in urine or stool may be suggested by the production of a red–purple colour in the specimen by the addition of dilute sodium hydroxide. Phenolphthalein in urine can be detected by extracting 10 ml urine with an equal volume of diethyl ether. After removal and extraction of the ether phase with 2 ml 0.1 *M* NaOH, a pink–red colour in the aqueous phase will occur in the presence of phenolphthalein (FANTUS and DYNIEWICZ 1938). The addition of excess 10 *M* NaOH to the aqueous phase leads to disappearance of this colour, as also does back titration with HCl at pH 9.2 (KRAMER and POPE 1964). Phenolphthalein excreted in urine is mainly in the conjugated form, chiefly sulphate, but also glucuronate. These do not turn pink on the addition of alkali unless free phenolphthalein is liberated by hydrolysis by boiling the urine with HCl. However, other substances such as beetroot, rhubarb and bromsulphophthalein can cause a reddish or purple colour in this test. This has on occasions led to patients being wrongly accused of surreptitious laxative abuse and thus it was desirable for more specific tests to be developed. While the tests we have mentioned are qualitative, a quantitative spectrophotometric assay for phenolphthalein in serum and urine has been developed (MORRIS and POWELL 1979) and shown to be sensitive to 10^{-5} M phenolphthalein. Both the free and conjugated forms can be measured.

There are a number of methods for the detection of bisacodyl and the anthraquinones in faeces and urine (FAIRBAIRN and SIMIC 1964; JANSEN and KAMP 1976; KASPI et al. 1978; VYTH and KAMP 1979). However, a much broader screening method to detect phenolphthalein, bisacodyl, bisoxatin, danthron, oxyphenisatin, and rhein in urine has been described (DE WOLFF et al. 1981). The first four were also detectable in faecal samples. Rhein is a metabolite of many vegetable laxatives such as senna, cascara, aloes, and rhubarb (VYTH and KAMP 1979) and its detection now permits the recognition of ingestion of vegetable laxatives as well as all the diphenolic and anthraquinones, except sodium picosulphate. A 20 ml sample from a 24 h urinary collection is treated with β-glucuronidase, subjected to column extraction and then high pressure thin layer chromatography using two different systems. All six of the laxatives were detectable in the urine 18 h after the administration of a single dose and all except oxyphenisatin and bisoxatin were still present 32 h after ingestion. Rhubarb ingestion and the administration of 73 other drugs were tested and did not interfere in either of the two chromatographic systems, thus confirming the high specificity of this method.

β) *Osmotic Laxatives*. Measurement of stool osmolality and electrolytes may reveal an "osmotic gap" (KREJS and FORDTRAN 1978), when the osmolality of the faecal fluid is greater than the sum of the measured electrolytes in the stool (twice the sum of the concentrations of Na^+ and K^+). A normal stool osmolality in the presence of a large osmotic gap suggests that the diarrhoea is osmotic and may be due to ingestion of saline purgatives (READ et al. 1980).

Faecal inorganic sulphate excretion is raised following sodium sulphate (Glauber's salt) ingestion (METCALFE-GIBSON et al. 1967). In normal subjects and patients with diarrhoea due to causes other than laxative consumption, excretion is less than 4.5 mequiv./l (GOIFFON et al. 1961; PHILLIPS et al. 1965; WRONG et al. 1965). However, this measurement is very difficult and few laboratories will perform it. A simple ward test to detect excess sulphate in the stool is to add barium chloride to it. A white precipitate of barium sulphate may occur if the faecal sulphate concentration is raised. Measurements of daily urinary magnesium (normal <16 mequiv.) and sulphate (normal <56 mequiv.) excretion (LONG 1961; WOOTON 1964) may also prove helpful. All these chemical tests should be performed several times, either to confirm a positive result or so as not to miss intermittent laxative consumption.

b) Locker Search

Although not always fruitful (FRENCH et al. 1956), there are many instances where laxatives have been discovered following a search of the patient's possessions (BUNIM et al. 1958; CUMMINGS et al. 1974). The Medical Defence Union in the United Kingdom comments "It is legally quite unjustifiable to search a patient's possessions without his knowledge and consent although it is difficult to see how a patient could sue for this and what offence is committed which is triable in a Magistrates' Court" (CUMMINGS 1974).

However, if these patients are to be identified, the clinician may well have to resort to devious tactics. At least two experienced staff should conduct the search, which is best performed as soon as possible after admission, before the patient has had time to choose a suitable hiding place. Ideally the patient should be put in a side room and then taken elsewhere in the hospital at short notice. This permits the search to be performed discreetly and thus reduces the chance of other patients passing on the information that the staff have been busy behind the curtains, thus alerting the suspicion of the patient under investigation and reducing the possibility of discovery. If laxatives are found, it should then be possible to check that the supply decreases with time (BUNIM et al. 1958).

5. Management

In view of the sporadic nature of the condition and in the absence of any large long-term follow-up study, the best way to manage this condition is unresolved (CUMMINGS et al. 1974). Confrontation has brought mixed results. Suicide gestures have been reported both in surreptitious abusers (CUMMINGS et al. 1974) and in a mother administering laxatives to her child (ACKERMAN and STROBEL 1981). Patients may deny abuse (READ et al. 1980), admit it but with total indifference (KRAMER and POPE 1964) or accept that they have been caught out and stop taking laxatives (HEIZER et al. 1968; KRAMER and POPE 1964; LITCHFIELD 1959; MÅRTENSSON 1953; RAMIREZ and MARIEB 1970; READ et al. 1980). At follow-up they may continue to use laxatives (HOUGHTON and PEARS 1958) or develop substitution symptoms.

The hypokalaemia should be corrected cautiously and sodium bicarbonate should also be administered to prevent a precipitous fall in serum bicarbonate on restoration of the body potassium (HOUGHTON and PEARS 1958; OWEN and VERNER 1960). Spironolactone may help in the treatment of secondary hyperaldosteronism (FLEISCHER et al. 1969; CUMMINGS 1974). The oedema which can develop in the period immediately after stopping laxatives (COGHILL et al. 1959; HEIZER et al. 1968; SCHWARTZ and RELMAN 1953) is thought to be due to a large but transient sodium retention (ELKINTON et al. 1951), due to the impaired ability of the kidney to excrete a sodium load in potassium deficiency (BLACK and MILNE 1952) and can be helped by salt restriction. Outpatient support, monitoring the serum electrolytes for biochemical evidence of continued consumption, should be provided (HOUGHTON and PEARS 1958; CUMMINGS 1974).

Establishing the diagnosis is important in that it should prevent further unnecessary investigation. It should also prompt an assessment of the patient's psyche (KRAMER and POPE 1964), lead to an enquiry into possible factitious symptoms in other family members (ACKERMAN and STROBEL 1981) and to the institution of appropriate psychotherapeutic care.

E. Summary

Cathartic drugs have been in use for several thousand years. Only in recent years has light been thrown on the mechanism of action of different laxatives, leading to revised ideas on their classification. They are freely available, both on prescription and as over-the-counter medicines. When used properly, bulk laxatives may be beneficial in a variety of colorectal disorders, such as constipation, diverticular disease and irritable bowel syndrome. Prophylactic use should be encouraged to prevent excessive straining during defaecation following myocardial infarction, anorectal surgery and childbirth. The osmotic and contact cathartics have a special use in bowel preparation for surgical, endoscopic and radiological procedures and when rapid purgation is required, as in poisoning and helminthic infections.

Two types of laxative abuse are described, namely habitual abuse and surreptitious abuse. Phenolphthalein and the anthraquinone derivatives have been most abused in this respect. Long-term anthraquinone use may lead to melanosis coli and cathartic colon, with typical histological and radiological features. Surreptitious abuse presents as a factitious illness with diarrhoea, hypokalaemia, abdominal pain and thirst, as well as melanosis coli. Over 90% of cases occur in women, many of whom work in a paramedical situation.

Wider recognition of the range of normal bowel habit and a cultural change with rejection of Victorian mores and concepts of "intestinal autointoxication" have led to a decrease in inappropriate laxative consumption. However, they are still widely prescribed and bought. There is a need for stricter control of their purchase. Although it was as long ago as 1937 that Witts drew attention to the dangers associated with the use of laxatives, his lesson still needs to be preached today.

References

Abramowitz EW (1950) Phenolphthalein today: critical review. Am J Dig Dis 17:79–82

Ackerman NB Jr, Strobel CT (1981) Polle syndrome: chronic diarrhea in Münchhausen's child. Gastroenterology 81:1140–1142

Aitchison JD (1958) Hypokalaemia following chronic diarrhoea from overuse of cascara and a deficient diet. Lancet 2:75–76

Alvarez WC (1924) Intestinal autointoxication. Physiol Rev 4:352–375

Anonymous (1962) The treatment of constipation. Lancet 1:1010–1011

Anonymous (1966) A case of purgative addiction. Br Med J 1:1344–1348

Anonymous (1972) Laxative jaundice. Br Med J 1:325

Anonymous (1973 a) Bulk "laxatives" in medicine and surgery. Drug Ther Bull 11:77–80

Anonymous (1973 b) Laxatives and dietary fiber. Med Lett Drugs Ther 15:98–100

Anonymous (1973 c) In England now. Lancet 2:1079

Asbeck F, Hirschmann WD, Deck K, Castrup HJ (1972) Letaler Krankheitsverlauf bei einer Patientin mit anorexia nervosa, Aikohot und Laxantien-Abusus. Internist (Berlin) 13:63–65

Asher R (1951) Münchausen's syndrome. Lancet 1:339–341

Ayvazian LF, Steward DS, Merkel CG, Frederick WW (1967) Diffuse lipoid pneumonia successfully treated with prednisone. Am J Med 43:930–934

Bartle HJ (1928) The sigmoid: anatomy, physiology, examination and pathology. Med J Rec 127:521–524

Benson JA, Culver PJ, Ragland S, Jones CM, Drummey GD, Bongas E (1957) The D-xylose absorption test in malabsorption syndromes. N Engl J Med 256:335–339

Berning H, Fischer R (1961) On the chronic abuse of laxatives and its effects on mineral metabolism. Dtsch Med Wochenschr 86:2153–2156

Bigard MA, Gaucher P, Lassalle C (1979) Fatal colonic explosion during colonoscopic polypectomy. Gastroenterology 77:1307–1310

Binder HJ, Donowitz M (1975) A new look at laxative action. Gastroenterology 69:1001–1005

Black DAK, Milne MD (1952) Experimental potassium depletion in man. Lancet 1:244–245

Block LH (1947) Management of constipation with a refined psyllium combined with dextrose. Am J Dig Dis 14:64–74

Bockus HL, Willard JH, Bank J (1933) Melanosis coli: the etiologic significance of the anthracene laxatives: a report of 41 cases. JAMA 101:1–6

Boyd JT, Doll R (1954) Gastrointestinal cancer and the use of liquid paraffin. Br J Cancer 8:231–237

Bretagne JF, Vidon N, L'Hirondel C, Bernier JJ (1981) Increased cell loss in the human jejunum induced by laxatives (ricinoleic acid, dioctyl sodium sulphosuccinate, magnesium sulphate, bile salts). Gut 22:264–269

Brocklehurst JC, Kahn MY (1969) A study of faecal stasis in old age and the use of Dorbanex in its prevention. Geront Clin (Basel) 11:293–300

Browne JCM, Edmunds V, Fairbairn JW, Reid DD (1957) Clinical and laboratory assessments of senna preparations. Br Med J 1:436–439

Bruckstein AH (1978) Laxatives and cathartics, uses and abuses. NY State J Med 78:1078–1082

Bueckner HA, Strug LH (1956) Lipoid granuloma of lung of exogenous origin. Dis Chest 29:402–415

Bunim JJ, Federman DD, Black RL, Schmid R, Sokoloff L, Shurley J (1958) Factitious diseases: clinical staff conference at the National Institute of Health. Ann Intern Med 48:1328–1341

Burkitt DP, Meisner P (1979) How to manage constipation with high-fiber diet. Geriatrics 34 (2):33–35, 38–40

Burkitt DP, Walker ARP, Painter NS (1972) Effect of dietary fibre on stools and transit-times, and its role in the causation of disease. Lancet 2:1408–1411

Burman D, Stevens D (1977) Münchausen family. Lancet 2:456

Busse WW, Schoenwetter WF (1975) Asthma from psyllium in laxative manufacture. Ann Intern Med 83:361–362

Chaudhary NA, Truelove SC (1962) The irritable colon syndrome. Q J Med 31:307–322

Cochran KM, Nelson L, Russell RI, Godding E (1977) Laxatives and gastric mucosal damage – the danger of dioctyl sodium sulphosuccinate. Gut 18:A 422

Coghill NF, McAllen PM, Edwards F (1959) Electrolyte losses associated with the taking of purges investigated with aid of sodium and potassium radioisotopes. Br Med J 1:14–19

Conn JW (1965) Hypertension, the potassium ion and impaired carbohydrate tolerance. N Engl J Med 273:1135–1143

Connell AM, Frankel H, Guttmann L (1963) The motility of the pelvic colon following complete lesions of the spinal cord. Paraplegia 1:98–115

Connell AM, Hilton C, Irvine G, Lennard-Jones JE, Misiewicz JJ (1965) Variation of bowel habit in two population samples. Br Med J 2:1095–1099

Cummings JH (1974) Laxative abuse. Gut 15:758–766

Cummings JH, Sladen GE, James OFW, Sarner M, Misiewicz JJ (1974) Laxative-induced diarrhoea: a continuing clinical problem. Br Med J 1:537–541

Darrow DC, Schwartz R, Iannucci JF, Coville F (1948) Relation of serum bicarbonate concentration to muscle composition. J Clin Invest 27:198–208

de Graeff J (1961) Severe potassium deficiency due to misuse of laxatives. Ned Tijdschr Geneeskd 105:200–202 de Graeff J, Schuurs MAM (1960) Severe potassium depletion caused by the abuse of laxatives: one patient followed for 8 years. Acta Med Scand 166:407–422

Delchier JC, Métreau JM, Lévy VG, Opolon P, Dhumeaux D (1979) L'oxyphénisatine, laxatif responsable d'hépatites chroniques et de cirrhoses – toujours commercialisé en France. Nouv Presse Med 8:2955–2958

de Wolff FA, de Haas EJM, Verweij M (1981) A screening method for establishing laxative abuse. Clin Chem 27:914–917

Donaldson AN (1922) Relation of constipation to intestinal intoxication. JAMA 78:884–888

Dujovne CA, Shoeman LW (1972) Toxicity of a hepatotoxic laxative preparation in tissue culture and excretion in bile by man. Clin Pharmacol Ther 13:602–608

Duncan AS (1957) Standardized senna as a laxative in the puerperium. Br Med J 1:439–441

Elkinton JR, Squires RD, Crosley AP Jr (1951) Intracellular cation exchanges in metabolic alkalosis. J Clin Invest 30:369–380

Elston CW (1966) Pneumonia due to liquid paraffin: with chemical analysis. Arch Dis Child 41:428–434

Exton-Smith N (1972) Constipation in geriatrics. In: Jones FA, Godding EW (eds) Management of constipation. Blackwell, Oxford, p 157

Fairbairn JW, Michaels I (1950) Vegetable purgatives containing anthracene derivatives. II. The evaluation of senna pod and its preparations. J Pharm Pharmacol 2:807–812

Fairbairn JW, Simic S (1964) Estimation of C-glycosides and O-glycosides in cascara (Rhamnus purshiana D.C., bark) and cascara extract. J Pharm Pharmacol 16:450–454

Fairbairn JW, Moss MJR (1970) The relative purgative activities of 1,8-dihydroxyanthracene derivatives. J Pharm Pharmacol 22:584–593

Fantus B, Dyniewicz JM (1938) Phenolphthalein studies; elimination of phenolphthalein. JAMA 110:796–799

Fingl E (1980) Laxatives and cathartics. In: Goodman LS, Gilman A (eds) The pharmacological basis of therapeutics, 6th edn. Macmillan, New York, pp 1002–1012

Fisher RE (1938) Psyllium seeds: intestinal obstruction. Calif W Med 48:190

Fleischer N, Brown H, Graham DY, Delena S (1969) Chronic laxative-induced hyperaldosteronism and hypokalaemia simulating Bartter's syndrome. Ann Intern Med 70:791–798

Fleisher D, Ament ME (1977) Diarrhea, red diapers and child abuse. Clin Pediatr 17:820–824

Forbes G, Bradley A (1958) Liquid paraffin as a cause of oil aspiration pneumonia. Br Med J 2:1566–1568

Fordtran JS, Ingelfinger FJ (1968) Absorption of water, electrolytes and sugars from the human gut. In: Code CF (ed) Intestinal absorption. American Physiological Society, Washington, DC, pp 1457–1490 (Handbook of physiology, vol 3)

Frame B, Guiang HL, Frost HM, Reynolds WA (1971) Osteomalacia induced by laxative (phenolphthalein) ingestion. Arch Intern Med 128:794–796

Freiman DG, Engelberg H, Merrit WH (1940) Oil aspiration (lipoid) pneumonia in adults: clinicopathologic study of 47 cases. Arch Intern Med 66:11–38

French JM, Gaddie R, Smith N (1956) Diarrhoea due to phenolphthalein. Lancet 1:551–553

Gastard J, Goiffon B (1960) Apropos du dépistage des fausses diarrhées entretenues par la phénolphthaléine. Arch Mal Appar Dig 49:627–629

Ghadially FN, Parry EW (1966) An electronmicroscope and histochemical study of melanosis coli. J Pathol Bacteriol 92:313–317

Godding EW (1975a) Constipation and allied disorders. 3. Therapeutic agents – chemical laxatives. Pharm J 215:60–62, 81–84

Godding EW (1975b) Constipation and allied disorders. 2. Therapeutic agents – hydrophilic bulking agents. Pharm J 215:34–36

Goiffon R, Goiffon B, Fron G (1961) Contribution à l'étude des électrolytes des selles. III. Mesure des anions. Gastroenterologia (Basel) 96:312–325

Goldfinger P (1969) Hypokalemia, metabolic acidosis and hypocalcemic tetany in a patient taking laxatives. J Mt Sinai Hosp 36:113–116

Goldman JL (1937) Esophageal obstruction from a hydroscopic gum laxative (saraka) JAMA 108:1408–1409

Goldstein GB, Lam KC, Mistilis SP (1973) Drug-induced active chronic hepatitis. Am J Dig Dis 18:177–184

Gossain VV, Werk EE (1972) Surreptitious laxation and hypokalemia. Ann Intern Med 76:671

Goulston SJM, McGovern VJ (1969) The nature of benign strictures in ulcerative colitis. N Engl J Med 281:290–295

Graham-Stewart CW (1963) What causes haemorrhoids? A new theory of etiology. Dis Colon Rectum 6:333–344

Grauwels J (1962) Diarrhée chronique entretenue par la prise clandestine de laxatifs. Acta Gastroenterol Belg 25:858–866

Halmi K, Brodland G, Loney J (1973) Prognosis in anorexia nervosa. Ann Intern Med 78:907–909

Halpern A, Selman D, Shaftel N, Shaftel HE, Kuhn PH, Samuels SS, Birch HG (1960) The peripheral vascular dynamics of bowel function. Angiology 11:460–479

Harvey RF, Read AE (1973a) Effect of cholecystokinin on colonic motility and symptoms in patients with the irritable bowel syndrome. Lancet 1:1–3

Harvey RF, Read AE (1973b) Saline purgatives act by releasing cholecystokinin. Lancet 2:185–187

Haward LRC, Hughes-Roberts HE (1962) The treatment of constipation in mental hospitals. Gut 3:85–90

Heilbrun N (1943) Roentgen evidence suggesting enterocolitis associated with prolonged cathartic abuse. Radiology 41:486–491

Heilbrun N, Bernstein C (1955) Roentgen abnormalities of the large and small intestine associated with prolonged cathartic ingestion. Radiology 65:549–556

Heizer WD, Warshaw AL, Waldmann TA, Laster L (1968) Protein-losing gastroenteropathy and malabsorption associated with factitious diarrhea. Ann Intern Med 68:839–852

Herland AL, Lowenstein A (1957) Physiologic rehabilitation of the constipated colon in pregnant women: use of a standardized senna derivative. Q Rev Surg Obs Gynecol 14:196–202

Honig PJ, Holtzapple PG (1975) Hypocalcemic tetany following hypertonic phosphate enemas. Clin Pediatr 14:678–679

Houghton BJ, Pears MA (1958) Chronic potassium depletion due to purgation with cascara. Br Med J 1:1328–1330

Hubacher MH, Doernberg S (1964) Laxatives. II. Relationship between structure and potency. J Pharm Sci 53:1067–1072

Hurst AF (1919) Constipation and allied intestinal disorders, 2nd edn. Oxford University Press, London, pp 336–339

Hurst AF (1937) Constipation. In: Rolleston H (ed) The British encyclopaedia of medical practice, vol 3. Butterworth, London, pp 376–384

Hyland CM, Foran JD (1968) Dioctyl sodium sulphosuccinate as a laxative in the elderly. Practitioner 200:698–699

Illingworth RS (1953) Abnormal substances excreted in human milk. Practitioner 171:533–538

Jalan KN, Walker RJ, Prescott RJ, Butterworth STG, Smith AN, Sircus W (1970) Faecal stasis and diverticular disease in ulcerative colitis. Gut 11:688–696

Jansen JW, Kamp PE (1976) Het aantonen van bisacodyl in faeces en urine. Pharm Weekbl 111:164–166

Javert CT, Macri C (1941) Prothrombin concentration and mineral oil. Am J Obstet Gynecol 42:409–414

Jewell FC, Kline JR (1954) The purged colon. Radiology 62:368–371

Jones FA (1967) Cathartic colon. Proc R Soc Med 60:503–504

Jones FA, Godding EW (1972) Management of constipation. Blackwell, Oxford

Kaspi T, Royds RB, Turner P (1978) Qualitative determination of senna in urine. Lancet 1:1162

Kaupke C, Sprague T, Gitnick GL (1977) Hypernatremia after the administration of lactulose. Ann Intern Med 86:745–746

Kendall AC (1954) Fatal case of encephalitis after phenolphthalein ingestion. Br Med J 2:1461–1462

Korelitz BI, Janowitz HD (1960) Dilatation of the colon, a serious complication of ulcerative colitis. Ann Intern Med 53:153–163

Kramer P, Pope CE (1964) Factitious diarrhea induced by phenolphthalein. Arch Intern Med 114:634–636

Krejs GJ, Fordtran JS (1978) Physiology and pathophysiology of ion and water movement in the human intestine. In: Sleisenger MH, Fordtran JS (eds) Gastrointestinal disease, 2nd edn. Saunders, Philadelphia, pp 297–313

Krejs GJ, Walsh JH, Morawski SG, Fordtran JS (1977) Intractable diarrhea. Intestinal perfusion studies and plasma VIP concentrations in patients with pancreatic cholera syndrome and surreptitious ingestion of laxatives and diuretics. Am J Dig Dis 22:280–292

Kurlandsky L, Lukoff JY, Zinkham WH, Brody JP, Kessler RW (1979) Münchausen syndrome by proxy: definition of factitious bleeding in an infant by ^{51}Cr labelling of erythrocytes. Pediatrics 63:228–231

Large PG, Mukheiber WJ (1956) Injury to rectum and anal canal by enema syringes. Lancet 2:596–599

Laughlen GF (1925) Studies on pneumonia following nasopharyngeal injections of oil. Am J Path Bost 1:407–414

Lee DL (1979) Münchausen syndrome by proxy in twins. Arch Dis Child 54:646–647

Lennard-Jones JE, Langman MJS, Jones FA (1962) Faecal stasis in proctocolitis. Gut 3:301–305

Lennon GG (1957) Senna as a laxative. Br Med J 2:1438

Lesna M, Hamlyn AM, Venables CW, Record CO (1977) Chronic laxative abuse associated with pancreatic islet cell hyperplasia. Gut 18:1032–1035

Levine D, Goode AW, Wingate DL (1981) Purgative abuse associated with reversible cachexia, hypogammaglobulinaemia and finger clubbing. Lancet 1:919–920

Linquette M, Belbenoit C, May JP, Meerovich R (1964) Hypokaliemie par abus de laxaties. Retentissement renal. Lille Med 9:46–48

Litchfield JA (1959) Low potassium syndrome resulting from the use of purgative drugs. Gastroenterology 37:483–488

Long C (1961) Biochemists' handbook. Spon, London

Lou TC (1949) Biological assay of vegetable purgatives; senna leaf and fruit and their preparations. J Pharm Pharmacol 1:673–682

Love DR, Brown JJ, Fraser R, Lever AF, Robertson JIS, Tinsbury GC, Thomson S, Free M (1971) An unusual case of self-induced electrolyte depletion. Gut 12:284–290

McConnell TH (1971) Fatal hypocalcemia from phosphate absorption from laxative preparation. JAMA 216:147–148

MacHardy G, Balart LA (1970) Jaundice and oxyphenisatin. JAMA 211:83–85

Mahler RF, Stanbury SW (1956) Potassium – losing renal disease. Q J Med 25:21–52

Manning AP, Heaton KW, Harvey RF, Uglow P (1977) Wheat fibre and irritable bowel syndrome. Lancet 2:417–418

Marshak RH, Gerson A (1960) Cathartic colon. Am J Dig Dis 5:724–727

Mårtensson J (1953) Hypopotassaemia with paresis following the abuse of laxatives (in Swedish). Nord Med 49:56–57

Meadow R (1977) Münchausen syndrome by proxy: the hinterland of child abuse. Lancet 2:343–345

Meisel JL, Bergman D, Graney D, Saunders DR, Rubin CE (1977) Human rectal mucosa: proctoscopic and morphologic changes caused by laxatives. Gastroenterology 72:1274–1279

Metcalfe-Gibson A, Ing TS, Kuiper JJ, Richards P, Ward EE, Wrong OM (1967) In vivo dialysis of faeces as a method of stool analysis. II. The influence of diet. Clin Sci 33:89–100

Meulengracht E (1938) Osteomalacia of the spine following the abuse of laxatives. Lancet 2:774–776

Meulengracht E (1939) Osteomalacia of the spinal column from deficient diet or from disease of the digestive tract. III. Osteomalacia e abuse laxantium. Acta Med Scand 101:187–210

Misiewicz JJ, Waller SL (1966) Cathartic colon. Lancet 1:1263

Moriarty KJ, Fairclough PD, Clark ML, Dawson AM (1982) Inhibition of glucose and water absorption in the human jejunum by dioctyl sodium sulphosuccinate: a prostaglandin-mediated phenomenon? Gut 23:A443

Morris SM, Powell DW (1979) Spectrophotometric assay of phenolphthalein in biological fluids. Anal Biochem 95:465–471

Morson BC (1971) Histopathology of cathartic colon. Gut 12:867–868

Morson BC, Dawson IMP (1979) Gastrointestinal pathology. Blackwell, Oxford, pp 695–697

Naess K (1970) Oxyphenisatin and jaundice. JAMA 212:1961

Nixon HH (1961) Discussion on megacolon and megarectum with the emphasis on conditions other than Hirschsprung's disease. Proc R Soc Med 54:1037–1040

Owen EE, Verner JV Jr (1960) Renal tubular disease with muscle paralysis and hypokalemia. Am J Med 28:8–21

Painter NS (1972) Irritable or irritated bowel. Br Med J 2:46

Painter NS, Almeida AZ, Colebourne KW (1972) Unprocessed bran in treatment of diverticular disease of colon. Br Med J 2:137–140

Pearse AGE (1972) Histochemistry, theoretical and applied, 3rd edn. Churchill-Livingstone, Edinburgh, p 1091

Pearson AJG, Grainger JM, Scheur PJ, McIntyre N (1971) Jaundice due to oxyphenisatin. Lancet 1:994–996

Perkins JG, Petersen AB, Riley JA (1950) Renal and cardiac lesions in potassium deficiency due to chronic diarrhea. Am J Med 8:115–123

Phillips RA, Love AHG, Mitchell TG, Neptune EM Jr (1965) Cathartics and the sodium pump. Nature 206:1367–1368

Pick L (1911) Über die Melanose der Dickdarmschleimhaut. Berl Klin Wochenschr 48:840, 884

Pick N (1891) Colon pigmented black throughout with lead. Trans Path Soc Lond 42:109

Pickering LK, Kohl S (1981) Münchausen syndrome by proxy. Am J Dis Child 135:288

Piepmeyer JL (1974) Use of unprocessed bran in treatment of irritable bowel syndrome. Am J Clin Nutr 27:106–107

Pietsch JB, Shizgal HM, Meakins JL (1977) Injury by hypertonic phosphate enema. Can Med Assoc J 116:1169–1170

Pike BF, Phillippi PJ, Lawson EH (1971) Soap colitis. N Engl J Med 285:217–218

Plum GE, Weber HM, Sauer WG (1960) Prolonged cathartic abuse resulting in roentgen evidence suggestive of enterocolitis. Am J Roentgenol 83:919–925

Plumley PF (1973) Radical surgery in the treatment of cathartic colon. Proc R Soc Med 66:243–244

Ramirez B, Marieb NJ (1970) Hypokalemic metabolic alkalosis due to Carter's little liver pills. Conn Med 34:169–170

Rawson MD (1966) Cathartic colon. Lancet 1:1121–1124

Read NW, Harford WV, Schmulen AC, Read MG, Santa Ana C, Fordtran JS (1979) A clinical study of patients with fecal incontinence and diarrhea. Gastroenterology 76:747–756

Read NW, Krejs GJ, Read MG, Santa Ana C, Morawski SG, Fordtran JS (1980) Chronic diarrhea of unknown origin. Gastroenterology 78:264–271

Reynolds TB, Peters RL, Yamada S (1971) Chronic active and lupoid hepatitis caused by a laxative, oxyphenisatin. N Engl J Med 285:813–820

Reynolds TB, Lapin AC, Peters RL, Yamahiro HS (1970) Puzzling jaundice: probable relationship to laxative ingestion. JAMA 211:86–90

Ritchie JA, Truelove SC (1980) Comparison of various treatments for irritable bowel syndrome. Br Med J 281:1317–1319

Rowland CG, Rogers AG (1959) Rectal perforations after enema administration. Can Med Assoc J 81:815–818

Sagild U, Andersen V, Andreasen PB (1961) Glucose tolerance and insulin responsiveness in experimental potassium depletion. Acta Med Scand 169:243–251

Salm R, Hughes EW (1970) A case of chronic paraffin pneumonitis. Thorax 25:762–768

Schmid W (1952) Zum Wirkungsmechanismus diatetischer und medikamentöser Darmmittel. Arzneim Forsch 2:6–20

Schrodt GR (1963) Melanosis coli: a study with the electron microscope. Dis Colon Rectum 6:277–283

Schwartz WB, Relman AS (1953) Metabolic and renal studies in chronic potassium depletion resulting from overuse of laxatives. J Clin Invest 32:258–271

Sharaiha Z, Graham DY (1981) In vivo comparison of phenolphthalein and phenolphthalein glucuronide effect on rat ileum and colon. Gastroenterology 80:1281

Shields R, Mulholland AT, Elmslie RG (1966) Action of aldosterone upon the intestinal transport of potassium, sodium and water. Gut 7:686–696

Silk DBA, Gibson JA, Murray CRH (1975) Reversible finger clubbing in a case of purgative abuse. Gastroenterology 68:790–794

Sladen GE (1972) Effects of chronic purgative abuse. Proc R Soc Med 65:288–291

Smith B (1967) Myenteric plexus in Hirschsprung's disease. Gut 8:308

Smith B (1968) Effect of irritant purgatives on the myenteric plexus in man and the mouse. Gut 9:139–143

Smith B (1972) Pathology of cathartic colon. Proc R Soc Med 65:288

Smith D (1967) Severe anaphylactic reaction after a soap enema. Br Med J 4:215

Soper HW (1938) Phenolphthalein. Am J Dig Dis 5:297

Souter WA (1965) Bolus obstruction of gut after use of hydrophilic colloid laxatives. Br Med J 1:166–168

Speare GS (1951) Melanosis coli: experimental observations on its production and elimination in 23 cases. Am J Surg 82:631–637

Staffurth JS, Allott EN (1962) Paralysis and tetany due to simultaneous hypokalemia and hypocalcemia, with other metabolic changes. Am J Med 33:800–806

Stanbury SW (1958) Some aspects of disordered renal tubular function. Adv Intern Med 9:231–282

Steigmann F, Barnard RD, Dyniewicz JM (1938) Phenolphthalein studies: phenolphthalein in jaundice. Am J Med Sci 196:673–688

Stewart MJ, Hickman EM (1931) Observations on melanosis coli. J Path Bact 34:61–72

Swerdlow DB, Labow S, D'Anna J (1974) Tetany and enemas: report of a case. Dis Colon Rectum 17:786–787

Taylor EW, Bentley S, Youngs D, Keighley MRB (1981) Bowel preparation and the safety of colonoscopic polypectomy. Gastroenterology 81:1–4

Thompson WG (1979) Catharsis. In: Thompson WG (ed) The irritable gut. University Park Press, Baltimore, pp 107–124

Thompson WG, Heaton KW (1980) Functional bowel disorders in apparently healthy people. Gastroenterology 79:283–288

Todd IP (1973) Cathartic colon: surgical aspects. Proc R Soc Med 66:244–245

Tolman KG, Hammar S, Sannella JJ (1976) Possible hepatotoxicity of doxidan. Ann Intern Med 84:290–292

Travell J (1954) Pharmacology of stimulant laxatives. Ann NY Acad Sci 58:416–425

Turell R (1960) Laceration to anorectum incident to enema. Arch Surg 81:953–954

Vaisrub S (1978) Baron Münchausen and the abused child. JAMA 239:752

van Rooyen RJ, Ziady F (1972) Hypokalaemic alkalosis following the abuse of purgatives: case report. S Afr Med J 46:998–1003

Vecht-van den Bergh R (1979) Anorexia nervosa op oudere leeftijd. Ned Tijdschr Geneeskd 123:105–108

Verity CM, Winckworth C, Burman D, Stevens D, White RJ (1979) Polle syndrome: children of Münchausen. Br Med J 2:422–423

Voinchet O, Mouchet A (1974) Obstruction de l'oesophage par mucilage. Nouv Presse Med 3:1223–1225

Von Vámossy Z (1900) A phenolphthaleinröl mint a törköly-bor indicatoráról. Orv Hetil 44:144–146

Vyth A, Kamp PE (1979) Detection of anthraquinone laxatives in the urine. Pharm Weekbl (Sci Ed) 1:84–87

Waldmann TA (1961) Gastrointestinal protein loss demonstrated by Cr-51-labelled albumin. Lancet 2:121–123

Wands JR, Weiss SW, Yardley JH, Maddrey WC (1974) Chronic inorganic mercury poisoning due to laxative abuse. Am J Med 57:92–101

Williams CT (1867) Black deposit in the large intestine from the presence of mercury. Trans Path Soc London 18:111–116

Wittoesch JH, Jackman RJ, McDonald JR (1958) Melanosis coli: general review and a study of 887 cases. Dis Colon Rectum 1:172–180

Witts LJ (1937) Ritual purgation in modern medicine. Lancet 1:427–430

Wolff HP, Vecsei P, Krück F, Roscher S, Brown JJ, Düsterdieck GO, Lever AF, Robertson JIS (1968) Psychiatric disturbances leading to potassium depletion, sodium depletion, raised plasma renin concentration, and secondary hyperaldosteronism. Lancet 1:257–261

Wooton IDP (1964) Micro-analysis in medical biochemistry, 4th edn. Churchill, London

Wrong O, Metcalfe-Gibson A, Morrison RBI, Ng ST, Howard AV (1965) In vivo dialysis of faeces as a method of stool analysis. I. Technique and results in normal subjects. Clin Sci 28:357–375

Young JF, Brooke BN (1968) Enema shock in Hirschsprung's disease. Dis Colon Rectum 11:391–395

Zurrow HB, Sergay H (1966) Lipoid pneumonia in a geriatric patient. J Am Geriat Soc 14:240–243

CHAPTER 31

Intestinal Permeability Studies in Humans

K. Ewe, R. Wanitschke, and M. Staritz

A. Introduction

The intestinal mucosa separates the intestinal lumen from the interior milieu of the body. Substrate which enters the body has to pass this barrier. Anatomical and functional factors determine the permeability of the mucosa for the various substrates which may be different in site, extent or species. The permeation through the mucosa is achieved by several mechanisms such as active, facilitated or passive transport, persorption or pinocytosis; substances may also move from the blood to the intestinal lumen following physicochemical laws. Details of the processes pertaining to intestinal permeability are mainly derived from animal experiments and can only partially be applied to humans. However, there are several techniques which permit study of human intestinal permeability. These methods and their results will be discussed in this chapter.

B. Methods for Studying Intestinal Permeability in Humans

In humans, the possibilities of studying intestinal permeability are limited for obvious reasons, especially if specific transport mechanisms are involved. Traditional tolerance tests or balance studies can give only crude and approximate estimates of intestinal permeability. There are three main methods which are employed to study these questions more specifically:

(a) intestinal perfusion; (b) use of test molecules with different physicochemical properties, and (c) transmucosal electrical potential difference (PD).

The most direct way to approach these problems is the intestinal perfusion technique which has been applied extensively to study the many problems involved in intestinal permeability. The permeation of unmetabolized test molecules through the mucosa permits one to draw conclusions with regard to intestinal permeability if one relates the transfer to their physicochemical properties. Still another possibility of determining the characteristics of intestinal permeability in humans is the measurement of transmucosal electrical PD which reflects ion movement and may change with alterations of permeability caused by physiological conditions such as changes in luminal contents or else by drugs or diseases.

I. Intestinal Perfusion

The principle of the intestinal perfusion method is the determination of changes in substrate concentration at the beginning and the end of the test segment. From the disappearance (or appearance) rate the transfer of solute can be calculated. This can be achieved by transintestinal intubation (BLANKENHORN et al. 1955). Tubes are placed at the site of perfusion. Polyvinyl tubing can be cemented together and tubes of various numbers of lumina, diameter and arrangements can be constructed. When these tubes were used originally to measure absorption, an intestinal loop was occluded by two balloons and the test solution was instilled into the occluded segment, but the contents may leak past the balloons and it was difficult to empty the segment completely within a reasonable period of time. This difficulty was overcome by the introduction of nonabsorbable markers which permit one to calculate net fluid and solute movement from an aliquot of perfusate, and complete recovery of the instilled fluid is not necessary.

This technique was introduced by SCHEDL and CLIFTON (1961 a, b) (Fig. 1). A transintestinal tube was used which was interrupted at the perfusion site by a solid

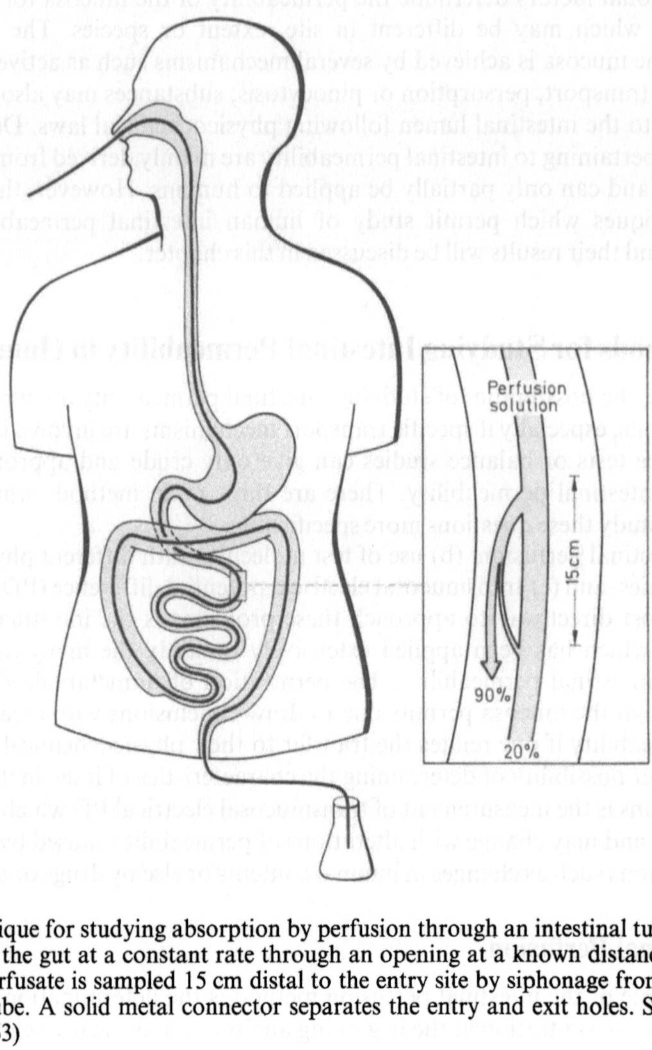

Fig. 1. Technique for studying absorption by perfusion through an intestinal tube. The solution enters the gut at a constant rate through an opening at a known distance from the nose. The perfusate is sampled 15 cm distal to the entry site by siphonage from the distal end of the tube. A solid metal connector separates the entry and exit holes. SCHEDL and CLIFTON (1963)

metal connector. The solute was perfused in the aborad direction and approximately 20% was recovered 15 cm caudally through the distal part of the tube. Later on, different types of tubes were proposed; e.g., with a proximal occluding balloon and others with a mixing segment.

Several problems emerge from intestinal perfusion (FORDTRAN 1966, 1969; LEVITT 1977; SLADEN 1968; SOERGEL 1971; WHALEN et al. 1966).

1. To express results of transport and permeability correctly it is necessary to relate the experimental data to mucosal surface area. This can be estimated only approximately by taking the length of the perfused segment because of some "sleaving" and telescoping, depending on the tone and contraction of the intestine.
2. Perfusate will flow in either direction, orad and aborad, and the length of the absorbing intestinal segment will be underestimated. Regurgitation may influence the results significantly as has been shown experimentally by MODIGLIANI et al. (1971, 1978).
3. The surface area of the perfused segment depends on the part of the bowel which is perfused apart from its length. The ratio of mucosal surface area of jejunum to ileum for a given length is about 2:1 (FISHER and PARSONS 1950).
4. The unstirred water layer is influenced by the perfusion rate. The increase of flow rate of the perfusate reduces the thickness of the unstirred layer, raising the substrate concentration at the mucosa and hence its absorption (DIETSCHY et al. 1971; MODIGLIANI and BERNIER 1971; REY et al. 1974).
5. Contamination of the perfusion area may occur from gastric, biliary, pancreatic and intestinal secretion. This will influence the values of flow rate, net water movement and ion composition of perfusate. In addition, secretagogue bile acids may influence net electrolyte and water movement (MEKHJION et al. 1971) although WINGATE et al. (1973 b) have shown that physiological amounts of lecithin in the bile abolish their effects on intestinal transfer.
6. In a perfused segment, concentration changes caused by solute transport proceed in an exponential rather than in a linear fashion, especially if substances are rapidly absorbed or secreted. This is usually not taken into account by conventional calculations.

These points have to be considered when results obtained by the perfusion technique are interpreted.

1. Types of Perfusion Tube

At present two main perfusion methods are employed in the small intestine: a multilumen tube with a proximal occluding balloon and a triple lumen tube including a mixing segmemt.

a) Multilumen Tube with a Proximal Occluding Balloon

We have introduced a multilumen tube which overcomes contamination by means of a proximal occluding balloon (Fig. 2; EWE and SUMMERSKILL 1965).

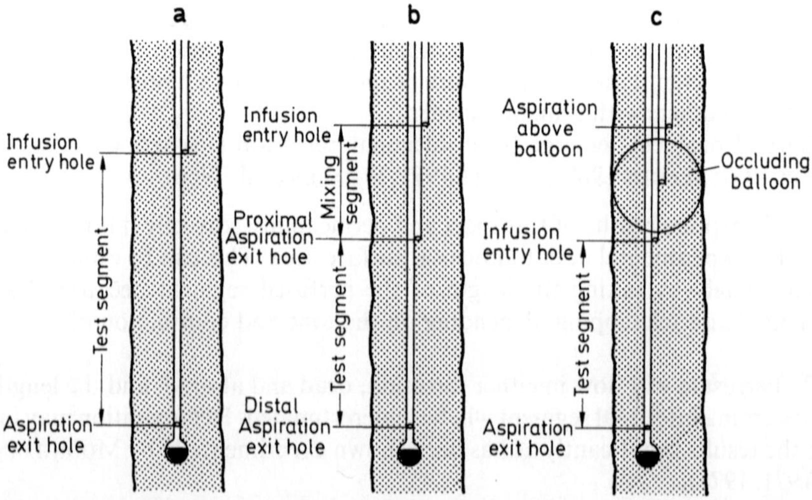

Fig. 2 a–c. Schematic view of human small intestinal absorption measurements by (**a**) double-lumen tube; (**b**) triple-lumen tube with mixing segment; and (**c**) double-lumen tube with proximal occluding balloon. MODIGLIANI et al. (1973)

Proximal to the balloon the contaminants are removed through one lumen of the tube. Although the balloon adds to the discomfort when swallowing the tube, it is usually not noticed once the tube is in place, especially if a vent ensures a constant pressure of 40 mmHg in the balloon, even if a bowel contraction occurs. This method also prevents proximal reflux (MODIGLIANI and BERNIER 1971). Concentration and composition of perfusate can thus be kept constant at the site of perfusion. Whether motility is stimulated by the balloon and blood supply of the perfused segment is influenced has been discussed, but comparison of results with the balloon inflated or deflated tends to show no difference (PHILLIPS and SUMMERSKILL 1966).

b) Triple Lumen Tube

The triple lumen tube allows the perfusate and contaminating fluids to mix in a "mixing segment", usually 10–15 cm in length (COOPER et al. 1966; FORDTRAN 1969; FORDTRAN et al. 1965; WHALEN et al. 1966). An aliquot sample is taken at the distal end of the mixing segment which at the same time is the starting point of the test segment of length 20–30 cm. From the difference in composition of the sample between the distal end of the mixing segment and of the distal part of the test segment the values of substrate transport and permeability are calculated. This method takes into account the contamination from above. The tube is simple, and conditions are comparatively physiological as gastrointestinal secretions are present in the intestine normally. To obtain reproducible results an equilibrium time of at least 30 min, optimally 60 min, is required (WHALEN et al. 1966). The major disadvantage of this method is that the composition of the perfusate will change in the mixing segment before it reaches the test segment and flow rate, which is composed of perfusion rate plus fasting intestinal contents, cannot be controlled exactly. When both methods – the triple lumen tube and the balloon tube – were tried in the same individuals, no significant difference was found in electrolyte and water movement (MODIGLIANI et al. 1978).

c) Perfusion of the Colon

Unlike the small intestine where only a segment is studied, usually the total colon is perfused when studying colonic transport and only occasionally segmental perfusion is performed (BILLICH and LEVITAN 1969; LEVITAN et al. 1962). The tube is monitored radiologically into the cecum which requires 1–3 days as a rule. Multilumen tubes are used by some, with openings above the distal end for proximal sampling of ileal contents (AMMON and PHILLIPS 1973; DEVROEDE and PHILLIPS 1969; MEKHJIAN et al. 1971) or an occluding balloon is attached above the distal perfusion openings which is held in place by the ileocecal valve and prevents contamination from above and also propulsion of the tube into the colon (EWE and HÖLKER 1974). The perfused solution is collected via a rectal catheter inserted 5–10 cm above the anal verge. Because of the length of the colon and its haustration and retrograde peristalsis, steady state conditions are usually not achieved before 1 h when a perfusion rate of 10 ml/min is used (DEVROEDE and PHILLIPS 1969) and small amounts of perfused drug (bisacodyl) were still present in the samples which were collected 2 h after bisacodyl-free solution was perfused (EWE and HÖLKER 1974). The same volume marker, polyethylene glycol (PEG) 4,000, is used as in small intestinal perfusion to account for net water movements.

2. Nonabsorbable Perfusion Marker

A reference marker is essential for the determination of intestinal permeability because luminal contents cannot be recovered completely. An ideal intestinal fluid marker has to possess several properties: it has to be nonabsorbable, it must be inert, stable and not be degraded nor trapped by mucus or substrate. It should not influence intestinal absorption or secretion nor motility and it should be measurable accurately and easily. It should not separate from the perfusate as is the case when water-soluble markers are used together with fat (WIGGINS and DAWSON 1961).

No ideal marker is known today but, PEG 4,000 fulfils most of these criteria. It is not absorbed to any significant extent, it is water soluble and does not bind to mucus (FORDTRAN 1966; JACOBSON et al. 1963; SCHEDL and CLIFTON 1962; WIGGINS and DAWSON 1961). It mixes with biological material for which it was originally used by HYDEN (1955). The accuracy of PEG as a volume marker was studied by various investigators in animal experiments and found to be satisfactory (JACOBSON et al. 1963; SCHEDL et al. 1966). The turbidimetric method for its quantitative determination is relatively complicated, but the method was greatly simplified by the introduction of ^{14}C (WINGATE et al. 1972) or ^{3}H-labelled PEG (KRAG et al. 1975). The commonly used concentration of PEG is 5 g/l. DAVIS et al. (1980) described an influence of this and higher concentrations on electrolyte and water movement which was attributed to an osmotic effect, although this is difficult to explain as for instance 4 g/l PEG 4,000 should constitute only 1 mosmol.

Other markers were used such as polyvinylpyrrolidone (PVP), which binds to mucus (SCHEDL and CLIFTON 1962), or phenol red, which is less stable and is absorbed more than PEG. Moreover, bile contamination of perfusate requires correction by measuring it at three different wavelengths (SCHEDL and CLIFTON 1961 b). Other markers which are less commonly used are bromsulphtalein, indocyanine green and chromic chloride (DONALDSON and BARRERAS 1965; FORDTRAN et al. 1961; WORNING and AMDRUP 1965).

II. Intestinal Permeability Studied by Test Molecules

Although only global information on intestinal permeability can be derived from the passage of test molecules through the mucosa and their excretion in the urine, this method is widely used in clinical practice because of its practicability, the D-xylose and vitamin B_{12} absorption test being the most popular. In addition, uptake and excretion of other macromolecules has been studied to define permeability characteristics of the small intestine in health and disease. Some studies on intestinal secretion of macromolecules have been performed which follow the opposite way, namely from blood to the gut lumen.

An ideal "intestinal permeability probe" as formulated by CHADWICK et al. (1977 a) should have the following properties:

1. Its transmucosal transport should follow first-order kinetics.
2. It should be excreted rapidly, completely and unchanged in the urine after absorption.
3. It should be nontoxic, not degraded by intestinal bacteria, and not metabolized after absorption.
4. It should be a mixture of inert water-soluble molecules of varying sizes.
5. It should be measurable with sensitivity, precision, accuracy and ease in biological fluids.

No ideal marker exists, and their advantages, disadvantages and use in permeability testing will be discussed in the following section.

1. D-Xylose

D-Xylose is a pentose which is absorbed by the same transport mechanism as hexoses such as glucose and galactose, but its affinity for this carrier system is much less. Because of the relative impermeability of the intestine for xylose it discriminates more clearly between normal and abnormal absorption than would other test substances which are absorbed more efficiently and whose absorption would not be impaired with moderate degrees of malabsorption. Approximately 60% of D-xylose is absorbed when 25 g is given in 500 ml solution within 5 h, as has been estimated by an intestinal intubation and nonabsorbable marker (PEG) technique (FORDTRAN et al. 1962). It was found that 90% of the total xylose absorption occurred in the upper 160 cm of the jejunum and, thus, this test reflects the absorptive capacity of the upper part of the gut. Xylose is metabolized to a certain extent, and only about half of what has been absorbed or has been given intravenously is excreted in the urine. Normal renal function is a prerequisite for its reliability. The slight decrease in D-xylose excretion in the older age group can be attributed to a mild reduction of renal function in the elderly (KENDALL 1970). Another source of error may be bacterial overgrowth in the jejunum as D-xylose is metabolized by bacterial enzymes (GOLDSTEIN et al. 1970).

After an oral load of 25 g xylose in 500 ml fluid, an average of 6.7 g (26.6%) will be excreted in the urine, as calculated from 12 reports (EWE 1976). In nontropical sprue, D-xylose excretion is significantly decreased while excretion of larger test molecules is significantly increased. This apparent paradox will be discussed in Sect. B.II.3.b. Absorptive dysfunction of the lower ileum such as in Crohn's disease is not reflected by the D-xylose test (FOWLER and COOKE 1969; GERSON et al. 1973). Although the reliability of the D-xylose test has been questioned repeatedly (KRAWITT and BEEKEN 1975; SLADEN and KUMAR 1973), it is still commonly used for screening upper intestinal malabsorption.

2. Vitamin B_{12}

Unlike xylose, vitamin B_{12} is mainly absorbed in the distal part of the small intestine. It is the largest essential nutrient and has a molecular weight of 1,360. Its molecular diameter is about 10 Å, but it increases to approximatively 44 Å if it is attached to intrinsic factor. Permeability of the intestine for vitamin B_{12} is low, but it shares the peculiarity with bile acids of being absorbed in a part of the small intestine which is less permeable than the upper part. Table 1 (from WILSON 1962) demonstrates the differences in the capacity of human intestine to absorb different nutrients. How and where the large vitamin B_{12}–intrinsic factor complex penetrates the mucosal surface is not exactly known, however, the intrinsic factor probably does not pass into the enterocyte, but releases the vitamin before. If used as an absorption test (Schilling test), vitamin B_{12} has to be given together with 50 mg intrinsic factor to rule out intrinsic factor deficiency. Ileal resection and Crohn's disease are the most common causes which lead to vitamin B_{12} malabsorption. The length of diseased ileum correlates with vitamin B_{12} malabsorption; we found that vitamin B_{12} absorption was highly pathological and even below values observed in pernicious anaemia, if most of the terminal ileum was inflamed or resected (EWE et al. 1971). This was confirmed by GERSON et al. (1973) who determined as a cut-off point for pathological vitamin B_{12} absorption 90 cm of diseased or resected ileum.

A dose of 0.5–1 μCi vitamin B_{12} ^{57}Co is given orally in 50 ml water and 2 h later a flushing dose of 1,000 μg vitamin B_{12} is applied intramuscularly ^{57}Co is counted in 24-h urine samples. Normally 8%–30% is excreted which is one-third to one-quarter of the absorbed dose. Absorption of vitamin B_{12} is a good example of the dual mechanism by which a substance may permeate through the intestinal mucosa: by a specific carrier-mediated absorption which is very efficient and by a concentration-dependent passive mechanism. The latter allows absorption of about 1% from pharmacological doses in the milligram range.

While serum levels of radiocobalt-labelled vitamin B_{12} increased substantially after a delay of 4 h with the intrinsic factor-mediated transfer in the ileum, ab-

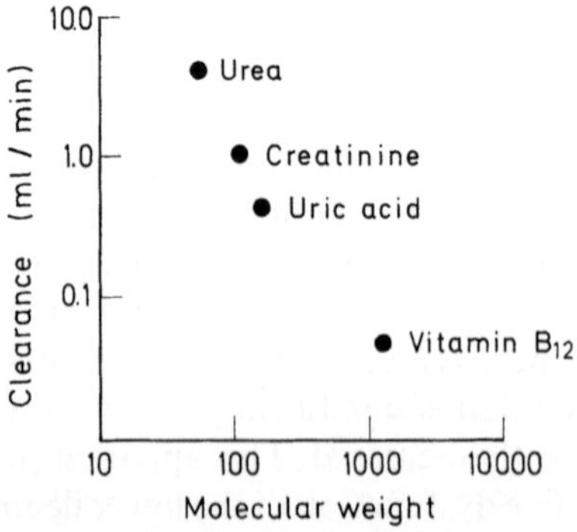

Fig. 3. Clearance compared with molecular weight (double-logarithmic plot). LOEHRY et al. (1973)

Table 1. Comparison of transport capacity for different nutrients

Substance	Absorptive capacity in humans	
	(g/day)	(m*M*/day)
Water[a]	18,000	1,000,000
Glucose[b]	3,600	20,000
Amino acids[c]	600	5,000
Triglycerides[d]	700	900
Cholesterol	4	10
Iron[e]	0.012	0.2
Vitamin B_{12}	0.000001	0.000001

[a] BORGSTRÖM et al. (1957) found 500 ml test meal diluted to 1,500–2,500 in duodenum and mostly resorbed at the level of the midgut. This amounted to absorption of about 1,500 ml in 4 h in one half of the intestine. This value was multiplied by 12 to obtain the value in the table

[b] 250 mg glucose fed to human subjects is probably completely absorbed in 3–4 h and probably only in the first half of the gut

[c] BORGSTRÖM et al. (1957) found 25 g protein completely absorbed in upper quarter of gut in 4 h. Average mole weight taken as about 120

[d] 30 g corn oil absorbed in upper quarter of gut in 4 h

[e] Of 100 mg dose, 12 mg absorbed

[f] Vitamin B_{12} absorbing mechanism is saturated at about 1.5 µg. It should be emphasized that these calculations are extremely rough approximations because of the many assumptions which must be made

sorption of vitamin B_{12} without binding to intrinsic factor occurred shortly after ingestion from a high dose of 100 µg in patients with pernicious anaemia, rising steadily over 4 h (DOSCHERHOLMEN et al. 1959). Therefore, vitamin B_{12} may be absorbed by either mechanism. A dose of 50 µg has been selected as a "watershed" between these processes (WITTS 1961). In the case of vitamin B_{12} absorption was 81% from 1 µg, 22% from 5 µg, 3% from 50 µg, and about 1% from 100 µg and above. Thus, both principles overlapped: specific, carrier-dependent transport prevailing at low substrate concentrations, and passive, concentration-dependent transfer at high concentrations. Transfer of vitamin B_{12} from blood to gut lumen is also low. This has also been shown in humans (LOEHRY et al. 1973). Vitamin ^{68}Co was given intravenously and collected from upper jejunum by intestinal intubation. When vitamin B_{12} clearance was compared with the clearance of smaller solutes such as uric acid or creatinine an inverse relationship between clearance and molecular size was demonstrated (Fig. 3; LOEHRY et al. 1973).

3. Other Test Substances

a) Polyethylene Glycol

Low molecular weight PEG 400 has been used as "an intestinal permeability probe" (CHADWICK et al. 1977 b). The molecular weight of PEG ranged from 242 to 594. A dose of 10 g was infused through a nasointestinal tube into the upper jejunum, ileum or colon, and 6-h urine samples were analysed quantitatively and qualitatively for PEG 400. The larger the molecule, the lower was the absorption in either part of the intestine (Fig. 4). There was, however, a striking difference

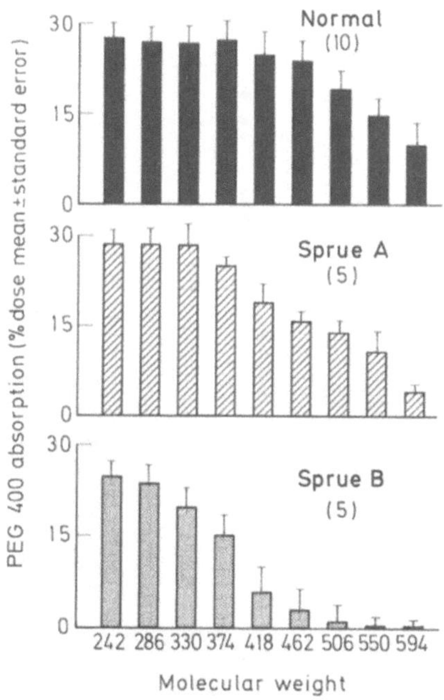

Fig. 4. Comparison of absorption and molecular weight for PEG 400 in ten normal subjects and ten patients with coeliac sprue. Percentage absorption of each molecular weight component was assessed by urinary recovery over 6 h after administration of 10 g PEG 400 by mouth. Group A patients had gained more than 5% in body weight and group B less than 5% after treatment with a gluten-free diet. CHADWICK et al. (1977 b)

between the different intestinal areas. For instance, absorption of larger PEG molecules (molecular weight 462–594) ranged from 19% to 9.5% in the jejunum, from 9.3% to 0.7% in the ileum and from 1.3% to 0% in the colon. Thus, permeability decreased markedly from the proximal to the distal part of the gut. Dihydroxy bile acids increased and nontropical sprue decreased permeability.

b) High Molecular Weight Mono- and Oligosaccharides

Oligosaccharides are very slowly metabolized after reaching the bloodstream. They are almost quantitatively excreted in the urine. This has been shown for stachyose, raffinose, lactulose, melibiose, lactose, paltinose, and sucrose in humans (MENZIES 1974). Human mucosa lacks hydrolytic activity for the disaccharides melibiose and lactulose, the trisaccharide raffinose, and the tetrasaccharide stachyose (MENZIES 1974; WHALEN et al. 1966), and these carbohydrates have therefore been used for testing intestinal permeability in health and disease as have mannitol and cellobiose (COBDEN et al. 1978; GORDON et al. 1972; HAMILTON et al. 1982; YOUNG et al. 1980). Again, permeability of these markers was dependent on molecular weight in healthy adults and a profile of restricted permeability could be described for these markers, including dextran (molecular weight 3,000) (WHEELER et al. 1978). If the same solutions were made hypertonic by adding glycerol, a large increase in permeability was found (Fig. 5). A similar increase in per-

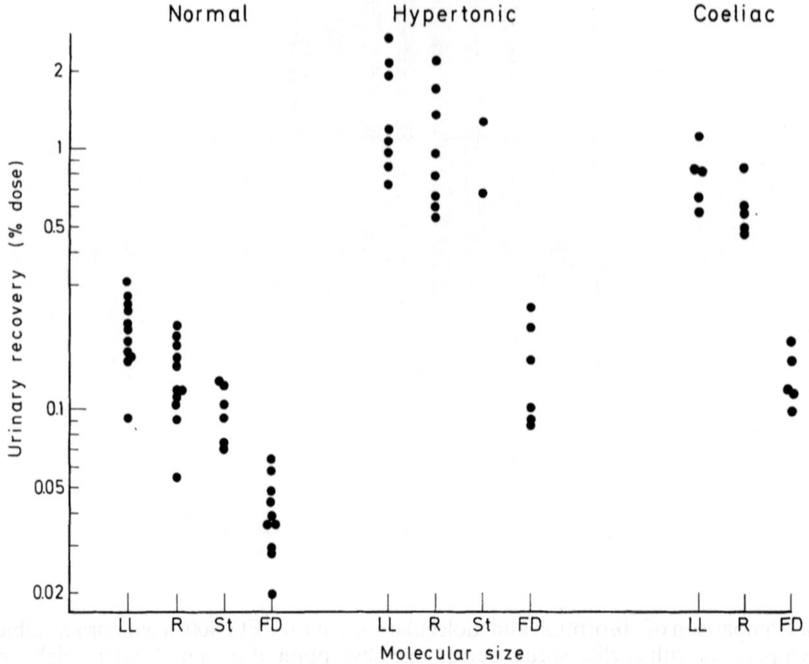

Fig. 5. Percentage urinary recovery of permeability markers over 5 h in normal subjects, hypertonic experiments and coeliac disease after oral ingestion. *LL*, lactulose; *R*, raffinose; *St*, stachyose; *FD*, fluorescein isothiocyanate dextran. WHEELER et al. (1978)

meability was seen spontaneously in patients with coeliac disease which will be discussed in Sect. E.I. Similarly, more mannitol (molecular radius 4 Å), namely about 20%, was excreted in the urine than was the disaccharide cellobiose (molecular radius 5 Å), of which only approximately 0.5% was excreted.

c) Test Molecules Used in Exudative Enteropathies

Gastrointestinal leakage of plasma proteins into the gut can be detected by a variety of labelled macromolecules such as dextran ^{59}Fe (HOYUMPA et al. 1976) and PVP I^{131} of PVP I^{125} (GORDON 1959) which are not split by digestive enzymes; or by isotopes of albumin ^{51}Cr (WALDMANN 1961), caeruloplasmin ^{67}Cu (WALDMANN et al. 1967) or albumin ^{95}Nb (JEEJEEHOY et al. 1965) which are poorly absorbed by the alimentary tract after being split off in the intestinal lumen.

Many diseases are potentially associated with exudative enteropathy (JARNUM 1962; JEFFRIES 1978), and mechanisms leading to protein loss vary considerably with different diseases. In most of them, exudation of protein is not based on increased intestinal permeability. In intestinal lymphangiectasia, for instance, protein exudation includes serum proteins of different molecular weights, immunoglobulins as well as albumin and even formed particles such as lymphocytes (STROBER et al. 1967), probably owing to damage and rupture of dilated intestinal lacteals. Protein exudation from ulcerative lesions such as in Crohn's disease or ulcerative colitis is another example of intestinal plasma protein loss independent of intestinal permeability.

On the other hand, in normal humans some plasma protein leaks into the gastrointestinal tract physiologically (for review see ALPERS and KINZIE 1973). It has been estimated by WETTERFORSS et al. (1960) that 6–8 g, i.e. 30%–50%, of the daily albumin catabolism takes place in the intestinal lumen, whereas other investigators conclude that the gut plays a less important role in plasma protein metabolism (FRANKS et al. 1963). Normally, there seems to be a high degree of selectivity of exudation of plasma proteins in relation to their molecular weight, as studied by intravenous injection of PVP ^{125}I and intestinal recovery by perfusion (KINGHAM and LOEHRY 1978). Smaller molecules of the PVP mixture (molecular weight 8,000–80,000) were cleared to a much greater extent than the larger molecules (see Sect. B.II.3.b). This selectivity was lost in patients with Crohn's disease and with sprue and exudative enteropathy. It is suggested that the abnormality of the epithelial cells leads to an increase in permeability, but not a change in selectivity. Changes of the basement membrane are believed to account for the loss of selectivity of the small intestinal protein exudation, as is the case in coeliac disease (KINGHAM and LOEHRY 1978).

III. Electrical Transmucosal Potential Difference

Ion movement across the gastrointestinal mucosa contributes to generate an electrical PD. Transport potentials arise from active ion transport, and diffusion potentials are formed by diffusion of ions down electricochemical gradients across membranes of different permeability characteristics for cations and anions (see Sect. C.II).

1. Origin of PD and Relation to Intestinal Permeability

The precise origin of the PD is not completely understood. It seems to be generated in the epithelial layer of the mucosa, predominantly by active ion transport across membranes of different permeabilities. It is generally accepted that Na^+ is the most important ion in this regard while anion secretion will further contribute to the negativey of the luminal site (ARCHAMPONG and EDMONDS 1972; COOPERSTEIN and BROCKMAN 1959; DALMARK 1970). The complexity of electrical phenomena is reflected by the fact that the interior of the cell is electrically negative with respect to both the serosal and the luminal membrane, but the integral transmucosal PD is luminal side negative and serosal side positive.

If permeability of the mucosa is high, ion selectivity decreases, ions will flow back along the electrical gradient, and the PD will be low. Electrical resistance of the mucosa is mainly related to the permeability of the paracellular shunt pathway which accounts for more than 90% of transmucosal conduction (SCHULTZ 1977). Therefore, the PD is low in the upper small intestine and rises distally. It is self-evident that the presence of a pathway that permits rapid transepithelial ionic diffusion essentially precludes the presence of large transepithelial electrical PDs secondary to transcellular active ion (primarily Na^+) transport and the development of significant sustained transepithelial ion gradients during the absorptive process. In humans, the PD in the jejunum with isotonic saline or in the resting state is around zero or slightly negative from the luminal to the serosal side and reaches -10 mV if glucose is added (FORDTRAN et al. 1968; TURNBERG et al. 1970; WINGATE et al. 1973a).

2. Methodology

PD is measured in humans either by catheters perfused by electrolyte solutions or by agar bridges, i.e. catheters filled with agar-agar which has been boiled with saturated KCl solution. The recording electrode is inserted into the lumen of the bowel. The reference electrode cannot be placed at the serosa of the intestine in humans for obvious reasons. GEALL et al. (1970) have established that peripheral blood is equivalent to the intestinal serosa as a site for the reference electrode. Other authors prefer subcutaneous placement of the reference electrode after previous infiltration of the skin with normal saline solution (ARCHAMPONG and EDMONDS 1972).

Factors which may disturb PD measurement and may give rise to artifacts are: motility moving the electrode in the lumen; air bubbles or other interruptions in the tube; and liquid junction potentials. The latter may originate if solutes of different ionic strength and concentration come into contact with each other. This is the case in the stomach, it may be of some inportance in the small intestine where the PD is low, but it does not play a role in the large intestine (READ and FORDTRAN 1978). Junction potentials may be corrected by a formular of BARRY and DIAMOND (1970).

3. Application of PD Measurements in Humans

Different parameters of small intestinal permeability have been studied in the small intestine in humans by measuring PD differences under various conditions.

Unstirred water layer thickness was estimated by PD measurements during kinetic studies of electrogenic glucose absorption (READ et al. 1977), and cation permselectivity from PD changes during osmotically induced intraluminal directed flow (GUSTKE et al. 1981) (see Sect. C.II). Because interpretation of small changes of the low PD in the jejunum is difficult and because of artifacts such as those caused by motility (BROWN et al. 1976), propantheline bromide has been used to abolish these unwanted effects (BROWN et al. 1976; READ et al. 1974, 1976).

Difficulties are considerably less in the colon and rectum. The lower colon is most impermeable to ions, and hardly any backdiffusion of sodium occurs in this part of the gut, in contrast to the upper small intestine (BILLICH and LEVITAN 1969; FORDTRAN et al. 1965). This is reflected by a high rectal PD of 25–40 mV (EWE and WANITSCHKE 1980). Factors affecting active or passive transfer mechanisms (i.e. permeability) such as diseases or drugs can be measured comparatively simply because of the high original PD and the easy access to this area.

C. Permeability Characteristics of the Human Gut

I. Studies Employing Intestinal Intubation and Perfusion

1. Intestinal Sampling After Test Meals

Intubation studies in humans have shown that the permeability of the proximal intestine must be very high. In these studies different kinds of meal were given and samples taken along the small intestine, net water movement being taken into account by using PEG as nonabsorbable marker.

After a slightly hypotonic steak meal (232 mosmol/kg) or a hypertonic milk and doughnuts meal (630 mosmol/kg) isotonicity was practically reached after the passage of the duodenum (FORDTRAN and LOCKLEAR 1966). Osmotically active organic constituents had been replaced mainly by NaCl in a concentration which reached plasma levels at the proximal jejunum (Fig. 6). BORGSTRÖM et al. (1957) followed the disappearance of different constituents of a test meal containing corn oil (74 g), skimmed milk powder (126 g) and glucose (138 g). They found that 20% of glucose was absorbed after passing the duodenum, but practically all glucose had disappeared by the time the mid-small bowel had been reached. The same applied to fat and protein (BERGSTRÖM et al. 1957; FORDTRAN and LOCKLEAR 1966).

Recently a liquid formula diet of various amounts of carbohydrates (polycose, a glucose polymer, sucrose and glucose) and osmolalities (337, 519, 669 mosmol/kg) was tested. Most carbohydrates were hydrolysed and absorbed in the duodenum (65%–82%) and all but about 10% was absorbed in the proximal 30 cm of jejunum (RUPPIN et al. 1981).

2. Determination of the Reflection Coefficient

Nonlipid solutes and water may penetrate the intestinal mucosa by two main routes: (a) through aqueous channels or "pores"; and (b) by a membrane carrier system. The anatomical site of the paracellular shunt pathway through channels or "pores" is generally believed to be located at the tight junction between two

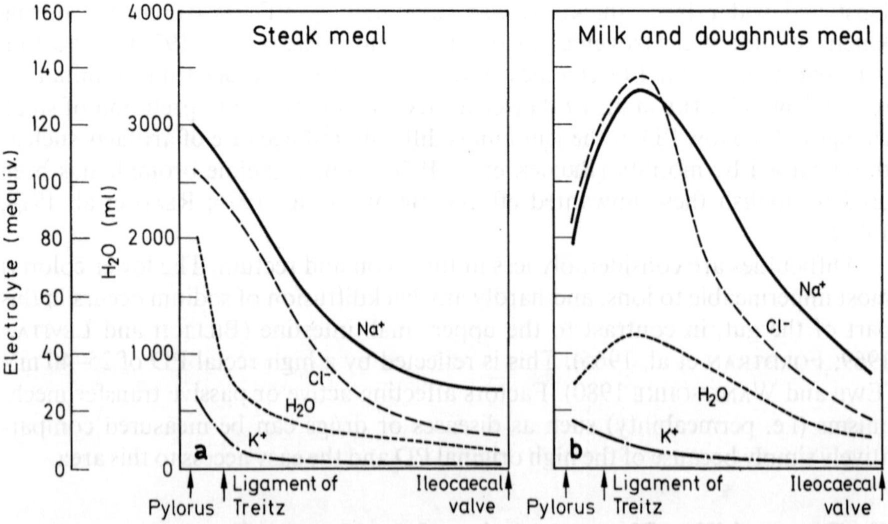

Fig. 6 a, b. Amounts of electrolytes and water passing different levels of the small intestine after a steak meal (**a**) and a doughnut meal (**b**). After FORDTRAN and LOCKLEAR (1966)

adjacent enterocytes (FORDTRAN and DIETSCHY 1966; WHALEN et al. 1966). In humans, the effective pore size has been calculated for different levels of small in testine and colon by perfusing solutions of various nonlipid-soluble solutes and different reflection coefficients (BILLICH and LEVITAN 1969; FORDTRAN et al. 1965).

The theoretical basis for this calculation rests on the demonstration of the ability of these osmotically active solutes to exert an effective pressure gradient across a membrane in relation to the molecular radius of the solute and the radius of water-filled channels or pores across this membrane. Calculated and measured osmotic pressure of a semipermeable membrane should be identical, and the reflection coefficient $R_f = 1$ if the radius of the solute exceeds the radius of the channel. If the solute moves as freely as water, R_f will approach 0. If some of the solute passes the membrane, the effective osmotic pressure will be smaller than calculated (SOLOMON 1960). The effective osmotic pressure divided by the theoretical osmotic pressure has been defined as the reflection coefficient by STAVERMAN (1951).

FORDTRAN et al. (1965) have determined water movement in response to osmotic gradients created by perfusing practically nonabsorbable mannitol or smaller nonlipid solutes such as urea, erythritol and NaCl. From the difference in bulk water flow for mannitol and the smaller solutes the individual reflection coefficients can be calculated. A further relationship exists between reflection coefficient and membrane pore radius (RENKIN 1954; SOLOMON 1960).

Reflection coefficients were low in the upper jejunum (FORDTRAN et al. 1965): the volume (ml) of water "pulled" in 1 min by 1 mosmol from hypertonic urea, erythritol and NaCl solution divided by the corresponding rate (ml/min) per mosmol of hypertonic mannitol (R_f) was 0.48 for urea; 0.64 for erythritol and 0.58 for NaCl. R_f approached 1.0 in the ileum (0.89 urea; 0.89 erythritol; 0.95 NaCl).

The pore radius calculated from these results was 6.7–8.8 Å for the jejunum and 3.0–3.8 Å in the ileum. The difference in pore size was also reflected by a ninefold higher net water flow into the jejunum than into the ileum secondary to the same osmotic gradient. In a similar study analogous diameters were calculated by SOERGEL et al. (1968) namely 7.9 Å and 2.9 Å for the pore radius of the upper and lower small intestine. In contrast to these results, the differences in the rates of unidirectional diffusion of water were not much different in the jejunum and ileum (WHALEN et al. 1966). One reason for this discrepancy could be that the diffusion of water is proportional to the second power, but bulk flow is proportional to the fourth power of the radius of the pore, according to Poiseuille's Law (FORDTRAN et al. 1965; PAPPENHEIMER et al. 1951).

To calculate the pore radius in the colon, a similar study was performed by BILLICH and LEVITAN (1969). The results confirmed the observation dating back to GOLDSCHMIDT and DAYTON (1919), that the colon is less permeable than the small intestine. Urea was not absorbed, and the reflection coefficient in the colon was 1.0 for mannitol and urea as well. As the molecular radius of urea is 2.3 Å, it may be concluded that the equivalent pore size of the human colon is less than 2.3 Å.

The difference in filtration coefficient for hypertonic solutions of 800 mosmol containing mannitol and 140–150 mequiv./l NaCl points into the same direction: It amounted to 0.044 ml min^{-1} $mosmol^{-1}$ in a 20-cm jejunal and 0.005 ml min^{-1} $mosmol^{-1}$ in a 20-cm ileal test segment (FORDTRAN et al. 1965), but only 0.0007 ml min^{-1} $mosmol^{-1}$ for the whole colon (BILLICH and LEVITAN 1969). Na^+ was absorbed against a lumen–blood gradient of 140 mequiv./l in the colon (BILLICH and LEVITAN 1969) and of 110 mequiv./l in the ileum, but of only 17 mequiv./l in the jejunum (FORDTRAN et al. 1968).

Little is known about the permeability characteristics of different parts of the colon (BILLICH and LEVITAN 1969). It seems that the permeability of the proximal colon approaches that of the terminal ileum (BILLICH and LEVITAN 1969; LEVITAN et al. 1962), whereas the rectosigmoid is "tight". In the study of BILLICH and LEVITAN (1969) some preliminary data were given concerning this question: In the perfused colon with a total length of 75–85 cm, 65% of the total decline of osmolalities of a hypertonic test solution occurred over the first 10 cm, 87% over 20 cm, and 97% over the proximal 40 cm.

3. Polyethylene Glycol 400 Perfusion

These differences in permeability of different parts of the human intestine were confirmed by a different technique using low molecular weight polyethylene glycols perfused at different levels of the gut (CHADWICK et al. 1977b). PEG 400 (molecular weight 252–594) was perfused through a 30-cm segment of upper jejunum, proximal ileum, and the whole colon. The larger the molecule, the lower was the absorption in either part of the intestine. There were, however, striking differences along the intestinal tract (Fig. 7). For instance, absorption of larger molecules of the PEG mixture (molecular weight 462–594) were 19.0%–9.5% in the jejunum, 3.0%–0.7% in the ileum and 1.3%–0% in the colon. Thus, permeability decreased markedly from the proximal to the distal part of the gut.

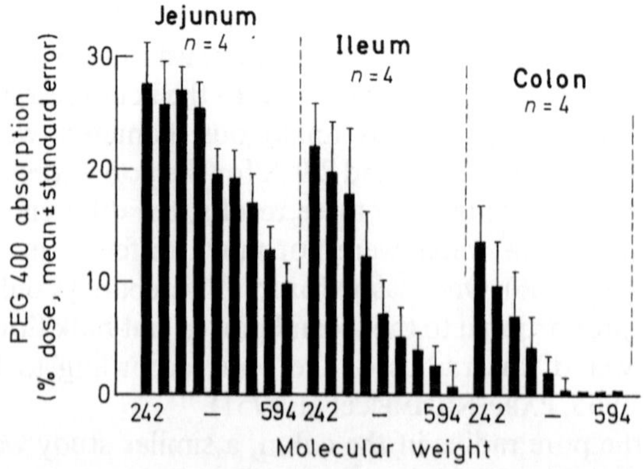

Fig. 7. Comparison of absorption and molecular weight in humans for PEG 400 after regional infusions via nasointestinal tube at the proximal jejunum (ligament of Treitz), proximal ileum (180 cm from the nose), and caecum. Percentage absorption of each molecular weight component was assessed by urinary recovery over 6 h after bolus infusion of 10 g PEG 400 in four normal subjects. CHADWICK et al. (1977 b)

II. Selectivity of Cation Permeability

Another feature of the tight junction complex relating to intestinal permeability is cation selectivity. Section C.II was concerned with solute movement, regardless of its electrical charge. It has been shown in animal experiments that the intestine is more permeable to cations than to anions (FRIZZEL and SCHULTZ 1972; WRIGHT and DIAMOND 1968). It has been postulated that the lining of the tight junctions or "pores" or "channels" contain fixed negative charges such as carboxylic and phosphate groups which repel anions and facilitate cation permeation.

In humans, selectivity of cation permeability of jejunum and ileum has been calculated from the effects of passive ion diffusion on transmucosal electrical PD. Different rates of solute flow through the mucosa were evoked by using various isotonic (280 mosmol/kg) and hypertonic (908 mosmol/kg) solutions containing either NaCl or mannitol or both (GUSTKE et al. 1981).

The ratio of permeability $p_{\text{anion}}:p_{\text{cation}}$ was 0.816 : 1 for the jejunum and 0.220 : 1 for the ileum. This indicates that anion movement through the mucosa is restricted as compared with cations and that the discrimination is much more pronounced in the ileum than in the jejunum.

III. Transcellular Intestinal Permeability

Permeability of the mucosa for a large variety of substances depends, among other factors, on their mode of transport. Different transport mechanisms and carrier systems have been proposed which are discussed in more detail elsewhere in this book. To demonstrate the possibilities of characterizing transport mechanisms in humans, some examples are given in Sect. C.III.1.

The term "active transport" implies that the substrate to be transported is taken up by some kind of a transport system generally referred to as a "carrier". Receptor sites of the carrier are usually limited in number and saturable, similar to enzymes. Hence, many attempts at quantitative expression of carrier-mediated intestinal absorption are based on terms drawn from enzymology.

1. Calculation of Intestinal Absorption Kinetics in Humans

Perfusion studies permit one to determine net water movement and concentration changes of substances in the lumen and to calculate the rate of absorption over a defined area of intestine at a known period of time. From these data it is possible to calculate intestinal absorption kinetics in humans. The mathematical model commonly used is that of Michaelis and Menten who applied this kind of analysis to the study of sucrose hydrolysis by invertase. The term "Michaelis–Menten kinetics has long been used in enzymology and was first adopted for intestinal transport by FISHER and PARSONS (1953).

If v (g cm^{-1} min^{-1} or mol cm^{-1} min^{-1}) is the rate of this process, v_{max} the maximum rate possible and C the substrate concentration, the relation between these factors can be expressed by the equation

$$v = \frac{v_{max}\, C}{C + Km},$$

where K_m is a constant. To illustrate this relationship, the results of the perfusion study of HOLDWORTH and DAWSON (1964, 1965) on glucose, galactose and fructose absorption is demonstrated (Fig. 8). At the lower end of the curve, absorp-

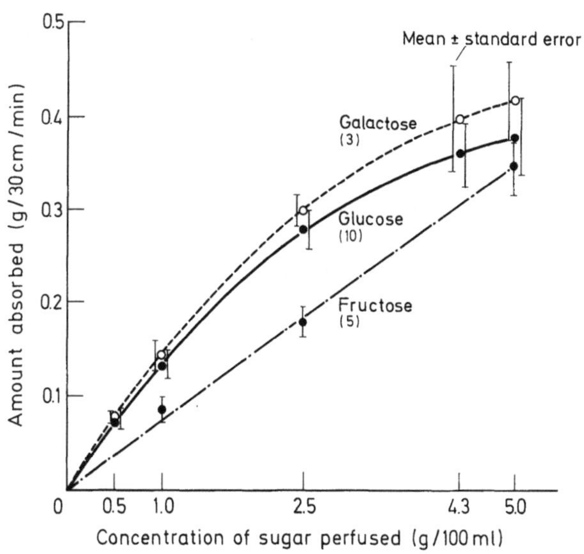

Fig. 8. Absorption of glucose, galactose, and fructose in normal subjects. Figures in parentheses indicate number of subjects in each group (intestinal perfusion; flow rate 20 ml/min). HOLDWORTH and DAWSON (1965)

tion rate v is nearly proportional to concentration C for all three sugars, a relationship called "first-order kinetics". At the top of the curve, absorption rate remains concentration dependent for fructose, but is becoming independent of concentration for glucose and galactose, a relationship called "zero-order kinetics". Hence, there is a gradual transition from first-order kinetics at low concentration to zero-order kinetics at high concentrations for glucose and galactose, while first-order kinetics is maintained by fructose.

Another quantity which can be derived from the Michaelis–Menten curve is the concentration of substrate which enables the process to proceed at half-maximum concentration K_m and the maximum rate itself v_{max}. These two values, K_m and v_{max}, are often used to characterize transport systems. The most popular way to determine the values of K_m and v_{max} is the plot of the reciprocals of rate and concentration introduced by LINEWEAVER and BURK (1934)

$$\frac{1}{v} = \frac{1}{C} \frac{k}{v_{max}} + \frac{1}{v_{max}}.$$

It is claimed by some authors that unstirred layer effects influence transport and permeability kinetics: "The application of the Michaelis–Menten equations with use of reciprocal plots to derive values for K_m and J^n is not only theoretically incorrect but, in addition, this manipulation introduces yet other errors into the determination of K_m and J^n" (THOMSON and DIETSCHY 1977).[1]

2. Examples of Determining Absorption Kinetics in Humans

From the given example (Fig. 8) the Lineweaver–Burk plot can be derived (Fig. 9) and v_{max} and K_m can be determined. From this experiment v_{max} of glucose was 0.67 g and that of galactose 1.0 g/30 cm/min. The concentration necessary to

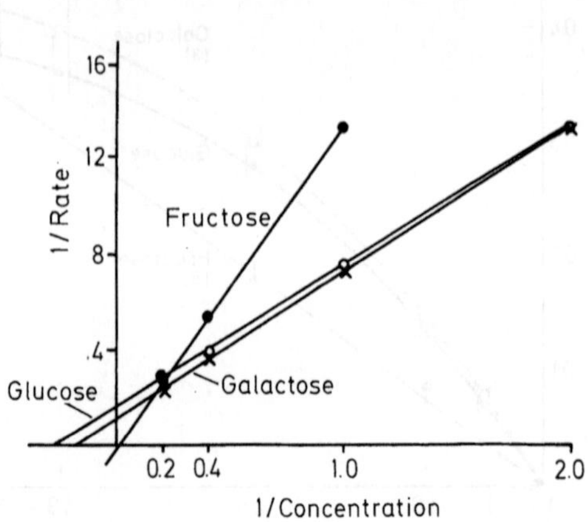

Fig. 9. Lineweaver–Bork plot for absorption of fructose (*curve A*), galactose (*curve B*), and glucose (*curve C*), calculated from Fig. 8

1 In this context, J is an absorption rate rather than a flow rate

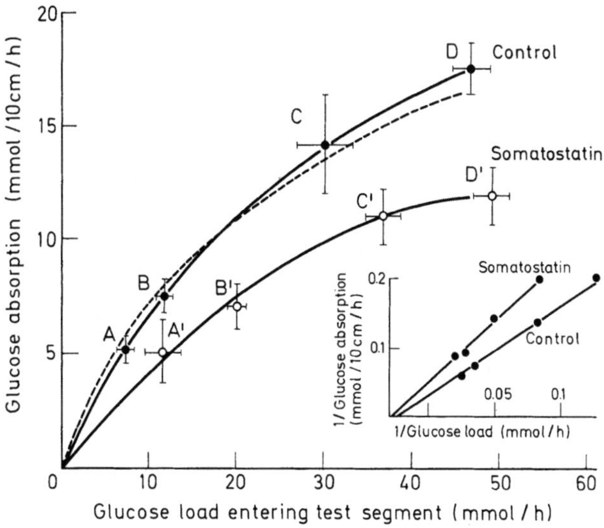

Fig. 10. Kinetic curves for glucose absorption from 10-cm test segments of human jejunum. Each point represents the mean ± standard error of five observations. Lineweaver–Burk analysis showed a reduction of v_{max} for glucose absorption (27.8 and 15.2 mmol/10 cm/h for initial control and somatostatin periods, respectively, while K_m values were similar (31.6 and 24.1 mmol/h). *Broken curve* glucose absorption during final control periods, indicating that glucose absorption returned to normal after somatostatin administration. *Inset* linear transformation of the glucose absorption curves. KREJS et al. (1980)

reach half the maximum absorption rate K_m for glucose was 3.3 g and 5 g/100 ml for galactose. Fructose was absorbed passively in this experiment.

Another application of this type of approach to transport phenomena in humans is to study the competition of various substrates for the same carrier (competitive inhibition) or other effects, such as pharmacological or hormonal influences on absorption characteristics. An example of this type of study is taken from an article on the effect of somatostatin on glucose absorption (Fig. 10; KREJS et al. 1980).

The shapes of the curves from control and somatostatin periods were similar, suggesting a similar K_m, but v_{max} was reduced from 27.8 in control to 15.2 mmol/10 cm/h (somatostatin) as determined by Lineweaver–Burk plot (K_m control 31.6 mmol/h; K_m somatostatin 24.1 mmol/h). Analysis of covariance between the slopes was statistically different. A selective reduction in mucosal surface area by decreasing villous movement was suggested as the most likely explanation for these results.

The third example is given to demonstrate what seems to be a general biological principle. At low concentration substrate may be transported against electrochemical concentration gradients by an active mechanism following Michaelis–Menten kinetics. At high concentrations an additional passive component overlaps the hyperbolic curve, resulting in a curvilinear type of absorption curve. This phenomenon has been demonstrated, e.g. for calcium absorption (EWE 1972b,

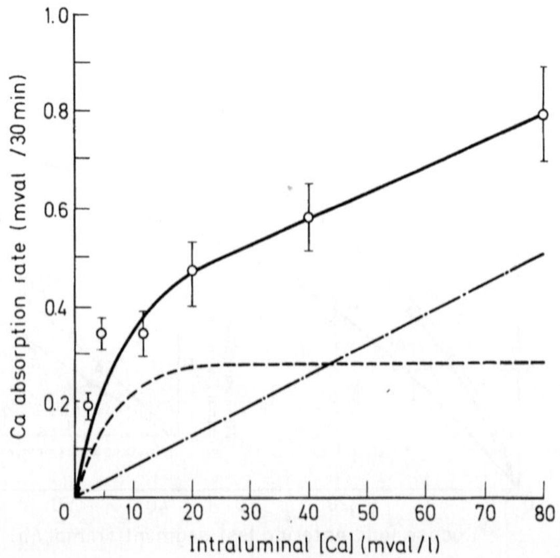

Fig. 11. Calcium absorption in the human upper jejunum. *Full curve* shows experimentally determined absorption curve derived by a double-balloon catheter technique which is also shown analysed into active (*broken curve, long dashes*) and passive components (*broken line, short dashes*). Ewe (1974)

1974). The cut-off point dividing active and passive components was calculated at 6.4 mequiv./l from intubation studies in humans for a 30-cm segment of upper jejunum (Fig. 11). Similar curves and conclusions were derived from animal studies (Ewe 1972a; Wasserman and Taylor 1969; Zornitzer and Bronner 1971).

IV. Unstirred Water Layer and Intestinal Permeability

Maximum transport rate, apparent Michaelis constant, permeability coefficient, and other factors of intestinal permeability are influenced by unstirred water layers adjacent to the mucosal surface and hence, by the flow rate of solute through the intestinal lumen. The effective thickness of the unstirred layer has been calculated by the induction of an osmotic or diffusional electrical PD (Dainty and House 1966; Diamond 1966).

In humans, the thickness of unstirred layer in the jejunum was estimated during kinetic studies of electrogenic glucose absorption (Read et al. 1974, 1977). The transmucosal PD was measured in response to infusion of solutions containing various glucose concentrations. The thickness of the layer was 632 ± 24 μm (mean ± standard error) in healthy volunteers and was significantly thicker than in patients with active coeliac disease, i.e. with flat mucosa: 442 ± 23 μm. For comparison, in the rat small intestine in vitro, the thickness of the unstirred layer was 180–220 μm with an unstirred solution and 140–160 μm with a stirred solution (Hoyumpa et al. 1976; Sallee and Dietschy 1973; Wilson and Dietschy 1974), and in the rabbit jejunum in vitro 330 μm and 110 μm respectively (Westergaard and Dietschy 1974).

The unstirred layer was reduced by increasing the perfusion rate. Several studies in humans have shown that absorption rate increased with an increase in intestinal flow rate (DEVROEDE and PHILLIPS 1969; DRILLET et al. 1971; LOVE 1968; MODIGLIANI and BERNIER 1971; REY et al. 1974; SLADEN and DAWSON 1969). This interrelationship is important in the context of intestinal permeability. The permeation of a substance through the mucosa is characterized by the permeability coefficient which depends on the properties of the membrane, including the unstirred layer as well as those of the substance. Unstirred layer effects have been observed predominantly in highly permeable substances (SALLEE and DIETSCHY 1973; WESTERGAARD and DIETSCHY 1974; WILSON and DIETSCHY 1974). The influence of an unstirred layer on the permeability of a substance following saturation kinetics depends on its concentration; at low concentration its absorption rate is reduced. At higher substrate concentration the transport system may be saturated in spite of the unstirred layer.

The assessment of the thickness of unstirred layers in humans in vivo is highly dependent on technical factors. Therefore, data from different studies differing in technical details can be compared only with caution. This may explain the variable results from ten studies on hexose absorption, as determined by perfusion in intestinal segments, compiled by FORDTRAN and INGELFINGER (1968).

A wide range of perfusion rates have been used, mostly in the vicinity of 10 ml/min, but also as low as 3.6 and as high as 30 ml/min. Little information is available about physiological flow rates after meals in the different parts of the intestine. With subjects who had been fed a steak meal, FORDTRAN and LOCKLEAR (1966) calculated from results of an intubation study that approximately 2,000 ml fluid enters the small intestine. In a similar study, BORGSTRÖM et al. (1957) found that this fluid will enter the upper jejunum within 3–4 h. If 2,000 ml passes the upper small intestine within approximately 200 min, an upper jejunal flow rate of 10 ml/min can be calculated. Thus, it appears that a perfusion rate of 10 ml simulates physiological conditions in the upper jejunum. As appreciable fluid absorption occurs in the upper jejunum and flow rate decreases rapidly in the lower part of the jejunum, a perfusion of about 2 ml/min would be physiological for the ileum. Under these conditions an unstirred layer thickness and related factors may be reasonably physiological.

V. Intestinal Permeability to Peptide Macromolecules

It is generally believed that the intestinal mucosa is impermeable to macromolecules from peptides and proteins. It is in terms of nutrition, but not biologically and immunologically. Ingested antigens, toxins, and antibodies may pass the mucosal barrier in quantities which may be important in the pathogenesis of local and systemic immunological and disease states (WALKER and ISSELBACHER 1974). Moreover, proteolytic and hydrolytic enzymes and hormones may pass the mucosa intact, the importance of this phenomenon is not fully understood yet. Various factors may influence the mucosal permeability to these peptide macromolecules.

No clear definition of the term "macromolecule" exists for peptides and proteins. The definition of polypeptides includes peptides consisting of 10–100 amino acids; more than 100 amino acids connected by peptide bonds are referred to as a protein. In terms of molecular weight this would amount to 1,000 and above for the polypeptide and 10,000 and more for proteins; arbitrarily, a molecular weight of 1,000 is taken as the lower limit for macromolecule (SEIFERT 1976).

1. Permeability of the Neonatal Small Intestine

It has been known for a long time that the neonatal mammalian small intestine is permeable to proteins, even at the size of immunoglobulins (for review see MORRIS 1968). This also applies to humans (IYENGAR and SELVARAJ 1972; LEISSRING et al. 1962; READ et al. 1974; ROTHBERG 1969; WALZER 1927), although there was some controversy as to the absorption of colostric globulins (NORDBRING 1957). The increased permeability lasts but a few days, and the "closure" of the intestinal tract for macromolecules is related to morphological and functional maturation of small intestinal epithelial cells (MORRIS 1968). In addition, gastric, and pancreatic secretions are being produced in increasing quantities at the same time, and along with them, protein digestion occurs and the amount of intact globulins decreases considerably in the intestine. However, small, immunologically effective quantities of peptide macromolecules also pass the small intestine in later life and can be detected by immunological techniques in humans (ANDRÉ et al. 1974; GRUSKY and COOKE 1955; KORENBLAT et al. 1968; SCHMID et al. 1969; WALZER 1927).

After adsorption to the microvillous membrane, the macromolecules are taken up by an invagination process called endocytosis and migrate through the cell in the form of small vesicles (phagosomes) towards the cell nucleus, where they coalesce with lysosomes to form large vacuoles (phagolysomes) (MORRIS 1968). Most of the protein is digested within these structures and leaves the cell at the basolateral membrane by a reverse endocytosis (exocytosis). Whether or not specific receptors mediate the uptake of peptide macromolecules is not clear.

2. Measurements of Intestinal Transfer of Intact Peptides and Proteins in Humans

WALZER (1927) used a passive cutaneous anaphylaxis technique to detect circulating food proteins. He took the serum of patients with food allergy and injected it intradermally into a normal person. If this person ate the protein against which the patient was allergic, a skin reaction developed. A prerequisite for this antigen–antibody reaction is the antigenicity of the ingested protein which has been absorbed unchanged.

KORENBLAT et al. (1968) showed that 15%–30% of normal adults develop milk precipitins after physiological load of oral milk protein or bovine albumin. SEIFERT (1976) used horse anti-human lymphocyte serum. The lymphocyte count after oral ingestion of the anti-lymphocyte serum dropped by 10%–30%. HEINRICH et al. (1979) found that pancreatic enzymes were also reabsorbed and reutilized in humans, a process which has been called enteropancreatic circulation.

3. Factors Influencing Transfer of Peptide Macromolecules

Permeability of the intestinal mucosa to peptide macromolecules may be influenced by various factors and may even be the cause of disease. Secretory IgA is the predominant immunoglobulin present in intestinal secretions and on the glycocalyx mucous coat of the human enterocyte (TOMASI et al. 1965). There is ample evidence that this group of immunoglobulins acts to protect the intestinal epithelium from uptake of antigenic and toxic macromolecules (BUCKLEY and DEES 1969) as well as bacteria (WILLIAMS and GIBBONS 1972) and viruses (OGRA andKARZON 1970). Another factor affecting transport of intestinal macromolecules is mucosal viability. In humans, absorption of ingested protein such as egg albumin increases with acute gastroenteritis as compared with periods free of disease (GRUSKY and COOKE 1955).

An alteration in the natural barrier to intestinal uptake of antigens may also contribute to food allergies. An altered mucosal epithelium after gastroenteritis may predispose susceptible individuals to sensitizing quantities of allergens (SEWELL et al. 1963), or an altered secretory immune system may also allow for uptake of critical amounts of sensitizing proteins (AMMANN and HONG 1971).

VI. Persorption of Particles

It has been shown in Sect. C.V that large molecules may permeate the intestinal wall, probably be pinocytosis. But even large solid particles, of diameter in the micrometer range, may pass the mucosal barrier; this was first described by HERBST (1844). This process which has been studied extensively by VOLKHEIMER (1964, 1977) is called "persorption". After oral application of diatoms, pollen,

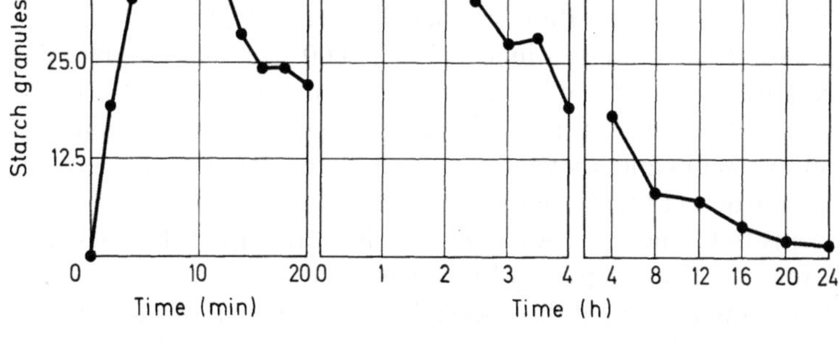

Fig. 12 a–c. Corn starch granules in the venous blood of young test subjects after ingestion of 200 g corn starch. First peak appears 6 min after ingestion (**a**); second peak after 90 min (**b**); only a few isolated starch granules remain in the blood 24 h after ingestion (**c**). VOLKHEIMER (1977)

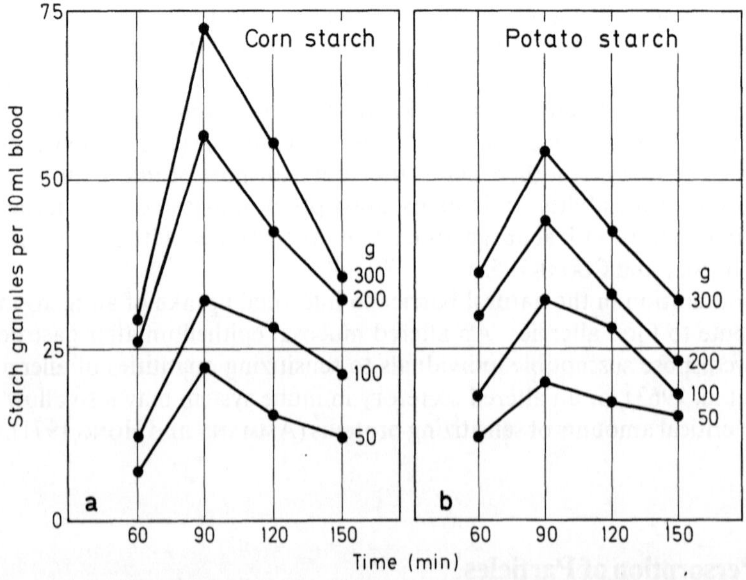

Fig. 13a, b. Starch granules in the venous blood of young test subjects after ingestion of various amounts of corn starch (**a**) and potato starch (**b**). Amount ingested is indicated for each curve. Volkheimer (1977)

spores, cellulose particles, plant cells, and starch granules, these substances were regularly demonstrable in blood and urine by light microscopy. Because of their relatively small number it is necessary to examine blood or urine in a counting chamber for up to 5 h per sample.

When 200 g corn starch is given orally to healthy volunteers and 10 ml blood is drawn at intervals of 2, 30, or 240 min, granules can be discovered in the blood (Fig. 12). A first peak is reached after 6 min and a second after 90 min. The number of starch granules in the blood is directly related to the ingested load (Fig. 13). Neostigmine, nicotine, and caffeine increased starch persorption whereas atropine and barbiturates decreased it. Corn and potato starch was excreted in bile taken from patients with a T-tube in situ as early as 10 min after ingestion and had their maximum concentration in urine 3 h after oral intake.

The rate of persorption is estimated 1 in 50,000 ± 25,000 (standard deviation) of ingested particles capable of persorption, i.e. 10^6 from 50×10^9 in 200 g corn starch and 5×10^4 from 2.5×10^9 in 200 g potato starch. Permeation of particles of a size up to 100 μm and above is not possible transcellularly because the diameter of these particles exceeds that of the mucosal cell severalfold. The site of penetration seems to be the extrusion zone of cells at the tip of the intestinal villi as studied histologically in animals by Volkheimer (1977).

The clinical implication of this special kind of intestinal permeability is not yet known. No information exists on the influence of intestinal disease on persorption. Its immunological significance is not appreciated nor is its importance for environmental medicine, if one considers for instance that PVC particles and asbestos fibres are absorbed.

D. Influence of Drugs on Intestinal Permeability

Many studies have been performed on the absorption and pharmacokinetics of drugs (see FORTH and RUMMEL 1975), but little is known about the effects of drugs on intestinal permeability in humans. Drugs may influence Na^+, K^+-ATPase activity, may change cAMP concentration in the enterocyte, and may alter intestinal permeability at the tight junctions or elsewhere. Thus, they may affect intestinal transfer in several ways.

I. Influence on Electrolyte and Water Transfer

By intestinal perfusion and rectal PD measurements, several drugs which influenced intestinal electrolyte and water transfer were studied by our group. Laxatives (EWE 1977; EWE and HÖLKER 1974) will be discussed elsewhere. Cardiac glycosides (digoxin and meproscillarin) and certain diuretics (ethacrynic acid) changes net absorption of NaCl and water into secretion and enhanced K^+ secretion in the colon. These effects were in the same range as laxatives (Fig. 14; WANITSCHKE and EWE 1983). In parallel, rectal PD fell significantly under the influence of lipid-soluble digitoxin and meproscillarin, but not with the more water-soluble digoxin (Fig. 15; EWE and WANITSCHKE 1983). Normally, these drugs are absorbed in the small intestine and do not reach the colon in sufficiently high concentrations to evoke secretions, i.e. diarrhoea.

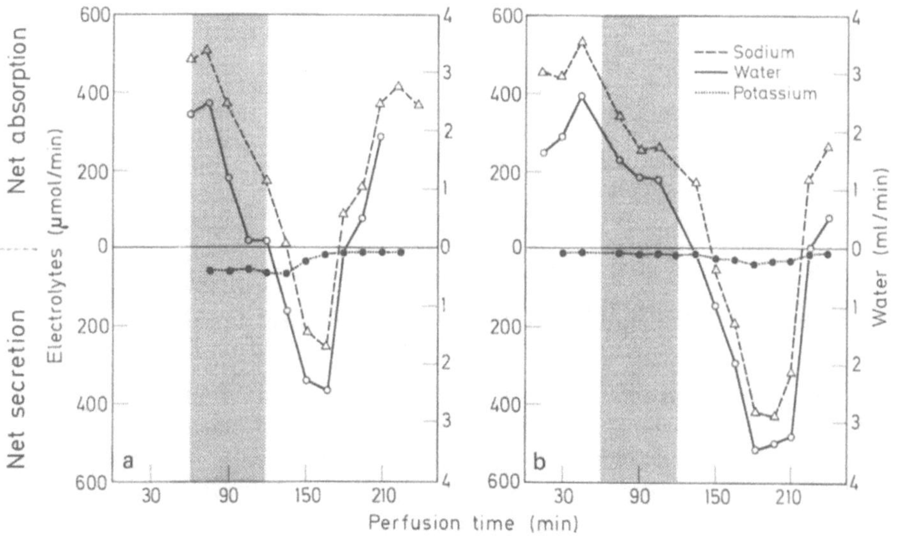

Fig. 14 a, b. Effects of 10^{-5} mol/l digoxin (**a**) and 2.8×10^{-4} mol/l ethacryinic acid (**b**) on water and electrolyte balance in the human colon. Perfusion of the whole colon (NaCl 138, $NaHCO_3$ 25, KCl 5 mequiv./l, PEG 4,000 5 g/l). Perfusion rate 5 ml/min. WANITSCHKE and EWE (1983)

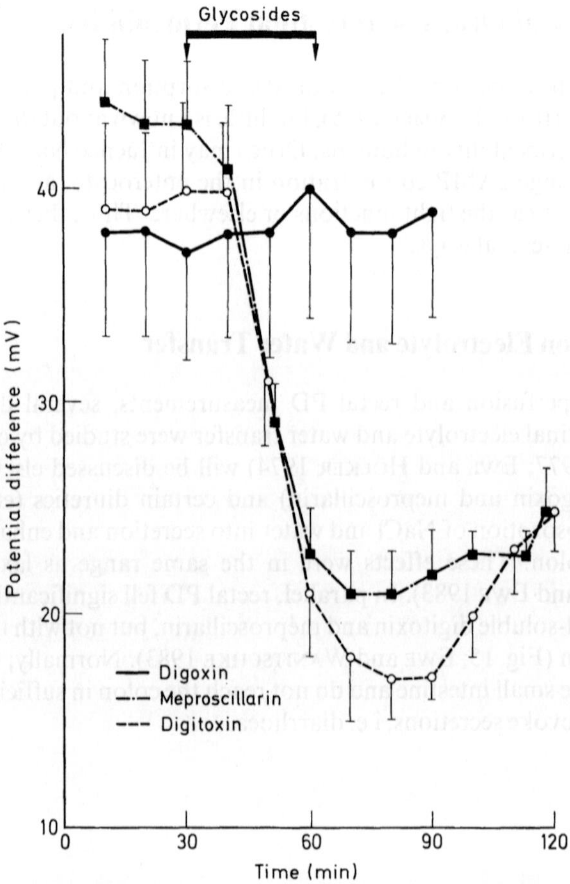

Fig. 15. Effect of cardiac glycosides on electrical potential difference measured between the rectum (direct electrode) and blood (electrode in cubital vein) by means of polyvinyl tubes continuously perfused with isotonic NaCl. The rectum was perfused (for composition and rate see Fig. 14) and meproscillarin (0.5 mg-%), digitoxin (2.5 mg-%) and digoxin was added over a 30-min period. EWE and WANITSCHKE (1980)

II. Change in Intestinal Permeability by Cytostatic Treatment

Chemotherapeutic agents may damage the gastrointestinal mucosa and thereby influence the intestinal permeability. When patients with metastatic colon carcinoma under therapy with 5-fluorouracil were given large marker molecules (PVP ^{14}C, average molecular weight 11,000) and the nonabsorbable antibiotic tobramycin (molecular weight 467), urinary excretion of these compounds increased reproducibly up to 20-fold which was apparent at days 8–15 of treatment (SIBER et al. 1980). Tobramycin excretion in the urine was 8.5 times higher than PVP excretion, but the ratio of both markers remained constant (SIEBER et al. 1980). Therefore, increased intestinal permeability during cytostatic therapy may be of clinical importance when "nonabsorbable" antibiotics or toxins may pass the damaged mucosa.

E. Intestinal Permeability in Disease

Normal intestinal permeability depends on intact morphological and functional conditions and may therefore be influenced by diseases. In humans, several diseases have been investigated in this regard using various techniques.

I. Coeliac Disease

Nontropical sprue is the disease most thoroughly and intensively studied for derangements in permeability, and more detailed information may be obtained in addition to biopsy (ANONYMOUS 1981). Some interesting results have emerged from these studies.

In coeliac disease, the damage caused by gluten mainly attacks the tips of the villi resulting in a "flat" mucosa while crypt cells are less involved and regenerate hyperactively. How does this affect permeability? Conventional tests of absorption such as the D-xylose absorption test are pathological in coeliac disease and reflect the damage of the absorbing part of the mucosa. Applying intestinal perfusion techniques, it can be demonstrated that malabsorption occurs for various substrates such as electrolytes and water (FORDTRAN et al. 1967; WENSEL et al. 1969), calcium (WENSEL et al. 1969), pentoses and hexoses (COBDEN et al. 1978, 1980; FORDTRAN et al. 1967; GERSON et al. 1974; MENZIES 1974; MENZIES et al. 1979; READ et al. 1976; SCHEDL and CLIFTON 1961a; WHEELER et al. 1978), amino acids and peptides (ADIBI et al. 1974; SILK et al. 1974a), and folic acid (GERSON et al. 1974). In contrast, the ileum absorbs normally or may even compensate for the malabsorption by adaptation (SILK et al. 1974b). This is in accordance with the morphological finding that maximal mucosal damage is located in the proximal small intestine (STEWARD et al. 1967).

Several attempts have been made to characterize in more detail the nature of the derangement observed in the sprue syndrome and to answer the question whether the malabsorption is simply due to the decreased mucosal area or whether specific alterations of permeability and transport processes are also involved. FORDTRAN et al. (1967) applied the principle of restricted diffusion (RENKIN 1954) based on the simultaneous measurement of diffusion rates of solutes with different molecular diameters in patients with sprue (see Sect. C.I.2). The larger the pore size through which the solutes permeate, the smaller the discrimination and vice versa. Three pairs of solutes were studied: urea/tritiated water; erythritol/urea; L-xylose/urea. The diffusion ratio in control subjects was 0.8; 0.5; 0.3 respectively for the three pairs. The diffusion ratio in sprue patients was only 0.2 for urea/water, and could not be calculated for the other two substances because absorption rates were negligibly low. The increased discrimination ratio and negligible absorption of larger molecules was interpreted to be the consequence of a marked decrease in effective pore size besides the decreased surface area and impaired transport process (sodium and water in this study).

These results were confirmed by CHADWICK et al. (1977b) using a different approach to this problem. Low molecular weight polyethylene glycols (PEG 400) were applied to control subjects and patients with coeliac sprue. Intestinal permeability was markedly decreased in the patients with the most active disease as compared with normal volunteers (see Fig. 4). The patients with moderate disease showed intermediate profiles. Patients of the most severely diseased group hardly excreted any of the larger molecules of the PEG mixture in the urine.

In contrast to these findings other authors found an increase of intestinal permeability for large molecules in sprue (Cobden et al. 1978, 1980; Menzies 1974; Menzies et al. 1979; Wheeler et al. 1978). An oral load of test molecules of different molecular weight was given to the patients: lactulose, raffinose, stachyose, and dextran (Wheeler et al. 1978), cellobiose and mannitol (Cobden et al. 1978, 1980), and L-rhamnose and lactulose (Menzies et al. 1979).

When the solution was made hypertonic, permeability increased considerably in normal subjects, as shown by an increased urinary excretion of test molecules and the decrease of restricted diffusion ratios. In patients with sprue a spontaneous increase of permeability occurred, and alteration in the profile of restriction was found, even when isotonic solutions were given. For instance, mannitol (molecular radius 4 Å) was absorbed and excreted in the urine to a lesser degree than in normal subjects (0.79% versus 19.6%), whereas cellobiose (radius 5 Å) was absorbed and excreted to a higher extent in patients with sprue: 0.97% versus 0.32% (Cobden et al. 1978, 1980).

How can these contradictory observations be reconciled, i.e. malabsorption of smaller substances and increased absorption of larger molecules as compared with normals? Part of the difference may be due to the different techniques, e.g. perfusions of a diseased segment of the upper jejunum or urinary excretion of marker molecules which may have passed the whole small intestine, including distal parts which are usually less involved. On the other hand these results have been taken to formulate a concept of intestinal permeability which at least partially explains the different experimental findings (Chadwick et al. 1977b; Cobden et al. 1978; Fordtran and Ingelfinger 1968; Wheeler et al. 1978).

The increase of restricted diffusion discrimination (low ratio of larger to smaller molecules) using comparatively small test molecules (Fordtran et al. 1967) and the decrease (high ratio of large to smaller molecules) using large test molecules (Cobden et al. 1978, 1980; Menzies et al. 1979; Wheeler et al. 1978) in patients with sprue was thought to be due to a change not only in pore size, but also in number. While from these and other experiments (Chadwick et al. 1977b; Loehry et al. 1973) it was decided that the distribution of "pores" (or pore equivalents) in the small intestine remains constant (i.e. many small pores; a moderate number of medium-sized pores and a small number of large pores), but the absolute number of pores of all sizes progressively decreases down the length of the small intestine. This relation is disturbed in the sprue syndrome. The small pores through which small solute (Fordtran et al. 1967) and mannitol (Cobden et al. 1978, 1980) or rhamnose (Menzies et al. 1979) permeate, decrease in number and diameter, but the few larger pores increase or are newly formed (extrusion zones) through which the larger molecules such as dextran (Wheeler et al. 1978), collobiose (Cobden et al. 1978, 1980), and lactulose (Menzies et al. 1979) may pass.

II. Inflammatory Bowel Disease

1. Crohn's Disease

When intestinal permeability was tested in a patient with Crohn's disease by using the technique of low molecular weight PEG 400 absorption (CHADWICK et al. 1977 a), it was found that the urinary excretion curve was shifted towards the larger molecules of the mixture as compared with normal subjects. This was taken as a sign of increased permeability (SUNDQUIST et al. 1980). This finding was confirmed by applying another method using test molecules of different sizes (COBDEN et al. 1978, 1980), namely cellobiose and mannitol, as discussed for the sprue syndrome. Cellulose: mannitol ratios were abnormally high in patients with proximal or midbowel Crohn's disease, whereas those with the disease confined to the ileum and/or colon had normal ratios. This method also gave normal results in ulcerative colitis (UC). One patient with jejunal disease had an abnormal ratio which became normal after small bowel resection, but later recrudescence of the disease was reflected by a corresponding change of test molecule ratio (COBDEN et al. 1980).

Perfusion studies were performed in the ileum in patients with mild disease of the terminal ileum and caecum. Some had diarrhoea, others had not. Patients without diarrhoea absorbed electrolytes, glucose, xylose, glycochenodesoxycholic acid (GCDC) and water, whereas patients with diarrhoea secreted electrolytes and water and absorbed significantly less glucose, xylose, and GCDC (B. KRAG and E. KRAG 1976; E. KRAG and B. KRAG 1976).

It seems that functional disturbances of the intestine do not necessarily correlate with morphological changes, as the radiological findings in both groups were similar. It was concluded that apparent changes in permeability are of physiological importance in the pathogenesis of diarrhoea observed in patients with Crohn's disease.

2. Ulcerative Colitis

Permeability was increased in UC and Crohn's disease of the colon when EDTA ^{51}Cr or vitamin B_{12} ^{57}Co (RASK-MADSEN et al. 1973) or PVP ^{125}I (average molecular weight 33,000, range 8,000–85,000) (RASK-MADSEN 1973 a) was instilled into the inflamed colon. Several studies deal with the permeability of electrolytes and water in UC. When unidirectional fluxes of $^{24}Na^+$, $^{42}K^+$, and H_3O were determined by colonic perfusion (HARRIS and SHIELDS 1970; RASK-MADSEN 1973 b) or by instillation into the rectosigmoid (LEVITAN and BRUDNO 1967), the lumen–plasma flux was low and the plasma–lumen flux was increased with the relationship of water and Na^+ absorption preserved. This is also compatible with the idea of increased permeability of the inflamed mucosa with and without altered activity of the Na^+-pump since the electrical gradient diminished with unchanged plasma concentration of Na^+ and K^+ (RASK-MADSEN and BRIX-JENSEN 1973).

An intact epithelium is a prerequisite for normal transmucosal PD. Several studies on patients with inflammatory bowel disease of the colon and rectum showed a reduced or even inverted (luminal positive, serosal negative) PD in some cases with acute exacerbation (EDMONDS 1970; EDMONDS and PILCHER 1973; RASK-MADSEN 1973 b; RASK-MADSEN and BRIX-JENSEN 1973; RASK-MADSEN and

Dalmark 1973; Rask-Madsen et al. 1973; Ruddel et al. 1977). The PD correlated with increased leakiness of the mucosa to Na^+; it was usually restored to normal when the patient was successfully treated with salazosulfapyridine and/or corticosteroids.

Deranged permeability of the intestinal mucosa to macromolecules has been proposed to play a role in the pathogenesis of inflammatory bowel diseases (Shorter et al. 1972). Sensitization by macromolecules or nonenteropathogenic gram-negative bacteria may occur during the neonatal period of susceptible infants when the mucosal barrier is incomplete. Reexposure to intestinal antigens or to bacteria may occur in later life when a temporary breakdown of the mucosal barrier results from acute gastroenteritis (Grusky and Cooke 1955; Perlmann et al. 1967). This reexposure evokes the local primary cellular immune-mediated hypersensitivity reaction, resulting in inflammatory bowel disease.

3. Other Diseases

In patients with eczema and food allergy, absorption of large test molecules (PEG 4,000) was greater than in normal subjects, while absorption of smaller molecules (PEG 600) was unchanged. Interestingly, in patients, more PEG 4,000 was recovered in the second 12-h urine sample than in the first sample after ingestion. This could point to an abnormal permeability in the more distal small intestine or even in the colon (Jackson et al. 1981).

Permeability was normal in different gastroenterological diseases such as pancreatic disease, blind loop syndrome, gastric surgery, or lactase deficiency, when screened by the cellobiose : mannitol excretion ratio (Cobden et al. 1980). Human subjects with cholera were given labelled mannitol intravenously. They had no increased mannitol clearance into the gut. This is consistent with a normal filtration or permeability and points to a secretory process (Gordon et al. 1972).

Hormones or hormone-like substances may influence intestinal physiology by various mechanisms, for instance effects on motility, changes in blood supply, or transport mechanisms mostly of electrolytes and water (for review see Barbezat 1973; Ewe 1975). Diarrhoea was attributed to elevated levels of VIP, GIP, calcitonin, and certain prostaglandins in patients with endocrine active tumors. Perfusion studies have confirmed the stimulatory effect of absorption of Na^+ by mineralocorticoids and the inhibitory action on sodium net absorption of others such as gastrin, secretin, CCK, glucagon, GIP, VIP (for review see Ewe 1975).

Interpretation of results in relation to clinical importance is difficult to assess because pharmacological doses were often used, purity of hormones was not always maintained, interaction with other hormones could not be ruled out and techniques were often different. When all the hormones mentioned (except VIP) were given simultaneously in physiological doses, basal net absorption of electrolytes and water was reversed to net secretion as tested by intestinal perfusion (Poitros et al. 1980). The secretagogue effects of VIP (Krejs and Fordtran 1980), calcitonin (Gray et al. 1976), and somatostatin (Krejs et al. 1980) have been confirmed.

Bile acids and fatty acids may reach the colon in sufficiently high concentrations to affect permeability when the ileum is diseased or resected, resulting in bile acid or fatty acid malabsorption. Perfusion studies have shown that free and conjugated dihydroxy bile acids (MEKHJIAN et al. 1971; WINGATE et al. 1973b) and hydroxy fatty acids (AMMON and PHILLIPS 1973) caused reversible secretion of electrolytes and water, explaining the so-called chologenetic diarrhoea with increased colonic oxalate absorption through the more permeable colonic mucosa. This is discussed in detail in Chap. 29.

References

Adibi SS, Fogel MR, Agraval RM (1974) Comparison of free amino acid and dipeptide absorption in the jejunum of sprue patients. Gastroenterology 67:586–591
Alpers DH, Kinzie JL (1973) Regulation of small intestinal protein metabolism. Gastroenterology 64:471–496
Ammann AJ, Hong R (1971) Selective IgA deficiency: presentation of 30 cases and a review of the literature. Medicine 50:223–236
Ammon HV, Phillips SF (1973) Inhibition of colonic water and electrolyte absorption by fatty acids in man. Gastroenterology 65:744–749
André L, Lambert R, Bazin H, Heremans JF (1974) Interference of oral immunization with the intestinal absorption of heterologues albumin. Eur J Immunol 4:701–705
Anonymous (1981) Sugering the Grosby capsule. Lancet 1:593–594
Archampong EG, Edmonds DJ (1972) Effect of luminal ions on the transepithelial electrical potential difference in human rectum. Gut 13:559–565
Barbezat GO (1973) Stimulation of intestinal secretion by polypeptide hormones. Scand J Gastroenterol 8 [Suppl 22]:1–21
Barry PH, Diamond JM (1970) Junction potentials, electrode standard potentials and other problems in interpreting electrical properties in membranes. J Membr Biol 3:93–122
Billich CO, Levitan R (1969) Effects of sodium concentration and osmolality on water and electrolyte absorption from intact human colon. J Clin Invest 48:1336–1347
Blankenhorn DH, Hirsch J, Ahrens EH (1955) Transintestinal intubation: technique for measurements of gut length and physiological sampling at known loci. Proc Soc Exp Biol Med 88:356–362
Borgström B, Dahlquist A, Lundh G, Sjövall J (1957) Studies of intestinal digestion and absorption in the human. J Clin Invest 36:1521–1536
Brown BH, Holdsworth CD, Levin RJ, Read NW, Smallwood RH (1976) The relationship between intestinal motility and fluctuations in transmural potential difference in the human jejunum. J Physiol (Lond) 259:20P–30P
Buckley RH, Dees SC (1969) Correlation of mild precipitins with IgA deficiency. N Engl J Med 281:465–469
Chadwick VS, Phillips SF, Hofmann AF (1977a) Measurements of intestinal permeability using low molecular weight polyethylene glycols (PEG 400). I. Chemical analysis and biological properties of PEG 400. Gastroenterology 73:241–246
Chadwick VS, Phillips SF, Hofmann AF (1977b) Measurements of intestinal permeability using low molecular weigth polyethylene glycols (PEG 400). II. Application to normal and abnormal permeability states in man and animals. Gastroenterology 73:247–251
Cobden I, Rothwell J, Axon ATR (1980) Intestinal permeability and screening tests for coeliac disease. Gut 21:512–518
Cobden I, Dickinson RF, Rothwell J, Axon ATR (1978) Intestinal permeability assessed by excretion ratios of two molecules: results in coeliac disease. Br Med J 2:1060
Cooper H, Levitan R, Fordtran JS, Ingelfinger JF (1966) A method for studying absorption of water and solute from human small intestine. Gastroenterology 50:1–7
Cooperstein JL, Brockman SK (1959) The electrical potential difference generated by the large intestine: its relation to electrolyte and water transfer. J Clin Invest 38:435–442
Dainty J, House CR (1966) "Unstirred layer" in frog skin. J Physiol (Lond) 182:66–78
Dalmark M (1970) The transmucosal electrical potential difference across the human rectum in vivo following perfusion of different electrolyte solutions. Scand J Gastroenterol 5:421–426

Davis GR, Santa Ana CA, Morawski SG, Fordtran JS (1980) Inhibition of water and electrolyte absorption by polyethylene glycol (PEG). Gastroenterology 79:35–39
Devroede GJ, Phillips SF (1969) Studies of the perfusion technique for colonic absorption. Gastroenterology 56:92–100
Diamond JM (1966) A rapid method for determining voltage-concentration relations across membranes. J Physiol (Lond) 183:83–100
Dietschy JM, Sallee VL, Wilson FA (1971) Unstirred water layers and absorption across the intestinal mucosa. Gastroenterology 61:932–934
Donaldson RM, Barreras RF (1965) Intestinal absorption of trace quantities of chromium. J Lab Clin Med 66:866–867
Doscherholmen A, Hagen PS, Liu M, Olin L (1959) Delay of absorption of radiolabeled cyanocobalamin in the intestinal wall in the presence of intrinsic factor. J Lab Clin Med 54:434–439
Drillet F, Rey F, Rey J (1971) Influence of the flow rate of perfusion on the in vivo kinetics of glucose and amino acid absorption. Acta Paediatr Scand 60:371
Edmonds CJ (1970) Electrical potentials of the sigmoid colon and rectum in irritable bowel syndrom and ulcerative colitis. Gut 11:867–874
Edmonds CJ, Pilcher D (1973) Electrical potential difference of sodium and potassium flux across rectal mucosa in ulcerative colitis. Gut 784–789
Ewe K (1972a) Calcium transport in rat small intestine in vitro and in vivo. Naunyn Schmiedebergs Arch Pharmacol 273:352–365
Ewe K (1972b) Calcium absorption in health and disease. In: Frick P et al. (eds) Ergebnisse der inneren Medizin und Kinderheilkunde, vol 33. Springer, Berlin Heidelberg New York, pp 231–269
Ewe K (1974) Die intestinale Calcium-Resorption und ihre Störungen. I. Physiologie der intestinalen Calcium-Resorption. Klin Wochenschr 52:57–63
Ewe K (1975) Der Einfluß von Hormonen auf intestinale Transfervorgänge von Wasser und Elektrolyten. Arzneim Forsch 25:499–506
Ewe K (1976) Resorptionsprüfungen. In: Forell MM (ed) Verdauungsorgane. Springer, Berlin Heidelberg New York (Handbuch der inneren Medizin, vol 3/6)
Ewe K (1977) Influence of diphenolic laxatives on water and electrolyte permeation in man. In: Kramer M, Lauterbach F (eds) Intestinal permeation, IGS 391. Excerpta Medica, pp 420–425
Ewe K (1980) Effect of rhein on the transport of electrolyte, water and carbohydrates in the human jejunum and colon. Pharmacology 20 [Suppl 1]:27–35
Ewe K, Hölker B (1974) Einfluß eines diphenolischen Laxans (Bisacodyl) auf den Wasser- und Elektrolyttransport im menschlichen Colon. Klin Wochenschr 52:827–833
Ewe K, Summerskill WHJ (1965) Transfer of ammonia in the human jejunum. J Lab Clin Med 65:839–847
Ewe K, Wanitschke R (1980) The effect of cathartic agents on transmucosal electrical potential difference in the human rectum. Klin Wochenschr 58:299–306
Ewe K, Romahn A, Oberhausen EA (1971) Vitamin B 12-Resorption und ihre Beeinflussung durch Intrinsic Factor bei Normalen und Ileumresezierten. In: Amon R, Ritter U (eds) Aktuelle Berichte aus dem Gebiet der Verdauungs- und Stoffwechselkrankheiten. Thieme, Stuttgart, pp 210–213
Fisher RB, Parsons DS (1950) The gradient of mucosal surface area in the small intestine of the rat. J Anat 84:272–282
Fisher RB, Parsons DS (1953) Glucose movements across the wall of the rat small intestine. J Physiol (Lond) 119:210–223
Fordtran JS (1966) Marker perfusion techniques for measuring intestinal absorption in man. Gastroenterology 51:1089–1093
Fordtran JS (1969) Segmental perfusion techniques. Gastroenterology 56:987–988
Fordtran JS, Dietschy JM (1966) Water and electrolyte movement in the intestine. Gastroenterology 50:263–285
Fordtran JS, Ingelfinger FJ (1968) Absorption of water, electrolyte, and sugars from the human gut. In: Code CF (ed) Alimentary canal. Am Physiol Soc, Washington, pp 1457–1490 (Handbook of physiology, vol 3/6)

Fordtran JS, Locklear TW (1966) Ionic constituents and osmolality of gastric and small intestinal fluids after eating. Am J Dig Dis 11:503–521
Fordtran JS, Levitan R, Bikerman V, Burrows BA (1961) The kinetics of water absorption in the human intestine. Trans Assoc Am Physicians 74:195–205
Fordtran JS, Rector FC, Carter NW (1968) The mechanisms of sodium absorption in the human intestine. J Clin Invest 47:885–900
Fordtran JS, Soergel KH, Ingelfinger FJ (1962) Intestinal absorption of D-Xylose in man. N Engl J Med 267:274–279
Fordtran JS, Rector FC, Locklear TW, Ewton MF (1967) Water and solute movement in the small intestine of patients with sprue. J Clin Invest 46:287–298
Fordtran JS, Rector FC, Ewton MF, Soter N, Kinney J (1965) Permeability characteristics of the human small intestine. J Clin Invest 44:1935–1944
Forth W, Rummel W (1975) Pharmacology of intestinal absorption. In: Forth W, Rummel W (eds) Gastrointestinal absorption of drugs, vol 1. Pergamon, Oxford (International encyclopedia of pharmacology and therapeutics)
Fowler D, Cooke WT (1969) Diagnostic significance of D-Xylose excretion test. Gut 1:67–70
Franks JJ, Mosser EL, Austadt GL (1963) The role of the gut in the albumin catabolism. I. Studies in jejunoilectomized rabbits. J Gen Physiol 46:415
Frizzell RA, Schultz SG (1972) Ionic conductance of extracellular shunt pathway in rabbit ileum. Influence of shunt on transmural sodium transport and electrical potential differences. J Gen Physiol 59:318–346
Geall MG, Code CF, McIlrath DC, Summerskill WHJ (1970) Measurement of gastrointestinal transmural electrical potential difference in man. Gut 11:34–37
Gerson CD, Cohen N, Janowitz HD (1973) Small intestinal absorptive function in regional enteritis. Gastroenterology 64:907–912
Gerson CD, Cohen N, Brown N, Lindenbaum J, Hepner GW, Janowitz HD (1974) Folic acid and hexose absorption in sprue. Am J Dig Dis 19:911–919
Goldschmidt S, Dayton AB (1919) Studies in the mechanism of absorption from the intestine. I. The colon. A contribution to the one-sided permeability of the intestinal wall to chloride. Am J Physiol 48:419
Goldstein F, Karacoday S, Wirts CW, Kowlessar OD (1970) Intraluminal small-intestinal utilization of D-Xylose by bacteria. Gastroenterology 59:380–386
Gordon RS (1959) Exsudative enteropathy. Abnormal permeability of the gastrointestinal tract demonstrable with labelled polyvinyl pyrrolidone. Lancet 1:325–326
Gordon RS, Gardner JD, Kinzie JL (1972) Low mannitol clearance into cholera stool as evidence against filtration as the source of stool fluid. Gastroenterology 63:407–412
Gray TK, Braman P, Juan D, Morawski G, Fordtran JS (1976) Ion transport changes during calcitonin-induced intestinal secretion in man. Gastroenterology 71:392–398
Grusky FL, Cooke RE (1955) The gastrointestinal absorption of unaltered protein in normal infants and in infants recovering from diarrhea. Pediatrics 16:763–768
Gustke RF, McCormick PG, Ruppin H, Soergel KH, Whalen GE, Wood CM (1981) Human intestinal potential difference: recording method and biophysical implications. J Physiol (Lond) 321:571–582
Harris J, Shields R (1970) Absorption and secretion of water and electrolytes by the intact human colon in diffuse untreated proctocolitis. Gut 11:27–33
Heinrich HC, Gabbe EE, Brüggemann J, Icagic F, Classen M (1979) Enteropancratic circulation in man. Klin Wochenschr 67:1295–1297
Herbst G (1844) Das Lymphgefäßsystem und seine Verrichtung. Vandenhoeck, Göttingen
Holdworth CD, Dawson AM (1964) The absorption of monosaccharides in man. Clin Sci 27:371–379
Holdworth CD, Dawson AM (1965) Glucose and fructose absorption in idiopathic steatorrhea. Gut 6:387–391
Hoyumpa AM, Nichols S, Schenker S, Wilson FA (1976) Thiamine transport in thiamine-deficient rats; role of the unstirred water layer. Biochim Biophys Acta 436:438–447
Hyden S (1955) A turbidimetric method for determination of higher polyethylene glycols in biological material. Ann Agr Coll 22:139–145

Iyengar L, Selvaraj RJ (1972) Intestinal absorption of immunoglobulins by newborn infants. Arch Dis Child 47:411–414

Jackson PG, Lessof MH, Baker RWR, Ferrett J, McDonald DM (1981) Intestinal permeability in patients with eczema and food allergy. Lancet 1:1285–1286

Jacobson ED, Brody DC, Broitman SA, Fordtran JS (1963) Validity of polyethylene glycol in estimating intestinal water volume. Gastroenterology 44:761–767

Jarnum S (1962) Protein-losing gastroenteropathy. Blackwell, Oxford

Jarnum S, Westergaard H, Yssing M, Jensen H (1968) Quantitation of gastrointestinal protein loss by means of Fe^{59}-labelled iron dextran. Gastroenterology 55:229–241

Jeejeehoy KN, Singh B, Mani RS, Sanjawa SM (1965) The use of ^{95}Nb-labelled albumin in the study of gastrointestinal protein loss. In: Birke G et al. (eds) Physiology and pathophysiology in plasma protein metabolism. Huber, Bern, pp 61–67

Jeffries GH (1978) Protein metabolism and protein losing enteropathy. In: Sleisenger MH, Fordtran JS (eds) Gastrointestinal disease, 2nd edn. Saunders, Philadelphia, pp 354–367

Kendall MJ (1970) The influence of age on the xylose absorption test. Gut 11:498–501

Kingham JGC, Loehry CA (1978) Selectivity of small intestinal exudate in celiac disease and Crohn's disease. Dig Dis Sci 23:33–38

Korenblat RE, Rothberg RM, Minden P, Farr RS (1968) Immune response of human adults after oral and parenteral exposure to bovine serum albumin. J Allergy Clin Immunol 41:226–235

Krag B, Krag E (1976) Regional ileitis (Crohn's disease). II. Electrolyte and water movement in the ileum during perfusion with bile acids. Scand J Gastroenterol 11:487–490

Krag E, Krag B (1976) Regional ileitis (Crohn's disease). I. Kinetic of bile acid absorption in the perfused ileum. Scand J Gastroenterol 11:481–486

Krag E, Krag B, Lenz K (1975) A comparison of stable and H-labelled polyethylene glycol 4,000 as non absorbable water phase markers in the human ileum and faeces. Scand J Gastroenterol 10:105–108

Krawitt EL, Beeken WK (1975) Limitations of the usefulness of the D-Xylose absorption test. Am J Clin Pathol 63:261–263

Krejs GJ, Fordtran JS (1980) Effect of VIP infusion on water and ion transport in the human jejunum. Gastroenterology 78:722–727

Krejs GJ, Browne R, Raskin P (1980) Effect of intravenous somatostatin on jejunal absorption of glucose, amino acids and electrolytes. Gastroenterology 78:26–31

Leissring JC, Anderson JW, Smith DW (1962) Uptake of antibodies by the intestine of the newborne infant. Am J Dis Child 103:160–165

Levitan R, Brudno S (1967) Permeability of the rectosigmoid mucosa to tritiated water in normal subjects and in patients with mild idiopathic ulcerative colitis. Gut 8:15–18

Levitan R, Fordtran JS, Burrows BA, Ingelfinger FK (1962) Water and salt absorption in the human colon. J Clin Invest 41:1754–1759

Levitt MD (1977) Use of the constant perfusion technique in the nonsteady state. Gastroenterology 73:1450–1454

Lineweaver H, Burk D (1934) The determination of enzyme dissociation constants. J Am Chem Soc 56:658–666

Loehry CA, Kingham J, Baker J (1973) Small intestinal permeability in animals and man. Gut 14:683–688

Love AHG (1968) Absorption characteristics of the human small intestine during segmental perfusion. J Physiol (Lond) 197:38P–39P

Mekhjian H, Phillips SF, Hofmann AF (1971) Colonic secretion of water and electrolyte induced by bile acids: perfusion studies in man. J Clin Invest 50:1569–1577

Menzies IS (1974) Absorption of intact oligosaccharide in health and disease. Biochem Soc Trans 2:1042–1047

Menzies IS, Pounder R, Sukha H, Laker MF, Bull J, Wheeler PG, Creamer B (1979) Abnormal intestinal permeability to sugars in villous atrophy. Lancet 2:1107–1109

Modigliani R, Bernier JJ (1971) Absorption of glucose, sodium, and water by the human jejunum studied by intestinal perfusion with a proximal occluding balloon and at variable flow rates. Gut 12:184–193

Modigliani R, Rambaud JC, Bernier JJ (1973) The method of intraluminal perfusion of the human small intestine I: principle and technique. Digestion 9:176–192
Modigliani R, Ramboud JC, Bernier JJ (1978) Validation of the use of a tube with a proximal occlusive balloon for measurement of intestinal absorption in man. Dig Dis Sci 23:720–722
Morris IG (1968) Gamma globulin absorption in the newborn. In: Code CF (ed) Alimentary canal. Am Physiol Soc, Washington, pp 1491–1512 (Handbook of physiology, vol 3/6)
Nordbring F (1957) The failure of newborn premature infants to absorb antibodies from heterologous colostrum. Acta Paediatr Stockholm 46:569–578
Ogra PL, Karzon DT (1970) The role of immunoglobulins in the mechanism of mucosal immunity to virus infection. Pediatr Clin North Am 17:385–400
Pappenheimer JR, Renkin EM, Borrero LM (1951) Filtration, diffusion, and molecular sieving through peripheral capillary membranes. A contribution to the pore theory of capillary permeability. Am J Physiol 167:13–46
Perlmann P, Hammerstrom S, Lagercrantz R, Gustafsson B (1967) Antibodies to colon in rats and human ulcerative colitis. Cross reactivity with Escherichia Coli 0:14 antigen. Proc Soc Exp Biol Med 125:975–982
Phillips SF, Summerskill WHJ (1966) Occlusion of the jejunum for intestinal perfusion in man. Mayo Clin Proc 41:224–231
Poitros P, Modigliani R, Bernier JJ (1980) Effect of combination of gastrin, secretin, cholecystokinin, glucagon, and gastric inhibitory polypeptide on jejunal absorption in man. Gut 21:299–304
Rask-Madsen J (1973a) Sieving characteristics of inflamed rectal mucosa. Gut 14:988–989
Rask-Madsen J (1973b) Simultanous measurement of electrical polarization and electrolyte transport by the entire normal and inflamed human colon during in vivo perfusion. Scand J Gastroenterol 8:327–336
Rask-Madsen J, Brix-Jensen P (1973) Electrolyte transport capacity and electrical potentials of the normal and inflamed human rectum in vivo. Scand J Gastroenterol 8:169–175
Rask-Madsen J, Dalmark M (1973) Decreased transmural potential difference across the human rectum in ulcerative colitis. Scand J Gastroenterol 8:321–326
Rask-Madsen J, Hammergaard EA, Knudsen E (1973) Rectal electrolyte transport and mucosal permeability in ulcerative colitis and Crohn's disease. J Lab Clin Med 81:342–353
Read NW, Fordtran JS (1978) The role of intraluminal junction potential on the generation of gastric potential difference in man. Gastroenterology 76:932–938
Read NW, Holdworth CD, Levin RJ (1974) Electrical measurement of intestinal absorption of glucose in man. Lancet 2:624–627
Read NW, Levin RJ, Holdsworth CD (1976) Electrogenic glucose absorption in untreated and treated coeliac disease. Gut 17:444–449
Read NW, Barber DC, Levin RJ, Holdsworth CD (1977) Unstirred layer and kinetic of electrogenic glucose absorption in the human jejunum in situ. Gut 18:865–876
Renkin EM (1954) Filtration, diffusion, and molecular sieving through porous cellulose membranes. J Gen Physiol 38:225–243
Rey F, Drillet F, Schmitz J, Rey J (1974) Influence of flow rate on the kinetics of the intestinal absorption of glucose and lysine in children. Gastroenterology 66:79–85
Rothberg RM (1969) Immunoglobulin and specific antibody synthesis during the first weeks of life in premature infants. J Pediatr 75:391–399
Ruddell WSJ, Blendis LM, Lovell D (1977) Rectal potential difference and histology in Crohn's disease. Gut 18:284–289
Ruppin H, Bar-Meier S, Soergel KH, Wood CM (1981) Effects of liquid formular diets on proximal gastrointestinal function. Dig Dis Sci 26:202–207
Sallee VL, Dietschy JM (1973) Determinants of intestinal mucosal uptake of short and medium chain fatty acids and alcohols. J Lipid Res 14:475–484
Schedl HP, Clifton JA (1961a) Kinetics of intestinal absorption in man: normal subjects and patients with sprue. J Clin Invest 40:1069

Schedl HP, Clifton JA (1961 b) Small intestinal absorption of steroids. Gastroenterology 41:491–499

Schedl HP, Clifton JA (1962) Polyvinylpyrrolidone I^{131} as an indicator of net intestinal water flux: its binding by intestinal mucus. Proc Soc Exp Biol Med 110:381–384

Schedl HP, Clifton JA (1963) Cortisol absorption in man. Gastroenterology 44:134–145

Schedl HP, Miller DM, White D (1966) Use of polyethylene glycol and phenol red as unabsorbed indicators for intestinal absorption studies in man. Gut 7:159–163

Schmid WC, Phillips SF, Summerskill WHJ (1969) Jejunal secretion of electrolytes and water in nontropical sprue. J Lab Clin Med 73:772–783

Schultz SG (1977) Some properties and consequences of low resistance paracellular pathway across the small intestine: the advantage of being "leaky". In: Kramer M, Lauterbach F (eds) Intestinal permeation. Excerpta Medica, Amsterdam, pp 382–391

Seifert J (1976) Enterale Resorption großmolekularer Proteine bei Tieren und Menschen. Z Ernährungswiss [Suppl] 18:1–72

Sewell P, Cooke WT, Cox EV, Meynell MJ (1963) Milk intolerance in gastrointestinal disorders. Lancet 2:1132–1135

Shorter RG, Huizenga KA, Spencer RJ (1972) A working hypothesis for the etiology and pathogenesis of nonspecific inflammatory bowel disease. Dig Dis Sci 17:1024–1031

Siber GR, Mayer RJ, Levin MJ (1980) Increased gastrointestinal absorption of large molecules in patients after 5-flurouracil therapy for metastatic colon carcinoma. Cancer Res 40:3430–3436

Silk DB, Kumar PJ, Perrett D, Clark ML, Dawson AM (1974 a) Amino acid and peptide absorption in patients with coeliac disease and dermatitis herpetiformis. Gut 15:1–8

Silk DBA, Kumar PJ, Webb JPW, Lane AE, Clark ML, Dawson AM (1974 b) Ileal function in patients with untreated adult coeliac disease. Gut 16:261–267

Sladen GE (1968) Perfusion studies in relation to intestinal absorption. Gut 9:624–628

Sladen GE, Dawson AM (1969) Effects of flow rate on the absorption of glucose in a steady state perfusion system in man. Clin Sci 36:133–145

Sladen GE, Kumar PJ (1973) Is the xylose test still a worthwhile investigation? Br Med J 3:223–226

Soergel KH (1971) Intestinal perfusion studies: values, pitfalls, and limitations. Gastroenterology 61:261–263

Soergel KH, Whalen GE, Harris JA (1968) Passive movement of water and sodium across the human small intestinal mucosa. J Appl Physiol 24:40–48

Solomon AK (1960) Measurement of the equivalent pore radius in cell membranes. In: Kleinzeller A, Kotyk A (eds) Membrane transport and metabolism. Academic, New York, p 94

Staverman AJ (1951) The theory of measurement of osmotic pressure. Rec Trav Chim 70:344–352

Stewart JS, Pollock DA, Hoffbrand AV, Mollin DL, Booth CC (1967) A study of proximal and distal intestinal structure and absorptive function in idiopathic steatorrhoea. Q J Med 36:425–444

Strober W, Wochner RD, Carbone PP, Waldmann TA (1967) Intestinal lymphangiectasia: a proteinlosing enteropathy with hypogammaglobulinemia, lymphopenia and impaired homograft rejection. J Clin Invest 46:1643–1656

Sundquist T, Magnusson K-E, Sjödahl R, Stjernström I, Tageson C (1980) Passage of molecules through the wall of the gastrointestinal tract. Gut 21:208–214

Tomasi TB, Tan EM, Solomon A, Pendergast RA (1965) Characteristics of on immune system common to certain external secretions. J Exp Med 121:101–124

Thomson ABR, Dietschy JM (1977) Deviation of the equations that describe the effects of unstirred water layers on the kinetic parameters of active transport processes in the intestine. J Theor Biol 64:277–294

Turnberg LA, Bieberdorf FA, Morawski SG, Fordtran JS (1970) Interrelationship of chloride, bicarbonate, sodium, and hydrogen transport in the human ileum. J Clin Invest 49:557–567

Volkheimer G (1964) Durchlässigkeit der Darmschleimhaut für groß-korpuskuläre Elemente (Herbst-Effekt). Z Gastroenterol 2:57

Volkheimer G (1977) Persorption of particels: Physiology and pharmacology. Adv Pharmacol Chemother 14:163–167
Waldmann TA (1961) Gastrointestinal protein loss demonstrated by ^{51}Cr-labelled albumin. Lancet 2:121–123
Waldmann TA, Morell GA, Wochner RD, Strober W, Sternlieb I (1967) Measurement of gastrointestinal protein loss using ceruloplasmin labelled with ^{67}copper. J Clin Invest 46:10–20
Walker WA, Isselbacher KJ (1974) Uptake and transport of macromolecules by the intestine: possible role in clinical disorders. Gastroenterology 67:531–550
Walzer M (1927) Studies in absorption of undigested protein in human beings. I. A simple direct method of studying the absorption of undigested proteins. J Immunol 14:143–149
Wanitschke R, Ewe K (1983) Drugs and the colon. In: Bustos-Fernándes L (ed) Colon-structure and function. Plenum, New York, pp 275–292
Wasserman RH, Taylor AU (1969) Some aspects of the intestinal absorption of calcium with special reference to vitamin D. In: Comar CL, Bronner F (eds) Mineral metabolism. III. Calciumphysiology. Academic, New York, pp 321–403
Wensel RH, Rich C, Brown AC, Volwiler W (1969) Absorption of calcium measured by intubation and perfusion of the intact human small inestine. J Clin Invest 48:1768–1774
Westergaard H, Dietschy JM (1974) Delineation of dimensions and permeability characteristics of two major diffusion barriers to passive mucosal uptake in rabbit intestine. J Clin Invest 54:718–732
Wetterforss J, Gullberg R, Liljedahl S-O, Plantin L-O, Birke G, Olhagen B (1960) Role of stomach and small intestine in albumin breakdown. Acta Med Scand 168:347–362
Whalen GE, Harris JA, Geenen JE, Soergel KH (1966) Sodium and water absorption from human small intestine. The accuracy of the perfusion method. Gastroenterology 51:975–984
Wheeler PG, Menzies IS, Creamer B (1978) Effect of hyperosmolar stimuli and coeliac disease on the permeability of the human gastrointestinal tract. Clin Sci Mol Med 54:495–501
Wiggins HS, Dawson AM (1961) An evaluation of unabsorbable marker in the study of fat absorption. Gut 2:373–376
Williams RC, Gibbons RJ (1972) Inhibition of bacterial adherence by secretory immunoglobulin A; a mechanism of antigen disposal. Science 177:697–699
Wilson FA, Dietschy JM (1974) The intestinal unstirred layer: its surface area and effect on active transport kinetics. Biochim Biophys Acta 363:112–126
Wilson TH (1962) Intestinal absorption. Saunders, Philadelphia, p 10
Wingate DL, Hayward MG, Johnson CM, Marczewski AG, Petty RG, Wilson EJ (1973a) Physiological changes in human transjejunal potential difference. Scand J Gastroenterol 8:473–489
Wingate DL, Phillips SF, Hofmann AF (1973b) Effect of glycine-conjugated bile acids with and without lecithin on water and glucose absorption in perfused human jejunum. J Clin Invest 52:1230–1236
Wingate DL, Sandberg RJ, Phillips SF (1972) A comparison of stable and ^{14}C-labelled polyethylene glycol as volume indicator in the human jejunum. Gut 13:812–815
Witts LJ (1961) Some aspects of the pathology of anaemia. II. Investigation of Castle's hypothesis. Br Med J 404–410
Worning H, Amdrup E (1965) Experimental studies on the value of the reference substances polyethylenglycol, bromsulphthalein and ^{51}Cr as indicators of the fluid content in the intestinal lumen. Gut 6:487–493
Wright EM, Diamond JM (1968) Effects of pH and polyvalent cations on the selective permeability of gallbladder epithelium to monovalent ions. Biochim Biophys Acta 163:57
Young TK, Lee SL, Tai LN (1980) Mannitol absorption and excretion in uremic patients regularly treated with gastrointestinal perfusion. Nephron 25:112–116
Zornitzer AE, Bronner F (1971) In situ studies of calcium absorption in rats. Am J Physiol 220:1261–1266

Subject Index

Handbook of Experimental Pharmacology

Continuation of "Handbuch der experimentellen Pharmakologie"

Editorial Board
G. V. R. Born, A. Farah,
H. Herken, A. D. Welch

Springer-Verlag
Berlin
Heidelberg
New York
Tokyo

Volume 25
Bradykinin, Kallidin and Kallikrein

Volume 26
Vergleichende Pharmakologie von Überträgersubstanzen in tiersystematischer Darstellung

Volume 27
Anticoagulantinen

Volume 28: Part 1
Concepts in Biochemical Pharmacology I

Part 3
Concepts in Biochemical Pharmacology III

Volume 29
Oral wirksame Antidiabetika

Volume 30
Modern Inhalation Anesthetics

Volume 32: Part 2
Insulin II

Volume 34
Secretin, Cholecystokinin Pancreozymin and Gastrin

Volume 35: Part 1
Androgene I

Part 2
Androgens II and Antiandrogens/Androgene II und Antiandrogene

Volume 36
Uranium - Plutonium - Transplutonic Elements

Volume 37
Angiotensin

Volume 38: Part 1
Antineoplastic and Immunosuppressive Agents I

Part 2
Antineoplastic and Immunosuppressive Agents II

Volume 39
Antihypertensive Agents

Volume 40
Organic Nitrates

Volume 41
Hypolipidemic Agents

Volume 42
Neuromuscular Junction

Volume 43
Anabolic-Androgenic Steroids

Volume 44
Heme and Hemoproteins

Volume 45: Part 1
Drug Addiction I

Part 2
Drug Addiction II

Volume 46
Fibrinolytics and Antifibronolytics

Volume 47
Kinetics of Drug Action

Volume 48
Arthropod Venoms

Volume 49
Ergot Alkaloids and Related Compounds

Volume 50: Part 1
Inflammation

Part 2
Anti-Inflammatory Drugs

Volume 51
Uric Acid

Handbook of Experimental Pharmacology

Continuation of "Handbuch der experimentellen Pharmakologie"

Springer-Verlag
Berlin
Heidelberg
New York
Tokyo

Volume 52
Snake Venoms

Volume 53
Pharmacology of Ganglionic Transmission

Volume 54: Part 1
Adrenergic Activators and Inhibitors I

Part 2
Adrenergic Activators and Inhibitors II

Volume 55
Psychotropic Agents

Part 1
Antipsychotics and Antidepressants

Part 2
Anxiolytics, Gerontopsychopharmacological Agents and Psychomotor Stimulants

Part 3
Alcohol and Psychotomimetics, Psychotropic Effects of Central Acting Drugs

Volume 56, Part 1+2
Cardiac Glycosides

Volume 57
Tissue Growth Factors

Volume 58
Cyclic Nucleotides

Part 1: **Biochemistry**

Part 2: **Physiology and Pharmacology**

Volume 59
Mediators and Drugs in Gastrointestinal Motility

Part 1: **Morphological Basis and Neurophysiological Control**

Part 2: **Endogenous and Exogenous Agents**

Volume 60
Pyretics and Antipyretics

Volume 61
Chemotherapy of Viral Infections

Volume 62
Aminoglycoside Antibiotics

Volume 63
Allergic Reactions to Drugs

Volume 64
Inhibition of Folate Metabolism in Chemotherapy

Volume 65
Teratogenesis and Reproductive Toxicology

Volume 66
Part 1: **Glucagon I**
Part 2: **Glucagon II**

Volume 67
Part 1
Antibiotics Containing the Beta-Lactam Structure I

Part 2
Antibiotics Containing the Beta-Lactam Structure II

Volume 68, Part 1+2
Antimalarial Drugs

Volume 69
Pharmacology of the Eye

Volume 71
Interferons and Their Applications

MIX
Papier aus verantwortungsvollen Quellen
Paper from responsible sources
FSC® C105338
FSC
www.fsc.org

If you have any concerns about our products,
you can contact us on
ProductSafety@springernature.com

In case Publisher is established outside the EU,
the EU authorized representative is:
Springer Nature Customer Service Center GmbH
Europaplatz 3, 69115 Heidelberg, Germany

Printed by Libri Plureos GmbH
in Hamburg, Germany